# Norman Geschwind

## Selected Publications on Language, Epilepsy, and Behavior

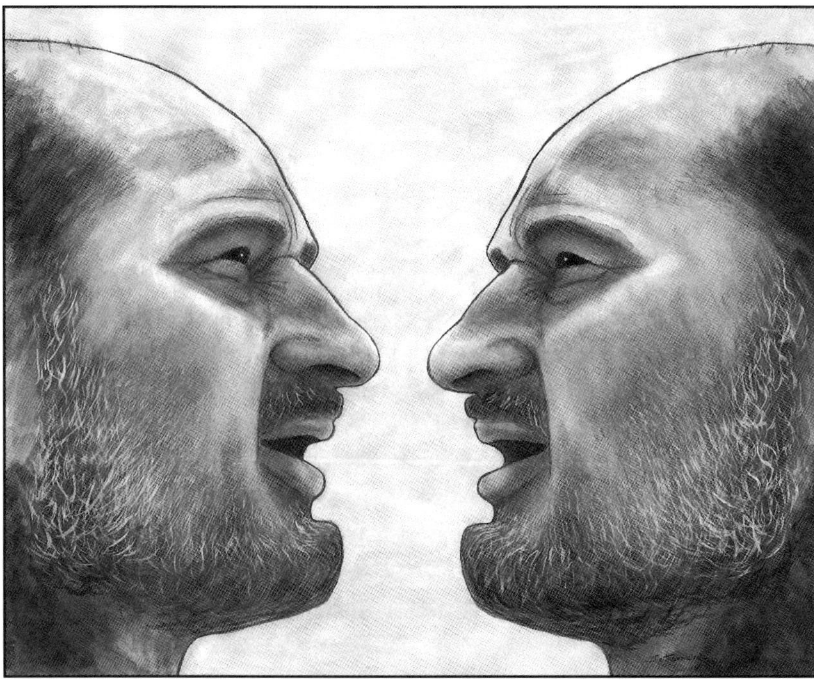

**Left Brain, Right Brain: Dr. Norman Geschwind's Vase**

*by Jacqui Streeton (the Thornbird)*

# Norman Geschwind

## Selected Publications on Language, Epilepsy, and Behavior


*Orrin Devinsky, M.D.*

Professor of Neurology, New York University School of Medicine, New York; Chief of Neurology and Head, NYU-HJD Epilepsy Center, Hospital for Joint Diseases, New York

*Steven C. Schachter, M.D.*

Assistant Professor of Neurology, Harvard Medical School, Boston; Director of Clinical Research, Comprehensive Epilepsy Center, Department of Neurology, Beth Israel Deaconess Medical Center, Boston



**Butterworth-Heinemann**

Boston Oxford Johannesburg Melbourne New Delhi Singapore

Every effort has been made to ensure that the drug dosage schedules within this text are accurate and conform to standards accepted at time of publication. However, as treatment recommendations vary in the light of continuing research and clinical experience, the reader is advised to verify drug dosage schedules herein with information found on product information sheets. This is especially true in cases of new or infrequently used drugs.

Recognizing the importance of preserving what has been written, Butterworth–Heinemann prints its books on acid-free paper whenever possible.

**Library of Congress Cataloging-in-Publication Data**

Geschwind, Norman

Norman Geschwind : selected publication on language, epilepsy, and behavior / Orrin Devinsky, Steven C. Schacter.

p. cm.

Includes bibliographical references.

ISBN 0-7506-9753-9 (hardcover)

1. Geschwind, Norman. 2. Neurology. 3. Language disorders. I. Devinsky, Orrin. II. Schacheter, Steven C. III. Title.

[DNLM: 1. Geschwind, Norman. 2. Neurologic Manifestation—collected works. 3. Brain Diseases—collected works. 4. Brain—physiology—collected works. 5. Brain—physiopathology—collected works. WL 7 G389n 1997]

RC339.52.G47A25 1997

616.8—dc21

DNLM/DLC

for Library of Congress 96–37401

CIP

**British Library Cataloguing-in-Publication Data**

A catalogue record for this book is available from the British Library.

The publisher offers special discounts on bulk orders of this book.

For information, please contact:

Manager of Special Sales

Butterworth–Heinemann

313 Washington Street

Newton, MA 02158–1626

Tel: 617-928-2500

Fax: 617-928-2620

For information on all medical publications available, contact our World Wide Web home page at: http://www.bh.com/bh/

10 9 8 7 6 5 4 3 2 1

Printed in the United States of America

# Contents

# Preface

Few individuals create disciplines. Many make significant contributions, identify new disorders, new techniques, new models. Many discover new treatments, new clinical findings, new interpretations of old data. Normal Geschwind created behavioral neurology as we now know it.

He was largely responsible for the resurgence of interest in brain-behavior relationships, for the introduction of a behavioral neurology section at the American Academy of Neurology, for redirecting psychiatric thought away from psychoanalysis and towards the brain, and for providing our generation, and future generations, with the structure and confidence to approach neurobehavioral problems.

Prior to Geschwind, many in neurology considered the corpus callosum to be a structural beam; the aphasias an amorphous, confusing mass for which localization had little meaning, clinical examination shed little insight, and classification was hopeless; there was no concept of "disconnection" between cortical and subcortical areas; apraxia loosely applied to problems from eyelid closure to gait but had lost its original and valid neurobehavioral-localizing meaning - most neurologists had never seen "apraxia" in their training or practice; developmental disorders affecting language and behavior were in the province of psychology, outside the boundaries of neurology; behavioral changes in temporal lobe epilepsy were viewed from a wholly negative and limited perspective; and the anatomical presence and meaning of hemispheric asymmetry was largely lacking.

Norman Geschwind breathed fire into the air of neurobehavioral disorders. He rekindled the great discoveries of the late 19th and early 20th century European neurologists. He added his own synthesis and observations and force of will to see this fledgling of behavioral neurology grow into one of the most dynamic in neurology. Most of the great behavioral neurologists, and those who have been trained by them, have been touched by the fire of Norman's mind.

Selecting which articles to reproduce was a difficult task. Due to space constraints we have not included "Disconnexion Syndromes in Animals and Man." It is a classic article that deserves reading by anyone with a serious interest in behavioral neurology.

OD
SCS

# Acknowledgments

We thank Pat Geschwind for her support and permission to reproduce these articles. We thank all of the co-authors and publishers who also graciously provided consent for these articles to see fresh light. Susan Pioli and Jana Friedman of Butterworth-Heinemann have been steady supporters who have helped see this project from its inception to completion. Helene Abramson helped coordinate much of the work obtaining permissions and organizing this project.

Finally, we thank Norman Geschwind, for all that he gave us, and for all the inspiration his spirit continues to give.

# Norman Geschwind

## Selected Publications on Language, Epilepsy, and Behavior

# PART I

# Disconnection Syndromes

## *Orrin Devinsky*

Norman Geschwind's most powerful and persisting influence on neurology was his work on disconnection syndromes in animals and man. His contribution in this area was twofold: (1) resurrecting the German and French literature from the late 19th and early 20th centuries that had been buried by neglect and misinterpretation, and (2) adding new carefully studied cases that revealed how anatomy—neuronal masses and fiber pathways—could shed light onto the mechanisms of behavior.

In 1961, Edith Kaplan evaluated a man who had a left frontal resection for a glioblastoma. Postoperatively, he developed a marked grasp reflex in the right hand, but not the left. For Kaplan, this case provided an opportunity to test the assertions made by Bouman and Grünbaum that the grasp reflex caused characteristic mechanical defects in writing.[1] Kaplan found that the man could write normally with his right hand but aphasically with his left hand. She was astonished to find aphasic writing restricted to the left hand. She could have told a thousand neurologists about this case, and it would have remained one of those curiosities that doesn't seem to fit into the comfortable pigeon-holes of knowledge, but she told Norman Geschwind. She related this case history to Geschwind a week after he had read Dejerine's description of callosal syndromes in man. The timing was fortuitous, but Pasteur's dictum applied—chance favors the prepared mind.

They presented two cases to the Boston Society of Neurology and Psychiatry on December 14, 1961. The first case was that of pure word blindness (alexia) without agraphia from a lesion of the left visual cortex and splenium. The second case was the man who had a left frontal resection referred to above. A brief report of the meeting was published in The New England Journal of Medicine,[2] and then a complete article was published in Neurology[3] (reproduced following this preface). In the brief communication, Geschwind and Kaplan anonymously reported that callosal syndromes were well known before 1940. Akelitis' studies of patients following callosal section for intractable epilepsy seemingly refuted previously well-documented clinical-neuropathologic cases of callosal syndromes. However, Sperry and coworkers demonstrated dramatic results after callosal sections using new examination techniques.[4]

In 1961, Geschwind met Oliver Zangwill at a meeting on dyslexia in Baltimore. "He listened patiently to the exposition of my ideas on the significance of the cortico-cortico connections for the higher functions. A short time later, while on a trip to Boston, he suggested to me that I should prepare an extended account of these ideas."[5] The result was the two part opus, "Disconnexion Syndromes in Animals and Man" published in Brain in 1965.[6,7] The length of these papers and inclusion in a prior volume of Geschwind's collected works,[1] regrettably led us to exclude them from the current volume.

The roots for Geschwind's disconnection syndromes, as well as his major contributions in aphasia, lie in late 19th century Germany. Wernicke's life and contributions were a source of great interest to Geschwind.[8,9,10] Wernicke wrote his classical treatise, "The Symptom Complex of Aphasia: A Psychological Study on an Anatomical Basis," in 1874, at age 26 years.[11] Wernicke begins his monograph with a tribute to Meynert:

> "Meynert's theory of the connections of the brain contains the foundations of a precise physiology of the central nervous system. It provides only a broad, general outline, to be sure, but one of such brilliant inner truth that it can even now be applied without hesitation to individual cases.
>
> The present case is an attempt to make practical use of Meynert's neuroanatomical teachings in an area in which fundamental principles of this kind are badly needed but up to now have scarcely been applied—the normal speech process and the disturbances of this process, which are known as aphasia."

In the introduction to his classic work on fluent aphasia with paraphasia from posterosuperior temporal lesions, Wernicke adds,

> "The surface of the brain is a mosaic of very simple elements of this kind, which are characterized by their anatomical connections with the periphery of the body. Everything beyond these elementary functions, such as the linking of different sense impressions to form a concept, thought, and consciousness, is a function of the fiber tracts that connect different cortical regions with each other, i.e., a function of the association systems, to use Meynert's terminology."

Geschwind's disconnection syndromes revived Meynert's attention to anatomy and cortical-cortical connections. In turn, Meynert and Wernicke relied on Burdach (1825), Flechsig (1872) and other anatomists who carefully mapped the association bundles comprising much of the cerebral white matter and their patterns of myelination.[11] Wernick'e 1874 monograph established that posterior superior temporal lesions caused an aphasic syndrome with fluent speech and paraphasia. However, Meynert previously identified the adjacent temporal cortex (Heschl's gyrus) as the termination for the auditory pathways and that lesions in the posterior superior temporal gyrus cause an aphasia distinct from the disorder following destruction of Broca's area.[10] Wernicke created a new approach to behavioral analysis, postulating conduction aphasia (fluent paraphasic speech with preserved comprehension—he did not predict impaired repetition—see Introduction to Aphasia and Apraxia) from lesions disconnecting Wernicke's and Broca's aphasia. He predicted the lesion would lie in the insula. Subsequent clinical-pathological cases confirmed Wernicke's prediction of conduction aphasia, but von Monakow's studies identified the lesion in the inferior parietal region, disrupting the arcuate (superior longitudinal) fasciculus, not in the insula.[10] More than a century later, the insula region, as well as the inferior parietal region, would find support in neuroimaging studies.

The integration of Meynert's anatomical approach with Wernicke's psychological (behavioral) studies led to a productive period in Continental neurology. Broca's localization of the motor speech area was supplemented by attention to connections and associations of different cortical areas. Lesions of these fiber bundles caused specific deficits. Dejerine described the first callosal syndrome in 1892—alexia without agraphia.[12] Liepmann, Wernicke's disciple, reported the first neuropathological study of a unilateral lesion causing pure word deafness at the turn of the century.[13,14] This disconnection syndrome resulted from a lesion that isolated Wernicke's area from auditory inputs of both hemispheres. Liepmann reported the case of Regierungsrat, in which the patient's clinical defects (including the newly coined syndrome, apraxia) were explained on the basis of several lesions disconnecting cortical areas.[13] The patient died two years later, and the neuropathology confirmed the predicted lesions sites.[14] The following year (1907), Liepmann and Maas published the case of Ochs, in whom apraxia resulted from a callosal lesion.[15] These authors, as well as Geschwind, applied Flechsig's rule to their interpretations: primary receptive areas have no direct neocortical connections except with immediately adjacent sensory association areas.[16]

The intrahemispherical and callosal disconnection syndromes were reconfirmed by neurologists and accurately summarized by authorities such as Kinnier Wilson (1908) over the next thirty years, but these syndromes were relegated to oblivion.[17] Holistic neurologists such as Head,[18] Marie,[19] von Monakow,[20] and Goldstein[21] confirmed cases of disconnection syndromes. Yet they denied the value of localization—tossing out the overzealous microlocalization of Kleist[22] together with the accurate localizations described by Wernicke, Dejerine, and Liepmann. Karl Lashley's holistic Gestalt psychology viewed the cerebral cortex as an equipotential mass.[23] Thus, as Dejerine and Liepmann exited academia, Akelaitis' published that callosal lesions in epilepsy patients cause no deficits,[24,25] thus hammering nails into the coffin of disconnection syndromes. Norman Geschwind removed the nails. As great minds do so well, they simultaneously look backwards and forwards while fully attending to the material that lies in front of their eyes.

In his 1974 book, "Norman Geschwind: Selected Papers on Language and the Brain," Geschwind ends the preface to his disconnection papers with the comment that he has revised many of his ideas and plans on publishing these revisions in book form.[1] When I was a first year medical student, Geschwind granted my unreasonable request for a weekly tutorial with him. I would read and then meet him to discuss my attempt to comprehend some aspect of behavioral neurology. My understanding of neurophysiology and neuroanatomy and neurology was quite meager; I struggled for some time to fully follow his orations. After several months, I came to one of those Friday sessions to disagree with Geschwind. He asked me to read about right parietal lesions, the syndrome of left-sided neglect, and the associated confabulatory responses. In Part II of his disconnection paper, Geschwind seemed to stretch the disconnection theory too far. "The right hemisphere is probably always at a disadvantage in relation to the left since the pathway from any part of it to the speech area is probably at least one neuron longer than the pathway from the corresponding part of the left hemisphere."[7] Geschwind then went on to note that the Jackson,[23] Penfield[26] and others found that deja vu most often resulted from right-seizure foci. ". . . this tendency of the minor hemisphere to give rise to such illusions is not the result of emotion or memory in the minor hemisphere but another example of the increased tendency to confabulatory response in cases of lesions of the association cortex on the right side." I suggested that in the title of that section, "The Problem of Right Parietal Dominance," was the solution to the problem. The right parietal lobe was dominant for surveying and attending to space and the body. He opened his eyes wide, paused as I trembled inside—perhaps this would be our last session. He then launched into a 40 minute monologue from which I could comprehend momentary bits and pieces. He circled back to the right parietal lobe, smiled, and said he thought that I was right. He had revised his ideas significantly. He liked my idea, but broke my heart when he told me it was not new.

Geschwind never revised his Disconnection Syndromes in an article or book. The lure of a new, uncharted area—the developmental aspects of the brain and how immunity, hormonal influence, and cerebral development interact—would largely occupy Geschwind's thoughts during the next, final decade of his life.

The outline of his two part opus, "Disconnexion Syndromes in Animals and Man," concludes this preface.

*Part I*

Introduction
Acknowledgments

I. Anatomical background: Flechsig's rule
 Connexions of the visual association areas

II. Agnosias in Animals
 Removals of temporal neocortex: the visual-limbic disconnexion syndrome
 The effects of the extent of the lesion

## References

1. Geschwind, N. Preface, Chapter II. *Selected Works of Norman Geschwind on Language and Behavior.* Boston: Boston Univ Press, 1974.
2. Geschwind, N, Kaplan, E. Random Reports: Human Split-Brain Syndromes. New England Journal of Medicine, 1962; 266,1013. (Published anonymously)
3. Geschwind, N, and Kaplan, E. A Human Cerebral Deconnection Syndrome: A Preliminary Report. Neurology, 1962;12,675-685.
4. Gazzaniga, MS, Bogen, JE, and Sperry, RW. Some functional effects of sectioning the cerebral commissures in man. Proc Nat Acad Sci, 1962;48,1765-1769.
5. Geschwind, N. Preface, Chapter II. *Selected Works of Norman Geschwind on Language and Behavior.* Boston: Boston Univ Press, 1974, p 105.
6. Geschwind, N. Disconnexion Syndromes in Animals and Man. I. Brain, 1965; 88(2),237-294.
7. Geschwind, N. Disconnexion Syndromes in Animals and Man. II. Brain, 1965; 88(3);585-644.
8. Geschwind, N. Carl Wernicke, The Breslau School and The History of Aphasia. In EC Carterette (ed.), *Brain Function, Volume III: Speech, Language, and Communication.* Berkeley: University of California Press, 1963, pp 1-16.
9. Geschwind, N. Wernicke's Contribution to the Study of Aphasia. Cortex, 1967; 3,449-463.
10. Geschwind, N. The Work and Influence of Wernicke. In RS Cohen and MW Wartofsky (eds.), *Boston Studies in the Philosophy of Science, Vol IV.* Dordrecht-Holland: D. Reidel, 1969, pp 1-33.
11. Wernicke, C. The symptom complex of aphasia: A psychological study on an anatomical basis. In RS Cohen and MW Wartofsky (eds.), *Boston Studies in the Philosophy of Science, Vol IV.* Dordrecht-Holland: D. Reidel, 1969, pp 34-97.
12. Dejerine, J. Contribution a l'etudie anatomo-pathologique et clinique des differentes varietes de cecite verbale. C R Soc Biol (Paris), 1892;44,61-90.
13. Liepmann, H. *Das Krankheitsbild der Apraxie (Ômotorischen Asymbolie),* Berlin, 1900.
14. Liepmann, H, and Storch, E. Mschr Psychiat Neurol, 1902;11,115-128.
15. Liepmann, H, and Maas, O. Fall von linksseitiger Agraphie und Apraxie bei rechtsseitiger lahmung. J Psychol Neurol, 1907;10,214-227.
16. Flechsig, P. Developmental (myelogenetic) localization of the cerebral cortex in the human subject. Lancet, 1901;2,1027.

17. Wilson, SAK. A contribution to the study of apraxia with a review of the literature. Brain, 1908;31,164-216.
18. Head, H. *Aphasia and Kindred Disorders of Speech.* Cambridge: Cambridge Univ Press, 1926.
19. Marie, P, and Chatelin, C. Les trouble visuels dus aux lesions des voies optiques intracerebrales et de la sphere visuelle corticale dans les blessures du crane par coup de feu. Rev Neurol (Paris) 1915;22,882-925.
20. von Monakow, C. Die Lokalisation im Grosshirn. The mechanism of vision, XVIII. Effects of destroying the visual associative areas of the monkey. Genet Psychol Monogr, 1914;37,107-166.
21. Goldstein, K. *Language and Language Disturbances: Aphasic Symptom Complexes and Their Significance for Medicine and Theory of Language.* New York: Grune & Stratton, 1948.
22. Kleist, K. *Gehirnpathologie.* JA Barth: Liepzig, 1934.
23. Lashley, KS. *Brain Mechanisms and Intelligence.* Chicago: University of Chicago Press, 1929.
24. Akelaitis, AJ. Studies on the corpus callosum. Study of language functions (tactile and visual lexia and graphia) unilaterally following section of the corpus callosum. J Neuropath Exp Neurol, 1943;226-262.
25. Akelaitis, AJ. A study of gnosis, praxis and language following section of the corpus callosum and anterior commissure. J Neurosurg, 1944;1,94-102.
26. Mullan, S, and Penfield, W. Illusions of comparative interpretation and emotion: Production by epileptic discharge and by electrical stimulation in the temporal cortex. Arch Neurol Psychiatry, 1959;81,269-284.

# CHAPTER 1

# A Human Cerebral Deconnection Syndrome: A Preliminary Report

*Norman Geschwind and Edith Kaplan*

We propose in this paper to present a patient whose clinical picture appears to us to be most simply explainable by a partial deconnection of the two cerebral hemispheres. He appears to behave as if there were 2 nearly isolated half-brains, functioning almost independently.

In the early years of this century, several cases were described which showed some of the phenomena that are present in our patient. Sittig[1] reviews these cases in his monograph on apraxia. The earlier workers generally described these cases as showing apraxia and apractic agraphia of the left side and left-sided astereognosis and attributed these findings to lesions of the corpus callosum.

In the 1940s, considerable doubt was cast on the role of the corpus callosum by the extensive studies of Akelaitis[2] and his co-workers on humans whose corpora callosa had been sectioned surgically (to prevent the interhemispheric spread of seizures) and who subsequently presented virtually no abnormalities. Earlier physiological work in animals also failed to show convincing disturbances. Bremer, Brihaye, and André-Balisaux[3] have reviewed this literature. By contrast, in the last five years, the work of Sperry[4] and his co-workers has convincingly proved that in animals, section of the callosum produces behavior which is most simply explained as resulting from deconnection of the 2 hemispheres. It was Sperry's work which alerted us to the possibility of deconnection syndromes in man.

Our patient shows behavior similar to that described by the earlier workers. In addition, we have observed several manifestations not previously mentioned. Detailed anatomical confirmation of the localization of the lesion is not yet available. The patient continues to be studied actively at this time. However, in view

---

Reprinted with permission from *Neurology*. 1962; 12: 675-685.

of the unusual character of these findings, we are presenting this brief clinical description as a preliminary report in the hope of stimulating other workers to look for similar cases and to investigate their anatomical substratum. A more detailed report of this patient will be published at a later date.

## CASE REPORT

P.J.K., (BVAH U-53490), a 41-year-old white, married police officer, was admitted to the Boston V.A. Hospital, Neurology Section, on March 2, 1961. One month before admission the patient had begun to develop dull headaches, primarily over the left orbit, lasting several hours, recurring 3 to 4 times a week, and frequently associated with nausea and vomiting. The members of the family had over the previous few months noticed increasing behavioral changes manifested by indifference; apathy; forgetfulness; diminished alertness; confusion for dates, events, and people; diminution in personal neatness; and increased friction in interpersonal relations, particularly at work.

The patient had no significant history of birth or childhood illness. He had been graduated from high school at 18, had served in the Navy from 1941 to 1945, and since 1949 had been a policeman. Past history and family history were otherwise not relevant.

General physical examination revealed a well-developed, well-nourished man. The temperature was 98.60 F., blood pressure was 110/90, and pulse, 80. There were no significant abnormalities in the remainder of the general examination.

Neurological examination revealed a patient who was alert, cooperative, and oriented in all spheres. He exhibited inappropriate jocularity against a background of general apathy. He had no insight into his illness and appeared unconcerned about it. He kept repeating questions as if he did not quite understand them. He could remember only 1 of 3 items after five minutes. He repeated 6 digits forward and 4 backward. He made many errors in subtracting sevens serially from 100. His proverb interpretations were very poor, being little more than restatements without interpretation. He did simple written arithmetic correctly but failed on more complex material such as multiplying 214 by 35. When asked to draw a clock face at a certain hour, he frequently reversed the large and small hands.

The patient was right-handed. Except for a few paraphasias and some hesitancy in naming objects, speech was normal. He drew a rough map of the United States on which his localization of many cities and states was correct except for New Mexico which was included twice in different parts of the Southwest. There was no right-left disturbance.

On examination of the cranial nerves, the optic disks were indistinct but without papilledema. Visual fields to confrontation showed a questionable binasal lower quadrant defect, but this was not confirmed by perimetry. The right pupil was slightly larger than the left, but both showed normal responses to light and convergence. Optokinetic reflexes were present bilaterally. There was questionable flattening of the left nasolabial fold. Cranial nerves were otherwise intact.

Motor examination showed normal bulk, tone, strength, and coordination throughout. Deep tendon reflexes were 1+ to 2+ throughout but equal on both sides. Abdominals were 2+ bilaterally. Plantars were flexor, and grasping, sucking, and snout reflexes were said to be absent. Sensory examination showed no abnormality of touch, pin-prick, position sense, vibration, two-point discrimination, or stereognosis. Stance and gait were both normal.

Laboratory examination showed a hematocrit of 45 percent and a hemoglobin of 14.3 grams. White blood count was 6,200 with a normal differential. Corrected sedimentation rate was 15 mm per hour; fasting blood sugar, 94 mg; blood urea nitrogen, 23 mg; prothrombin time, 100 percent; bleeding time, 1 minute; and coagulation time, 18 minutes. Spinal fluid showed an opening pressure of 160 mm and a closing pressure of 80 mm. The fluid was clear and colorless with no cells. Protein was 60 mg; sugar, 110; chloride, 118 mEq; colloidal gold, 011232100; and zinc sulfate test, 4+. Serology was negative in spinal fluid and blood.

The electrocardiogram was normal. Visual fields by perimetry were normal. X-rays of the chest and skull were felt to show no definite abnormality. A pneumoencephalogram with 20 cc of air was consistent with a left frontal space-occupying mass. A left carotid arteriogram was consistent with a left frontal mass, probably a glioma.

Psychological testing on March 8, 1961, revealed a Wechsler Adult Intelligence Scale full scale I.Q. of 81 with a verbal I.Q. of 79 and a performance I.Q. of 87. On the Wechsler Memory Scale, he achieved a score of 87. Memory for visual forms showed impairment but copying was normal. The results of psychological testing were regarded as clearly consistent with intellectual deterioration.

On March 16, 1961, the patient underwent a left frontal craniotomy. On inspection, all of the visible left frontal lobe was markedly softened. A cyst deep in this lobe was aspirated through the middle frontal gyrus. A frontal amputation was performed revealing tumor in the depths. Because of edema, the anterior border of the corpus callosum was not identified. A large branch of the anterior cerebral artery on the medial surface of the frontal lobe was amputated. This was thought to be most likely the frontal polar artery. The ventricular system was not entered. The patient received 3 liters of blood and tolerated the procedure well.

The pathologist described the specimen as left frontal lobe, weighing 107 gm, and identified the tumor microscopically as a glioblastoma multiforme.

Postoperatively, the patient showed a dense right hemiplegia and a marked aphasia. He improved steadily and was returned to the Neurology Service. On the 49th postoperative day, neurological examination revealed a patient disoriented in time, but correctly oriented to place and person. He was apathetic but smiled most of the time. He confabulated in response to questions about the reasons for his admission to the hospital. There was impairment of recent memory, calculation, and abstraction. His speech showed at most a few mild paraphasic errors. He followed complex commands poorly. There was a dense weakness of the right leg and moderate weakness of the hand and arm with equal involvement of flexors and extensors. The finger-nose test was well done.

There was a mild tremor in the outstretched fingers of the right hand as well as a marked grasp reflex. The tendency to grasp was most marked when the zone between thumb and forefinger was stroked. Traction on the arm further intensified the grasp. When the examiner's hand was brought near the palmar surface of the patient's right hand without actual contact, the patient's hand followed the examiner's.

In the left limbs, tone, power, and coordination were completely normal, and there was no trace of grasping in either the left hand or foot. Deep tendon reflexes were symmetrically hyperactive and both plantars were flexor.

Sensory examination on the right showed a mild loss of position sense in the fingers and a denser loss in the foot. Vibration and stereognosis were intact and localization of touch was grossly accurate. Two-point discrimination was mildly impaired and pin-prick appeared to be mildly diminished. On the left side, sensory examination was at first very confusing because the patient gave extremely variable reports. However, when for reasons which will become apparent later, technics for testing sensation on the left side were developed in which the patient was required to respond nonverbally (for example, pointing up and down in position sense testing, tapping once or twice for two-point discrimination), it could be shown that position sense, vibration, two-point discrimination, pinprick, and touch localization were all normal in the left arm and leg. Discussion of stereognosis in the left hand will be deferred to the section on Results of Special Studies.

On May 22, 1961, it was discovered by one of us (E.K.) that he could not write with his left hand. At this time a program of special investigations was instituted, the results of which are given later.

Psychological testing on May 28 and September 13 showed no essential differences from preoperative testing.

The patient remained in the hospital until September 4, 1961, by which time he had improved considerably. He was oriented in all spheres but still had little insight into his illness and showed unchanged intellectual impairment. The right hemiplegia had improved markedly. In the right arm there was only mild weakness of abduction of the right shoulder; in the right leg there was only mild weakness in flexion and extension at the knee and inability fully to dorsiflex the ankle. The patient could now walk unaided. The grasping responses were markedly diminished in all respects except that with the diminution of the paralysis of the right leg, a mild grasp reflex had now become apparent in the right foot. Improvement observed during follow-up after discharge from the hospital will be discussed below.

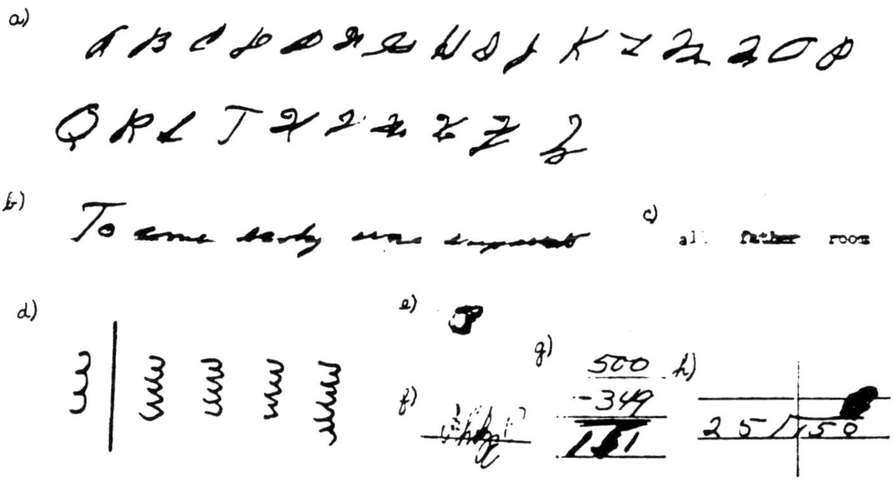

FIGURE 1. Samples of performances with the right hand, demonstrating the effect of the grasp reflex: (a) the alphabet; (b) the sentence, "To come early was impossible" written to dictation; (c) the words, "all," "father," and "room" typed with the right index finger; (d) to the left of the vertical line examiner's model three-looped figure, to the right of the line patient's successive attempts to copy the model; (e) the number "3" written to dictation; (f) the patient's preoperative writing of his first name; (g) and (h) the heavily written numbers are the patient's solutions to the problems written by the examiner (preoperative).

## Results of Special Studies

When it was discovered that the patient was unable to write correctly with his left hand, a program of carefully planned testing was set up. The results of these examinations are now given.

At the time of testing the patient showed no evidence of aphasia in his spontaneous speech although there was a mildly halting quality to his language productions. The patient showed no evidence of word-finding difficulty. There was at most a mild difficulty in comprehension of complex spoken or written material which was felt to be consistent with his intellectual impairment. He correctly repeated numbers, letters, words, and sentences presented verbally.

*Writing with the right hand* When asked to write with this hand, the patient produced normal sentences and made no errors in spelling. There were certain characteristic disturbances in the motor performance (Figure 1). His writing tended to get smaller with letters closer together; eventually one letter would be written over the preceding one (Figure 1b). In writing single letters or numbers he tended to keep going over the outline (Figure 1e). He would add extra loops when writing 3s or ms or three-looped figures (Figure 1d). Review of his preoperative writing revealed that similar defects had been present although they had passed unnoticed (Figure 1f, g, h). Bouman and Grünbaum[5] in their study of patients with grasp reflexes described similar graphic disturbances.

Similarly, letters, numbers, words, and sentences were correctly written to dictation. He copied all forms of written material correctly. When presented with printed material, he would copy it in script, which is the typical response of normal people to this task.

In typing with the right hand (using one finger), he produced his name and words to dictation with no errors (Figure 1c).

*Writing with the left hand* By contrast, when asked to write with this hand he made many errors. In writing the alphabet, he produced many incorrect or completely unrecognizable letters (Figure 2a). On dictation, he would generally write a clearly recognizable letter or number but usually not the one demanded. When asked to write words and sentences to dictation, he would usually produce an unrecognizable scrawl (Figure 2b). On occasion, however, the response consisted of well-written but clearly incorrect words such as yonti for yesterday (see also Figure 2e, 2f). He copied printed and written material correctly but would reproduce printed material with block letters and not script. There was no trace of the motor difficulties seen in the productions of the right hand (Figure 2c).

In typing with his left hand, he could not produce his own name correctly nor could he type words correctly to dictation (Figure 2d).

When he had seen the incorrect productions of his left hand, he was quite astonished. However, spontaneous attempts to correct generally resulted in repeated difficulty (Figure 2d).

*Object and letter identification with the right hand* With his eyes closed, the patient correctly and rapidly named objects and cardboard letters placed in his right hand. Similarly, he could, after the object was taken away, correctly draw the object which had been in his hand. If letters or numbers were traced on his right hand, he generally named them correctly.

*Object and letter identification with the left hand* By contrast, when objects, numbers, or letters were placed in the left hand, the patient (with eyes closed) generally named them incorrectly. The errors usually bore no resemblance to the stimulus object. For example, a ring was identified as "an eraser," a watch as "a balloon," a padlock as "a book of matches," and a nail as "an elastic." The errors were not constant. Thus on another occasion he called a ring "a package of some sort;" a screw driver on one test was "a spoon" and on another "a piece of paper."

It was striking to observe that when handling the objects he would move them actively about within his fingers and would focus on their salient features. For example, he inserted his finger into a thimble, ran his thumb over the teeth of a comb, rubbed the bristles of a tooth brush, and retracted the point of a ballpoint

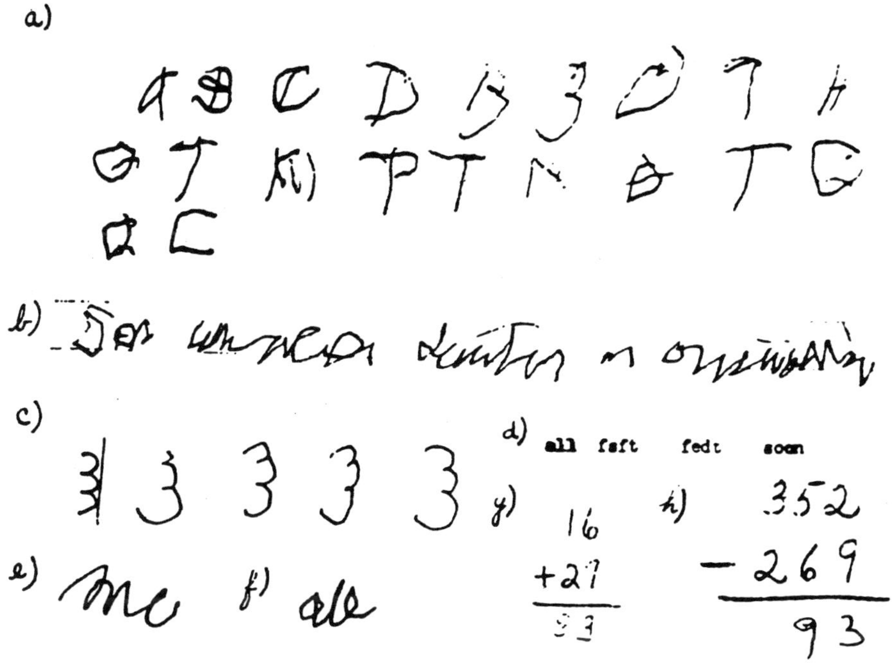

FIGURE 2. Samples of performances with the left hand, demonstrating errors in language and calculation along with the absence of disturbances due to grasp reflex: (a) the alphabet; (b) the sentence, "To come early was impossible" written to dictation; (c) to the left of the vertical line examiner's model three-looped figure, to the right of the line patient's successive copies of the model; (d) attempts with left index finger to type the words, "all," "father," "father" (the second being a spontaneous attempt to correct the first error), and "room;" (e) attempt to write "run" to dictation; (f) attempt to write "go" to dictation; (g) and (h) the patient's solutions to the problems set by the examiner.

pen. Despite his appropriate handling of the dominant features of these objects, he misnamed them all.

When it was made clear to him that he was to show how the object placed in his hand was to be used, the subject (with eyes closed) proceeded with little hesitation to manipulate the item correctly, usually giving simultaneously an incorrect verbal account. Thus, given a hammer, he made hammering movements correctly while saying "I would use this to comb my hair with it." Given a key, he went through the motions of inserting it into a lock and turning it but said that he was "erasing a blackboard with a chalk eraser." Holding a pair of scissors correctly, he made cutting movements in the air but said that "I'd use that to light a cigarette with." When his eyes were open he correctly identified the objects in his left hand.

Still another method was employed to study identification with the left hand. The patient, with eyes closed, was given an object in this hand. The object having been taken away, the left hand of the patient (whose eyes still were closed) was placed in a box containing a number of items including the test object. He selected the correct object. Similarly, with eyes open, he would without hesitation point to the object in a group without touching it. He was also able to make a correct drawing with his left hand of an object that had been previously placed in this hand and then removed.

*Objects placed in one hand with identification by the other hand* If an object or letter was placed in the left hand behind the patient's back, he generally was unable with the right hand (a) to select it correctly from a group of objects presented to him either visually or tactually, (b) to write the name of the object, or (c) to draw a picture of the object. For example, a letter which would have been drawn correctly with the right hand after having been held in the right hand was drawn incorrectly with the right hand if the letter was placed in the left hand. Similarly, if objects were placed in the right hand, the patient was usually incapable of performing any of these maneuvers with his left hand.

These results contrast with data given earlier in which we demonstrated that if an object was placed in one hand, it could afterward be identified by drawing or selection by the same hand. In addition, we may note here that if letters were traced on the left hand, the patient could afterward trace them correctly on the ground with his left foot. If letters were traced on the right hand, he could not reproduce them correctly with the left foot. The right foot could not be tested in this way because of paralysis.

*Ability to perform commands* When the patient was asked to perform actions with his right hand, he did so correctly and without hesitation. For example, he could draw a square, wave goodbye, salute, and pretend to brush his teeth or comb his hair.

When asked to perform actions with his left hand, he made many errors, and even the correct responses were performed with a considerable delay. Thus, when asked to draw a square, he drew a circle. When asked to draw a triangle (which he had done earlier with his right hand without hesitation), he paused, asked if the examiner meant the figure with three corners, and finally drew the figure. When asked to point to the examiner with his left index finger, he pointed to his own eye with his left index and middle fingers. Immediately afterward he performed this action correctly with his right hand. Requested again to perform with his left hand, he pointed to the floor with his index finger. When asked to show how he would brush his teeth with his left hand, he on one occasion made the motions of lathering his face and on another went through the motions of combing his hair.

When asked to imitate the examiner's movements or to manipulate objects, the patient performed correctly with *either* hand.

*Transfer of learning* We attempted to perform a version of Sperry's[4] experiment on transfer of learning. We intended to have the patient learn (when blindfolded) a simple maze with the index finger of one hand, and then test the index finger of the other hand. In our normal controls such learning always transferred in 1 or 2 trials. However, this experiment could not be carried through successfully. The patient learned the maze with his left hand but was totally incapable of running the maze with the right hand. This failure to perform with the right hand appeared to be due to the grasping responses. The patient would either hold his finger fixed at one point or, in an effort to free it, suddenly jerk his finger erratically out of the maze.

*Bilateral movements* The patient could make circles in the air with both hands, tap with both hands, or perform alternating movements with both arms. It was observed, however, that in these symmetrically performed activities the two hands would on most occasions move at first at the same speed but after a time become desynchronized; on other occasions they moved at different speeds right from the onset.

Previously learned movements requiring the cooperation of both hands such as threading a needle, catching a ball, tying shoelaces, and dressing himself were performed without difficulty.

*Parietal lobe testing* On the right side we have already noted evidence of mild position sense and two-point discrimination loss. On the left side both of these functions were normal. Pin-prick was identified correctly on both sides, but there was more withdrawal on the left. Touch and vibration were normal on both sides. Stereognosis, when appropriately tested for, was fully normal on both sides. Localization of touch was normal on both sides. Bilateral simultaneous stimulation gave highly variable results, but there was no consistent evidence of extinction on either side.

Using his right hand, he could correctly point out fingers on both hands and other body parts on both sides. With his left hand, he made many errors on this test but no more than in performing any other movements to verbal command with this hand. He could correctly name parts of the examiner's body. With his right hand he made only 1 error out of 8 in a screening test of right-left orientation (indicating body-parts on the examiner and on himself). With his left hand, on the same test, he made 6 errors but again his difficulty was no more profound than in performing other verbal commands with this hand.

He showed no evidence of topographic disorientation. On one occasion he was being taken from his home to the hospital in the car of one of the authors. He suggested a complicated short-cut and correctly gave all the directions for following it. He had no difficulty finding his way around the hospital. On a map he correctly located Europe, the Atlantic Ocean, the Mississippi River, the Rocky Mountains, New York, Chicago, San Francisco, and Miami.

In setting a clock face he often reversed the large and small hands but made no other errors. He copied complex stick figures perfectly with the model present.

On one occasion he pointed out correctly to the examiner that he had been given one stick too few to complete the design. He made 50 percent errors with the model absent. He performed normally on the Block-Design subtest of the Wechsler Adult Intelligence Scale. He drew and copied figures with either hand although on the right the proportions were poorer and he tended to make extra strokes. There was no evidence of neglect of either half of space in his drawings.

The patient dressed himself correctly and without difficulty. There was no neglect of the left side of the body. If neglect existed at all, it was manifested only on the right. He complained that his right hand was dead or useless and would use his left hand preferentially in many tasks (for example, in picking up objects from the floor). Objects placed in the left hand were always handled vigorously and correctly. The left arm showed no evidence of catatonic postures nor any responses of avoidance.

Simple written calculations were correct with the right hand, but he failed on more complex problems. With the left hand his calculations were grossly incorrect, even on the simplest problems (Figure 2g, h). His calculation difficulty with the right hand ran parallel to his poor performance on tests of abstraction, such as proverb interpretation and similarities.

*Course since discharge* The patient has been observed frequently in follow-up. At the time of this writing (two months after discharge), there have been some changes in the clinical picture. There have been some signs of progression in that the position sense loss in the right fingers is clearly worse, and he shows difficulties in identifying block letters placed in this hand. He makes many more errors in right-left testing. On a more complex test of finger identification than was used in the earlier testing, he still performs correctly with the right hand. He made 2 errors out of 10 on the most difficult subtest. This test is one in which the patient was asked to show on his body a pair of fingers simultaneously pointed to by the examiner on a model hand.

By contrast, his writing with the left hand has improved in that he produces fewer illegible words, but the words produced are still usually grossly incorrect. He makes fewer errors now in following verbal commands with the left hand.

## Discussion

In the early 1900s several cases sharing certain similarities with our patient were reported. In general, these cases were described as showing an apraxia of the left side, agraphia of the left arm alone, and astereognosis on the left. Along with these findings, there were generally associated a hemiplegia, worse in the leg, and a powerful grasp reflex on the same side as the predominantly crural hemiplegia. We have critically examined these reports, and in a later paper we will present our analysis of them in detail. We would stress here that in our opinion some of these cases, when viewed in isolation, would be difficult to interpret. Thus, in Liepmann and Maas's[6] famous case, Ochs, there was a dense hemiplegia involving the right arm as well as the leg. Since no testing for praxis or writing could be done except very rudimentarily on the right, one might have doubts as to the unilaterality of the apraxia and agraphia. Our view as to the possible difficulty of drawing conclusions from such a case coincides with that of Hécaen and Gimeno-Alava.[7] In Goldstein's[8] case other difficulties arise. Here the right side was perfectly normal, and apraxia, agraphia, and astereognosis were reported on the left. However, this patient had a left hemiplegia, worse in the leg, and a remarkably intense grasp reflex of the left hand. We agree with Denny-Brown[9] that careful study is needed to insure that apparent dyspraxic difficulties are not due to a grasp reflex.

Despite these difficulties, there are cases such as those of Van Vleuten[10] and Maas[11] in which the hemiplegia involved the right leg and not the right arm; where, despite the grasp reflex in the right hand, there were no right-sided agraphic or apraxic difficulties; and where the otherwise normal left side was reported to show agraphia, apraxia, and astereognosis.

The feature common to these early reports was a lesion in the distribution of the anterior cerebral artery, in some cases vascular, in some tumor, and in particular, in all instances involving corpus callosum. In many of these cases the localization was confirmed at post-mortem examination; in the others the pattern of crural monoplegia with a marked grasp reflex in the homolateral hand (such as had generally been present in the autopsied cases) led to a similar clinical localization.

The early workers interpreted their data as being due to callosal deconnection. They believed that the left hemisphere was the leading hemisphere for movement and that the right hemisphere could not function properly in isolation. In the same manner, they felt that the left hemisphere was dominant for stereognosis and that the astereognosis of the left hand could be interpreted as due to separation of the right somesthetic cortex from the left.

Cases of this type have been described much more infrequently in recent years. Other cases of left-sided apraxia have been noted in which the associated clinical symptomatology has been quite different and strongly suggestive of right parietal disease.[7]

Our own case shows clear clinical affinities with the early group in its association of what superficially appear to be purely left-sided difficulties together with right crural monoplegia and a right grasp reflex. Had we not introduced certain new methods of study, we might have interpreted the findings as those of left-sided apraxia, apractic agraphia, and astereognosis.

Our data clearly rule out astereognosis in the left hand. As long as verbal responses were avoided, identification was perfect. The patient was thus simply unable to name objects or letters placed in the left hand. It is important to stress that unless a patient is tested in this way, one can neither ascribe the difficulty to a right parietal lesion nor use the term "astereognosis."

Our patient's agraphia of the left hand cannot be regarded as being secondary to elementary movement difficulties. The patient drew very well with this hand, and indeed his drawing was better with this hand than with the right. The written productions often consisted of perfectly formed letters or numbers which were incorrect. His difficulties in forming words appeared equally in writing, using anagram letters, or typing.

In addition, our testing showed certain unusual features in the apparently apraxic manifestations. Thus the poor performance of commands by the left side would appear to fit the classical picture. However, we could apparently induce an apraxic difficulty of the right side by placing objects (concealed from vision) in the left hand and asking him to draw or otherwise identify them with the right hand. This was parallel to the inability to identify with the left hand, either by touch or pointing or drawing, objects that had been held (concealed from vision) in the right hand.

Certain interpretations of the data can be excluded. The possibility of hysteria or malingering must always be considered in cases with unusual manifestations, but this seems highly unlikely here. Classical hysterical manifestations were totally absent; the pattern of ability and disability was too complex, especially considering the patient's limited intellectual abilities; many features showed an affinity to the above-mentioned classical clinical pictures which could hardly have been known to the patient; and prolonged careful observation of his behavior militated against this interpretation. Similarly, the patient's intellectual impairment could not explain the differences on the two sides of the body. We will later discuss a possible indirect role of intellectual deterioration in the clinical picture.

The data do not support a parietal lobe syndrome either right- or left-sided as the cause of the difficulties. He showed some mild position sense and two-point discrimination loss on the right but no astereognosis on either side. There was no loss of two-point discrimination or position sense on the left. Dressing and topographic difficulties were absent; copying difficulties were not present; and there was no finger agnosia or other autotopagnosia. In particular, we were very careful to verify the absence of neglect of the left arm (if anything, there was a preference for this arm) or of the left half of space, and there was no evidence of avoiding responses or catatonic postures on the left. The course since discharge also supports this view. There has been evidence of progression of left parietal lobe signs: that is, increased position sense loss in the right hand, the appearance for the first time in this hand of an inability to identify block letters, and increased difficulties in right-left orientation. Yet this has been accompanied by an amelioration of many of the distinctive features of this case: improved writing and increased ability to follow verbal commands with the left hand.

Could the disturbances of the left arm be due to unsuspected involvement of the right hemisphere? We have already excluded the possibility of right parietal disturbance. Against the notion that there is involvement of motor regions of the right cerebrum is the total absence of left-sided weakness, grasping, or incoordination. On the right side, where such signs were present, the left-sided deficits were conspicuously absent. Even if there were some heretofore unknown higher order reflex disturbance (similar to grasping or avoiding) in the left arm, it could hardly explain the aphasic nature of his writing difficulties and his inability to name objects placed in the left hand; nor could it explain the failures of the right hand to reproduce or identify material placed in the left hand.

It appears to us that the simplest description of this patient's most striking disturbances is that he behaved as if his two cerebral hemispheres were functioning nearly autonomously. Thus we found that so long as we confined stimulation and response within the same hemisphere, the patient showed correct performance. If an object was placed in one hand when the patient had his eyes closed, the patient could manipulate it correctly. With the same hand he could select it afterward correctly from a group either tactually or visually or could draw it. By contrast, if the object was placed in one hand and any of the above responses demanded from the other hand, the performance was usually incorrect.

We interpret the difficulties in responding to or using language on the left in a similar way. Postoperatively, the patient was severely, although transiently, aphasic at the time that he had a dense right hemiplegia. This places his speech area almost certainly in the left hemisphere. His difficulties in producing language with the left hand or in responding to verbal commands requiring the use of the left side can be interpreted as resulting from deconnection of the right hemisphere from the speech area. The patient correctly named objects placed in the right hand and wrote correctly with the right hand both spontaneously and to dictation. Verbal commands were performed correctly with the right hand. By contrast, he generally was incorrect in naming objects in the left hand and wrote incorrectly with the left hand both spontaneously and to dictation. Verbal commands were frequently performed incorrectly with the left hand.

While the early cases were described as being apraxic in the left arm, we feel that a more precise delineation is possible in our patient. The patient showed no difficulties of performance of complex movements as long as stimulus and response were limited to the same hemisphere. The left hand showed difficulties only when the information had to be transferred from the left hemisphere, for example, in performing verbal commands, or drawing or otherwise identifying with the left hand objects held in the right (concealed from vision). But as we have shown, the right hand was equally poor in performing movements whose stimulus came from the right hemisphere, for example, in drawing objects held in the left hand. In other words, apparently apraxic difficulties could be induced in either hand.

Where is the lesion producing this disturbance? The interpretation that this functional deconnection of the two cerebral hemispheres is a result of damage to the corpus callosum appears to us to be the most likely one. It is in harmony with the earlier anatomical observations and is concordant with the evidence that puts a lesion into the distribution of the anterior cerebral artery. It is consistent with the observations of Sperry[4] and his students on the physiological functions of this commissure.

Sperry[4] used transfer of learning technics to show callosal deconnection. Such experiments were not possible in our patient. However, our evidence of lack of interhemispheric transfer is as direct as that which Sperry obtained by use of learning technics. In fact, certain of our experiments would be difficult to do with animals, for example, drawing with one hand an object held with the other. Similarly, experiments on transfer of language are possible only in man.

It is difficult to be certain of the pathological nature of the involvement. At first, infiltration by tumor would appear to be most likely. However, we do not know whether any of the findings of deconnection were present before operation. Furthermore, there has been steady improvement over the six months since operation in the right hemiplegia and grasp reflex and in the signs of deconnection. This would appear to us to be too long to be accounted for by surgical trauma or edema. The patient underwent an extensive frontal lobe resection and some branches of the anterior cerebral artery were ligated. We think it possible that the vessel supplying the corpus callosum on the left was either tied off or developed a thrombosis in response to surgical trauma. No postoperative angiogram was done so that we cannot at this time affirm the correctness of this hypothesis.*

The evidence also suggests that the lesion does not involve the posterior callosum. The patient read words tachistoscopically presented in either visual field as quickly as normals. It is interesting to compare the patient of Trescher and Ford,[12] the posterior end of whose callosum had been sectioned surgically. The patient could not read letters in the left visual field. In addition she could not name letters placed in the left hand but could name objects. The authors regarded this as a specialized tactile agnosia rather than as astereognosis on the basis of the excellent preservation of two-point discrimination and position sense and the dissociation between letters and objects. We feel it likely that if nonverbal identification of letters by the left hand had been tested, these authors would have found it intact and would have been able to strengthen their argument. The detailed differences between anterior and posterior callosal lesions will not be dealt with extensively at this point. This problem is dealt with more fully elsewhere (Geschwind[13]).

The one feature of the case that may at first appear to be somewhat perplexing is the retained ability of the patient to perform certain learned activities that require the cooperation of the two hands, such as threading a needle. It can readily be demonstrated, however, that two normals, one using the right hand and the other using the left, can combine to perform successfully such activities. It seems obvious that each hemisphere of the patient had learned its role in such

*The patient died on June 3, 1962 (after the submission of this paper). Dr. José Segarra, chief of neuropathology at the Boston Veterans Administration Hospital, examined the brain grossly on June 21, 1962, and found evidence which supports the validity of the hypothesis suggested in the text. There was massive involvement of the left hemisphere by tumor which had extended downward into the basal ganglia, but no tumor was present on the right side. The corpus callosum showed no infiltration by tumor but was, on the contrary, markedly thinned in its anterior two-thirds. The superior and medial surface of the left hemisphere extending back to the paracentral lobule was completely infarcted. The callosal and hemispheric lesions corresponded to the territory of the anterior cerebral artery.

Microscopic sections are now being prepared and a detailed description of all the pathologic findings will be presented in a later publication.

tasks, and that if two normals can cooperate in performing an activity, two isolated cerebral hemispheres can do so equally well.

The most serious objection to our interpretation is the negative results obtained by Akelaitis[2] and his co-workers in their studies of humans with callosal sections. We are not certain of the reasons for these discrepancies but would suggest certain possibilities. Most, although not all, of Akelaitis' patients were young and had epilepsy dating from childhood. It is possible that early hemispheric lesions inhibit the development of unilateral dominance for language. Second, youth alone may be important, just as the young compensate for cerebellar removals while adults do not; it is possible that alternative pathways may be more readily available or more easily developed in the younger patient with a callosal section. It may also be significant that Akelaitis' patients, with only one exception, were epileptics of some years' duration. It is conceivable that the occurrence of multiple seizures might facilitate the availability of alternative pathways. Another possibility is that partial deconnection may be more seriously disturbing in man than total separation. Further, it is possible that only a small number of humans are as heavily dependent on the callosum as are lower animals, so that the syndrome might be seen only in such subjects. Finally, it should be considered that, in the presence of intellectual deterioration, the patient is somehow less able to compensate for the destruction of the callosum (just as denial of hemiplegia in right parietal syndromes is more likely to occur in the presence of intellectual impairment). We cannot with assurance support any of these hypotheses.

Much of the early physiological work on the corpus callosum received its impetus from clinical observations. The physiological studies by Sperry and his co-workers are now in turn acting as a stimulus to clinicians to reinvestigate this problem. Human material offers certain special advantages, particularly the unilaterality of the speech area, that permit studies to be done that are not open to the animal investigator. We hope that further clinical researches in man will help to clarify some of these problems.

## Summary and Conclusions

A case of a 42-year-old man with a glioblastoma multiforme, who postoperatively was found to present many unusual findings, is reported. The patient's routine neurological examination showed a right hemiplegia worse in the leg with a very marked grasp reflex in the right hand and mild position sense loss on the right side. There were definite signs of intellectual deterioration.

Writing with the left hand was incorrect, both spontaneously and to dictation, while writing with the right hand was normal except for some disturbances caused by the grasp reflex. He named objects placed in the left hand (concealed from vision) incorrectly; he could select them afterward with his left hand by touch or pointing; and he could draw the object afterward with his left hand. Even while giving an incorrect verbal description, he could demonstrate correctly the use of the object being held in the left hand. If an object was placed in one hand (concealed from vision), he could not select it from a group or draw it with the other hand. He frequently performed verbal commands incorrectly with his left hand.

The authors feel that the simplest explanation of the phenomena is that the patient behaved as if his two cerebral hemispheres were disconnected and that the probable cause of this was a lesion of the corpus callosum. Alternative hypotheses and objections are considered, and a brief review is given of relevant earlier clinical observations as well as of the recent work of Sperry on callosal deconnection in animals.

## References

1. Sittig, O.: Über Apraxie, Berlin, Karger, 1931.
2. Akelaitis, A. J.: A study of gnosis, praxis and language following section of the corpus callosum and anterior commissure. J. Neurosurg. 1:94, 1944.
3. Bremer, F., Briplate, J., and Andre-Balisaux, g.: Physiologie et pathologie du corps calleux. Schweiz. Archiv. Neurol. Psychiat. 78:31, 1956.
4. Sperry, R. W.: Cerebral organization and behavior. Science 133:1749, 1961.
5. Bouman, L., and Grünbaum, A. A.: Über motorische Momente der Agraphie. Mschr. Psychiat. Neurol. 77: 223, 1930.
6. Liepmann, H., and Maas, O.: Fall von linksseitiger Agraphie und Apraxie bei rechtsseitiger Lähmung. J. Psychol. Neurol. (Lpz.) 10:214, 1907.
7. Hecaen, H., and Gimeno-Alava, A.: L'apraxie idéomotrice unilatérale gauche. Rev. Neurol. (Par.) 102:648, 1960.
8. Goldstein, K.: Zur Lehre von der motorischen Apraxie. J. Psychol. Neurol. (Lpz.) 11:169, 270, 1908.
9. Denny-Brown, D.: The nature of apraxia. J. Nerv. Ment. Dis. 126:9, 1958.
10. Van Vleuten, C. F.: Linksseitige motorische Apraxie. Z. Psychiat. 64:203, 1907.
11. Maas, O.: Ein Fall von linksseitiger Apraxie und Agraphie. Neurologisches Centralblatt 26:789, 1907.
12. Trescher, J. H., and Ford, F. R.: Colloid cyst of the third ventricle. Arch. Neurol. Psychiat. 37:959, 1937.
13. Geschwind, N.: The anatomy of acquired reading disorders. In Reading Disabilities, Baltimore: Johns Hopkins Press, 1962.

We wish to express our appreciation to several members of the Boston V.A. Hospital, and particularly to Dr. Harold Goodglass, director of research, Psychology Section, for his help and especially for his advice on testing procedures. We also wish to thank Dr. F. A. Quadfasel, chief of neurology, for his criticism and his profound knowledge of the earlier literature. We also wish to express our appreciation to the residents who took care of the patient, Drs. Merrill Reiss and Seymour Strum.

Supported in part by research grants from the National Institutes of Health to the Section of Psychology, Massachusetts Institute of Technology (M-1802) and to the Department of Psychology, Clark University (M-4187), Worcester, Massachusetts.

# PART II

# Language Disorders

## *Orrin Devinsky*

Geschwind revolutionized the conceptual framework of aphasic disorders. He read and appreciated the insights of the late 19th century German neurologists, which required a complete revision of the Queen Square British neurology he had been taught. Yet he contributed only a limited number of truly new observations. His brilliance for intensive and original investigation of a single case reached its pinnacle in aphasic patients. Geschwind created order from chaos. He linked function with anatomy. His classification was comprehensible to medical students. A decade before, senior neurologists considered aphasias as a single complex of overlapping and indivisible defects. He turned the amorphous mass of expressive disorders (a term he despised since even to hyperfluent Wernicke, aphasics expressed themselves abnormally, with paraphasias, neologisms, and tangential responses) into a logical order that could be systematically examined and mechanistically understood. Geschwind classified aphasias into fluent and nonfluent groups, which largely corresponded with lesions anterior (nonfluent) and posterior (fluent) to the central sulcus. He then renewed interest in testing repetition, a simple maneuver permitting identification of conduction or transcortical aphasias. Lichtheim, in 1885, described the importance of repetition in language assessment.[1] However, its meaning was subsequently lost or misplaced. For many 20th century neurologists before Geschwind, preserved repetition was incorrectly considered a function of the right hemisphere, despite its recognized preservation in transcortical sensory aphasia (e.g., Nielsen's classic monograph, "Agnosia, Apraxia, Aphasia: Their value in Cerebral Localization," 1936).[2]

Geschwind's insights into aphasia were based on the German literature from the late 1800s and early 1900s. Geschwind's two papers, reproduced here, "The Paradoxical Position of Kurt Goldstein in the History of Aphasia," (1964)[3] and "Wernicke's Contribution to the Study of Aphasia," (1967)[4] are classics. They are more than historical stories of aphasia, they are paradigmatic chapters in the history of science. Geschwind explored the social milieus (e.g., competition in the many independent German states) leading to the great discoveries and the factors that led to neurologists to abandon the truth (e.g., victory in WWI causing an assumption of superiority in academia without critical evaluation of the evidence, a preconceived framework into which observations were fit).

Geschwind's interest was not limited to the aphasias—it spanned from the evolution of language (see paper reproduced here, "The Development of the Brain and the Evolution of Language" (1964)[5]) [6,7] to biological foundations of handedness[8–14] (see paper reproduced here, "Language and Cerebral Dominance" (1975)[12]) to disorders masquerading as language disorders (see papers reproduced here, "Nonaphasic Disorders of Speech" (1964) [15] and "The Varieties of Naming Errors" (1967).[16] Geschwind synthesized his approach to understanding the anatomy of language, mechanisms underlying language disorders, examination of aphasic patients, and classification of aphasias in a remarkable series of papers and chapters, published in prominent journals (e.g. New England Journal of Medicine, Science, Scientific American—see papers reproduced here, "Aphasia" (1971) and "The Neural Basis of Language" (written with Damasio, 1984))[17–22] and textbooks (e.g., Handbook of Perception, Beeson and McDermitt's Textbook of Medicine).[23–25] These contributions define the modern approach to understanding, examining, diagnosing, and classifying patients with aphasia.

Geschwind recognized the role of the neocortical language areas as well as the white matter tracts that connect them. Again, his rediscovery of disconnection syndromes brought two aphasic syndromes back to clinical neurology: conduction aphasia[26–28] and the transcortical aphasias.[26,27,29] In Wernicke's classic 1874 monograph,[30] he postulated the existence of conduction aphasia (Leitungsaphasie) from a disconnection of the white matter fibers connecting Wernicke's and Broca's area (which he postulated ran through the insula, but was later convinced by von Monokaw (1908) that it ran through the arcuate fasciculus).[31] Wernicke predicted that patients with conduction aphasia would have fluent speech with paraphasias, strongly resembling the speech in patients with posterior superior temporal lesions. However, those with conduction aphasia would recognize their language errors as they had normal comprehension. Wernicke did not predict impaired repetition with conduction aphasia. Lichtheim (1885) correctly identified repetition defect as a cardinal feature of conduction aphasia and reported a case with this finding.[1] The transcortical aphasias stood as a striking contrast to conduction aphasia. The term *transcortical aphasia* was coined by Wernicke and later described patients with preserved repetition but impaired spontaneous speech (transcortical motor aphasia), impaired comprehension (transcortical sensory aphasia) or both (mixed transcortical aphasia).[29] The transcortical aphasias were summarized by Goldstein in his early and later writings.[32,33] Geschwind and colleagues' description of a man with isolation of the speech cortex following carbon monoxide poisoning[29] helped re-establish the existence and importance of the transcortical aphasias.

Current contributors to aphasia were trained or profoundly influenced by Geschwind. As he did in other areas, Geschwind refocussed our thoughts on the clinical details—what the patient can and cannot do, a sytematic approach to evaluate patients, an individual approach to see each patient, first compassionately as a human, and secondly, as an invaluable experiment of nature, teaching us something if we can only be granted the curiosity, intelligence, patience, and perseverance to see what lies in front of us. Geschwind had all those qualities, in abundance. Geschwind redirected our thoughts away from speculation and philosophical and psychological aspects of language and back towards a neuro-anatomical model. How does the brain work this phenomenon we call language? What is the role of different areas? What role do the connections between different areas play? By combining his clinical genius and his fascination for mechanism and anatomy, Geschwind brought the aphasias from a collection of bizarre symptom concatenations to a comprehensible group of language disorders.

## References


1. Lichtheim, L. 1885. On aphasia. Brain, 1885;7,433-484.
2. Nielsen, JM. *Agnosia, Apraxia, Aphasia: Their Value in Cerebral Localization.* New York: Hoebner, 1936, pp.88-89.
3. Geschwind, N. The Paradoxical Position of Kurt Goldstein in the History of Aphasia. Cortex, 1964;1,214-224.
4. Geschwind, N. Wernicke's Contribution to the Study of Aphasia. Cortex, 1967;3, 449-463.
5. Geschwind, N. The Development of the Brain and the Evolution of Language. In CIJM. Stuart (ed.), *Monograph Series on Languages an Linguistics, Vol. 17.* Washington: George Washington University Press, 1964, pp. 155-169.
6. LeMay, M, and Geschwind, N. Hemispheric Differences in the Brains of Great Apes. Brain, Behavior, and Evolution, 1975;11(1),48-52.
7. Geschwind, N. Anatomical Evolution and the Human Brain. Bulletin of the Orton Society, 1972;2,7-13.
8. Geschwind, N, and Levitsky, W. Human Brain: Left-Right Asymmetries in Temporal Speech Region. Science, 1968;161(837),186-187.
9. Geschwind, N. The Anatomical Basis of Hemispheric Differentiation. In JG Beaumont and S Dimond (eds.), *Hemisphere Function in the Human Brain.* London: Paul Elek, 1974, pp. 7-24.
10. Geschwind, N. Anatomical Asymmetry as the Basis for Cerebral Dominance. Fed Proc, 1978;37(9),2263-2266.
11. Geschwind, N. Anatomical and Functional Specialization of the Cerebral Hemispheres in the Human. Bull Mem Acad R Med Belg, 1979;134(6),286-297.
12. Geschwind, N. Language and Cerebral Dominance. In DB Tower (ed.), *The Nervous System, Vol. 2.* New York: Raven Press, 1975, pp. 433-439.
13. Geschwind, N, Galaburda, A, and LeMay, M. Morphological and Physiological Substrates of Language and Cognitive Development. In R Katzman (ed.), *Congenital and Acquired Cognitive Disorders. Research Publication: Research in Nervous and Mental Diseases, Vol 57.* New York: Raven Press, 1979, pp. 31-42.
14. Geschwind, N. Asymmetries of the Brain—Newer Developments. Bull Orton Society, 1979;29,67-73.

15. Geschwind, N. Non Aphasic Disorders of Speech. Int J Neurology, 1965;4(3),207-214.
16. Geschwind, N. The Varieties of Naming Errors. Cortex, 1967;3,97-112.
17. Geschwind, N. The Organization of Language and the Brain. Science, 1970; 170(961),940-944.
18. Geschwind, N. Aphasia. N Eng J Med, 1971;284,654-656.
19. Geschwind, N. Language and the Brain. Sci Am, 1972;226(4),76-83.
20. Geschwind, N. Linguistic Distinctions in Aphasia. Contemporary Psychology, 1981;26,833-834.
21. Geschwind, N. Aphasia Part 1: Examination of the Aphasic Patient. Neurol Neurosurg Update, 1982;3(6).
22. Geschwind, N. Aphasia Part 2: Diagnosis, Prognosis, and Treatment. Neurol Neurosurg Update, 1982;3(7).
23. Goodglass, H, and Geschwind, N. Language Disorders (Aphasia). In EC Carterette and M.P. Friedman (eds.), *Handbook of Perception, Vol. 7.* New York: Academic Press, 1976, pp. 390-428.
24. Geschwind, N. Disturbances of Language, Perception and Memory. In CS Keefer and RW Wilkins (eds.), *Medicine: Essentials of Clinical Practice.* Boston: Little, Brown & Company, 1970, pp. 973-980.
25. Geschwind, N. Focal Disturbances of Higher Nervous Function. In P Beeson and W. McDermott (eds.), *Textbook of Medicine.* Philadelphia: W.B. Saunders, 1971, pp. 99-102.
26. Geschwind, N. Disconnexion Syndromes in Animals and Man. I. Brain, 1965; 88(2),237-294.
27. Geschwind, N. Disconnexion Syndromes in Animals and Man. II. Brain, 1965; 88(3),585-644.
28. Benson, DF, Sheremata, WA, Bouchard, R, Segarra, JM, Price, D, and Geschwind N. Conduction aphasia: A clinicopathological study. Arch Neurol, 1973;28,339-356.
29. Geschwind, N, Quadfasel, FA, and Segarra, JM. Isolation of the Speech Area. Neuropsychology, 1968;6,327-340.
30. Wernicke, C. The symptom-complex of aphasia. In A Church (ed.), *Diseases of the Nervous System.* New York: Appleton, 1908, pp. 265-324.
31. von Monakow, C. *Die Lokalisation im Grosshirn und der Abbau der Funktion durch Kortikale Herde,* Wiesbaden: Bergmann, 1914.
32. Goldstein, K. "Die transkortikalen aphasien." Jena (Pt II), 1917.
33. Goldstein, K. *Language and Language Disturbances: Aphasic symptom complexes and their significance for medicine and theory of language.* New York, Grune & Stratton, 1948.

# CHAPTER 2

# The Development of the Brain and the Evolution of Language

*Norman Geschwind*

Most students of the problem are agreed that there is something special about human language. The major alternative views may be summed up in two simple categories: (1) There is nothing *qualitatively* distinctive about human language; man only possesses *more* language than lower animals. The opposing group of views state: (2) Only man has language. Both approaches leave us with difficulties. If man has more of something than a monkey, then just what particular function of the monkey's is it that is being multiplied in man? If only man has language, then what is the essence of this new addition to the armamentarium of the activities of animals?

The first group of theorists are likely not to worry about the details of what it is in the animal that is multiplied in man. They tend to express their ideas as *Gedanken* experiments: Tell me what you want the animal to do, and I can devise a training procedure to do it. The second group tend to phrase the differences in terms that are sometimes as ethereal as those of the first group are uncompromisingly untheoretical and practical.

Regardless of their particular position, the adherents of each of these views have shared in common either an inability or a lack of interest in specifying what change in the design of the human brain permits these quantitative or qualitative distinctions. This paper represents an attempt to bridge this gap in some small way. The linguist, even if he accepts the views presented here, may well find them disappointingly meager. The first day of this conference has been devoted to a series of papers representing much of the forefront of pure linguistic theory, and the overwhelming stress has been placed on aspects of syntax. The linguist would

---

Reprinted with permission from C.I.J.M. Stuart (ed.) Monograph Series on Languages and Linguistics, Vol. 17. Washington: Georgetown University Press, 1964, 155–169.

certainly wish to know in what way the human brain has become adapted to the production of syntactic speech. Instead he will have to be satisfied—if indeed he is satisfied at all—by a theory of object-naming. Let me, therefore, hasten to state that I make no pretensions for what I say except insofar as it applies to object-naming. On the other hand, an interest in object-naming is not ill-placed since much of the practical use of language rests on the basis of this rather unglamorous activity. Even object-naming in itself has its more interesting sides. Thus, workers in childhood development have tended to neglect the acquisition of names since this has been regarded as the simple enlargement of the lexicon, and have concentrated on the evolution of grammar. Yet the problem of the lexicon goes beyond the mere filling of the dictionary randomly. Thus the naming of colors, which to the adult appears like a remarkably simple task, is often acquired late, long after the child can name remarkably complicated objects. The ramifications of this extend still further into language performance. Thus there are reasons for regarding it as not unlikely that the time of acquisition of color-naming and of reading should be highly correlated.

There is perhaps one more reason to stress object-naming. While the mechanism suggested here for the naming of things throws no direct light on the acquisition of grammar, it does throw into relief some different ways of looking at the acquisition of grammar which may well be experimentally useful.

It is perhaps appropriate to put in one final comment on this type of theorizing. The linguist may wonder whether such a theory, even if correct, is any concern of his. Let me suggest some reasons which justify interest by linguists in this type of theory. In the first place, it is reasonable that anything which throws some light on the nature of language should be of interest to the linguist. A second reason is that the linguist has the ability to provide help to the student of the nervous system. The theory of object-naming to be propounded here has certain implications which might conceivably be more effectively tested in a non-Indo-European language.[1]

There is a third reason which is perhaps the most cogent one for the linguist to take some interest in these matters. I gathered from various sources, for example, from the proceedings of this conference a year ago, that the status of linguistic theories continues to be a difficult problem. In a sense, the difficulty reduces to that of deciding whether the best theory is simply the most economical set of axioms from which the language behavior can be deduced, i.e., in essence a condensed description. If this is true, then theoretical linguistics might appear to be only a more efficient form of description. I would wish, cautiously, to make the suggestion, that perhaps a further touchstone may be added: to what extent

---

[1] For example, the theory deals with the problem of color-naming as a corollary. The theory predicts that color-naming, if learned in a certain way, should be affected by certain lesions of the nervous system. In a hypothetical language in which there were no color-names, but in which the color of an object was stated as the color of some other well-known object, the theory would predict that this lesion should not have the same effect. A linguist is more likely to avoid the naive error that color-naming is done in the same way in all languages.

does the theory tie in with other, non-linguistic information, for example, the anatomical aspects of language? In the end, such bridges link a theory to the broader body of scientific knowledge. I would personally not see much virtue in the views of those theoreticians who feel that language and its disturbances must be viewed *separately* on the linguistic and biological levels. Let us now return to the main topic of this paper.

In order to specify what the differences are between man and subhuman primates, let me first discuss some of the features of learning in these non-human forms. I hope I may be forgiven for some preliminary remarks about some elementary anatomical and physiological aspects which may not be familiar to all of you. If the discussion *appears* very remote from our topic, please rest assured that it is all really germane.

Lying along the inner surface of the temporal lobes of the brain are a group of structures of extremely complex anatomy. For the sake of simplicity I will loosely use the term "limbic system" to refer to these and to their major connections in the **hypothalamus** and other structures lower in the brain. Included in the anatomical organization of this region are those parts of the brain which when stimulated give rise to sensations of taste or smell, and to certain emotions such as fear and their corresponding motor activities. For simplicity, we may divide those aspects of the limbic system of interest to us into two groups: (1) **Limbic motor responses**—these are highly organized, essentially inborn motor sequences which mediate the motor responses involved in fear, rage, and sexual activities. (2) **Limbic sensory responses**—these are the subjective feelings of smell, taste, hunger, and thirst and the corresponding feelings of satiation, sexual sensations, anger, and fear. It is not at all inaccurate to say that the limbic system mediates both the inborn motor sequences involved in those elementary activities intimately related to the survival of the organism or the species and the subjective experiences related to these activities.

Let us now consider by contrast the remaining "non-limbic" portions of the surface of the brain which, in fact, make up the bulk of the exposed surface of the hemispheres in the primates, including man. In particular, we will concentrate on the sensory portions of this non-limbic brain. There are three sensory regions which are to be specified here: the **visual cortex,** the **auditory cortex,** and the **somesthetic cortex** (which eventually receives the sensory information from the skin, muscles, bone, joints, and tendons—the term "touch" can loosely be used to designate this group of sensations). These three regions may be said to mediate the "non-limbic" modalities of sensation.

The zones we have so far considered, that is, the "limbic" regions on the medial surface of the temporal lobe, and the primary centers for the "non-limbic" sensations of vision, audition, and somesthesis, constitute only a small fraction of the surface of the hemisphere. These four regions, together with the classic **motor cortex,** are all, in the terminology of the great German neuroanatomist Flechsig, "primordial zones," that is, regions which mature early in the development of the individual. The most commonly used criterion for such maturation is the degree of myelination of the nerve fibers in these regions. These primordial zones also differ quite markedly from each other in cellular architecture.

If we contemplate the brain of a subprimate mammal, such as a rabbit or a cat, we find that these primordial zones make up the majority of the cerebral mantle. As we move up the phylogenetic scale we find the striking fact that these zones become increasingly separated by new areas of cortex. The cortex separating the primordial zones occupies a greater percentage of the surface in the primates and achieves its greatest extent in man, where it clearly occupies most of the surface of the hemispheres. It is indeed the development of this **association cortex** which is responsible for the higher functions of the nervous system. The association cortex matures later in the life of the individual. Flechsig called these regions "intermediary zones" to indicate their later myelination. The different parts of the association cortex are more like each other in structure than are the different primordial zones.

Let us now turn to the problem of the connections between these different regions of the cerebral mantle. Flechsig (1901) stated an important principle for the brain of man which has in recent years been re-emphasized for the brain of the subhuman primate by Bailey and von Bonin (1951). The principle asserts that in man the primordial zones, i.e., the regions of early maturation, do not have any significant number of direct connections between them. Thus there are no significant direct interconnections between the limbic regions, the motor cortex, the auditory, somesthetic, and visual cortexes.[2]

Each primordial zone has a significant number of connections only to the immediately adjacent association cortex. The association cortex itself may have long connections to other regions. Let us now consider the connections of the non-limbic sensory modalities. In particular, let us consider the connections of the visual cortex which are the best known and may serve as a paradigm for the others.

The primary visual cortex makes connections to the immediately adjacent visual association cortex. The visual association cortex has three important sets of connections, the first two of which I mention only in passing, and the third of which is immediately germane to our argument: (a) connections to the visual association cortex of the opposite side via the corpus callosum, (b) connections to the association cortex anterior to the classic motor cortex, and (c) the largest connection and the one of most concern to us runs from the visual association cortex to the outer and inferior surfaces of the temporal lobe.

Why should the largest connection of the visual cortex eventually reach this portion of the temporal lobe? If we consider in turn this region of the temporal lobe, we find that it makes connections with the limbic structures on the inner

---

[2] This principle holds to its full extent in man, the monkey, and chimpanzee, and probably in the other primates, at least the higher ones. It does not hold completely in sub-primate forms: for example, it is clearly not true of the cat's brain. It is therefore important to distinguish the species involved and not to generalize too readily to the human brain from that of lower forms, particularly when these lower forms are sub-primates.

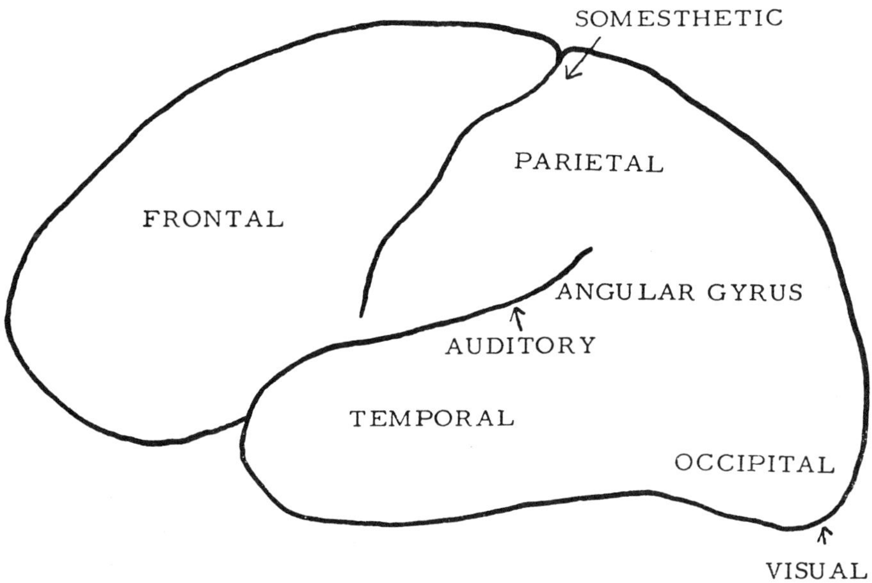


FIGURE 1. View of lateral (outer) surface of human left cerebral hemisphere. The frontal, parietal, temporal, and occipital lobes are indicated. In addition, the arrows point to the primary somesthetic, auditory, and visual regions of the cortex. The region of the angular gyrus is also shown. Fuller explanation is given in the text.

surface of the temporal lobe. In fact, the limbic structures themselves constitute one of the primordial zones, and therefore do not receive long connections directly from any other region of the cerebral cortex, but receive connections only from the nearby association cortex. The lateral and inferior temporal lobe is thus the association cortex for the limbic structures.

Let us now sum up briefly the point to which these considerations have led us. The visual cortex has its main connections to the limbic system. These are not direct connections but go by way of the association cortex adjacent to the visual cortex and the association cortex on the lateral and basal surfaces of the temporal lobe. We are now prepared—at last—to consider the functional significance of these anatomical connections.

In order to approach this problem, let us ask ourselves how a monkey would respond with a rage response to the sight of an object (such as a net) which he has learned to dislike. The impulse must travel over the pathway I have just specified from the visual cortex to the limbic structures and there arouse the inborn rage response. Suppose this pathway is broken at some point? The monkey will no longer respond with rage to this visual stimulus. We will have produced a visual-limbic disconnection.

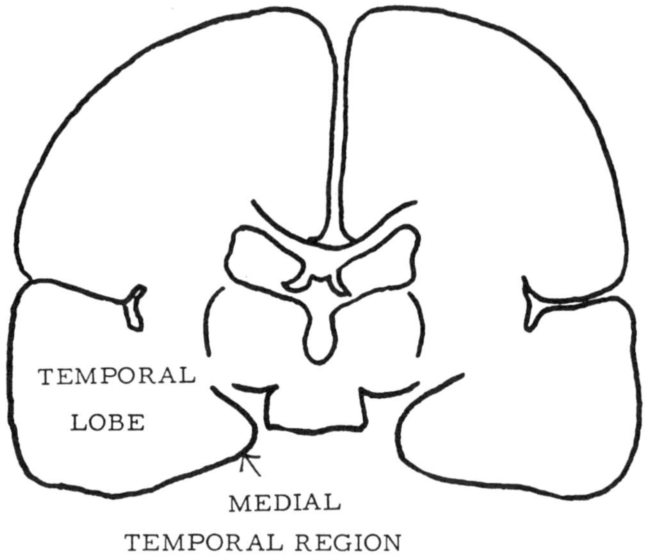


FIGURE 2. Cross-section in the vertical plane through the human brain. The temporal lobe is indicated. The medial temporal region (whose importance is discussed in the text) is also shown.

Consider now an example which is far more important for our purpose. How do we teach a monkey presented visually with, let us say, a circle and a cross, to press the lever under the circle rather than that under the cross? We do this by what the psychologists call *reinforcing* one or another response. We may reinforce positively, i.e., reward the response we wish the animal to make, or we may reinforce negatively, i.e., punish the response to be rejected. I do not wish to go into the complexities of the question of reinforcement. For the sake of simplicity, we may say that the primary reinforcers are limbic sensations, i.e., the rewards are such things as the taste of food, the satisfaction of hunger or thirst; the punishments are such things as the arousal of fear.

In effect, then, the visual learning paradigm in the monkey may be reduced to a simple formula: the animal learns to form associations of a visual stimulus to a "limbic" stimulus. In more general terms, learning in the monkey consists in forming associations between a "non-limbic" stimulus and a "limbic" stimulus. This is true for vision, audition, and somesthesis. From the point of view of evolution, this is reasonable: a stimulus in a non-limbic sensory modality is learned readily only to the extent that it arouses a sensation important to the survival of the individual animal or the species.

In order to look a bit more deeply at learning in the monkey, let us now turn to a somewhat different test situation, the one reported by Ettlinger (1960). Here the monkey is taught to choose one of two patterns presented visually, let us say, a circle rather than a cross, by the technique already mentioned of rewarding the choice of one item. After the monkey has learned this to a high degree so that he chooses the rewarded circle on nearly all occasions, another experiment is performed. The monkey is now permitted to palpate two solid figures, a circle and a cross respectively, which are concealed from vision. The animal is again rewarded for choosing the circle rather than the cross. Curiously enough, he shows no evidence of carry-over from the identical task done visually. The tactile task is treated by the monkey as a totally new one.

How are we to interpret this experiment and others which have essentially the same result? Ettlinger and others have argued that cross-modal transfers do not tend to occur in animals. But our previous discussion has already stressed that *all* learning in the monkey is cross-modal since the process of learning depends on the formation of associations between non-limbic and limbic sensations which is certainly a cross-modal task. The essence indeed of these experiments is that the animal has failed to form an association between two non-limbic modalities.[3]

The same task is, of course, remarkably easy in man who makes the transfer immediately in at least this particular experiment. What is the reason for the ease with which humans do this task which is so difficult for the monkey? Some authors say that man does it by means of verbal mediation. In other words, when one learns to choose a circle over a cross, one learns to choose the "circle." When the task is done we again choose the object which we have named "circle." The monkey's failure at these particular cross-modal tasks is thus attributed to his failure to use language.

A moment's reflection, however, shows that this argument which appears so plausible at first glance, has in fact been stated backwards. In order to call a seen object a circle, we must have learned to associate the visual stimulus with the auditory stimulus "circle." In other words, to say that the ability to perform cross-modal associations depends on the ability to name misses the real point which is, as it were, the reverse: *The ability to name depends on the ability to form non-limbic cross-modal associations,* particularly *visual-auditory and tactile-auditory.*[4] One may go further: *The ability to develop language in man probably depends on his ability to form cross-modal associations* between two non-limbic modalities. One might raise the objection, however, that a deaf man might learn language without using cross-modal associations at all. Could he not learn to read by being shown the picture of the object which corresponded to

---

[3] An objection might be raised that Ettlinger's experiment actually relates to cross-modal *transfer,* not cross-modal *association.* This problem is too complex to discuss fully at this point. Transfer is probably the simpler of the two, and therefore the failure of transfer probably also implies difficulty in association. In any case, other evidence, e.g., from conditioning experiments, also points to the difficulty of non-limbic intermodal *associations* in subhuman forms.

[4] It is true that in adult man, some visual-tactile associations may be done indirectly by the linking up of two separate cross-modal associations (visual-auditory and tactile-auditory). Each of these components is, however, itself an elementary non-limbic cross-modal association.

each new written word? Indeed he probably could. In order, however, for him to be able to name (in writing) things with which he palpated he would at least have to be able to form tactile-visual associations. There is, however, a further consideration. Even a visual-visual association is a link between two non-limbic stimuli, and it is questionable that even this would readily be acquired by the monkey.

We have asserted then the thesis that man develops language because he can form associations between two non-limbic stimuli. Couldn't limbic stimuli be useful as language? The answer of course is no: a monkey would have a great deal of difficulty arousing in another animal a smell or taste, or a feeling of hunger or thirst. We communicate by producing non-limbic stimuli—auditory, visual, or tactile.

What is the basis for the difference in the ability of man and the monkey to form pure non-limbic associations? Let us return to our anatomical considerations. As we have pointed out, there are three main connections from the visual association areas of a monkey—one to the symmetrical region of the opposite side, one to the motor association area, and the largest to the lateral and basal temporal lobe which is the association cortex for the limbic system. Thus none of the *main* connections are designed to mediate visual-auditory associations. There are, however, definite connections between some of the visual and auditory association areas, as shown for example in the experiments of Sugar, French, and Chusid (1948). These experimenters found clear evidence of fibers running from the auditory association cortex to the visual association cortex but none in the reverse direction; in other words they found no evidence for fibers which could mediate the arousal of auditory memories from a visual stimulus. Even the auditory to visual fibers they found constitute a group far smaller than the fiber systems mediating visual-limbic associations. The monkey brain thus probably contains visual, auditory, and somesthetic regions which, operating on the whole independently, feed into the limbic system stimuli which are used only to the extent that they more or less immediately affect survival.[5]

Even if a small number of fibers exist which have not been discovered between the visual and auditory regions, this would not affect the argument. The more information that must be carried between two cortical regions, the more fibers necessary to carry them. The more associations formed, the more cells are needed to store the memories. The monkey does not appear to have a sufficient basis anatomically to form extensive non-limbic intermodal associations. That a limited number of such associations could be performed perhaps with extensive training is probably correct, but there is probably an inherent limit to the speed of formation or the variety of such associations. One might say that the monkey lacks adequate "memory space" and "channel capacity" for this type of association.

---

[5] There is a possible exception in the "curiosity" drive which has been studied by such workers as Butler (1953) and which does not appear to be quite so "primitive" as the other limbic reinforcers. Even this drive is very likely to depend on the limbic system.

It might be worth digressing for a moment to consider the great strain put on the facilities of a brain by a demand for non-limbic intermodal associations. Consider the situation that visual, auditory, and somesthetic association areas discharge independently into the limbic system via association cortex. In order to add visual-auditory and visual-tactile associations to the visual-limbic associations, one would probably have to add at least twice as many fibers and cells as are now used for the visual-limbic connections alone. The probable minimum net effect of such an extensive addition of non-limbic intermodal fibers is therefore to triple the array of cells and fibers needed in the visual association system. It is no surprise that this uneconomical situation does not appear even in the subhuman primates.

What then of the human brain? What correlates with the newly acquired or at least greatly increased ability to form non-limbic intermodal associations and thus to develop language?

It is obvious that there has been marked development of the human brain in comparison to that of even the highest apes (Connolly, 1950). Thus the gorilla has the largest brain of any of the anthropoids, but it never even reaches half the weight of an average adult human brain. In addition, the **cerebellum** makes up a higher percentage of the brain in the anthropoid apes so that the cerebral hemispheres of man (which constitute the part which is of concern to us) are relatively even larger than the discrepancy in whole-brain weights would suggest. Furthermore, a fully adult gorilla is a considerably larger animal than a human. An orangutan which when fully grown may weigh as much as a small human adult has a brain which is about one quarter as heavy as the human brain at maturity.

The human brain at birth is perhaps 40% of its adult size, while that of the ape's is nearly 70% of full-grown size. This suggests that much of the human brain is evolutionarily late since it matures so late in the life of an individual. This supposition is amply borne out by closer inspection. The great increase in the size of man's brain is primarily in the association areas, rather than in the primary receptive areas. This growth is reflected in the **frontal pole,** the **temporal lobe,** and in the **inferior parietal region.** The greatest relative growth of the human brain compared to that of the subhuman primates is in the inferior parietal region, and it behooves us to look at this zone more carefully.

The impressive development of the inferior posterior parietal region (the region of the **angular gyrus**) is so great that some authors (e.g., Goldstein, 1927) even assert that this region is almost unique to man. Even those who deny this, such as von Bonin and Bailey (1961), still stress that it is this region of the brain which has expanded most markedly in man compared to any of the apes. Its advanced state is testified to by the fact that it is one of the last regions to myelinate and was called by Flechsig one of the "terminal zones" in contrast to the earliest myelinating "primordial zones" and the "intermediary zones" which myelinate at an intermediate period. According to Dr. Paul Yakovlev, this region does not mature in its cellular structure until three or four years or even much later in childhood.

This region is ideally located for the purposes of our theory. It is placed between the association cortexes of the three non-limbic modalities: vision, audition, and somesthesis. It is thus admirably suited to play the role of acting as the way-station by which associations may be formed between these non-limbic modalities. This area may well be termed "the association cortex" of the association cortexes. By providing the basis for the formation of non-limbic associations, it provides the anatomical basis for language—or at least for object-naming. Other authors have stressed the importance of the posterior parietal region for language,[6] but I hope that I have been able to give a physiological basis to this localization.

There are many problems associated with the discussion I have just presented. Indeed, rather than use the word 'problems,' I would perhaps have been more correct in saying that it raises many possibilities for further investigation. Much of the data now available does support the view advanced here. I will cite only a few examples of such data.

(Note to the reader: The following section contains rather technical material which can be omitted without violence to the main trend of the argument.)

Very large lesions of the angular gyrus region produce an aphasic picture in which the patient speaks volubly but communicates little information. The speech is in particular remarkably poor in the names of objects. The reason for this clinical picture is readily deducible. The connections from the rest of the brain to the auditory association area are cut off. On the other hand since the auditory association area and the motor speech region and their connections are intact, the patient can still produce the automatisms of language freely—these are those aspects of language not demanding intermodal transfer for their use at a given instant. The comprehension of language is seriously impaired since the arousal of associations in other modalities by the auditory speech patterns is also cut off by the lesion. These patients, despite severe comprehension defect, may show perfect repetition because they have preserved the connections between the auditory association cortex and the motor speech region.

Even more revealing as to the importance of intermodal associations are certain more limited lesions. Thus in certain partial lesions of the angular gyrus (first described by Dejerine, 1891) there may be an isolated loss of the ability to comprehend written language and to write (the so-called "pure alexia with agraphia"), while all other aspects of language are intact. The functions of the angular gyrus in auditory-visual associations may be quite dramatically brought out by considering an even more restricted lesion, that of the so-called "pure word-blindness without agraphia" (Dejerine, 1892; Geschwind, 1962). Here the left primary visual cortex is destroyed. The patient can thus see only with his right visual cortex. In addition, however, there is usually a destruction of the posterior end of the corpus callosum. This acts to cut off the right visual region from the left angular gyrus region, and thus the patient cannot understand written language. All other aspects of language are intact.

---

[6] See for example the discussion in Critchley (1953).

> The disturbances in these patients can be summarized as follows: they lose the ability to comprehend written language, to read music, and to name colors (but they can still match colors correctly and show other evidences of correct color perception by *non-verbal* means—see discussion in Geschwind, 1964). They tend to preserve the ability to name objects and to read numbers. How does one make sense of this constellation of impaired and preserved visual tasks? Reading is learned nearly always after speaking. While one learns in speaking to name objects with which one has had both tactile and visual experience, learning to read is almost exclusively dependent on pure visual-auditory connections (particularly after the earliest stages). When these pure connections are cut off the patient can no longer read. He can still copy the words he cannot read (which effectively rules out almost any perceptual theory of this disturbance) because visuo-motor connections in the right hemisphere are still intact. He can name objects because these arouse tactile associations further forward in the right hemisphere, and a connection can be made to the speech regions across an intact part of the corpus callosum lying forward of the damaged part.
>
> Color-naming and music-reading are lost with word-reading because they are very pure visuo-auditory tasks—we can identify an apple by its form or texture, but we cannot identify a color by these. Finally, number-reading is preserved because numbers are usually associated with a powerful somesthetic reinforcement (counting on the fingers) through a considerable part of childhood, a form of reinforcement not available for words.

The thesis presented here is that the development of object-naming depends on the presence of anatomical structures in man which are absent or poorly developed in the monkey. The assertion that object-naming depends on visual-auditory transfers is of course an old one in linguistics. Wittgenstein (1953) opens his *Philosophical Investigations* with a quotation from St. Augustine's *Confessions:* "When they (my elders) named some object and accordingly moved towards something, I saw this and grasped that the thing was called by the sound they uttered when they meant to point it out. . . ."

Can we expand the theory presented here to more than object-naming, and can we somehow use the same approach to help us with grammar? We may appropriately quote Wittgenstein's comment on the above passage, "Augustine does not speak of there being any difference between kinds of word. If you describe the learning of language in this way you are, I believe, thinking primarily of nouns like "table," "chair," "bread," and of people's names, and only secondarily of the names of certain actions and properties; and (*sc.* you are thinking) of the remaining kinds of words as something that will take care of itself." But, of course, Wittgenstein implies, and we must agree, that the other words will not take care of themselves. How would you teach a child the use of the word "if" by the method described by Augustine?

I do not have a solution to offer at this moment. It would be difficult to conceive of grammar as depending on intermodal transfers in the straight-forward manner that object-naming does. Grammar appears at first glance to be something that grows up within the auditory association system itself, to depend on intramodal, auditory-auditory associations (which can then be transferred *en bloc* to written language by use of the cross-modal association system we have discussed).

This answer is, needless to say, hardly satisfactory, but our earlier discussion may give a clue as to some useful future approaches. We began this paper by stressing the exact method by which a monkey learns to choose a circle over a cross. Similarly, we have discussed the exact mechanism of object-naming in man. We can answer questions as to how we would teach certain things to a monkey and how we could teach a child the name of an object. Let us consider the possible applications of the method to grammar. We have some important facts, gleaned in important studies in recent years, on the child's acquisition of grammar. These facts, however, are still concerned mostly with the age of acquisition of certain grammatical features, their order of acquisition, and the learning of distinctions between features that might at first be accepted as equivalent. To some extent we can specify what rule the child follows at each age. I would suggest, as a supplement and by no means a substitute to these very important studies, that some attention be paid to the actual act of learning by the child and that some experiments be devised to study the elementary situations in which children learn to use certain words. At its origin, grammar may well be acquired by mechanisms as naive as those of object-naming. Once these elementary associative steps are passed, the acquisition of the more complex structures presents less difficulty. It is the very first steps which are the vital ones. Once speech is developed, it can develop an autonomy from the outside world that is all too familiar. If our studies on learning by monkeys and object-naming in man are to be of use, they should teach us to study not what grammatical rule is acquired by the child at a given age but *how* he has acquired this rule and how we could teach it to him.

## Summary

Certain aspects of the anatomy of the nervous system in man and other primates were reviewed. The distinction was pointed out between the **limbic system** (those structures lying in general in the "core" of the brain and involved in the motor and sensory aspects of feeding, drinking, elimination, aggression, flight, and reproduction) and the **non-limbic** regions of the brain. It was pointed out that, anatomically, the major connections in sub-human primates from the non-limbic zones (vision, touch, audition) are to the limbic regions and that therefore learning in these animals should consist mostly of associations of non-limbic to limbic stimuli. By contrast, the non-human primates lack adequate anatomical structures for the development of associations between non-limbic modalities, and in fact such associations are not formed readily in them.

It was then pointed out that object-naming is in fact acquired by learning an association between two non-limbic stimuli (visual-auditory) and that the development of language in man has in fact been dependent on his acquisition of the ability to form non-limbic cross-modal associations. Reasons were given for the view that this ability depends on the great development of the **posterior parietal region** in man (the **angular gyrus region**).

There was some brief discussion of evidence in favor of this theory and a very brief mention of the possibilities of extension of this kind of theory to other aspects of linguistic behavior. In particular, stress was placed on the importance of studying the process by which a child learns a grammatical rule and experimentally devising techniques for teaching these aspects of language in order to learn the mechanisms of acquisition.

## References

Bailey, P. and von Bonin, G., *The Isocortex of Man* (University of Illinois Press, 1951).

Bonin, G. v. and Bailey, P. in *Primatologia,* edd. Hofer, H., Schultz, A. H. and Starck, D., Vol. II/2, (1961) Lieferung 10.

Butler, R. A., *J. Comp. Physiol. Psychol.,* 46, (1953), 95.

Dejerine, J. *Mém. Soc. Biol.,* 3, (1891), 191.

Dejerine, J. *Mém. Soc. Biol.,* 4 (1892), 61.

Ettlinger, G. *Behaviour,* 16, (1960), 56.

Flechsig, P. *Lancet,* II, (1901), 1027.

Geschwind, N. in *Reading Disability,* ed. J. Money (Baltimore, Johns Hopkins Press, 1964).

Geschwind, N. (1964) "Disconnection Syndromes in Animals and Man." In Press.

Goldstein, K. (1927) in *Handbuch der Normalen und Pathologischen Physiologie,* volume 10, Berlin (Springer).

Sugar, O., French, J. D. and Chusid, J. G. *J. Neurophysiol.,* 11, (1948), 175.

Wittgenstein, L., *Philosophical Investigations,* translated by G. E. M. Anscombe (New York, 1953).

Some of the work discussed was done under a grant (MH 08472-01) from the National Institute of Mental Health to the Department of Neurology, Boston University Medical School.

# CHAPTER 3

# Non-Aphasic Disorders of Speech

*Norman Geschwind*

The separation of aphasic from non-aphasic disorders of language has a significance which extends well beyond the simple desire of the scholar for neat ordering of his data. This distinction is of importance for the clinician who may, in the presence of such disorders, mistakenly assume the presence of disease of the classical speech regions in the left hemisphere and thus be led to an incorrect localization with resultant errors in investigation and management. Organic and psychiatric disease may be confused to the disadvantage of the patient. The physician may be misled by the malingerer to the disadvantage not of the patient himself but of those whom he is desirous of misleading.

The practical uses of this knowledge would alone justify calling it to the attention of physicians. To the researcher in the field of aphasia, the question has an importance transcending practical application in the clinic. The mistaken identification of a non-aphasic disorder as aphasic can lead the investigator to many errors. He may be led to compare the behavior of patients who in fact are not similar. The student of clinico-anatomic correlations may be particularly confused by his post-mortem findings. Thus, in some clinics cases of "aphasia" without post-mortem, lesions in the classical locations are frequently found. In at least two instances with which I am familiar, these cases should have been either recognized or strongly suspected to be non-aphasic speech disorders.

Let us outline here the groups of patients who will be of concern to us. We wish to distinguish first those patients who manifest speech disturbances on a functional psychiatric basis from those with neurological disease. Among those with neurological disease, we wish to separate those with diffuse disturbances of the brain from those with focal abnormalities in the speech regions.[1]

---

[1] It is worth commenting here that we are not concerned with the common difficulties in localization which result from distant effects of a primary disease process, such as occur particularly with space-

Reprinted with permission from *International Journal of Neurology*. 1964;4(3):207-214.

We will organize our material according to the clinical pictures presented by the patient.

Various aspects of the problem of non-aphasic speech disturbance have concerned students of aphasia since its beginnings. Thus, Wernicke (1874) pointed out in his classic monograph the common error of confusing fluent paraphasic speech with the productions of psychotics. Critchley (1964) has recently discussed this problem. A problem of particular interest in classical neurology was that of anomia or amnesic aphasia. One group of neurologists regarded isolated naming difficulties as resulting from localized lesions in the left posterior parietal region (a view held for example by Head, 1926, despite his well-known prejudices against localization); while another group insisted that anomia was the result of diffuse disease. Some neurologists (e.g., Gloning, Gloning, and Hoff, 1963) have supported the existence of both localized and unlocalized anomias. As will be shown later, it is likely that there exist both localized und unlocalized anomias, but their clinical pictures differ. It is primarily to the work of Weinstein and his associates (Weinstein, 1958; Weinstein and Kahn, 1955; Weinstein and Keller, 1964) that we are indebted for the clarification of the syndrome of non-localizable anomia.

## I. Mutism: Patients Who Say Nothing

As I learned several years ago from Dr. Macdonald Critchley, mutism is uncommon among aphasics, and the most limited aphasic usually has at least one utterance. The occasional aphasic who is mute usually exhibits certain other characteristics which are helpful clinically. Thus he nearly always attempts to communicate in some way, e.g., by gestures or grunts, although he may not succeed. His writing is usually impaired to roughly the same extent as his speech.

Patients with certain psychiatric syndromes may present with mutism. The patient mute as the result of depression will nearly always have a history of increasingly depressive behavior and will manifest many of the other characteristics of that disorder. Schizophrenia and hysteria may present with mutism. The age of the patient is a valuable aid here since the majority of the aphasias occur in an older age group, while schizophrenia and hysteria are disorders which almost always appear before the age of 30. Schizophrenic or hysterical mutism may well appear in patients who already have a long history of behavior disturbance, while most aphasias tend to be of acute onset in people who have

---

taking lesions. No neurologist is surprised to see a hemiplegia in the presence of a large cerebral tumor, regardless of its location, because of the effects of displacement of nervous structures, traction on blood vessels, herniations and cerebral edema. Similarly, a focal aphasic syndrome may occur in the presence of large space-taking masses and provide only poor information as to the site of the primary disease. What we are concerned with primarily here is the distinction between clinical syndromes which occur with delimited disease and those which require more diffuse involvement.

been behaviorally normal. Both the schizophrenic and the hysteric patient may write normally despite their mutism. Hysteria is less likely to present with mutism than with aphonia, i.e., a loss of voice. This type of patient (who whispers but produces correct language) should present no diagnostic problem.

There are also neurological causes of non-aphasic mutism. Thus mutism may reveal itself in cases of widespread involvement of the brain by the metabolic disturbances of medical illnesses, such as high fever, dehydration, uremia or congestive heart failure, in intoxications, or in widespread involvement of the nervous system itself, for example, diffuse dementing disorders.

In these cases (of dementia), the advent of mutism signifies not the involvement of the speech areas or their connections but rather that the dementing process has gone so far that in effect the patient has nothing more to say.

Mutism may also result from focal pathology. There is a small group of patients who present with the acute onset of a right hemiplegia and total mutism but with retained ability to write. Following Bastian (1898), we have designated these patients as aphemic rather than aphasic. The reason for calling this disorder non-aphasic is based on the fact that those patients we have seen with this syndrome have manifested no positive signs of aphasia as soon as there was some recovery of speech. With only slight recovery of speech, these patients show not the usual picture of a Broca's aphasia with markedly telegraphic speech but rather markedly effortful speech without agrammatism or other aphasic features. A more common picture is that of the patient with bilateral lesions leading to a classic pseudo-bulbar dysarthria. This disturbance is, however, uncommonly so severe as to produce a total state of mutism. The ability to write may of course be totally preserved in this situation. The other obvious signs of pseudo-bulbar palsy make this diagnosis easy. Mutism may be seen in the patient with multiple lacunar infarcts in the basal ganglia. It is also seen sometimes in patients who have undergone thalamotomies, particularly after bilateral operations.

More challenging are those cases of mutism without pseudo-bulbar signs or hemiplegias. These are the cases which show the syndrome of akinetic mutism, and their failure to speak is not isolated but is only one aspect of a general failure to act. Occasionally such patients will whisper faintly although they will not speak. They differ from the hysterical aphasic, however, in that it takes great effort to bring the akinetic mute to whisper weakly, while the hysterical aphasic may be quite prepared to produce considerable speech in a loud whisper. The akinetic mute may be particularly confusing for several reasons. Occasionally, he will not speak spontaneously, but will, like some mute schizophrenics, show echolalia (this disturbance will be discussed later on in this paper). He may show a great variability in behavior, occasionaly spontaneously producing a perfectly good sentence, and then lapsing back into mutism. In some instances, he may show some spontaneous speech, but this may manifest the non-aphasic naming disturbances to which we will return later. Akinetic mutism can occur in disease of the upper brain stem or may result from bilateral involvement of the frontal lobe anterior to the motor regions.

Mutism in children is a more difficult problem than in the adult. As we have noted, acquired aphasias in the adult rarely lead to mutism, but they do so commonly in the child. Even lesions which in the adult usually lead to fluent paraphasic speech, (i.e., temporal and/or parietal lesions), are likely to lead to mutism in childhood. The difficulty is further compounded by the fact that mutism tends to be more prominent as a manifestation of psychiatric disease in the child than it is in adults. In children, extreme caution is needed in distinguishing the aphasic from the non-aphasic.[2]

## II. Echolalic Disturbances

Stengel (1947) has written an excellent article on the functional characteristics of echolalia. Echolalia is rare in aphasias, at least in those aphasics with lesions in the classical Broca's or Wernicke's areas or their connections. It can occur in those syndromes which were called "trans-cortical aphasias" by the classic neurologists. It was on this group of cases that Kurt Goldstein (1917) wrote an extensive and detailed monograph. By trans-cortical aphasias were meant a group of disturbances in which repetition was very well preserved, in contrast to other disturbances in the production or comprehension of speech. The trans-cortical aphasias constitute a bridge between the aphasic and non-aphasic disorders of organic origin. Thus trans-cortical motor aphasia (in which repetition is excellent despite a lack of spontaneous speech) was thought by Goldstein to imply a lesion lying anterior to an intact Broca's area. Such patients may be nearly or totally mute except in repetition of the examiner's speech. Trans-cortical sensory aphasia (in which repetition is excellent in the face of grossly impaired comprehension) was thought by Goldstein to occur in patients with an intact speech area. Wernicke's and Broca's areas and the connections between them are preserved in this condition. The connections, however, of this intact speech area to the remaining cortical regions are destroyed by a large lesion in the posterior parietal region. We have seen one patient, followed on this service for several years, who exhibited this syndrome in life and showed at post-mortem the findings I have just cited.

As we have noted, echolalia may occur in the trans-cortical aphasias but is uncommon or at least not prominent in those patients with lesions directly involving the speech areas. Echolalia occurs in many but not all conditions where mutism may occur, e.g., in schizophrenics. It can be seen in certain general disturbances of the brain, such as recovery from coma (it was common when insulin coma was still widely used), or after head injury. It may be seen, as I have noted, in large frontal lesions. It occurs in a group of mental defectives who learn language but make little use of it as a propositional tool.

[2] I am not raising here the problem of the child who never learns to speak at all.

It should be noted that the properties of the echolalia itself are of little help in assessing the underlying cause. As Stengel brought out so well in his article, most cases of echolalia exhibit the same functional features regardless of their origin.

## III. Palilalic Disturbances

The tendency to palilalia, i.e., to repetition by the patient of words or phrases, is well recognized in certain psychotic patients. An aphasic with markedly limited speech may have a single recurrent utterance, but the palilalic psychotic may demonstrate his tendency in a large variety of phrases.

Palilalia in neurological disease is usually not associated with aphasia. Patients with Parkinsonism may demonstrate this abnormality. Palilalia is a particularly dramatic characteristic of the speech of the general paretic, although it is difficult to detect once the patient has developed a full blown babbling dysarthria. The classical test employing such phrases as "Methodist Episcopal" or "hippopotamus" is very effective in eliciting palilalic responses such as "hippopopotototamus." Less dramatic palilalia may be seen in other patients with progressive frontal disease. Palilalia, however, need not be confined to syllables as it is ordinarily in paretic speech but may involve whole words or phrases. Any variety of palilalia may occur paroxysmally in seizures involving the supplementary motor area (which lies in the frontal parasagittal region anterior to the motor cortex) as was pointed out in an excellent paper by Alajouanine and his co-workers (1959).

Palilalia, particularly when marked, as in the "babbling dysarthria" of the general paretic, may lead the observer mistakenly to believe that he is dealing with one of the aphasias marked by fluency and paraphasia, as exemplified by the classic Wernicke's aphasia, in which the patient may also produce a stream of incomprehensible speech. The general paretic will of course show the other stigmata of his disease which considerably simplifies the differential diagnosis.

## IV. Other Causes of Fluent Incomprehensible Speech

As we have just noted, the marked palilalia of the general paretic may be confused with the classic Wernicke's aphasia. Other conditions may equally present with fluent incomprehensible speech that may be misleading. Thus, the pseudobulbar dysarthric patient, much more frequently than is appreciated, shows a *rapid* dysarthria which may be totally incomprehensible. If the patient is forced to slow down (which is often very difficult to achieve), the speech may be recognized as non-aphasic. Such patients normally write correctly.

What was once a more common problem was that of differentiating schizophrenic word-salad from the Wernicke type of aphasia. This problem has become less frequent in recent years for the reason that schizophrenic word-salad is far less common in well-run mental hospitals. Certain features make the differential diagnosis straightforward. In the first place fluent aphasias occur mostly in older patients and are less frequently seen in younger ones and never in children. Schizophrenia, by contrast, nearly always has its onset below the age of 40, an age at which fluent aphasias are rare. Furthermore, schizophrenic word-salad is almost never seen in the acutely schizophrenic patient but is most typically seen in the chronic back-ward patient with a long history of behavioral abnormality and mental hospitalization. The acute onset of fluent incomprehensible speech in older people is therefore almost invariably the onset of fluent aphasia and not of psychosis. Schizophrenic word-salad has certain other features which are helpful in differentiation. It is likely to be filled with Klang-associations and rhymes. It may take a highly regular form, such as adding a fixed nonsense syllable to the end of each word. Secondly, schizophrenic word-salad may be confined to speech while writing is intact, while aphasic patients with fluent speech never have normal writing. The word-salad of the schizophrenic may, in other situations, be present in writing as well as speech or indeed be confined to writing alone. Certain features of word-salad in writing immediately mark it off from aphasic agraphias. One of the major features is that the schizophrenic will tend to fill pages of writing. Such graphorrhea is extremely rare even in aphasics who manifest gross logorrhea. The fluent aphasic often has excellent orthography, and his writing may contain many paragraphic errors, but he will almost never run on for pages. In addition, written word-salad will tend to show the same features seen in spoken word-salad, i.e., Klang-associations, rhyming, or the tendency to addition of a fixed syllable to every word (an excellent example of such a patient is given by Bastian, 1898, who apparently did not fully recognize the origin of the disturbance). In addition, the writing may be arranged in carefully worked out bizarre geometrical patterns.

Yet another cause of fluent incomprehensible speech is glossolalia (Kelsey, 1964) or "the gift of tongues." Members of certain religious groups at times have episodes of speaking in strange tongues such as are recorded in the New Testament. These people are not in fact likely to represent a diagnostic problem since they do not ordinarily come to the attention of the physician. In any case, the alteration of speech is episodic with normal speech between the periods of glossolalia.

## V. Grammatical Disturbances

Grammatical disturbances in aphasia are most strongly linked to aphasias with anterior lesions, in particular to the classic Broca's aphasia. The patient, if he is capable of connected speech at all, is typically "telegraphic," that is to say, he tends to produce speech in which there is a marked tendency to omit the small "connective" words. Aphasic telegraphic speech is always slow in rate, usually associated with articulation defect and with a tendency to repeat words (Howes, 1964). I have seen one instance of hysterical pseudo-agrammatism in a patient who had been arrested for passing bad checks. While in jail he had developed a disturbance of speech and was transferred to a mental hospital. On examination, he spoke in much the same manner that Indians generally do in Western films, e.g., "Me don't know why me here. Me wake up in jail. Me come hospital." What was striking about this speech was that despite the extreme agrammatism, the rate was normal and the words were well articulated except for a marked stutter (which had developed at the same time as the agrammatism). The combination of *rapid* agrammatic speech together with stuttering was unique in my experience. In addition, he showed no hemiplegia (as is usually present in most aphasics with telegraphic speech since they have anterior lesions) but did manifest certain other signs strongly suggestive of a hysterical illness. He had a total island of amnesia for the passing of the bad checks and in addition had a Ganser syndrome, one of the classic forms of hysterical pseudodementia. The diagnosis of functional disease received strong support when the patient, a day or two later, showed rapid clearing of all of these signs when he was reassured by his wife that their child would not be taken away by the court in the event of his conviction.

## VI. Non-Aphasic Misnaming

As I have commented earlier, Edwin Weinstein and his co-workers (Weinstein, 1958; Weinstein and Kahn, 1955; Weinstein and Keller, 1964), have clarified this syndrome for us. The major diagnostic problem is that of distinguishing this disturbance from a classical amnesic aphasia, a disorder resulting from a localized abnormality in the left posterior parietal region, and often accompanied by neighborhood signs such as a Gerstmann's syndrome or a hemianopia.

Non-aphasic misnaming does not occur in patients who are fully alert, oriented, and who readily admit their disability, while anomic aphasia can certainly occur in such circumstances. The patient with non-aphasic misnaming may show evidence of gross confusion, drowsiness, memory disturbance, or signs of a widespread dementia; on the other hand, he may show only subtle alterations in his state of consciousness or general awareness but is never fully normal in these respects. His naming disturbance has certain characteristics. In some instances he may fail to name even very simple objects and may produce paraphasic errors. The aphasic who manifests such a marked degree of misnaming will show marked word-finding difficulty in his spontaneous speech with a strong tendency to circumlocution. In non-aphasic misnaming, however, there is often a marked discrepancy between the patient's failure to name or his incorrect misnaming and his production of normal speech. One of the striking features of this type of misnaming is that the patient may show a selective difficulty in naming things related to his illness. Thus the patient may name even quite complex objects correctly and yet fail to name things such as "hospital," "doctor," "nurse," "thermometer." This selective failure may at times mistakenly lead the physician to assume that the patient is disoriented. The selective misnamings of items related to the illness may have a gallows humor quality. Thus one patient of mine, asked where he was, said, "In a slaughter-house," and asked to indicate the occupation of one of his physicians, said that he was a "grinder." This type of selective misnaming is absent in the true aphasic. Indeed it has often been my impression that many aphasics perform better on subjects related to their illnesses. Non-aphasic misnaming may sometimes make it impossible to detect the presence of a concomitant mild aphasic anomia.

The patient with non-aphasic misnaming frequently shows marked denial of his illness, asserting that he is not ill or that he has come in for some trivial complaint, totally avoiding and frequently actively refusing to admit his major problems.

This clinical picture of non-aphasic misnaming is seen in such conditions as congestive heart failure, uremia, delirium tremens, terminal carcinomas, and other diseases with widespread effects on metabolism. Whether the same clinical picture can be reproduced by restricted focal lesions anywhere in the nervous system is not certain. In any case, because of the nature of the illnesses which generally produce this picture, such patients are more likely to be seen by the internist than by the neurologist.[3]

I have seen one patient who exhibited a hysterical anomia. She exhibited no impairments of intellect or consciousness but failed to name very simple objects. Had she been suffering from a true aphasic anomi,a her spontaneous speech would have been noticeably abnormal; instead, her spontaneous speech was perfectly normal without circumlocutions or word-finding difficulties even when she was discussing material which demanded the use of a quite sophisticated vocabulary.

## VII. Paroxysmal Speech Disorders

The presence of a clear-cut stable aphasic syndrome assures the examiner that he is dealing with disease affecting directly or indirectly (e.g., via pressure or edema) the speech regions of the brain. Difficulties in speech occurring paroxysmally as part of a seizure disorder may, however, be derived from much wider areas of the brain. Thus seizures in the classic speech areas usually produce arrest of speech (although as Foerster, 1936, pointed out, runs of fluent incomprehensible speech are in fact seen rarely). Penfield (cited by Serafetinides and Falconer, 1963) has obviously described what appears to me to be fluent aphasia following a seizure. Arrest of speech may, however, be seen from sites other than the classical speech regions, e.g., the supplementary motor area (Penfield and Roberts, 1952). Indeed

[3] In their earlier papers Weinstein and his colleagues tended to use the term "paraphasia" to denote non-aphasic misnaming. This usage is somewhat confusing since paraphasic speech certainly occurs in many aphasics with left focal retro-Rolandic lesions. In a more recent paper (Weinstein and Keller, 1964) this terminology is not used; this paper is essentially an excellent summary of the criteria used to distinguish the paraphasias in focal aphasic lesions from those due to disease outside the speech regions.

*transient* aphasias may be seen after cortical excisions in this neighborhood as Schwab (1927) pointed out. As Alajouanine and his co-workers (1959) pointed out, the presence of palilalia in the paroxysm is characteristic for seizures in this location. It seems likely that such disturbances occur from either the right or the left side.

Serafetinides and Falconer (1963) have recently asserted that what they refer to as "paroxysmal dysphasia" (restricting this term to speech arrest and not including fluent paraphasic speech) is overwhelmingly a sign of left-sided disease but that "ictal speech automatisms" (i.e., well-articulated phrases occur during a seizure) come more often from the right side. I suspect that a further distinction may be possible. I would guess that "automatisms" in which the patient produces paraphasic circumlocutory utterances (like the case of Penfield, cited earlier) would result predominantly from left-sided disease, while automatisms in which speech production was normal would result from right-sided lesions.

The author wishes to express his gratitude to his secretary, Mrs. Ceoria Coates, who typed the manuscript, and to Drs. Fritz Friedland and Claude Biquard who prepared the German and French summaries respectively.

## References

Alajouanine, T., Castaigne, P., Sabouraud, O., and Contamin, F. (1959): Palilalie paroxystique et vocalisations iteratives au cours de crises épileptiques par lésion intéressant l'aire motrice supplémentaire, Rev. Neurol., 101:685-697.

Bastian, H. C. (1898): "A Treatise on Aphasia and other Speech Defects," London (H. K. Lewis).

Critchley, M. (1964): The Neurology of Psychotic Speech, Brit. J. Psychiat., 110:353-364.

Foerster, O. (1936): Motorische Felder und Bahnen, in Handbuch der Neurologie, Bumke, O. and Foerster, O. (eds.), 6:1-357.

Gloning, I., Gloning, K., and Hoff, H. (1963): Aphasia, A Clinical Syndrome, in "Problems of Dynamic Neurology," (ed. Halpern), New York (Grune and Stratton).

Goldstein, K. (1917): "Die transkortikalen Aphasien," Jena (Gustav Fischer).

Head, H. (1926): "Aphasia and Kindred Disorders of Speech," Cambridge (Cambridge University Press).

Howes, D. H. (1964): Application of the Word-Frequency Concept to Aphasia, in "Disorders of Language," (eds. de Reuck and O'Connor), Boston (Little, Brown).

Kelsey, M. T. (1964): "Tongue Speaking," New York, (Doubleday and Company).

Penfield, W., and Roberts, L. (1959): "Speech and Brain-Mechanisms," Princeton (Princeton University Press).

Schwab, O. (1927): Uber vorübergehende aphasische Störungen nach Rindenexzision aus dem linken Stirnhirn bei Epileptikern, Deutsche Z. f. Nervenheilkunde, 94:177-184.

Serafetinides, E. A., and Falconer, M. A. (1963): Speech Disturbances in Temporal Lobe Seizures, Brain, 86:333-346.

Stengel, E. (1947): A Clinical and Psychological Study of Echo-Reactions, J. Ment. Sci., 93:598-612.

Weinstein, E. A. (1958): Changes in Language Pattern as Adaptive Mechanisms, in "Psychopathology of Communication," New York (Grune and Stratton).

Weinstein, E. A., and Kahn, R. L. (1955): "Denial of Illness," Springfield (Charles C. Thomas).
Weinstein, E. A., and Keller, N. J. A. (1964): Linguistic Patterns of Misnaming in Brain Injury, Neuropsychologia, 1:79-90.
Wernicke, C. (1874): "Der aphasische Symptomenkomplex," Breslau (Max Cohn und Weigert).

This work was supported in part by a grant (MH 08472-01, Professor Davis Howes, Principal Investigator) from the National Institutes of Health to the Boston University Medical School.

# CHAPTER 4

# The Paradoxical Position of Kurt Goldstein in the History of Aphasia

*Norman Geschwind*

Until approximately three years ago I had accepted what to a very great extent has become the "standard" history of aphasia. Broca's achievement was seen through a distant mist. Following his arousal of interest in the field came, we are generally told, the long Dark Ages. For the next 60 years the field was apparently dominated by a group of scholars, mostly German, who studied aphasia entirely from an anatomical point of view. Indeed, the argument often goes, it was a study from a point of view of fictional anatomy, barely, if at all, above the level of the phrenologists who had only so recently been deposed. Only Hughlings Jackson, unrecognized outside his own country, was said to be free from the overriding neurological mythology.

According to this standard history, by the mid-1920s the situation had changed and the classical school was in full flight. The battle had been led in France by Pierre Marie, in Switzerland by von Monakow, in Germany by Kurt Goldstein, and in England by Henry Head. The ideas, or what were thought to be the ideas of this group, soon gained domination in the English-speaking world. Head (1926) had been shrewd enough to point out that much of the great German growth of neurology had been related to their victory in the Franco-Prussian war. He was not shrewd enough to apply this valuable historical lesson to his own time and to realize that perhaps the decline of the vigor and influence of German neurology was strongly related to the defeat of Germany in World War I and the shift of the center of gravity of intellectual life to the English-speaking world, rather than necessarily to any defects in the ideas of the German scholars.

---

Reprinted with permission from CORTEX, Masson, S.P.A., Vol. I, 1964, pp. 214–224

Chaos, as is well known, was Head's word and if chaos was perhaps not present before Head, it was certainly fully evident after him. Somewhere about 1960 I awoke, perhaps belatedly, to my own profound confusion. I had regarded myself as a member of the philosophically sophisticated Jackson-Goldstein-Head group. Yet, I was persistently troubled by the fact that people who had left their mark so indelibly in many areas of neurology, such as Wernicke, Bastian, Dejerine, Charcot, and many others, could apparently have shown what was asserted to be the sheerest naivete and incompetence in the area of the higher functions. It seemed difficult to accept the view that men who had established long-honored clinical pictures should have apparently been so incapable of examining an aphasic, or that scholars who had made fundamental anatomical investigations of permanent worth should have been so perfunctory and sloppy in their descriptions of the brains of aphasics. I, along with several of my colleagues of the Aphasia Unit of the Boston V.A. Hospital, decided to reinvestigate the problem at its source. Rather than accept the authority of even so distinguished a group as Marie, von Monakow, Head, and Goldstein, we would go back to the original literature and see for ourselves whether indeed the evidence was so poor as had been suggested. This was no minor problem. Practically none of this literature was available in English, except occasionally in accounts by its detractors, and much of it is contained in old journals, many of which are no longer published, and often difficult to obtain. The picture that emerged from this study was not the classic one of the chaotic confabulations of a group of tedious imperceptive German scholars, but rather that of the healthy active disagreements of a lively science. The broadside accusations of carelessness, of inadequate examination, of unconcern with psychology were all unfounded, at least when the best of the classicists were involved. There certainly had been people in this era who had indiscriminately collected series of well- and ill-described cases, but the best had never done so.

Actually, my colleagues and I were now even more confused. We had, in fact, expected to find that most of the criticisms of the great reformers would be justified and we were quite unprepared to find the case to be so clearly otherwise. It, therefore, became necessary in turn to go back to the writings of the leaders of the "reform movement" in aphasia and to reread them as carefully as their predecessors.

Jackson, we rapidly found, did not represent a problem. His early disagreement with Broca was long since a dead issue. As for his later writings, we found that writers as diverse as Head (1926), Nielsen (1946), and Penfield and Roberts (1959) all quoted him with equal approval. Otto Sittig (1931) who was in major part responsible for the introduction of Jacksonian ideas into German-speaking neurology after World War I, quoted Jackson extensively and approvingly in his monograph on apraxia in which he also accepted the fundamental analyses and observations of Hugo Liepmann, one of the greatest of the classical localizationists.

Pierre Marie had inveighed against Dejerine in the early 1900s and had carried on a bitter battle against classical views. But when Marie and Foix (1917) published their diagram of the lesions producing different aphasic syndromes, it was little different in fact from the diagrams of Marie's predecessors. Foix, one of Marie's major pupils, certainly shows no anti-localizationist bias in most of his writings.

Von Monakow was another one of the reformers. Just before World War I, Hugo Liepmann (1914) wrote a long reply to von Monakow's chapter on apraxia (itself nearly 100 pages long) in which Liepmann had been seriously taken to task. Liepmann quotes page after page of gross misquotation and misunderstanding from von Monakow's work (having read Liepmann with care, I agree with his objections). But the unkindest cut of all for Liepmann was to find that after many pages of criticism, von Monakow himself came to the same conclusion! Thus Liepmann writes, "Von Monakow . . . finally . . . arrives at his verification of all my propositions relating to localization without commenting that they are mine." He then quotes von Monakow's list of sites of predilection of apraxia, which indeed do coincide with Liepmann's older list. The monograph on apraxia by Victoria (1938) based on von Monakow's work also comes to conclusions that had been clearly stated by Liepmann, although this author also is critical of Liepmann.

Henry Head (1926) is often remembered as a major reformer. Yet, after inveighing against the diagram makers and damning their diagrams, he ended his book with a very classical set of localizations for his four types of aphasia, each carefully provided with a new name so as effectively to obscure the fact that in most instances his findings coincided with those of earlier workers! Any reader who goes to the discussion of specific aphasic syndromes in Russell Brain's (1961) writings will find that for all of Brain's admiration for his teacher, this author clearly reveals a return to many of the older views which Head had so dearly wished to destroy. It is even remarkable to find that Head had substituted the word "schema" for the hated word "center" of some of the classical writers. Yet, the definition given by Bastian (1898), one of Head's favorite *bêtes noires*, for a "center," is little different from Head's definition of a schema!

Thus Bastian wrote, ". . . There must be certain sets of structurally related cell and fibre mechanisms in the cortex . . . Such diffuse but functionally unified nervous networks may differ altogether from the common conception of a neatly defined 'centre,' and yet for the sake of brevity it is convenient to retain this word and refer to such networks as so many 'centres' . . ."

I would not in what I have said so far wish to suggest that any of the authors I have mentioned were trivial or insignificant men, nor indeed that they did not contribute to the advance of knowledge of aphasia. I would only wish to suggest that they were not so revolutionary as they thought they were, and that for all their protests they were nearer to the classical tradition (which was in any case not at all monolithic as is often suggested) than they asserted that they were.

To me, however, the most interesting of the four reformers is Kurt Goldstein, who has actually had much more profound effects on thought about the higher functions, certainly in the United States and probably even in England, than any of the others, even including Head. There are several reasons why Goldstein has been so influential. For one thing he has long outlived the others who have receded into the classical past and has continued to work long beyond them—Goldstein's recent book (Goldstein, 1948) although based heavily on his earlier German monograph (Goldstein, 1927) on localization in the cortex, was still a presentation of his ideas more than twenty years after Head's two volumes. Furthermore, Goldstein's work in the twenties and thirties, after the other authors had left the scene, coincided with the great rise of holistic approaches in other fields, such as psychology, psychiatry, anthropology, and sociology and therefore found an audience receptive, particularly in the United States, to its general approach. In addition, although the others, particularly Marie and Head had stressed what they liked to call the "psychological" approach, Goldstein's work was much more closely tied to the academic psychology of his era in Germany and later in this country. His work has therefore come to be widely diffused to large numbers of undergraduate students of psychology in many American universities, a group generally poorly informed both as to the work of the other reformers and almost totally uninformed about the classical neurologists criticized by this group.

I was therefore most intrigued to review Goldstein's work in the light of the fact that he is often regarded as the greatest influence in the revolt against the classical school of thought about aphasia. I had, of course, read some time ago the monograph (Goldstein, 1948) on language disturbances but distrusted my memory of it. I had already been surprised in reading other writers, such as Lange (1936) and Isserlin (1936), that they frequently quoted Goldstein's opinions on matters of localization. I began by reading and later by re-reading the work on cerebral localization, published in 1927, in the peak period of Goldstein's productivity. The arrangement of this book is a familiar one. Most of the first half is devoted to a discussion of theoretical principles and at first glance sounds like what most of us have been accustomed to think of as Goldstein's views, critical of classical approaches and stressing organismic considerations.

Roughly the second half of the book constitutes the "Special Part." Goldstein opens this part by pointing out that it would be most desirable to deal with the syndromes of each cytoarchitectonic region. All through the Special Part he stresses the details of cytoarchitecture and indeed reference back to the theoretical section shows that even this section began with an extended presentation of cytoarchitecture and myelinogenesis and indeed a defense of the work of Flechsig.

We come next in the Special Part to a long, elaborate, highly classical discussion of the motor regions, with several citations to Goldstein's own observations, and certainly little or no intrusion of the considerations of the theoretical section. The following section is on the sensory regions, another superb but classical discussion. In this section he cites, for example, cases of isolated loss of sensation confined to the ends of the thumbs and says, "These circumscribed deficits correspond to circumscribed lesions in the posterior central gyrus." He even goes on to express the view that there is probably a detailed projection of the periphery on the sensory cortex. He took special care to refute the critics of such a projection, e.g., Bonhoeffer, a very classical neurologist.

The next section is on the visual system, again highly classical. Anyone who thinks that Goldstein did not believe in isolated defects should note his comment that "*we* have confirmed many times" what Liepmann occasionally observed, that isolated disturbances of color sense without visual field defect can occur particularly with lesions in the left hemisphere. His discussion of what he calls the first form of psychic blindness states that, "There is often bilateral disease of the occipital lobe. (If there is a unilateral lesion it lies) . . . always in the *left* hemisphere (in right-handers), and indeed it then involves either the calcarine cortex or the optic radiation and the callosal fibers, so that excitations from neither the right nor the left half of the retina can get to the left hemisphere . . ." This is, needless to say, a highly classical connectionistic interpretation. Goldstein then goes on to dismiss the idea that this disorder is the result of the field defects; he rejects Niessl von Mayendorf's assertion that psychic blindness is the result of lesions of the macular bundle bilaterally. He then says, "The simultaneous occurrence of diffuse cerebral damage, as von Monakow assumes, is *not* necessary (for this clinical picture). There can persist a lasting psychic blindness even in an (otherwise) intact youthful brain with a quite circumscribed lesion . . ." I am not myself sure that this view is necessarily correct, but I would hardly assume that it could be considered revolutionary by classical localizationists.

We turn to the section on aphasia, where perhaps we might expect a more "Goldsteinian" approach. At first it appears that we are about to break totally with the classicists. He writes ". . . in our opinion these (distinct forms of aphasia) do not exist in reality . . ." Yet, two pages later we find that this is not the case. (Let me stress that these quotations from Goldstein are not "taken out of context." I have in each instance been as careful as I could be to ascertain that these were Goldstein's personal views.) He writes of the "symptom-complex which is usually characterized as word-dumbness or subcortical aphasia and which I would characterize as the peripheral form of motor aphasia . . ." He notes that writing may be normal, that reading is undisturbed, and that the anatomical substrate is a lesion of the classic Broca's region. He argues that this region is slightly wider than the usual classical zone, but concludes that the pars triangularis and orbitalis of the third frontal convolution do not belong to this region. He disagrees with Pierre Marie's view that lesions of this region produce dysarthria and not aphasia, and goes on to agree with Niessl von Mayendorf's inclusion of the Rolandic operculum in the anterior speech area although he has some disagreements with him. He goes on to say that by "an exclusive lesion of $F_3$ with intactness of the central operculum, severe motor aphasia, even persistent can appear . . ." Any of this could have been written by the staunchest of the classicists.

He does mention in this section that the presence or absence of writing defect with a Broca's aphasia is not only a question of anatomy but may be dependent on whether the patient had always been accustomed to speak when writing or not. In fact, however, this type of "functional" explanation had already been widely used by such classical localizers as Charcot. Goldstein goes on a page or two later to attribute restitution of function in some cases of Broca's aphasia to the taking over by the right side of some of the functions previously carried on by the left.

I need not pile on the examples in too much detail. He speaks a few pages later of the transcortical aphasias and refers to his own book on this topic which is certainly rich in anatomical discussion. He goes on to discuss pure word-deafness and agrees with Liepmann's views on the anatomical mechanism of this disturbance. And so it continues for page after page.

Perhaps it will be argued that his views had not yet fully matured and that he had as yet not absorbed fully his own philosophy, as expressed so forcefully in his introduction to the 1927 monograph. Let us therefore turn to the Goldstein of 1948. Again much of the book is taken up with theory and indeed with theory of the type that we would expect. Even so, we find him saying on page 47, ". . . the assumption of different functions for the different layers of the cortex is most probably justified." On page 55 he refers to earlier work of his own (published first in 1908) which showed that "tactile agnosia in the 'minor' hand may result from a lesion of the corpus callosum." On page 82 we discover that "It was Bastian who introduced the functional factor into the theory of aphasia for the explanation of the different preservation of different performances . . ." But this is the Bastian whom Head had criticized as one of the worst of the classicists! On page 129 we read the astonishing statement that "the collection of cases by Henschen leaves no doubt about the significance (of the second frontal gyrus) for the development of this particular form of agraphia . . ." It is perhaps surprising to see Goldstein agreeing with Henschen when so confirmed a localizer as Sir Charles Symonds (1953) finds the evidence for pure agraphia poor! On the next page Goldstein writes, "My case leaves no doubt that the anatomic cause of (agraphia of the minor hand) is a destruction of the corpus callosum as Liepmann first showed . . ." By the time we get to the second half of this book we find most of the 1927 conclusions repeated. Certainly there are more holistic discussions in the text but without question there are innumerable areas of agreement with the classical neurologists.

Must we then ask, "Which is the real Kurt Goldstein?" I frequently find that when I quote Goldstein on localization someone asks me, "Do you mean *Kurt* Goldstein?" One man protested that he had read Goldstein's books and had never seen any of the things that I had mentioned. I asked whether he had read the second half of the 1948 book on language disturbances, in which the case records and the discussion of individual syndromes were concentrated. He admitted that he hadn't on the assumption that it was merely "technical detail." I am certain that, like this man, when I read this book for the first time I had omitted or glossed over the "technical detail."

Actually the discrepancy between the two Goldsteins is less great than one might assume. Careful re-reading of the theoretical section in the 1927 monograph shows that many of the "philosophical" principles are followed by so many qualifications that they need not conflict with any theory. Thus Goldstein writes, "Since in the organism one is dealing with a unitary system, a stimulus would have to manifest itself everywhere in an alteration of the same kind." But a paragraph later he goes on to say, "Usually the effect of the change following on an adequate stimulus does not show itself everywhere, but especially in a more or less circumscribed region of the body . . ." He gives the reasons for this. The first is, "The alteration in response to a stimulus in a large system does not occur everywhere simultaneously and with equal intensity, but occurs sooner and more strongly near the site of the stimulus than in more distant regions . . ." Another reason he gives for differential responses is that "different parts of the nervous system are differently attuned to the different types of stimuli . . ." hardly a statement to disturb even the most die-hard of localizationists. A few pages later he states that "all forms of damage to the nervous system can be regarded from the point of view that one is dealing with an *isolation* of a certain part. All lesions of the nervous system exclude a certain part of the system." But this would suggest that a view of the organism as a unity might not be too useful.

What conclusion are we to draw? Kurt Goldstein was and is a great figure and a great contributor to the study of the higher functions of the nervous system. But his contribution was not totally to destroy his predecessors, to abolish the diagrams, or to bring order into the chaos. Few scientists create revolutions and the revolution in aphasia occurred in the 1860s with Broca and in the 1870s with Wernicke. Most people who advance their field must disagree with their predecessors to some extent and in some measure destroy the past; they must also disagree with their contemporaries and so increase chaos. Usually a field is least usefully active when it is apparently least chaotic.

Goldstein, like Head, von Monakow, and Marie, made advances and indeed great advances in the study of the higher functions. But rather than being the initiator of a totally new approach, he was a brilliant developer and reviser of a magnificent understructure developed in the years before his arrival on the scene. Aphasia did not stop in 1920 but it certainly did not begin at that time. What I have tried to show in part is that our standard view of the history of aphasia is at least a seriously distorted one. At its worst, this view of history has closed certain useful avenues of approach and forced us to forget important truths that even the so-called reformers accepted. The widespread neglect of the important elucidation of the functions of the corpus callosum by such people as Dejerine, Liepmann, and Goldstein himself at the turn of the century is an excellent example of the damage done by this failure to appreciate the past; significant experimental and clinical study was almost certainly delayed for many years by this neglect of the classical localizers.

How then are we to regard Goldstein's position? His contribution as a localizer in the classical sense is in fact highly significant although rarely taught. He also made a contribution in other ways. We should recall that his stress on looking at the background of the patient and at the intensity of the lesion were already stated by some of his classical predecessors. It should be noted that few of them were as excessively localizationist as is often assumed—in fact, some of them were less localizationist than Goldstein in relation to their interpretation of many issues! Goldstein stressed more than his predecessors the reaction of normal parts of the nervous system to illness in one portion and highlighted the importance of looking at more than the obvious impairment of the patient. But these and others of his so-called principles should not be regarded as great philosophic truths. It is far better to say that he suggested some ways of looking at disease of the nervous system which are sometimes useful. Thus was Goldstein correct in stressing the "total response of the patient?" There is no yes or no answer. Instead, we should say: Some phenomena are clarified by regarding them from the point of view of organismic reactions, others are clarified by being regarded atomistically. The major source of error is the failure to look at each phenomenon from both points of view to see which is most appropriate.

Perhaps I could most appropriately close with a recent statement by Goldstein (1953) himself about Hugo Liepmann, Wernicke's great pupil, and probably the most brilliant of the classical localizers in his synthesis of anatomy and behavior, "Liepmann's work will remain one of the landmarks of our knowledge of the function of the brain. He is a worthy representative of a great creative epoch in neurology." Evidently Goldstein did not reject his predecessors as much as many other people thought he had.

## Summary

A widely-accepted version of the history of the study of aphasia states that before the First World War this discipline was dominated by a group of workers who, with occasional exceptions, were unsophisticated psychologically and who attempted on the basis of inadequate clinical and pathological data to fit aphasia into a narrow anatomical scheme. According to this view a group of reformers appeared, Marie, von Monakow, Head, and Goldstein, who destroyed this inadequate classical scheme.

In this paper this view is criticized, and it is pointed out that none of the reformers made as great a break with the past as is generally thought. The work of Kurt Goldstein is particularly discussed, and it is pointed out that it is readily apparent from Goldstein's own works that he accepted a majority of the classical teachings, indeed even in details. It is also pointed out that many of Goldstein's holistic theoretical views were in fact so extensively qualified as to make them compatible with almost any approach. There is some discussion as to the reasons for the widespread rejection of the classical views when even its apparently severest critics accepted so much of the classical teachings.

In concluding, it is pointed out that Goldstein is indeed a great figure in the history of aphasia, but that his contribution must be reassessed as a brilliant extension of the works of his illustrious predecessors, not as a completely new approach based on the destruction of older unsound views.

## References

Bastian, H. C. (1898) *Aphasia and Other Speech Defects.* H. K. Levis, London.
Brain, W. R. (1961) *Speech Disorders.* Butterworth, London.
Goldstein, K. (1927) *Die Lokalisation in der Grosshirnride,* in Handbuch der Normalen und Pathologischen Physiologie. Vol. 10. Springer, Berlin.
Goldstein, K. (1948) *Language and Language Disturbances,* Grune and Stratton, New York.
Goldstein, K. (1953) *Hugo Karl Liepmann,* in The Founders of Neurology, ed. by W. Haymaker. Charles C. Thomas, Springfield.
Head, H. (1926) *Aphasia and Kindred Disorders of Speech.* Cambridge University Press, Cambridge.
Isserlin, M. (1936) *Aphasie,* in Handbuch der Neurologie, ed. by O. Bumke and O. Foerster, Vol. VI, 627–806. Springer, Berlin.
Lange, J. (1936) *Agnosien und Apraxien,* in Handbuch der Neurologie, ed. by O. Bumke and O. Foerster, Vol. VI, 807–960. Springer, Berlin.
Liepmann, H. (1914) *Bemerkungen zu v. Monakows Kapitel "Die Lokalisation der Apraxie,"* "Mschr. Psychiat. Neurol.," 35, 490–516.
Marie, P., and Foix, C. (1917) *Les aphasies de guerre,* "Rev. Neurol.," 31, 53–87.
Nielsen, J. M. (1946) *Agnosia, Apraxia, Aphasia.* Hoeber, New York.
Penfield, W., and Roberts, L. (1959) *Speech and Brain-Mechanisms.* Princeton University Press, Princeton.
Sittig, O. (1931) *Uber Apraxie.* Karger, Berlin.
Symonds, C. P. (1953) *Aphasia,* "J. Neurol. Neurosurg. Psychiat.," 16, 1.
Victoria, M. (1938) *Teoria de las Apraxias.* Alfredo Frascoli, Buenos Aires.

The work presented in this paper was supported in part by a grant (MH08472) from the National Institutes of Health to the Boston University School of Medicine (David Howes, Principal Investigator).

# CHAPTER 5

# Wernicke's Contribution to the Study of Aphasia

*Norman Geschwind*

In this symposium we are honoring the memory of Kurt Goldstein. It is appropriate in this setting to discuss the contribution of Carl Wernicke to the study of aphasia, a field which concerned Goldstein throughout his life. Like Wernicke, Goldstein was born in a small town in Upper Silesia and received his medical education in Breslau, the provincial capital. During Goldstein's period as a medical student, Wernicke held the chair of neurology and psychiatry in the medical school, and it was from Wernicke that Goldstein first learned about aphasia. The influence of this period on Goldstein was great, and I shall comment upon this later.

I have in an earlier paper written about Wernicke's life and the lives of some of his most important pupils, as well as the general effect of the Breslau school on the history of aphasia (Geschwind, 1966). In this paper I will not review this earlier material extensively but rather will treat in detail Wernicke's contribution to the study of aphasia, in particular his classic work, "Der Aphasische Symptomencomplex" published in 1874.

In order to put this publication in perspective, let us briefly consider its background. Wernicke received his medical degree in 1870 at the age of 22 from the University of Breslau. He worked for six months in the ophthalmology clinic under Forster, who was probably the first to recognize the young man's exceptional talent. He then went off as an assistant to a surgeon in the Franco-Prussian war. On his return to Breslau he took up a post as assistant in the psychiatric clinic. Carl Weigert, the developer of the stain for myelin that led to such important advances in neuroanatomy, was a fellow assistant. During this time Fritsch and Hitzig reported their important discoveries on the localized excitability of

Reprinted with permission from CORTEX, Masson, S.P.A., Vol. III, 1967, pp. 449-363.

the cerebral cortex of man. Wernicke spent six months with the great neuroanatomist Meynert in Vienna and this was probably the most important influence of his life. Having returned from Vienna he soon afterwards published "Der Aphasische Symptomencomplex" which was completed in May, 1874, less than four years after his graduation and after only three years of training in neurology. He was only 26 years old in the month that he completed the manuscript.

The major influence on this work was the short period with Meynert who influenced not only Wernicke but also many others, including Flechsig, the pioneer of developmental studies of the brain, the great anatomist Forel, and Freud. Meynert was one of the very first to be concerned with the relationship of anatomy to function, an interest that he transmitted to Wernicke. Thus in his early work Meynert correlated the increased size of certain portions of the motor pathways in the brain stem and spinal cord of the kangaroo with the great preponderance of the hind-limbs in that animal, and showed the contrasting pattern in the bat with its predominance of the forelimbs, thus also establishing himself as one of the pioneers in comparative neuroanatomy. He correlated development with order of myelination, thus laying the ground for Flechsig's later work. He brought order into the fiber systems of the brain by distinguishing the projection pathways connecting the cortex to the lower centers, the association pathways connecting different regions of the same hemisphere, and the commissural systems joining corresponding points in the two hemispheres. He pioneered the study of cortical cytoarchitecture by being the first to point out regional differences of cellular architecture in the cortex. He was the first to point out that the anterior parts of the brain had motor functions while the posterior parts were sensory in nature. In reviewing these accomplishments it is easy to see why it was written of him that "Erst seit Meynert ist das Gehirn beseelt" ("Only since the work of Meynert has the brain been given life"). As I will point out later, Meynert made a specific contribution to the study of aphasia that has generally been overlooked and which influenced Wernicke's thoughts on aphasia.

In the short space of 13 years between the publications of Broca in 1861 and Wernicke in 1874, interest in aphasia had grown rapidly. Bastian and Hughlings Jackson were already active in England, as were also a large number of French and German writers, and the literature of the subject was already sizeable. Wernicke's contribution to this growing literature was entitled "Der Aphasische Symptomencomplex: eine Psychologische Studie auf Anatomischer Basis" ("The symptom-complex of aphasia: a psychological study on an anatomical basis"). In the very opening of the paper he points out that he will apply Meynert's teachings to the problem of language and aphasia. Following this brief introduction we come to the first section in which Wernicke immediately makes clear his theoretical position.

He begins this section by pointing out that the doctrine of the equopotentiality of the brain, which had been advocated by the great French physiologist Flourens, had been recognized as untenable for some time but that it was equally incorrect to substitute for it the view of the phrenologists who arbitrarily assigned individual territories of the cortex to mental functions (as arbitrarily defined by the terminology of ordinary speech). Wernicke thus rejected the approach to cerebral function which denies all localization, but he equally strongly rejected the approach which was to appear in more sophisticated form in other writings on aphasia, i.e., the one which assumed that for every specifiable language function there was a particular piece of cortex assigned to that function, the approach of such authors as Henschen and above all Kleist (who, although a student of Wernicke's, eventually adopted a theoretical view of quite different nature from his).

In rejecting these extreme approaches, which we may label as the holistic and mosaicist respectively, Wernicke offers his alternative: ". . . only the most elementary psychic functions can be assigned to defined areas of the cortex . . ." and as examples of such elementary functions he cites visual, olfactory, and tactile perceptions in the central projection areas of the respective sensory nerves. "Everything which goes beyond these simplest functions, the association of different impressions into a concept, thinking, consciousness, is an achievement of the fiber tracts which connect the different regions of the cortex to each other, the so-called association system of Meynert. We will see later to what extent these more complicated achievements are even now amenable to examination." This then is the underlying thesis: the higher mental functions are not properties of localized regions of the brain, but are constructed out of the association of different regions, and it is the anatomical connections of these regions which make possible these associations.

Wernicke now turns to developing his ideas in detail. It is a characteristic of all nervous tissue, he writes, to preserve the effects of stimulation beyond the duration of the stimulus itself. In peripheral nerves this effect is brief and accounts for some of the phenomena of after-images, but in the cortex these residua of previous excitations may remain for long periods and it is these residua for which the name "memory-images" is suggested.

Basing himself on what then were recent physiological and anatomical observations, Wernicke points out that the parts of the brain lying anterior to the central fissure of Rolando are motor regions, while the remaining portions of the hemispheres are sensory in function. Thus the memory images of movements must lie in the frontal lobe, those of sensations in the appropriate regions of the other lobes.

He now turns to the problem of volitional movement. This is distinguished from reflex movement in two ways: (1) It does not occur in immediate response to an outside stimulus but can result from the memory images of former perceptions which need not be aroused in all instances by an external stimulus. Hence, although volitional movements differ from reflex movements, they have an essential unity with them. (2) The volitional movement is adapted more closely to its goal. It is, so to speak, "preformed" being built up of memory images of previous movements.

Volitional movements are thus also reflex movements but are distinguished by their dependence on remembered stimuli arising within the cortex which arouse remembered movements stored elsewhere in the cortex. As the number of sensory and motor images increases, the more associational possibilities exist, the greater becomes the variety of movements, and the greater becomes the choice of movements which may be available in any given situation, the exact selection depending on all the factors involved at any one time. Thus writes Wernicke in closing Section I, "The only correct scientific definition of free will agrees most closely with this mechanical concept of the origin of spontaneous movement."

In Section II, Wernicke turns to the specific problem of aphasia. He comments that although Broca's views as to the importance of the posterior end of the third frontal convolution for language had encountered considerable opposition, the publication of so many cases in agreement with his ideas, and the lack of effective counter views had led to continuing acceptance of Broca's position. In the interim, however, Meynert had published a most important work in which he demonstrated that the central projection of the auditory nerve lay in the cortex of the Sylvian fissure, and to this cortical region he assigned the designation of *Klangfeld* (sound-field). He supported his view by numerous autopsy findings in aphasics in which either the insular region or the adjoining parts of the Sylvian fissure were altered. Many academic physicians had adopted this view since it corresponded to the vaguely felt need to bring hearing into association with the process of speech and because it helped to account for the fact that most cases of aphasia in which Broca's area was intact had changes in the region specified by Meynert, i.e. in the temporal operculum and adjoining regions.

I might comment here that the significance of Meynert's contribution to the study of aphasia has generally been overlooked. In the discussions of the history of aphasia that I have so far consulted, he is mentioned only as Wernicke's teacher. Nielsen (1946) in his bibliography cites two works by Meynert on aphasia published in 1866 but does not refer to these in the text. It is important to appreciate that it was apparently he who first convincingly showed that aphasia could occur in temporal lobe lesions. It was Wernicke's function to complete the cycle started by Meynert by showing how this fact achieved meaning in terms of Meynert's own studies of the brain, and to point out the important fact that this new localization corresponded to a clinical picture different from that seen in lesions of Broca's area.

Wernicke now develops his central argument. The frontal lobe was already known at that time to be motor in function. Hitzig (cited in a footnote on p. 7) had shown that stimulation of the lower end of the Rolandic cortex in monkeys led to movements of mouth and tongue. Broca's area must be the center for the representation (i.e., memory-images) of the movements of this region, while the first temporal gyrus lying at the central projection of the auditory nerve must be the center for the images of sounds. The fibers between these regions, which Wernicke thought to run in the insula, must be the mediators of the psychic reflex arc between the heard and spoken word. It should be pointed out that Wernicke (1908) was later to modify his view on the path between the two cortical speech areas and to accept von Monakow's view that it ran not in insula but in the arcuate fasciculus, arching from the posterior temporal region around the back end of the Sylvian fissure and then running forward in the white matter of the parietal lobe until it reached the posterior inferior frontal region.

Wernicke now gives his analysis of the types of aphasia to be expected from various lesions. Peripheral lesions of the auditory pathway, not involving the first temporal gyrus, lead to deafness but not to disturbances in speech production in the adult, who already has a rich store of earlier acquired sound images which he can reproduce at will. But if peripheral deafness occurs before there is a consolidated store of sound images, the child remains mute since he has acquired no store of sound images with which to arouse movements of speech. Sound thus has a special relationship to speech which is shared by no other sense organ. As Wernicke notes, mutism occurring in a deaf child is a common and easily understood disorder, but the rare situation of a child endowed with normal hearing who cannot learn to speak rightfully deserves the name of congenital aphasia.

Wernicke enlarges his discussion of deaf-mutism to include an intriguing suggestion whose speculative character he is quick to admit. Of what significance, he asks, is unilateral deafness in childhood? This would lead to deaf-mutism only if the right ear were affected and only the left hemisphere capable of acquiring language, which seems unlikely. But perhaps right-sided deafness leads the child to develop the right hemisphere more for language than the left since he is now depending on his left ear. Could, he asks, such a process account for the existence of people with speech in the right hemisphere? This argument of Wernicke's would have seemed totally untenable a few years ago since the representation of each ear in both cerebral hemispheres (unknown at the time Wernicke was writing his paper) would seem to invalidate it. However, the recent emphasis on the Broadbent technique (Kimura, 1961) has again highlighted the more intimate relationship of each ear to the opposite hemisphere and perhaps warrants re-consideration of this speculation of Wernicke's.

Wernicke continued his analysis of aphasia to discuss the effects of a lesion of the first temporal gyrus, which has come to be called Wernicke's area in his honor by later authors.[1] The sound images of the names of objects will be lost. From this region arise the fibers which run from the auditory to the motor region, but these are now destroyed. In addition the association fibers from this region by which other sensory images are aroused will be destroyed. "The patient is thus neither capable of repeating nor understanding the spoken word." The representations of speech movements are retained since these were learned earlier, and thus "the capacity to speak is preserved but with some limitation. For in the usual act of speaking the sound image always appears unconsciously to be innervated simultaneously (as is indeed readily understandable from the process of development of speech), to be so to speak simultaneously hallucinated, and thereby to exercise a continuing correction on the course of the movement repre-

---

[1] Some recent authors, e.g., Penfield and Roberts (1959), have used the term to designate an area far larger than that referred to by Wernicke, but this is not in keeping with classical usage.

sentations. The deaf person . . . still makes full use of this corrective mechanism." The patient is thus also aphasic in speech as a result of the loss of this unconscious correction exerted by the sound image. "The errors consist in the ready confusion of words . . . He uses the same words now correctly, now incorrectly . . ." In the milder cases it is names of objects and actions which are most affected but the conjunctions and other words necessary for sentence structure are preserved although these can be lost in more severe cases. But in all cases two cardinal features persist—the patient has many words, and he lacks comprehension of spoken language.

In order to understand Wernicke's next comment we must try to place ourselves in the position of his readers. Wernicke was describing what he thought to be a new clinical syndrome. Although he was not cognizant of the fact, Bastian (1869) and Schmidt (1871) had already described aphasias with comprehension disturbances, but these papers had gone unnoticed and it was Wernicke who was the first to succeed in calling receptive aphasias to the attention of the medical world. Wernicke had, however, gone further than these authors in linking incomprehension of language to a type of speech disturbance different from that of Broca's aphasia, i.e., to what we would now speak of as a fluent paraphasic disturbance. Finally he had linked this new syndrome to a localization different from that of the classical Broca's aphasia.

Wernicke writes, "That cases with such manifestations have not been observed, or at least not published, until now, rests not only on the rarity of such cases but also on the fact that thoroughly experienced and intelligent physicians regard this condition as a confusional state—as I myself have had the opportunity to experience. For the psychiatrically trained man who knows the clinical forms of confusional states, the diagnosis has not the least difficulty." It is perhaps unfortunate that nearly a hundred years after the publication of Wernicke's paper the error he pointed out is still a common one, and patients with a fluent paraphasic syndrome are still often misdiagnosed as confused or psychotic.

Wernicke continues to list some further features of his new syndrome. A large potential vocabulary is a cardinal feature of this form, in contrast to the situation in Broca's aphasia. There is no hemiplegia, in contrast again to Broca's aphasia. "Agraphia is present. Writing is a conscious movement which is learned with intimate dependence on the sound and is always executed under its direction. Self-observation teaches us (and clinical experience agrees with this) that between the movement of writing and the concept there is no direct connection such as must be assumed between the speech movement and the concept." Wernicke now argues, however, that the educated reader will not be alexic since he has learned to understand the written word without a rendering into spoken form, although he will read aloud aphasically. The uneducated, by contrast, who always reads aloud will be alexic. This supposition would probably not be accepted today. Wernicke goes on to point out that with other lesions in the visual regions, agraphia and alexia alone could occur.

A comment is appropriate here on this syndrome of fluent paraphasic speech and disturbance in writing with comprehension difficulty for spoken and written language which came to be known as Wernicke's aphasia. It should be noted that Wernicke did not use the term "word-deafness" which was introduced by later writers. Furthermore, a certain number of authors state incorrectly that Wernicke claimed that a lesion of the first temporal gyrus produced the syndrome of pure word-deafness, i.e., difficulty in comprehension of speech out of all proportion to disturbances in the other modalities. Wernicke did not describe this syndrome nor did he even envisage its existence in this paper. It was not until Lichtheim (1885) that the theoretical possibility of this syndrome was suggested, and only later was it described clinically by Liepmann who was one of Wernicke's assistants in Breslau (Liepmann, 1898). Furthermore, Wernicke did not conceive of the syndrome he described as being a composite one, i.e., he did not argue that four separate lesions were necessary to produce the full syndrome, but asserted instead that as a result of the way in which language is learned and used all modalities would be affected by a disturbance of the auditory memory images.

Wernicke now considered the effect of a lesion involving the fibers connecting the sound field to the area of representations of movement but leaving each one of these regions intact. Wernicke called the resulting disturbance conduction aphasia (Leitungsaphasie). The patient understands everything, and can speak freely, but his speech is altered in the same way as in the form of aphasia just described, resulting from a lesion of the auditory field. For although the sound images are preserved in conduction aphasia, they cannot exert an influence on the choice of words. The patient can judge, however, whether his own productions are correct or incorrect and shows concern over his errors. In pure form, the patient will show in speech a great similarity with the sensory aphasic, but his comprehension is intact. This form of aphasia will show disturbances in reading and writing depending on how these were learned in childhood.

Wernicke omits any mention of the feature that was later to be regarded as the characteristic component of conduction aphasia, i.e., the disturbance of repetition in the face of fluent, paraphasic speech and good comprehension. Goldstein (1927) was later to regard this form of aphasia as the most truly aphasic of all types. Accordingly, he gave it the name "central aphasia" but specifically equated it to the conduction aphasia of other authors.

Wernicke, like Goldstein later, thought that this form of aphasia resulted from a lesion of the insula, since he thought that the pathway from the posterior to the anterior speech regions travelled by way of the insula. Later authors, however, believed that the lesion for it lay in the arcuate fasciculus, which was shown to be the actual pathway between these regions, a view which, as we have already noted, Wernicke (1908) came to accept.

Wernicke lists finally the effects of destruction of Broca's area. The patient understands everything but is mute or employs only a few simple words, which he uses mostly for the designation of objects. Most previously described cases of aphasia belonged to this group. Wernicke thought that agraphia would not result unless the patient had been accustomed to speak to himself while writing. The patient will not understand written language unless he has always read aloud.

Finally he turns to lesions in the descending pathways from the frontal lobe. These he assumes could produce aphasia, but may not do so since the descending fibers may be rearranged so that individual parts of the speech act might be impaired, thus leading to dysarthria. Wernicke shows no knowledge in this analysis of the role of callosal connections or of the bilateral innervation of the speech musculature. His failure to appreciate these facts made him believe that a *complete* lesion of one cerebral peduncle could lead to aphasia. His pupil Bonhoeffer (1914) was to add refinement to this analysis by considering the role of callosal connections and bilateral innervation.

Wernicke closes this analysis by assuming that in many cases the patient improves because of eventual substitution by the other hemisphere, a view that has remained a source of unsettled controversy even today.

Wernicke now discusses the problem of those deaf-mutes who, by means of very highly complicated special teaching techniques, learn to produce speech. He argues that in such patients the auditory sound-field must play much less of a role than it does in the normal acquisition of speech. Such patients could therefore become aphasic, but their lesions would involve different parts of the brain from those which would have to be damaged in normals. In particular, lesions of the first temporal gyrus might well be ineffective in producing aphasia. He urges the importance of studying post-mortem material from deaf-mute aphasics. We see here again Wernicke's emphasis on the fact that aphasia is produced not by lesions of fixed language areas but rather by damage to those areas which in any individual have been used in acquiring speech.

Wernicke now turns to a discussion of "Asymbolie," a term introduced by Finkelnburg. He argues that loss of recognition of an object results from the loss of the optic, tactile, and auditory components which go to make up the concept. The patient so affected would differ from the aphasic in that he would indeed fail to understand the significance of objects he has perceived. Wernicke admits that current anatomical knowledge is insufficient to specify the locus of the lesions. We see here a discussion of what later was to be called agnosia, to the study of which Lissauer (1889), one of Wernicke's assistants, made significant contributions.

Section III of the paper gives histories and clinical findings of ten patients. The first case was that of Suzanne Adam, a 59-year old lady who showed very poor comprehension and repetition, fluent, mildly paraphasic speech, alexia and agraphia, without gross neurological findings otherwise. She showed marked improvement, except for her agraphia. She did not come to post-mortem examination. However, writes Wernicke, this case recalled to him another earlier case, who had not been so well studied because, he says, at the time he saw her he had not yet worked out a correct analysis of the symptom-complex of aphasia. This was the case of Susanne Rother, a 75-year old lady who had been regarded when first admitted as suffering from aphasia with confusion. Her speech, while not so plentiful as that of the first cited case, was fluent and paraphasic. (It should be noted that the word paraphasia was never used by Wernicke at this time and came into literature later. He speaks instead of misused and distorted words.)

She had severe comprehension deficit which made some people think she was deaf. At post-mortem the Sylvian branch of the left middle cerebral artery was occluded. There was softening of the first temporal gyrus, and this was the only focal lesion found in the hemispheres.

It is on this case 2, admittedly studied inadequately, that the Wernicke argument rests since the remainder of the cases discussed did not show the cardinal syndrome described in the paper, that of fluent paraphasic speech with comprehension difficulty. Case 8 (Louise Funke), however, came to post-mortem after the paper was completed, and her findings were given in a brief appendix to the paper. In life she had shown the use of only one word "ja" and understood nothing. At post-mortem a major branch of the Sylvian branch of the middle cerebral artery was thrombosed. There was a large Sylvian infarct which included both Broca's area and the first temporal gyrus. Wernicke writes, ". . . in both cases (this one and case 2) the first temporal gyrus and its anastomosis with the second were involved. Both suffered from sensory aphasia. Could this agreement be the result of a coincidence?"

On this meager anatomical evidence his argument rested. Like Broca's first case, it was a slim reed on which to found so thorough-going a theory of aphasia. Other authors have claimed that none of Wernicke's cases supported his assertions, but this seems difficult to accept since the clinical and post-mortem findings of case 2 and case 8 were clearly consistent with his thesis, although they were not sufficient to prove it. Henry Head (1926) dismissed Wernicke's conclusions, but without taking into account the results in cases 2 and 8. It is perhaps ironic that Head himself cites cases of his own which he could have advanced in support of Wernicke's localizations. Thus his case 14 was a case of syntactical aphasia, the lesion of which Head places "in and around the upper temporal gyri and the parts beneath them." He says of the case that ". . . his speech was jargon . . . his words poured out in phrases which . . . were in most cases incomprehensible. He could not repeat a sentence said to him . . . He was unable to find names for common objects . . . Comprehension of spoken words was obviously defective . . ." It is almost as if he were quoting directly from Wernicke. Why Head so summarily dismissed Wernicke when his own evidence supported him must remain a mystery.

Wernicke closes his paper with some further comments. Baginsky, he notes, had spoken of "centrifugal" and "centripetal" forms of aphasia. But, he says, it is one thing to create hypothetical centers and quite another to construct a theory by converting known anatomical data into psychological form. He stresses the necessity of further anatomical knowledge. In the appendix, he credits Hitzig with recently published views on aphasia similar to his own independently developed ideas.

At this point it is reasonable to consider why this paper had so great an influence. One might entertain various theories. A consideration of some features of Wernicke's career may help to clarify some of the possibilities. He was only 26 when the paper was written, without previous publications, unknown, without academic rank, of an undistinguished family, in a provincial university, and without the support of major well-known figures. One can effectively dismiss the view that it was sheer prestige, academic authority or influence which were the sources of the effect of this paper. The growing prestige of German science in general would not account for the selection of his work over that of other better known German authors. A general tendency to accept diagram-making would again not be an adequate explanation since many writers of the day were producing their own diagrams.

Nor could the effect of the paper be attributed solely to Wernicke's later career. In the first place it had achieved a wide influence long before he himself had attained advancement. His academic progress was disappointingly slow, and for several years in Berlin he was without academic connections. Having once been appointed to the professorship in Breslau, he failed to move on from there to any of the more distinguished chairs. Hence, he never achieved great political influence within the German academic world. Furthermore he did very little further work on aphasia, leaving this area primarily to others. He advanced many other areas of neurology in later years, but the aphasias and related disturbances were left to his students and others to prosecute. In fact, it is important to realize that he considered his major activity to be his psychiatric investigations eventually to be summarized in his text "Grundriss der Psychiatrie in klinischen Vorlesungen." But while his work on aphasia was so successful, his psychiatry was to have little influence, although his psychiatric writing appeared during his period of greatest prestige. The same distinguished students who carried on his ideas in aphasia made the gesture of supporting their teacher's psychiatric teachings, but without enthusiasm. Yet Wernicke's psychiatry was also based on a simple diagram which failed of acceptance. The accusation of "brain-mythology" was made about his psychiatric teaching, yet his anatomical ideas on aphasia succeeded despite the unsuccessful attempts to apply the same epithet to them. In fact, the most successful psychiatric investigator of the period was Emil Kraepelin, who differed fundamentally from Wernicke. His psychiatry was not based on anatomy, was without diagrams, and was thoroughgoingly based on clinical descriptions.

Since this was a period in which psychiatry and neurology were still intimately linked in Germany, the very same people who accepted Wernicke's diagrammatic anatomical approach to aphasia were simultaneously adopting a very different psychiatric teaching. This should make us wary of accepting any simple conclusion that there was a general tendency to accept anatomical explanations or simple diagrams without question. Furthermore, scientific controversy raged in the German academic life of that period and disagreements were aired freely and at great length.

Perhaps only a more thorough investigation will unearth the full reasons for the acceptance of Wernicke's first paper, and I can here only suggest some possibilities. In the first place his paper brought new clinical facts to attention. As I have already mentioned, Bastian and Schmidt were the first to call attention to the sensory varieties of aphasia (and Wernicke who had been unfamiliar with these works was later to give them full credit), but it was Wernicke's work which succeeded in disseminating knowledge of these forms. He stressed the existence of fluent aphasias in contrast to the previously well-known forms, and called attention to the error of diagnosing these as confusional or psychiatric syndromes. He brought all of these elements together into a syndrome described for the first time. Furthermore, he had resolved the problem of the existence of cases of aphasia without damage to Broca's area by showing that Meynert's demonstration of cases of aphasia with temporal lobe lesions was clarified by the existence of a syndrome of temporal aphasia different from that of frontal aphasia. He established the localization of his syndrome of sensory aphasia, to be confirmed by later authors. It is important in viewing the paper to see it in the context of its period. Neuroanatomy was only beginning. The exact course of the auditory pathways was still unknown, and Wernicke pointed out that the somesthetic pathways were still a mystery. Standards of clinical examination were hardly developed, and pathological examination was based on gross findings. This paper came at the beginnings but was to be one of the forerunners of the great revolution in neurology.

One final point is worth stressing in considering the response to this paper. Meynert had pioneered in the attempt to correlate the structure of the brain with its functions, and Wernicke attempted to carry this trend forward. Broca had first shown the importance of localized lesions in producing aphasia, and Meynert had probably been the first to bring some rationale to the localizations, but it was Wernicke's paper which made the first searching attempt to link the facts of anatomy with the facts of behavior in a way that permitted both prediction of syndromes and the organized testing of hypotheses. Like Meynert, he gave the brain life. It was this trend that was continued in the work of many students both in Germany and elsewhere, and in good part must have accounted for the influential effects of this pioneering paper. The work of his own students, such as Liepmann, and of others, such as Dejerine, who employing what was essentially the Wernicke model were able to apply it successfully to the analysis of other syndromes, must have continued to give viability to Wernicke's teachings.

Indeed we must remember that even such writers as Goldstein, apparently so different in theoretical outlook, did not, as I have pointed out elsewhere (Geschwind, 1964), wholly reject Wernicke's approach. Goldstein took over a major portion of Wernicke's teachings and his connectionistic approach, and indeed even employed this type of analysis in the approach to some problems. As I have said earlier he first learned about neurology from Wernicke. Over half a century later he would write the following words of this early experience, ". . . his way of examining patients and his demonstrations were so elucidating and stimulating that we who had the good fortune to attend his clinics were deeply influenced in our further consideration of neurological and psychiatric problems. We could never forget him. His influence can be seen in the work of each of his many pupils, not a small number of whom became men of stature in their own right in the profession . . ." (Goldstein, 1953).

## References

Bastian, H. C. (1869) *On the various forms of loss of speech in cerebral disease,* "British and Foreign Med. Chir. Rev.," April (full reference not available, cited by Wernicke, 1908).

Geschwind, N. (1964) *The paradoxical position of Kurt Goldstein in the history of aphasia,* "Cortex," 1, 214-224

Geschwind, N. (1966), *Carl Wernicke, the Breslau school and the history of aphasia,* in U.C.L.A. Symposia in the Medical Sciences, ed. by E. Carterette. University of California Press, Los Angeles.

Goldstein, K. (1927) *Die Lokalization in der Grosshirnrinde,* in Handbuch der Normalen und Pathologischen Physiologie, Vol. 10, ed. by A. Bethe, G. v. Bergmann, G. Embden and A. Ellinger Springer, Berlin.

Goldstein, K. (1953) *Carl Wernicke,* in Founders of Neurology, ed. by W. Haymaker. Thomas, Springfield.

Head, H. (1926) *Aphasia and Kindred Disorders of Speech.* Cambridge University Press, Cambridge.

Kimura, D. (1961) *Some effects of temporal lobe damage on auditory perception,* "Canadian J. Psychol.," *15,* 156–165.

Lichtheim, L. (1885) *On aphasia,* "Brain," 7, 433–484.

Liepmann, H. (1898) *Ein Fall von Reiner.* Franck und Weigert, Breslau.

Lissauer, H. (1889) *Ein Fall von Reiner Sprachtaubheit nebst einem Beitrage zur theorie derselben,* "Arch. Psychiat. Nervenkr.," *21,* 222–271.

Nielsen, J. M. (1946) *Agnosia, Apraxia, Aphasia.* Hoeber, New York.

Penfield, W., and Roberts, L. (1959) *Speech and Brain Mechanisms.* Princeton University Press, Princeton.

Schmidt (1871) in "Allg. Z. Psychiat.," *27,* 304 (full reference not obtainable, cited by Wernicke, 1908).

Wernicke, C. (1908) *The symptom-complex of aphasia,* in Diseases of the Nervous System, ed. by A. Church, Appleton, New York, pp. 265–324.

Some of the research reported here was supported in part by Grant NB 06209 from the National Institutes of Health, to the Boston University Medical School. Presented in part at the Memorial Symposium in honor of Kurt Goldstein which took place at the Fourth Annual Meeting of the Academy of Aphasia in Chicago on October 16, 1966.

# CHAPTER 6

# The Varieties of Naming Errors

*Norman Geschwind*

In this paper I shall be discussing anomia in the sense of the inability of the patient to name things shown to him, what can be called failure of naming on confrontation. This task makes up so large a part of the testing of aphasia that it deserves attention. It is sometimes even asserted that failure in this task occurs in all aphasics. While as a rough statement this may be true, it deserves modification before it can be accepted without reservation. Thus there are certainly aphasics in whom naming on confrontation is very good relative to the patient's abnormal spontaneous speech production, even if rarely fully normal. This is particularly true in some cases of Broca's aphasia, and Jakobson (1964) has made much of this in his description of polar types of linguistic disturbance in aphasia.

I would stress also that we are speaking of naming in the narrower sense and not of word-finding in the flow of speech. The reasons for the failure to find words in one situation while they can be found in another have not yet been adequately studied and will not be discussed here. Instead I shall simply confine myself to discussing four distinguishable varieties of failure of confrontation naming, which may have some theoretical importance in considerations of aphasia and are of significance in clinical diagnosis.

The localization of anomia has often been a disputed point. In classical writings there were two opposing views, one which asserted that anomia resulted from a lesion of the left parietotemporal region while the other claimed that it was the result of diffuse disorder of the brain. The proponents of each localization had supporting data for their point of view. Gloning, Gloning, and Hoff (1963) dealt with this question simply by accepting both types of localization. As I will try to show, this problem can be at least partially resolved by the demonstration that local and diffuse localization, respectively, correspond to different types of anomia.

---

Reprinted with permission from CORTEX, Masson, S.P.A., Vol. III, 1967, pp. 97–112

One must of course be sure that the failure to name an object is not the result of failure of perception. Thus if a patient calls a "pencil" a "fork" it is conceivable that this could be the result of perceptual distortion. A test which is often used to rule out perceptual error is to offer the patient names and to see if he chooses the correct one. This test can, however, serve to exclude perceptual disturbance but cannot be used to prove that it is present. Thus if the patient always selects the correct name from those offered to him he must in each instance have recognized the object. Failure to accept the name might, however, be due not to incorrect perception of the object but to incomprehension of the name. Other tasks must be used to insure the correctness of perception. Correct pantomine of the use of the object proves correct perception. Similarly, matching tasks may be used. If a patient calls a "pencil" a "fork" but invariably matches a pencil to another pencil or a picture of a pencil, one must rule out perceptual difficulty. Similarly, if the patient is shown an object and misnames it but then draws it correctly, we must again exclude perceptual disturbance.

The classic form of anomia is characterized by difficulty in naming on confrontation, while the patient usually but not always accepts the correct name. The patient may also show by many of the other maneuvers listed above that he recognizes the object. He may simply fail to produce the name, or he may produce an incorrect name or a circumlocutory description. Almost invariably, when confrontation naming is impaired, the patient's spontaneous language production is disturbed so that while speech is fluent, it may contain many paraphasias, circumlocutions, or "empty" words (such as "thing," "place," or "these"). The word-finding difficulty in spontaneous speech is not confined to the names of physical stimuli but also involves abstract nouns and adjectives and other parts of speech (Wepman et al., 1956; Howes, 1964). When in addition to these features the patient's comprehension and repetition of speech are normal we have the classical syndrome of anomic aphasia, the lesion of which usually lies in the left temporo-parietal region (the angular gyrus). If disturbances of either comprehension or repetition or of both are present in association with the above picture of fluent, paraphasic speech, the localizations are somewhat different, although in all instances the lesions lie behind the Rolandic fissure.

In this first group the anomic difficulty tends to be a rather general one. It involves all modalities and all types of stimuli. The intensity of the disturbance is not, however, necessarily equal for all stimuli, as has recently been shown in careful studies by Goodglass et al. (1966).

In contrast to the above type of anomia we have another more restricted form, of which I will cite two examples, both of which I have presented elsewhere (Geschwind, 1965), although I did not in my earlier discussion bring out some of the differences between this type and the classical form of anomia discussed in the preceding paragraphs.

An example of this variety of anomia was seen in the patient of Geschwind and Kaplan (1962) who had a proven infarction of the corpus callosum sparing only the splenium. He had no difficulty in naming objects visually and speech was normal. When blindfolded he misnamed objects held in the left hand. The misnamings were bizarre, e.g., "eraser" for a ring, "balloon" for a watch, "book of matches" for a padlock, "an elastic" for a nail, "piece of paper" for a screwdriver. Furthermore, he did not accept the correct name when it was offered to him. That there was no perceptual failure could, however, be proven by the fact that after feeling an object with the left hand while blindfolded he could, using the same hand, pick the object by touch alone out of a bag or select it from a group with eyes open. When blindfolded he would use the object correctly with the left hand, while simultaneously misnaming it. In addition he could afterwards draw the object correctly with the left hand. It is clear that perception was intact and that this must be a naming defect.

It might be objected that one could explain this disturbance as the result of a combination of a minimal sensory defect in the left hand with minimal general naming disturbance. This is similar to the explanation advanced by Critchley (1966) to account for cases of color-naming difficulty. This type of explanation can be shown, however, to be inadequate to account for the naming difficulty of our patient for objects held in the left hand. The patient had definite sensory loss in the *right* hand as manifested by position, vibration, and two-point testing. In the *left* hand he could be shown by non-verbal testing to have normal sensation. Yet he correctly named objects felt with the right hand but not those held in the left. This fact clearly rules out the explanation of sensory loss plus minimal naming difficulty, since naming of objects held in the right hand should then have been more seriously involved than that of objects held in the left hand. I suspect that this type of explanation will rarely if ever be justified in any case. It is difficult to believe that a combination of two borderline disturbances could produce so dramatic and delimited a syndrome as this patient demonstrated. This case similarly cannot be accounted for by dementia or uncooperativeness since these would fail to explain the unilaterality of the disturbance.

A second example of this variety of anomia illustrates an even more delimited syndrome. This is the color-naming defect which accompanies some cases of pure alexia without agraphia. Geschwind and Fusillo (1966) have recently described such a case in detail. Consistent results were found on repeated careful testing over a nine-month period. This patient had a right hemianopia. He could not read, but he named objects normally (only one error in object-naming was made in all the testing sessions). He misnamed colors, but his misnaming always consisted of other color-words. The responses were not consistent in that the same red might on one occasion be called "gray," on another "green." The answer "gray" was, however, more common than any of the other color-words. The patient failed to select the correct answer from a group. Furthermore, he failed in the task of selecting a named color from a group presented to him. On the other hand, perceptual deficit was ruled out by the fact that the patient matched hues correctly despite wide differences in brightness or saturation, that he could sort colored chips correctly, even sorting into separate piles chips of slightly different shades of the same hue. He correctly matched colored pieces of paper to uncolored pictures of objects. Finally he performed normally on two pseudo-isochromatic tests of color vision, the Ishihara and the American Optical Company tests.

Loss of memory for color names was ruled out by the fact that he correctly answered questions such as, "What is the color of a banana?" Kinsbourne and Warrington (1964) in an earlier publication described a similar, although not identical, case.

It is obvious that this too is a naming disturbance. Critchley (1966) has suggested, as was noted above, the possibility that this disorder is not a specific entity "but rather a very mild disorder of visual perception coupled with a minimal dysphasia." This explanation is difficult to accept in the face of the powerful evidences of normal color perception I have cited above, and does not account readily for the highly delimited character of the syndrome. Furthermore, many patients with the combination of an obvious mild anomia and a hemianopia do not show dramatic difficulty in color naming, although one would expect this to be a common effect of this combination if Critchley were correct. Furthermore, since some degree of color-blindness is presented in about 7% of males, one would expect this percentage of mildly aphasic patients to show dramatic color-naming difficulties. Yet color-naming disturbances are rare and are most likely to occur in association with another rare syndrome, that of pure alexia without agraphia which has a characteristic pathological picture (Geschwind, 1962).

Both of the cases described above have come to anatomical examination, the brains having been cut in whole-brain sections, with alternate sections stained for myelin and cells. In the case of Geschwind and Kaplan, the corpus callosum was infarcted and the splenium was spared. In the case of Geschwind and Fusillo, the left visual cortex and the splenium were destroyed. The tactile naming difficulty in the left hand in the first case was interpreted as the result of disconnection of the right somesthetic cortex from the speech area, and the second case was interpreted as the result of disconnection of the right visual cortex from the speech area. Since I have discussed these explanations in detail elsewhere (Geschwind, 1965) I will return to our central interest at this moment, the character of the anomia in these cases.

Difficulties in naming, predominantly in a single modality, have been mentioned by many authors, although these have frequently been treated as agnosias. Arguments against this interpretation have been summarized in Geschwind (1965) and will not be repeated here. Two excellent recent examples of dissociation between modalities are seen in the case of Ettlinger and Wyke (1961), who named better visually than by touch, and in the cases of Spreen, Benton, and Van Allen (1966), who cited two patients with predominantly visual and three with predominantly tactile anomia. Kaplan and Geschwind (unpublished) observed one patient with a predominantly tactile naming disturbance.

Let us look at the features of this second form of anomia which distinguish it from the classical form. In the first place the second type of anomia is remarkably delimited, being confined to the tactile modality in the left half of the body in the first case and to color-naming in the second. The classical type of anomia is more global in its effect. In the second place spontaneous speech was normal in both of these cases, and neither patient showed word-finding difficulty except on confrontation. Thus the second patient showed no difficulty in finding color words except when confronted with a color. This contrasts with the classical form of anomia in which even mild confrontation naming difficulty is almost always accompanied by word-finding difficulty in spontaneous speech as manifested by hesitation, particularly in finding substantive words (as against "grammatical" words), by an increased tendency to use "empty" words, by circumlocution, or by production of paraphasias.

A third difference is in the nature of the errors. The classic anomic may fail to name or may produce verbal paraphasias, combinatory paraphasias (e.g. "ring-key" for "key-ring"), phonemic paraphasias, or even grossly neologistic errors. Patients with the second variety of anomia usually produce no combinatory or phonemic paraphasias or neologisms. This is not the result of differential severity of naming disturbance since classic anomics even when mildly impaired may produce phonemic paraphasias, while the cases of the second type of anomia discussed above produced no phonemic paraphasias despite gross naming failure in the affected spheres.

The errors of our patient with the tactile naming disturbance in the left hand were in general "wildly" incorrect and not errors in sphere (i.e., related by sound or meaning) such as are often produced by the classic anomic. It may be argued that in the case of color-naming deficit, the patient did produce errors in kind since he always produced the name of some color. This, however, overlooks the fact that it was the method of testing which led to this result. We would ask the patient, "What color is this?" and he would therefore confine his reply to color names. It is obvious that our first patient also used the information from the question "What do you feel in your left hand?" to give names of small palpable objects. This is a much larger class than that of colors and permitted therefore apparently more random answers.

A fourth difference, one of major importance, is the fact that the patients with the second type of anomia showed not only disturbance in naming but also what might at first be thought of as comprehension disturbance. Thus these patients failed to choose the correct name from a group. The second patient could not select a named color from a group. This special type of comprehension disturbance was not recognized classically since it was taken as evidence of "agnosic" difficulty. We have, however, already shown that these failures were not due to perceptual disturbance, but we can also see that they are not failures of comprehension in the usual sense. Thus these patients both perfectly understood the names of objects and colors in such sentences as, "Tell me the name of something red" or "Are roses green?" A more accurate description would be to say that the patients could not match the sensory stimulus to the spoken name. The classic anomic is like the second variety of anomic in failing to produce the name when presented with the stimulus, but differs from the second variety in usually being able to choose the correct stimulus from a group when presented with the spoken name.

Another difference lies in the patient's response to his deficit. The classic anomic may admit to not knowing the name. On the other hand he may show various forms of denial. He may insist that he never knew the name, or that he has always called it by the term which he has just used, even when this is clearly incorrect. He may assert that he really knows the word, but I suspect that this "tip-of-the tongue" phenomenon is at least as often mistaken in the patient as it is in normals.

The second group of patients almost never admit to not knowing the correct name but will almost always produce a response. When pressed as to the reasons for the discrepancy between his response and the one designated by the examiner as the correct one, the patient may assert that he hasn't done this kind of thing in the past or that things "look different" to him from the way they look to the examiner. In short, the classic anomic acts as if his vocabulary and that of the examiner differ; the patient with the second type of anomia may act as if his perception and that of the examiner differ although perception can be shown to be intact by nonverbal methods.

We can summarize the two groups as follows. The classic anomic has difficulty in naming on confrontation which more or less involves all types of material and is more or less equal for all sensory modalities. The inadequacies of naming may consist of failure to produce a response, verbal paraphasias which are generally related by sound or meaning, phonemic paraphasias, or circumlocutory descriptions. There is usually difficulty in spontaneous speech, manifested by word-finding pauses or any of the other difficulties listed above. The patient can usually choose the correct name if offered to him by the examiner and can select a named object from a group. The patient ascribes his errors to differences in knowledge or usage of words. The lesions in these cases are in the dominant angular gyrus region.

Contrasted with this is the second type of anomia, best characterized as an *inability to match a stimulus to its spoken name,* i.e., the patient can neither produce the name when presented with the stimulus nor choose the correct stimulus when given a name. The difficulty is confined to a single modality, and even to a single class within that modality, and may be confined to one-half of visual space or one side of the body. Circumlocutory errors or phonemic paraphasias occur uncommonly if at all. The errors consist primarily of verbal paraphasias which are not related to the correct word by sound and are related only in the most general way by meaning. Spontaneous speech is normal even for the categories which are specially impaired in confrontation naming. The patient cannot usually choose the correct name of the item when it is offered to him; nor can he select a named item correctly from a group. Comprehension deficit in the usual sense, however, is ruled out because the patient shows normal understanding of the same words when he is obliged to give purely verbal responses. Perceptual deficit is ruled out by the patient's ability to carry out the various tests listed earlier in the paper. The patient may ascribe his errors to differences in perception between himself and the examiner. The lesions are those which produce disconnections from the speech area.

It is of some importance to consider the differences between these groups of anomic disturbances. To call one disturbance aphasic and the other perceptual or agnosic runs counter to the demonstrated fact that perception can be shown to be intact even in those patients suffering from the second group of disturbances who assert that their difficulty is perceptual. A point of great theoretical importance which arises out of a careful consideration of the differences between the two groups is that one can safely reject the thesis that classical anomic aphasia is the result of the accumulation of large numbers of separate naming disturbances. Since the isolated naming disturbances are likely to be of the second variety, a large number of these appearing together in the same patient would produce a picture quite different from classical anomia, as any consideration of the discussion above will clearly show. Thus phonemic paraphasic errors may be seen in classical anomia, which is also associated with difficulties in spontaneous speech but without comprehension deficit; in all of these ways it differs from the isolated naming disturbances. Classical anomia appears therefore to differ not only in degree but also in kind from the isolated naming disturbances.

It seems clear, however, that occasionally one must encounter patients with classical anomia who also have the admixture of one or more isolated naming disturbances, thus leading to an apparent selective impairment of certain types of naming. Unfortunately there is little documentation as to whether such patients show the specialized type of comprehension disturbances specified above for the second group. Thus in the studies of Goodglass et al. (1966) cited above, it may be that the increased difficulty in certain naming tasks in classical anomics may reflect admixtures of "disconnection" anomias. If this is the case then one should find difficulties in comprehension of the specialized type I have described in these categories above. It will be important to investigate this further in the future.

How can one account theoretically for these two varieties of anomia? The second type, i.e., the "disconnection" anomia, appears to be more readily accounted for than does classical anomia. Thus if a lesion cuts off most of the connections between the cortical representation of a given sensory modality and the speech area, it is easy to see that the patient will name incorrectly since the sensory information will fail to reach the speech area. It is also easy to see that the patient will have difficulty matching a name spoken by the examiner to the stimulus since there is no path from the speech area to the association cortex of the modality in question. The patient will make no errors in matching *within* the affected modality, nor will he have any troubles in purely verbal tasks. Spontaneous speech would be normal. The patient will often refer to his errors *as if* they were due to perceptual difficulty since the speech area which is giving the account is indeed not receiving the perceptual information. As stated above, the lesion by disconnecting the speech area from some given sensory region prevents the matching of a sensory stimulus to a speech stimulus, regardless of the order of presentation.

Classic anomia implies, however, a lesion in a more complicated system. This system can be conceived of as one which receives the sensory information and finds the spoken word appropriate to it. It is a system which may be thought of as containing the rules for finding a word given some of its attributes. Obviously it uses information from all modalities since it can "find" a word when presented with the actual object in one or more modalities, or on the other hand it can find the word when given its attributes in verbal form. As may have been noticed, this system is referred to as finding the *spoken* word corresponding to a set of attributes. It is my guess that it would act primarily to find the auditory form of words since it is this form which is first learned. Finding the written word would therefore be secondary to finding the auditory form.

It is reasonable that the region involved in the activity of finding a word given some of its attributes in one or more modalities is the angular gyrus since, as I have suggested elsewhere (Geschwind, 1964, 1965), this region is probably involved in the formation of associations between the various non-limbic sensory modalities (vision, somesthesis, audition). It is also easy to understand why damage to such a region should leave the grammatical structure of spoken language so well preserved. The "small" grammatical words depend little if at all for their evocation on attributes in different sensory modalities. More generally grammatical structure, e.g., rules of word order and their transformations, is almost certainly not dependent on such intermodal interactions but probably develop, like the small grammatical words, almost entirely within the auditory system.

It is reasonable that such a set of rules would be formulated in the large region of gray matter which is probably more or less equi-potential. It also must be so designed that it is easier to find the attributes given the word than to find the word given the attributes, since patients with lesions in this system comprehend the word more readily than they can find it. The system is therefore in some ways like a punch-card system. It also seems reasonable, however, to assume that in the most extensive cases of destruction of the area involved in this activity, significant comprehension deficits would occur although they are not seen in partial destruction. I have made the speculation elsewhere (Geschwind, 1965) that perhaps these more extensive cases correspond to the "syndrome of the isolated speech areas" but I will not go further into this problem at this point. In any case, it seems clear that we need further study of the anatomical connections of the angular gyrus region and further investigation of the classical anomias in order to learn the rules by which words are encoded in this region. It would also seem reasonable that the delimited anomias ultimately depend on disconnections of a particular sensory modality from the left angular gyrus.

Having discussed these two types of anomia, each with localizable lesions (in the left angular gyrus or in connections to the left angular gyrus respectively), let us consider now a third variety. As was pointed out earlier, classically there was a disagreement as to the localization of anomic aphasia. One group attributed it to focal disease in the angular gyrus region while others claimed that diffuse lesions of the brain were necessary. As I have already noted, both groups were in fact partially correct. It is clear, however, that what was not realized classically was the fact that the anomias in the two types of syndromes were different. Edwin Weinstein and his co-workers (e.g., Weinstein and Keller, 1964) have made the most significant contribution in presenting the characteristics of anomia which may occur in acute diffuse disease of the brain. It is quite clear that many neurologists have overlooked this syndrome. On the other hand, it is necessary to avoid the reverse error, i.e., that of mistaking focal aphasic disturbance for this condition of "non-aphasic misnaming."

Non-aphasic misnaming typically occurs in disorders which diffusely involve the nervous system, especially when the disturbance comes on fairly rapidly. It is thus very common in head injuries, subarachnoid hemorrhages, rapidly increasing intracranial pressure, and in toxic or metabolic disorders such as intoxications, withdrawal syndromes, uremia, or congestive heart failure. Thus in my experience, the syndrome of non-aphasic misnaming has only rarely been seen on the Aphasia Unit in the Boston Veterans Administration Hospital, is occasionally seen elsewhere on the Neurology Service, but is more often seen in the medical or neurosurgical wards. By contrast, misnaming in the aphasic, whether in classic anomic aphasia or as part of one of the other syndromes resulting from post-rolandic lesions, can occur in chronic, stable form over months or years in patients having focal unilateral lesions without evidence of widespread diffuse involvement.

Non-aphasic misnaming is perhaps a poor term for the syndrome as a whole since it highlights only one feature of the disorder. Depending on the particular variation seen in any one case, the examiner may be deceived into thinking that the patient is aphasic, or that he is suffering from a disturbance of memory or of perception, or indeed that the patient is deliberately being facetious (Weinstein terms this "ludic" behavior, and it clearly corresponds in good part to the classical moria or Witzelsucht). This is illustrated in the sort of reply that one often gets from such patients when the question, "What do I do?" is made by the examiner. A typical response is "You're someone who asks a lot of questions" or "You're an investigator of some kind." Characteristically the errors tend to "propagate." Thus the patient being asked where he is may say "In a bus," and may then say that the examining physician is the driver, that those around him are passengers, and that the bed he is in is used by the driver for resting. It is usually obvious once a sequence of questions is asked that ordinary aphasic misnaming is readily ruled out. Thus in aphasic misnaming, there is no tendency to "propagation" although perseveration, i.e., repetition of the same incorrect word, occurs frequently. On the other hand, perseveration can also occur in non-aphasic misnaming and may thus present a difficulty of interpretation. In aphasic misnaming the problem rarely arises that one has to consider the possibilities of memory loss, perceptual difficulty, or jocularity since these are easily ruled out. It is much more difficult to exclude these in non-aphasic misnaming since it often appears impossible to obtain the patient's cooperation. The aphasic with misnaming who has no comprehension deficit usually accepts correction by the examiner, but in non-aphasic misnaming this is often difficult or impossible to achieve.

The "connected" or "propagated" character of the errors may show up particularly in relation to the hospital and the patient's illness. He may call the hospital a "hotel," the doctors "bell boys," the nurses "chambermaids," and will not accept correction. One man dying with terminal cancer said that the building in which he was located was a "slaughter house" where "they hang up bodies" and that the examiner was a "grinder." He denied specifically that it was a hospital. This example of what Weinstein calls "tragic ludic behavior" (equivalent to "gallows humor") illustrates another characteristic of the syndrome, i.e., that it is often possible to demonstrate that the patient in fact knows the correct answers since his errors are so clearly motivated. This is well illustrated by Weinstein's patient who asserted that she was in the "Mount Cyanide Rest Home." She could have produced this pun only with the knowledge that she was in fact in the Mount Sinai Hospital. This motivated misnaming is not a feature of aphasic anomia in which the patient will usually show no increased difficulty in talking about his illness or the hospital and may even perform at his best when the examiner turns to these topics.

One feature which often characterizes non-aphasic misnaming is that spontaneous speech is usually (but not invariably) normal despite gross errors in naming. In aphasic anomia errors in confrontation naming are almost always accompanied by a disturbance in spontaneous speech in which word-finding pauses, empty phrases, paraphasias, and circumlocutions appear.

Some of the errors in non-aphasic misnaming may appear to be more "aphasic" than the "motivated" or "propagated" misnamings. In some instances rather bizarre errors occur, misnamings apparently totally unrelated by sound or meaning, but also not occurring in an obvious connected context. The differential diagnosis of these may be quite difficult. Thus while it is true that classic aphasic anomia usually leads to errors which are related in sound or meaning to the correct word, it is clearly the case that such bizarre errors do occasionally occur, particularly in that group of patients with the syndrome of the "isolated speech area" which Goldstein (1917) discussed and which I have commented on elsewhere (Geschwind, 1965). In these cases, however, the patient suffers from a gross comprehension disturbance, often with echolalic repetition, and can thus be easily distinguished from cases of non-aphasic misnaming.[1]

It is not possible at this time to give a more detailed account of the pathogenesis of non-aphasic misnaming. While it typically occurs in situations in which there is diffuse involvement of the nervous system, this does not necessarily rule out that it is some focal aspect of the diffuse involvement which is really important. It is true that a single stable unilateral lesion has not been shown to produce this syndrome. It is possible, however, that stable bilaterally symmetrical lesions in some particular area are necessary. Certainly many aspects of this syndrome are reminiscent of some of the features of chronic bilateral frontal disease, but it

---

[1] Dr. Ennio De Renzi has pointed out to me that the syndrome of non-aphasic misnaming is similar in many ways to that described by continental psychiatrists as disordered language in mental confusion. He points out that a further useful criterion is that aphasics will generally have more difficulty in naming uncommon as against common objects while the patient with non-aphasic misnaming may paradoxically do better in the naming of uncommon objects. This same association could of course be seen in patients with hysterical or malingered naming disturbances.

would not be possible with assurance to equate non-aphasic misnaming with frontal disease. Furthermore, it is possible that this syndrome may occur transiently with acute unilateral disease in some specific focus and disappear in time, but this would be difficult to disentangle from the more widespread effects of acute lesions. In addition the place of involvement may not be cortical but may be subcortical, as Weinstein himself has suggested. Unfortunately our knowledge of well-defined chronic behavioral syndromes from non-cortical lesions is confined to a small number of disturbances such as Korsakow's syndrome or akinetic mutism. A further possibility is that the name-finding system, of which we spoke earlier in this paper and which is located in the angular gyrus region, may be very readily disturbed by diffuse disease because it depends so heavily on multiple connections from many regions.

The diagnosis of non-aphasic misnaming presents many difficulties. While one may see a relatively "pure" example, e.g., the patient who is intoxicated, the differential is much more difficult when there is concomitant focal damage. The problem is compounded by the fact that the syndrome of non-aphasic misnaming may be superimposed on a mild focal anomic disturbance or on a Korsakow's syndrome. Examination is particularly difficult in such cases because the cooperation of the patient is often extremely difficult to obtain. Thus we have seen cases in which once the non-aphasic misnaming had cleared, it became obvious that the patient was suffering from a classical Korsakow's syndrome. In other cases with clearing of the picture of non-aphasic misnaming, we have observed a mild but definite aphasic anomia with an appropriate left posterior Rolandic lesion. This syndrome remains a major problem for students of the neurology of behavior and has been generally neglected except in the pioneering work of Weinstein.

We have now presented three situations in which misnaming may occur—classical anomic aphasia, those disconnection syndromes in which matching of a stimulus with its spoken name is impaired, and the syndrome of non-aphasic misnaming. We now turn to a fourth group of disturbances which includes hysterical and malingered anomias. In these cases the patient often fails to find the names of very simple objects presented to him. He usually shows great apparent concern over the failure. If the examiner insists that he is sure the patient can find the word, he often receives a response of annoyance or a protest that it is impossible to go on. These responses can also occur but are much less likely in aphasic anomia. The clue to the diagnosis in these cases is that despite a gross global defect of confrontation naming in all modalities, the patient's spontaneous speech is normal. Thus one patient whom I examined would fail to name as common an object as a pencil presented either visually or tactually and yet could tell us with perfect fluency in her spontaneous speech that her husband was an electronics engineer who was working on the design of digital computers. The anomia may be the only obvious abnormality or may occur against the background of a more outspoken hysterical pseudo-dementia, e.g., an outspoken Ganser syndrome. This "functional" misnaming syndrome is rare but failure to recognize it may have serious consequences.

## Summary

Four syndromes are discussed in which there occurs failure of naming on confrontation. The first is the anomia of posterior aphasia-producing lesions. The second is a much more delimited disturbance produced by lesions which isolate certain sensory regions from the speech area (probably from the left angular gyrus in particular) and which may be best characterized as failure to match certain sensory stimuli to their spoken names. The third syndrome is that of non-aphasic misnaming which occurs in disorders which diffusely involve the brain. The fourth is anomia occurring as a manifestation of hysteria or malingering. The clinical syndromes are outlined as well as the distinguishing features of the anomia in each type. Some of the theoretical problems raised by each form of anomia are also discussed.

## References

Critchley, M. (1966) *Acquired anomalies of colour perception of central origin,* "Brain," *88,* 711–724.

Ettlinger, G., and Wyke, M. (1961) *Defects in identifying objects visually in a patient with cerebrovascular disease,* "J. Neurol. Neurosurg. Psychiat.," *24,* 254.

Geschwind, N. (1962) *The anatomy of acquired disorders of reading,* in Reading Disability, ed. by J. Money. Johns Hopkins University Press, Baltimore, pp. 115–130.

Geschwind, N. (1964) *The development of the brain and the evolution of language,* in Monograph Series on Language and Linguistics, ed. by C.I.J.M. Stuart. Georgetown University Press, No. 17, pp. 155–169.

Geschwind, N. (1965) *Disconnexion syndromes in animals and man,* "Brain," *88,* 237–294 and 585–644.

Geschwind, N., and Fusillo, M. (1966) *Color-naming defects in association with alexia,* "A.M.A. Arch. Neurol.," *15,* 137–146.

Geschwind, N., and Kaplan, E. (1962) *A human cerebral deconnection syndrome,* "Neurology," *12,* 675–685.

Gloning, I., Gloning, K., and Hoff, H. (1963) *Aphasia—a clinical syndrome,* in Problems of Dynamic Neurology, ed. by L. Halpern. Grune and Stratton, New York, pp. 63–70.

Goldstein, K. (1917) *Die transkortikalen Aphasien.* Gustav Fischer, Jena.

Goodglass, H., Klein, B., Carey, P., and Jones, K. ((1966) *Specific semantic word categories in aphasia,* "Cortex," *2,* 74–89.

Howes, D. H. (1964) *Application of the word-frequency concept to aphasia,* in Disorders of Language, ed. by A.V.S De Reuck and M. O'Connor. Little, Brown, Boston, pp. 47–48.

Jakobson, R. (1964) *Towards a linguistic typology of aphasic impairments,* in Disorders of Language, ed. by A.V.S. De Reuck and M. O'Connor. Little, Brown, Boston, pp. 21–46.

Spreen, O., Benton, A. L., and Van Allen, M. W. (1966) *Dissociation of visual and tactile naming in amnesic aphasia,* "Neurol.," *16,* 807–814.

Weinstein, E. A., and Keller, N. J. S. (1964) *Linguistic patterns of misnaming in brain injury,* "Neuropsychologia," *1,* 79–90.

Wepman, J. M., Bock, R. D., Jones, L. V., and Van Pelt, D. (1956) *Psycholinguistic study of aphasia: a revision of the concept of anomia,* J. Speech and Hearing Disorders," *21,* 468–477.Dr. Norman Geschwind, V. A. Hospital, 150 South Huntington Ave., Boston, Massachusetts 02130.

Supported in part by Grants NB06209 and MH08472 from the National Institutes of Health to the Boston University Aphasia Research Center.

# CHAPTER 7

# Aphasia

*Norman Geschwind*

Aphasia, a common, distressing, and often permanent aftereffect of neurologic disease, has received little attention in recent years not only in general medical publications but even in the neurologic literature. This neglect has resulted from the idea that the aphasias are exotic disorders, of little practical value to the clinician, and not susceptible to experimental analysis, and that discussion of them demands a penchant for abstruse philosophical speculation. Limitations of space preclude dealing with all these misconceptions, and this article will concentrate only on the practical clinical uses of a knowledge of aphasia.

Most clinicians have been taught an apparently simple classification based on an expressive-receptive dichotomy. In this scheme a patient with trouble speaking has an expressive aphasia, implying a lesion in Broca's area, whereas if he cannot comprehend language, he suffers from receptive aphasia, implying a more posterior lesion. This classification is misleading and should be abandoned.

Because of limitations of space we will deal here only with the common aphasias that make up the overwhelming majority of cases seen in practice. We will omit the rare, interesting, and theoretically important conditions such as the pure alexias and pure word-deafness. In all the forms of aphasias discussed here there is disturbance of language output. It should be stressed that aphasia is by definition a disturbance of language. If a patient is totally mute one cannot be sure whether he is aphasic. A simple rule of thumb in those with disordered output is that however distorted the patient's speech may be, if when it is transcribed he is producing correct English sentences, he is not suffering from aphasia but rather from some form of articulatory disability.

The most important distinction in disorders of language output is that between fluent and nonfluent aphasias. Patients with the latter produce little speech, which is uttered slowly, with great effort and with poor articulation.

---

Reprinted with permission from *The New England Journal of Medicine*. 1971; 284 (12): 654-656.

Characteristically the speech of such patients lacks the small grammatical words and endings, so that it may take on the quality of a telegram. Asked about the weather, such a patient may say, "Sunny," and if urged to produce a full sentence he may say, "Weather—sunny."

By contrast, the patients with fluent aphasia effortlessly produce well articulated, long phrases or sentences with a normal grammatical skeleton, having normal rhythm and melody. Such patients often speak at a higher rate than normal. The speech is abnormal, however, since despite the many words produced, it is often remarkably devoid of content.

The abnormality of the speech output in the fluent aphasias is manifested primarily by failure to use the correct word, which is substituted for by circumlocutory phrases ("what you use to open a door"), by nonspecific words (like "thing"), or by incorrect words, so-called paraphasias, which are of two kinds. Verbal paraphasias consist of the substitution of one correct English word or phrase for another, sometimes related in meaning (e.g., "knife" for "fork"), sometimes totally unrelated (e.g., "Argentinian rifle" for "thumb"). Literal (or phonemic) paraphasias consist of the replacement of one or more sounds in otherwise correct words (e.g., "spoot" for "spoon"). In some cases the words produced are frankly neologistic (e.g., "flieber" or "sodent").

Lesions in Broca's area produce nonfluent aphasia. Because these lesions also generally involve the adjacent motor cortex, most patients with nonfluent aphasia suffer from an appreciable hemiparesis, which is usually greater in the arm. Even though these lesions destroy the face area of the motor cortex, facial weakness is usually less prominent than arm weakness, since even the lower half of the face has substantial bilateral innervation. By contrast, the presence of a fluent aphasia means that Broca's area is intact; the patient typically does not suffer from hemiplegia, and his lesion lies in either the temporal or the parietal lobes. This underscores the incorrectness of the commonly accepted notion, mentioned earlier, that disorder in speech output means "expressive aphasia," which in turn means a lesion in Broca's area.

There are several forms of fluent aphasia that are distinguished on the basis of the patient's ability to comprehend and to repeat spoken language. In Wernicke's aphasia the lesion lies in the posterior superior temporal region. These patients fail both to understand the examiner's words and to repeat them. The patient with conduction aphasia, whose lesion usually lies deep in the portion of the parietal lobe just above the Sylvian fissure, shows normal comprehension of spoken language but repeats the examiner's words incorrectly. The disability in repetition is most marked not for long words, but rather for short grammatical words, so that phrases such as, "He was here," are more difficult than words such as "presidential." "No ifs, ands, or buts" is the hardest of all phrases to repeat for such patients. The patient with anomic or amnestic aphasia also suffers from a fluent aphasia, in which comprehension and repetition are both preserved. When this occurs acutely as the result of vascular occlusion, the lesion most commonly lies in the region of the angular gyrus or the adjacent portion of the lower temporal lobe. In many cases, however, anomic aphasia is difficult to

TABLE 1. Differential Characteristics of Fluent Aphasias.*

| *Type of Aphasia* | *Comprehension* | *Repetition* |
|---|---|---|
| Wernicke's | – | – |
| Conduction | + | – |
| Anomic | + | + |
| Isolation | – | + |

*– indicates serious involvement, + little or no impairment; naming of objects is defective in all these aphasias.

localize since, particularly in its milder forms, it may be seen as a recovery stage from other types of aphasia and is also a frequent manifestation of metabolic or other widespread disorders of the brain. Finally, in a remarkable, although rare, condition the patient suffers from a fluent aphasia with a severe loss of comprehension but repeats even long phrases produced by the examiner with ease. In these cases the lesion surrounds but leaves intact the classic speech regions that lie above and below the Sylvian fissure. This has been termed "isolation of the speech area."

Testing the capacity to repeat phrases spoken by the examiner is of great importance in the differential diagnosis of the fluent aphasias (Table 1). Despite the major importance of this ability it is generally neglected in most texts on aphasia.

In some cases there is a massive lesion that destroys both Broca's area and Wernicke's area, so that the patient, who almost invariably has a severe hemiplegia, suffers from a grossly nonfluent aphasia combined with a severe loss of comprehension and repetition. This is a global aphasia.

Every patient who is aphasic in speech is also aphasic in writing (although there are rare patients who are aphasic in writing but not in speech). Therefore, if a patient is able to produce fully normal language in written form, but does not speak, one can safely conclude that he is suffering not from aphasia but from mutism. This implies that his lesion does not involve the speech areas, and furthermore that if any speech returns, it may be severely dysarthric but will not manifest difficulties in word finding or in grammar. Such a condition has often been seen in patients with Parkinson's disease who have undergone bilateral thalamic surgery. Aphasic patients are also occasionally mute in the acute stage, but in most cases, the ability to produce some words eventually returns.

Difficulty in naming objects is common in all the varieties of aphasia discussed above, and therefore does not distinguish a particular type. The term "anomic aphasia" should therefore be used only as we have employed it above, to describe a fluent aphasia with essentially normal comprehension and repetition. Tests of naming are generally not useful if the patient's speech is normal.

If a patient remains hemiplegic as the result of vascular disease for three weeks, one can predict that the chance for noteworthy recovery is minimal. On the other hand, some patients may recover spontaneously even from aphasias that persist well beyond this period. One should be wary about making a prognosis on aphasia before three months have elapsed. Controlled studies of speech therapy have shown that most of the recovery from aphasia is spontaneous, although specific therapy may have a small but definite effect, which is especially useful in severe cases of Broca's and conduction aphasia.

Fluent aphasia may be misdiagnosed since many physicians are unaware of the frequency of aphasia without a hemiplegia. The patient may be called psychotic or confused, particularly when there is a rapid outpouring of abnormal speech. In practice, the differential diagnosis is easy. Schizophrenic word salad occurs primarily in patients with chronic back-ward schizophrenia. The acute onset of abnormal speech in a middle-aged person is therefore almost invariably diagnostic of a fluent aphasia. If a patient with aphasic speech has no hemiplegia, one can usually, on this basis alone, conclude that one is dealing with a fluent aphasia.

Aphasias in association with lesions of the right hemisphere are extremely rare. Among right-handed persons they occur less than once in 100 cases, and even among those who are left-handed, at least 60 per cent of aphasias result from lesions in the left hemisphere.

In patients with metabolic disorder or raised intracranial pressure one occasionally observes aphasic disorders. Curiously enough, the aphasia caused by these nonspecific widespread disorders of the brain is nearly always of the anomic variety described earlier, whereas clear-cut aphasias of the other types are almost never seen. The aphasias seen after head injury and in the presenile dementias are also most frequently of the anomic type. By contrast, anomic aphasia is much less common with vascular disease than are Wernicke's, Broca's, or conduction aphasias. One must therefore be wary, on being confronted with an anomic aphasia, of ascribing it to vascular disease, especially in a patient who is somewhat drowsy, and one should always look carefully for metabolic disorder or some space-taking lesion within the brain.

We have placed emphasis in this article only on the practical usefulness of aphasia to the clinician. It is well to realize, however, that in the past few years there has been a resurgence of interest in the anatomic and physiologic mechanisms in the brain that underlie language dominance and the other higher functions. These studies are beginning to indicate the directions that may lead to physiologically based methods of improved therapy for the disorders of the capacities that are the most distinctive biologic attributes of man.

Some of the work reported here was supported in part by a grant (NS-06209) from the National Institutes of Health.

# CHAPTER 8

# Language and Cerebral Dominance

*Norman Geschwind*

Over the past 25 years, interest in the aphasias, in the neural organization of language, and in cerebral dominance and its biological foundations has grown steadily. The contrast between the high level of activity today and the low level of the late 1940s will perhaps be made clearer by a brief consideration of the earlier history of this field and of its state in 1950.

From the earliest beginnings of neurology in the 1860s, clinicians were involved in the investigation of the aphasias and related disorders. Broca and Wernicke specified some of the major principles that have guided study ever since—the presence of delimited regions in the brain, lesions of which led to disorders of language, and the major importance of the left hemisphere in these functions. Enthusiasm for these problems persisted almost unabated over the next 50 years. Nearly all of the major pioneers of neurology contributed to the knowledge of the cerebral organization of language. It is probably true that even today the overall level of activity in this field does not equal the peaks attained during this classical period.

After World War I there was a dramatic decline of interest among clinical neurologists in brain-behavior relationships, a decline that was particularly striking in the English-speaking world. The last great representatives of the classical tradition on the continent died in the 1920s, in France (Dejerine) and in Germany (Liepmann). In England, Head violently attacked the classical teaching, and his book was probably one of the major factors in the loss of interest in aphasia. American neurologists with few exceptions exhibited little activity in this area. Later in this period the work of Akelaitis and his co-workers convinced nearly all neurological scientists that lesions of the corpus callosum had no

---

Reprinted with permission from D.B. Tower (ed), *The Nervous System, Volume 2*. New York: Raven Press, 1975; 433-439.

marked effects upon behavior. It was characteristic of the period that no one reviewed adequately the earlier masterful descriptions of callosal syndromes by Liepmann, Dejerine, Goldstein, and others and that the conclusions of Akelaitis were therefore accepted without question.

Three other major figures were partly responsible for the decline of interest in the neurological approach to behavior. Freud was indirectly responsible by causing a shift of concern from physiological brain mechanisms of behavior to the psychological effects of early life experiences. Kurt Goldstein, who had come as a refugee to the United States, exerted a powerful influence on American psychology. Despite his own abiding personal interest in brain mechanisms, his teaching paradoxically reinforced the tendency to shy away from study of the brain. Even more influential perhaps was Karl Lashley, one of the pioneers in the study of changes in animal behavior through ablative experiments on parts of the brain. Despite Lashley's persistent personal concern with the brain, his work, also somewhat paradoxically, reinforced the general skepticism concerning the possibilities of relating brain mechanisms to language.

It should not be thought that neurological activity in disorders of language had totally come to a halt in the period between the two world wars. Pötzl and his students in Vienna maintained an active and productive unit. Luria in the Soviet Union carried out an elaborate series of investigations during World War II (although some of his results were first published in 1947 in Russian, they were not available in English until much later). What was characteristic of the 1920–1950 era was, however, a sharp decline in this area compared to the high level of the preceding 60 years, the isolation of the investigators from each other, and particularly a lack of knowledge of what was going on in other countries. Therefore, the discussions of the callosal syndromes by Sittig and Lange during this period simply went unnoticed in the English- and French-speaking worlds.

In brief, in 1950 there was a low level of activity in the fields of aphasia and dominance, widespread ignorance of earlier studies, a powerful tendency to reject those that had not been forgotten, and a general skepticism as to the possibilities of deepening one's understanding of the relationship of the brain to language. On the other hand, there was great excitement over the advances in animal work, as exemplified by the studies on the frontal lobe in Fulton's laboratory, and in particular Jacobsen's discovery of delayed response deficits, Lashley's many investigations, the description of the Klüver-Bucy syndrome, the Papez theory of emotion, and the newer knowledge of hypothalamic mechanisms of behavior that came from the work of Hess, Ranson, and Ingram. All of these appeared to promise a bright future for the study of brain mechanisms in animals, which compensated to some extent for the general wariness concerning the study of higher functions in man.

The last 25 years have, however, been attended by a great increase in studies of language and dominance, which has been reflected in the journals and in the programs of neurological meetings. The programs of the early meetings of the American Academy of Neurology had, at most, only a handful of papers on behavior. In the past few years, not only have there been special courses in this area, but the number of papers has increased so sharply as to warrant the setting aside of an entire morning session. Not only have the general neurological journals published many more papers, but three journals devoted primarily to the study of the human higher functions have come into being within the same period (*Neuropsychologia, Cortex,* and *Brain and Language*).

Let me now turn to a consideration of some of the advances in certain specific aspects of the specialization of the hemispheres.

## The Right Hemisphere

One of the most striking changes in the last 25 years has been in the increased awareness of the importance of the human right cerebral hemisphere. Classical doctrine had given it little importance for the higher functions. Not only was language placed in the left hemisphere but the discovery of the Gerstmann syndrome with its localization in the left temporo-parieto-occipital junction had apparently also given the left hemisphere predominance in other nonlinguistic areas, such as right-left discrimination, awareness of body parts, and calculations. The general belief that constructional disorder followed left hemisphere lesions made this half of the brain apparently dominant for spatial functions. The right hemisphere in classical doctrine had had three roles in the higher functions: (a) it was the site of speech in left-handers, (b) it could take over the function of speech after damage to the left hemisphere in children and in some adults, and (c) denial or unconcern was more common after left than right hemiplegia, as had been pointed out by Babinski.

The new knowledge upset the conventional teachings in many ways. Studies by Goodglass and Quadfasel, Zangwill, Hécaen, Luria, and the Glonings asserted that persistent serious aphasia in left-handers was, in fact, more common after left-sided than after right-sided lesions. However, it was not simply that the left-hander much more frequently had speech on the left than had been thought. The work of the Glonings strongly suggested that the left-hander is likely to become aphasic with lesions on either side, although he recovers better on the average from right-sided lesions. This is in striking contrast to right-handers, who almost never become aphasic from right-sided lesions. It was realized that the study of left-handers was complicated by the necessity to distinguish between "normal" and "pathological" left-handers, the latter group consisting of those who had shifted handedness as a result of early brain lesions, and who may make up a significant proportion of those operated for epilepsy. Hécaen's work called attention to a further distinction, that between those sinistrals with and without a family history of left-handedness, who appear to differ in their response to brain lesions. Furthermore, the problem of the definition of handedness has become a major one. There are still no universally accepted criteria for right- or left-handedness.

Studies of right parietal lesions led to striking findings by many of those cited as well as Milner, Bender, Denny-Brown, Benton, DeRenzi, and others. Constructional difficulty was, in fact, more frequent and more intense after right lesions than after left lesions. Right-sided lesions led to difficulties in a whole set of nonverbal perceptual functions, including those involving musical capacities, visual form, color, and stereoscopic vision. Neglect of one-half of space and unconcern or denial of hemiplegia were clearly more common with right-sided lesions. The list of right-sided talents has not been exhausted and some evidence such as that offered by Gainotti and Galin even suggests that the emotional responses of the two hemispheres differ, with right-sided lesions leading to a kind of personality change that had been classically associated with bilateral frontal disease.

There had even been a tendency, perhaps, to overstress some aspects of right hemisphere disorder. Thus some authors tend to consider right hemisphere lesions as being responsible for all spatial disorders, neglecting the frequent occurrence of constructional difficulties and spatial difficulties with left lesions. Some authors had strongly attacked the idea that the Gerstmann syndrome (acalculia, finger agnosia, right-left difficulty, and agraphia) had any special association with left parietal lesions, but others continued to advance evidence to defend the older view. Some authors had tried to ascribe prosopagnosia (facial recognition difficulty) to right hemisphere illness, but post-mortem findings had shown bilateral lesions in all cases.

In the last 15 years there has been renewed interest in the classical question as to the participation of the right hemisphere in recovery from lesions in the language areas of the left hemisphere. Of particular interest was the observation by such investigators as Landsdell and Milner that the use of the right hemisphere for language could interfere with the usual functions of that half of the brain. Thus the child who had developed right hemisphere speech as a result of an early lesion in the left hemisphere was likely to show impairment in the kinds of spatial and perceptual functions in which the right hemisphere normally plays a major role.

A particularly interesting study of right hemisphere language was presented by Smith. The patient was a man in his late 40s on whom Burklund had performed a complete left hemispherectomy for a glioblastoma. Although the patient was right-hemiplegic and aphasic, he was not totally mute nor totally lacking in comprehension, and the case represents an intriguing study of the linguistic capacities of the "minor" hemisphere.

## Denial Syndromes and Inattention

The rise in interest in right hemisphere disease led to a renewal of concern with denial of illness, so prominent a feature of the acute left hemiplegia. Although early in this period overwhelming emphasis had been placed on the right parietal lesion, Weinstein and Kahn called attention to the high frequency of denial in patients without right focal lesions but who are suffering from impairments in alertness or orientation. The greater prevalence of denial, however, in right than left focal lesions, still led many to argue for a special right hemisphere role in these syndromes.

Animal work raised the possibility that the tendency to attribute all sensory inattention to parietal lesions was perhaps too limited. Welch and Stuteville confirmed Kennard's older observation of inattention from unilateral frontal lesions in monkeys, and clinical evidence in man was also forthcoming. Experiments in animals showed unilateral inattention after unilateral hypothalamic lesions, whereas Heilman and Watson demonstrated the same phenomenon with unilateral cingulate lesions. These findings, combined with Flynn's studies of the effects on sensory fields of hypothalamic stimulation, have opened a new area of study of the interaction between limbic mechanisms and sensory attention that should have important effects on future investigations.

## Cerebral Dominance

In the preceding sections of this chapter some aspects of cerebral dominance were discussed. One of the important advances during this period was the development of techniques for studying dominance in a more direct fashion. Wada devised a widely used technique, the injection of sodium amytal into one carotid artery to determine cerebral dominance for speech. Bogen and Gordon recently applied this method to demonstrate the probable dominance of the right hemisphere for singing.

The technique of dichotic listening, adapted from the studies of Broadbent by Doreen Kimura, has proved to be of great value in her hands and in studies done by others. In its simplest form, the method consists of simultaneous presentation of different words to the two ears of the subject, who is asked to identify the words. Typically he shows greater accuracy in specifying the stimulus presented to the right ear. The introduction of this method has led to the steady development of an increasingly complex methodology which promises to continue to be productive.

Other techniques have also been devised for studying separate stimuli presented to the two hemispheres in modalities other than the auditory. The studies of Efron on the timing of simultaneous events by the two hemispheres represent another ingenious method that has not yet been adequately exploited. The study of changes in specific areas of intellectual functioning after unilateral electric shock is another technique that has given some interesting results. It has been found that verbal memory impairment is greater after ECT when both electrodes are placed over the left scalp than when the electrodes are placed on both sides in the conventional manner. Placement of both electrodes on the right side produces the least verbal memory disorder. Some authors claim that right-sided placement of both electrodes is also more effective in treating depression than is left-sided placement.

Whereas routine techniques of electroencephalography have made some contribution to the study of dominance, a very important new field has been opened by the application of evoked potential techniques to these problems. Grey Walter's studies of the conditioned negative variation, although not directed to the problem of dominance, were a major impetus to further work. McAdams and Whitaker claimed to find large potentials over Broca's area before speech production, whereas Morrell reported similar findings over posterior speech regions in response to words. Although this technique is still in its infancy, the possibilities for its future contributions seem almost unlimited.

Another avenue has been opened through the studies of anatomical asymmetries of the hemispheres. The generally prevailing view well into the 1960s was that anatomical asymmetries of the hemispheres were either absent or so limited in extent as not to be responsible for the dramatic functional asymmetries. However, following up the earlier studies of Pfeifer, Geschwind, and Levitsky showed the presence in adult brains of very large right-left asymmetries in the planum temporale (i.e., that area of the upper surface of the temporal lobe that lies behind Heschl's gyrus). The left planum temporale is part of the classical Wernicke's area, i.e., a region known to be of importance in speech. These results have been confirmed in three other series, those of Wada, Teszner, and Witelson and Pallie. Wada also showed that these asymmetries were present in the brain of newborns and fetuses. They are not, therefore, the result of postnatal environmental effects. The arteriographic study of LeMay and Culebras added further information. Their studies appear to confirm the old observation of Cunningham that the Sylvian fissure is angled upward more sharply on the right than on the left. They claimed to find the same asymmetry in the endocranial cast of the LaChapelle aux Saints skull, which is perhaps 30,000 years old. In addition, they showed that the left parietal operculum was better developed than the right. These studies, as well as others showing pneumoencephalographic differences on the two sides, promise to be useful in correlating structure with function in life. The new computerized radiological scanning techniques may well make possible extensive study of asymmetries by noninvasive methods in the living human.

## Callosal Syndromes

Perhaps in no other area had the striking neglect of older work been so obvious than in that of callosal syndromes. The important results of Dejerine and particularly of Liepmann were almost totally neglected 25 years ago. The few cases in which callosal disconnection signs had been shown after surgery of the splenium, such as those of Trescher and Ford in 1937 and Maspes in 1948, received as little attention.

Myers and Sperry called attention early in the period under discussion to the occurrence of callosal disconnection syndromes in animals. Geschwind and Kaplan presented in 1961 a case of callosal disconnection, confirmed by postmortem findings. The following year Gazzaniga, Bogen, and Sperry studied their first case of surgical separation of the commissures for intractable epilepsy and also found signs of hemispheric disconnection. Studies on patients with callosal lesions had a special importance and constituted one of the most striking features of this period. They provided a wealth of observations on the functions of the hemispheres and thereby contributed to ideas on dominance. They also opened up a new concern for both motor and sensory pathways, the relationships of which were to the ipsilateral rather than the contralateral side of the body. Probably no other area of study was more intriguing to those philosophers of science concerned with consciousness, volition, and the unity of man.

One other effect of these studies deserves emphasis. They were probably more effective than any other stimulus in again arousing interest in the anatomical connectivity of the cortex as an essential link in the attempt to explain behavior in relationship to the brain. Indeed, this period saw not only an increased volume of work on the cortical connections by such major contributors as Kuypers, Pandya and Van Hoesen, Jones and Powell, and Nauta, but also a renewed interest in these studies by other investigators who were not themselves anatomists. There was renewed concern with the interpretation of many clinical syndromes based on involvement of corticocortical connections.

Like most important advances, the study of callosal patients has opened up a tremendous number of questions. For example, the field of the apraxias (i.e., failure to carry out learned movements correctly despite intact comprehension and absence of elementary motor or sensory disorder) long neglected by most neurologists, has received a considerable impetus. Liepmann's old idea of cerebral dominance for learned movement has been revived with many additions. The study of pure alexia without agraphia, in which lesions of the splenium are usually present has similarly raised important questions about the mode of handling of different types of visual stimuli by the brain.

At the beginning of this period, callosal syndromes and lesions were regarded as rare, even by the few who were aware of the older literature on their existence. It came to be appreciated, however, that callosal lesions are very common. Destruction of any part of the cerebral cortex which gives rise to callosal fibers is as much a commissural lesion as is damage to the same fibers in the midpoint of their course. The facial apraxia that so commonly accompanies Broca's aphasia, is perhaps the most common of all callosal syndromes. It seems probable that although some of these callosal syndromes from cortical lesions have been recognized many others await discovery.

## Aphasia and the Biological Bases of Language

Classically, of course, aphasia was the most intensively studied disorder of the higher functions in man. But in the year 1947 it would have been difficult to find many studies being undertaken in the United States that were primarily concerned with brain mechanisms of language. Luria, Conrad, and Russell had studied penetrating brain wounds producing aphasia during World War II in the Soviet Union, Germany, and England. Penfield and Roberts published in the late 1950s their studies of stimulation of the brain, which added considerably to our knowledge of the cerebral organization of language. Following up Brickner's earlier work, they had confirmed the participation of the supplementary motor cortex in certain language activities. The very fact of the occurrence of aphasias from this region, described by such authors as Alajouanine and Petit-Dutaillis, and in this country by Rubens, introduced a new element in the physiology of language the significance of which has not yet been fully explored. Another important contribution was the demonstration by such authors as Ciemens that aphasias may follow lesions of the left pulvinar. These aphasias, like those of the supplementary motor areas, are transient, but the importance of these regions remains unclear, although perhaps they have great significance in the early acquisition of language.

Penfield's work called attention to ictal aphasias, and these were also studied by others. A fascinating area was opened up by the discovery of forms of epilepsy precipitated by language stimuli. Bickford described reading epilepsy, in which nonlinguistic visual stimuli are not epileptogenic, but other more unusual forms of language-induced epilepsy were described. Thus Asbury and Prensky described graphogenic epilepsy. Epilepsy induced by the patient's own speech was described by Geschwind and Sherwin. Forster described a patient whose seizures were induced only by the voice of one particular radio announcer.

The increasing interest in the anatomical bases of the aphasias affected relationships with other disciplines. Thus, several investigators have shown great interest in the differing linguistic disorders of aphasia depending on the site of the lesion. One might also mention the names of Luria, Jakobson, Hécaen, Goodglass, Howes, Lecours, Lhermitte, and Vignolo who, among many others, have studied these problems. At the beginning of the period, the simple "expressive-receptive" dichotomy which had come to dominate descriptions of aphasia in the period between the two wars, was still the most widely used linguistic classification. By the end of that period, increasing stress was being placed on the fluency or nonfluency of the aphasic utterances, on the details of preservation or loss of grammatical structure, and on the nature of the semantic errors.

During this period there was also an increased interest in the clinical picture of aphasia in relation to the underlying lesion with a corresponding increase in the publication of well-described cases, careful anatomical studies, and new approaches to interpretation. Many syndromes that had long been regarded as rare, or whose existence had been denied, began to be recognized more frequently, e.g., isolated word-deafness, the isolated alexias, and conduction aphasia. Interest in the isolated agraphias, which had long been one of the most difficult points of classical theory, was revived. Hécaen pointed out the increased frequency of pure agraphia in left-handers, while Chédru and Geschwind stressed the curious occurrence of isolated or nearly isolated difficulties of writing in confusional states. The occurrence of aphasia with left unilateral lesions in deaf-mute patients was pointed out again by such authors as Tureen and Douglas. The studies of Weinstein and co-workers had called attention to disorders of speech that appeared in patients with metabolic disorders or with head injury or raised intracranial pressure. It seemed possible that some of these required a different interpretation from the disorders occurring after lesions in the classical speech regions.

The anatomical investigations of the aphasias were advanced not only by a renewed interest in post-mortem studies but also by the application of *in vivo* methods. Hence, Benson and others studied the relationship of clinical picture to radioisotope scan localization. The advent of computerized radiological scanning techniques makes it likely that studies in life will multiply rapidly.

The increasing interest in language as a biological phenomenon aroused new interest in the evolutionary changes in the brain that might have accounted for the emergence of language. Especially challenging were the demonstrations by the Gardners and by Premack that chimpanzees apparently have linguistic abilities. These studies provide hope that certain experimental studies not possible in man may be carried out in animals.

## Dominance Effects in Memory

The advances in the study of memory mechanisms in the brain have been reviewed elsewhere in this volume. I will therefore confine this discussion to dominance effects in memory.

It has been recognized for some time that severe permanent memory disorders require lesions in both hemispheres, e.g., the bilateral medial temporal removals described by Scoville and Milner. However, evidence has appeared showing that specific memory disorders may occur after unilateral lesions. Thus, the studies of Meyer and Yates and of Milner and her co-workers have shown that in epileptic patients undergoing temporal lobe surgery those who have been subject to left-sided excisions usually show an impairment in verbal memory, whereas those undergoing right-sided excision show greater difficulty in memory for certain nonverbal stimuli, e.g., visual patterns. Geschwind and Fusillo described a patient who for several months manifested a severe memory disorder which eventually, however, disappeared almost entirely. At post-mortem examination, the brain showed a left medial temporal infarction. Similar clinical and pathological findings have been reported in later cases. These results combined with those of Milner suggest that the dominance effects in memory may be quite marked in normals, but that after unilateral damage a considerable but incomplete degree of compensation takes place.

## References

Because of necessary editorial limitations on the number of references, it is impossible to document fully the work of all those who have contributed to the resurgence of the neurological study of language and dominance. The bibliography that was chosen therefore consists primarily of review articles, monographs, and multiauthor reference works. The journals *Neuropsychologia* and

*Cortex* have for several years presented articles that deal with nearly all aspects of this field, many of which contain extensive bibliographies of earlier work.

Critchley, Macdonald (1953): *The Parietal Lobes.* Edward Arnold, London.

Dimond, S. J., and Beaumont, J. G., editors (1974): *Hemisphere Function in the Human Brain,* London.

Ettlinger, G., editor (1965): *Functions of the Corpus Callosum* (Ciba Foundation Study Group No. 20). Little, Brown, Boston.

Gazzaniga, M. S. (1970): *The Bisected Brain.* Appleton, New York.

Geschwind, N. (1974): *Selected Papers on Language and the Brain.* Reidel, Dordrecht and Boston.

Gloning, I., Gloning, K., and Hoff, H. (1968): *Neuropsychological Symptoms and Syndromes in Lesions of the Occipital Lobe and the Adjacent Areas.* Gauthier-Villars, Paris.

Goodglass, H., and Blumstein, S., editors. (1973): *Psycholinguistics and Aphasia.* Johns Hopkins Press, Baltimore.

Hécaen, H., editor. (1972): *Neuropsychologie de la Perception Visuelle.* Masson, Paris.

Hécaen, H., and Ajuriaguerra, J. de (1964): *Left-Handedness: Manual Superiority and Cerebral Dominance.* Grune & Stratton, New York and London.

Luria, A. R. (1970): *Traumatic Aphasia.* Mouton, The Hague and Paris.

Milner, B. (1973): Hemispheric specialization: Scope and limits. In: *The Neurosciences: Third Study Program,* edited by F. O. Schmitt and F. G. Worden, pp. 75–89. MIT Press, Cambridge, Mass.

Penfield, W., and Roberts, L. (1959): *Speech and Brain-Mechanisms.* Princeton University Press, Princeton, N.J.

Stein, D. G., Rosen, J. F., and Butters, N., editors. (1974): *Plasticity and Recovery of Function in the Central Nervous System.* Academic Press, New York.

Vinken, P. J., Bruyn, G. W., Critchley, M., and Frederiks, J. A. M., editors. (1969): *Handbook of Clinical Neurology, Vol. 3: Disorders of Higher Nervous Activity.* North-Holland Publ. Corp., Amsterdam.

Vinken, P. J., and Bruyn, G. W., Critchley, M., and Frederiks, J. A. M., editors. (1969): *Handbook of Clinical Neurology, Vol. 4: Disorders of Speech, Perception and Symbolic Behavior.* North-Holland Publ. Corp. Amsterdam.

Warren, J. M., and Akert, K., editors. (1964): *The Frontal Granular Cortex and Behavior.* McGraw-Hill, New York.

Weinstein, E. A., and Kahn, R. L. (1955): *Denial of Illness.* Charles C Thomas, Springfield, Ill.

Zangwill, O. L. (1960): *Cerebral Dominance and its Relation to Psychological Function.* Oliver & Boyd, Edinburgh and London.

# CHAPTER 9

# The Neural Basis of Language

*Antonio R. Damasio and Norman Geschwind*

## Introduction

Until the middle of the 1960s, the understanding of the anatomical basis of language in humans had grown on the strength of a handful of methods. The oldest and admittedly the most fruitful of them was the neuropathological study of focal cerebral lesions in patients with aphasia. A closely related method was the behavioral study of patients who had undergone surgical interventions, such as the ablation of a cerebral lobe or even an entire hemisphere. Other approaches were provided by (a) the electrical stimulation of the human cerebral cortex, in awake patients during surgical interventions, aimed at studying the effect of stimulation on language behaviors; (b) the use of established neuroradiological techniques, such as cerebral angiography and pneumoencephalography, for indirect localization of lesions related to language disturbance; and (c) the study of language behavior after transient hemispheric inactivation caused by a barbiturate injected into the carotid artery of one side (the Wada Test). Unquestionably, the advances brought about by the combination of those methods were remarkable. For instance, from about the middle of the nineteenth century and for a period of nearly 100 years, neurologists collected a large number of single case studies in which distinctive disturbances of the use of language were correlated with specifically located lesions found at autopsy. The analyses, however, went beyond mere correlation since investigators used the growing knowledge of the connectional patterns of the brain to develop flow-diagrams for various activities within and between hemispheres. The neuropathological substrate of many syndromes of aphasia and of such associated disturbances as pure alexia and the apraxias were described during that period, and the syndromes of callosal lesions were recognized and interpreted in terms of hemispheric disconnection. But the

Reprinted with permission from *Annual Review of Neuroscience,* Volume 7: 127-147, © 1984, by Annual Reviews Inc.

anatomical basis of several other language syndromes could not be defined on the basis of isolated and occasionally conflictual observations, and for decades the fruitful approach of anatomo-clinical correlation came to an impasse. One problem resided with the method of behavioral analysis, the quality and comprehensiveness of which varied from author to author and from decade to decade. In the postwar period it appeared that the problem might be solved with the introduction of more standard instruments of neuropsychological assessment. But by then the availability of autopsy material had declined so much that a significant number of observations capable of accounting for case-to-case variablity could not be attained. Yet another important problem was the prevailing antilocalizationist attitude, which succeeded in reducing the impact and even suppressing the facts and ideas of the early neurology of aphasia. Meanwhile, the study of patients following neurosurgical procedures continued to confirm and amplify many of the findings of the neuropathological studies, especially in relation to cerebral dominance for language. This was true for studies of callosally sectioned patients and also for the electrical stimulation of human cerebral cortex, which lent support to the concept of cerebral dominance, confirmed the existence of cortical areas specialized in language processing, and revealed the existence of additional cortical areas, e.g. supplementary motor area, involved in the process of language production. But the impasse was only broken in the past 15 years, during which the understanding of the anatomical basis of language has developed dramatically. The change can be traced to the following factors: (a) a gradual reversal in the attitude toward cerebral localization spearheaded by a reappraisal of the work of the classic aphasiologists and by the availability of a systematized theory on the anatomical basis of complex behavior (cf Geschwind 1965), (b) the development of relatively standard instruments of neuropsychological assessment, (c) the introduction of powerful new methods of radiological cerebral imaging, and (d) the study of cerebral asymmetries in man and in animals.

The panorama had begun to change by the late 1960s as a result of the introduction of radioisotope scanning, and it changed dramatically with the introduction, in 1973, of computerized tomography (CT). By the late 1970s the first studies of large series of brain-damaged patients with language disturbances began to be published. Current developments in other techniques of neuroimaging, such as tomographic regional cerebral blood flow (SPECT), positron emission tomography (PET), and nuclear magnetic resonance (NMR), together with more refined CT technology, hold promise for the continuation of anatomical studies in humans with neurological disease.

Also by the late 1960s, the first statistically confirmed findings of cerebral asymmetries in humans led to the discovery that specific cerebral areas, clearly related to language, were often larger in the dominant hemisphere. In recent years the presence of asymmetries has been repeatedly confirmed, for a variety of language-related cerebral structures, using diverse methods, and cerebral asymmetries have now been studied in animals as well, paving the way for animal models of cerebral dominance. This review concentrates on the advances brought about by the introduction of the new radiological methods and by the systematic study of cerebral asymmetry.

## Radioisotope Correlates of the Aphasias

Radioisotope brain scanning is an unsatisfactory technique for cerebral localization. Nonetheless, in the days prior to the advent of CT, radioisotope scans allowed relatively reliable localization of lesions in relation to the major quadrants of a hemisphere and also permitted the first indirect anatomical studies of large series of patients evaluated with standardized behavioral methods. Two studies using this method provided important information.

An association between the different linguistic characteristics of aphasic speech and the localization of the lesions had been suggested by several of the early writers on aphasia. Benson (1967) clarified that relationship in a study of 100 aphasic patients who were evaluated with radioisotope scans and with a rating scale for ten features of aphasic speech. The features were rate of speech, prosody, pronunciation, phrase length, effort, pauses, press of speech, perseveration, word use, paraphasia. The pattern of these features in the different aphasic syndromes was such that they formed two distinct clusters in the majority of patients. The patients belonging to one of these clusters had almost without exception lesions located anteriorly to the central sulcus. The patients belonging to the other cluster had lesions located posterior to the central sulcus. The speech of the anterior group was characterized by a low rate of verbal output, dysprosody, dysarthria, effort—in short, nonfluent speech. The other group with posterior lesions had normal or higher than normal verbal output, normal prosody and articulation, effortless and syntactically well-organized speech—in short, fluent speech, which was also abnormal because of incorrect choice of content words. Thus, this study helped to confirm the belief suggested by the descriptions of Wernicke himself, that linguistically different aphasic syndromes are strongly associated with remarkably different lesions within the dominant hemisphere.

The study by Kertesz et al (1977) attempted to identify the radioisotope correlates of the principal aphasia syndromes. In spite of a certain amount of overlapping of lesions due to the technical limitations of the method, the prevalent loci of Broca's aphasia, Wernicke's aphasia, and conduction aphasia (to be described below) were clearly distinguishable. Less consistent correlations were obtained for the transcortical aphasias.

## Computerized Tomography Correlates of the Aphasias

The era of computerized tomography (CT) began in 1973 and the first major studies on the aphasias began to appear in 1977. The technique is noninvasive and the results highly consistent. In vascular lesions, the best type of specimen for anatomical correlation, the images become remarkably stable within three to four weeks after onset and permit a detailed morphological study. Although CT cannot provide many of the fine macroscopic details of a postmortem examination and none of the microscopic ones, it permits inferences about anatomical structures that were, until now, only obtainable with autopsy. Thus, our concepts of the more frequent lesions associated with the aphasias have been sharpened. In addition, the anatomical bases of some previously unrecognized syndromes of aphasia have been described as well as alternative anatomical loci for some classical syndromes. Currently available information permits a fairly comprehensive mapping of different left hemisphere structures involved in the processes of speech and language. We discuss the progress made in the past four years in relation to each specific entity.

### Wernicke's Aphasia

In Wernicke's aphasia the salient distinguishing features are fluently aphasic speech of the type described above, poor repetition, and a significant auditory comprehension deficit. According to CT data, most patients with Wernicke's aphasia resulting from cerebrovascular disease have lesions that involve Wernicke's area (Brodmann's area 22, lying in the posterior aspect of the left superior temporal gyrus) to a greater or lesser extent. The only exception to this rule, in this as well as any other aphasia syndrome, are right-handed patients with inverted dominance ("crossed aphasia") and a minority of left-handed or ambidextrous patients. The primary left auditory cortex (areas 41, 42) is not involved necessarily (see Figure 1). The extent of the lesion is variable and parallels the presence or absence of associated linguistic disturbances (alexia, agraphia) and nonlinguistic disturbances (constructional apraxia, acalculia), as well as the severity of the auditory comprehension and speech defects. Not uncommonly the lesion extends into the parietal lobe, especially into the angular gyrus, Brodmann's area 39, and into the postero-inferior temporal lobe, the second and third temporal gyri in which areas 21, 20, and 37 are located (Damasio 1981). In patients with vascular lesions, CT suggests that the lesions of Wernicke's aphasia are the result of infarction or hemorrhage in the territory of posterior temporal branches of the middle cerebral artery; the angular gyrus artery may be involved as well. Occasionally, the lesions may be exclusively subcortical and may act by disrupting input and output of an otherwise intact auditory association cortex. The remarkable consistency of the anatomical findings in patients with the clinical syndrome of Wernicke's aphasia cannot be overemphasized. It lends support to the concept of Wernicke's area as a crucial processing center for language.

### Broca's Aphasia

In Broca's aphasia the salient features are nonfluent aphasic speech with poor repetition but with considerable preservation of auditory comprehension. Controversy regarding the anatomical correlates of Broca's aphasia has repeatedly

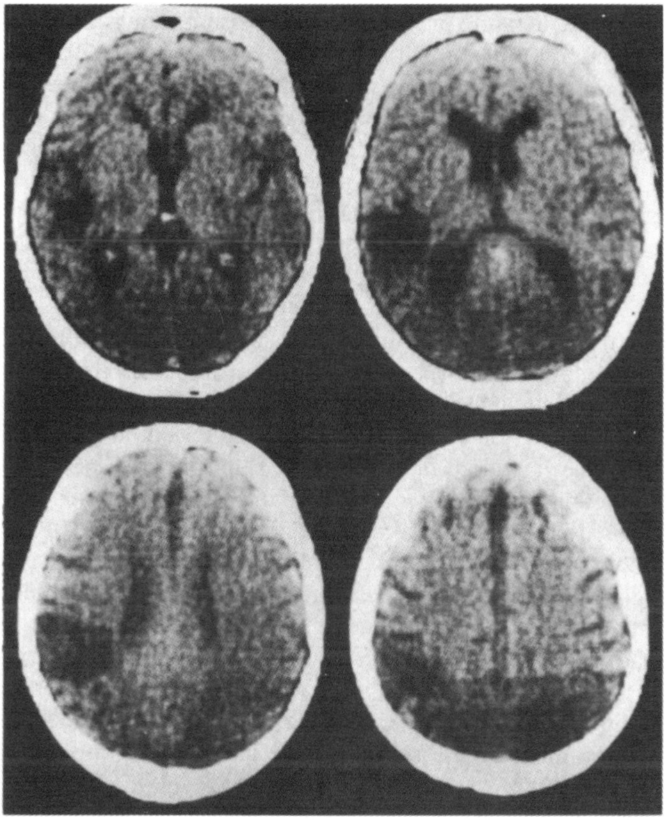

FIGURE 1. CT of a patient with Wernicke's aphasia. The photos show a low density image in the left temporo-parietal region, involving Wernicke's area. The lesion was caused by a nonhemorrhagic infarction.

been found in the literature on the anatomical bases of the aphasias. It formed the basis for the confrontation between Pierre Marie and Jules Dejerine in their renowned discussions at the Société de Medicine. It has been fueled by occasional descriptions of cases of Broca's aphasia in which it was reported that no lesion in Broca's area could be found, and by cases of lesions in Broca's area in patients who failed to show the typical clinical picture of Broca's aphasia. Curiously, this type of controversy has been much less common in relation to Wernicke's aphasia, and even the issues regarding conduction aphasia or the transcortical aphasias have been of a less conflicting nature. CT has now helped clarify the issue.

CT was crucial in finally revealing the limits of the lesion in Broca's original case, Leborgne, one of the bones of contention in the debate between Marie and Dejerine. The brain of that patient had never been cut but had been preserved as a museum specimen. Broca's description of the lesion had been made from inspection of the lateral surface of its left hemisphere. He emphasized the damage to the third left frontal gyrus, an area which he proposed as the seat of the faculty of articulate language. Marie disagreed, contending that the lesion most probably involved not only the third frontal gyrus but also the insula and basal ganglia, as well as Wernicke's area itself. In turn, Dejerine was convinced that the lesion spared both Wernicke's area and the basal ganglia region. Recently CT cuts of the Leborgne brain were obtained, in the horizontal level of Dejerine's classical cerebral sections. The results show that the truth lies in between. The lesion did spare Wernicke's area, as Broca and Dejerine claimed. But the involvement of the basal ganglia and insular cortex was massive (Castaigne et al 1980).

CT scan findings were also crucial in the study of Mohr and associates, who reviewed autopsy records of the Massachusetts General Hospital (Mohr 1976). Mohr concluded that infarction confined to the inferior frontal gyrus causes a brief period of mutism, which is later replaced by effortful speech, but that it does not cause a significant linguistic defect. On the other hand, he noted that a more severe syndrome characterized by persistent mutism, verbal stereotypes, and agrammatism is associated with a considerably larger infarct involving most of the frontal operculum and insula. Findings from four other studies (those of Naeser & Hayward, 1978; Kertesz et al, 1979; Damasio et al, 1979; and Damasio, 1981) support to a great extent Mohr's contention. Lesions confined to the midfrontal convolution and to the nearby motor area rarely produce the typical picture of persistent Broca's aphasia. More extensive lesions involving adjoining regions of the premotor cortex and of the orbital aspects of the frontal operculum commonly produce typical Broca's aphasia. Extensive lesions of the frontal operculum extending into the insula and into the basal ganglia are associated with severe language and motor deficits of the type described by Broca in his original case. On occasion, such lesions cause at first what amounts to a global aphasia, which may in time turn into a Broca-like aphasia (see Figure 2 for an example). At any rate, current CT evidence confirms the notion that Broca's aphasia is related to damage of the anterior language zone, and that it is not, as Marie and others would have it, the result of a combination of lesions in Wernicke's area and in the motor system. Past controversy clearly stems from the fact that the anatomo-clinical correlation in this syndrome is not as consistent as in Wernicke's aphasia, in itself an interesting issue quite worthy of further inquiry.

## Conduction Aphasia

Conduction aphasia resembles Wernicke's aphasia in the presence of mostly fluent abnormal speech and poor repetition, but relatively well-preserved auditory comprehension. The controversy surrounding conduction aphasia had to do with the distinctiveness of the entity that had been all but ignored in some classification systems. The entity was revived by Konorski et al (1961) and Geschwind (1965), who noted its importance for the understanding of the physiopathology of the aphasias. But although the syndrome became accepted, the matter of

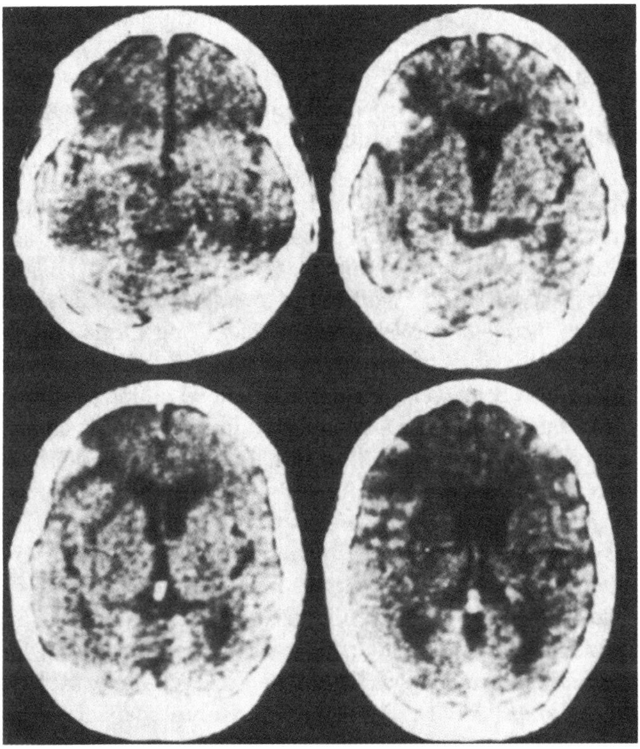

FIGURE 2. CT of a patient with Broca's aphasia. The photos show a high density image in the lower aspect of the left frontal operculum. The lesion was a nonhemorrhagic infarction and the high density quality was the result of "gray matter enhancement." Such a phenomenon is noted during the period of natural repair of a lesion when iodine contrast is injected intravenously prior to scanning.

whether or not it had an equally distinctive anatomical correlate rested on the study by Benson and associates (1973) in which the results of three postmortem cases were analyzed. More recently, CT scan findings from several studies, covering a large number of cases, have proved that conduction aphasia is commonly associated with an independent lesion located between the area frequently damaged in Wernicke's aphasia and the area in the frontal operculum commonly associated with Broca's aphasia and its variants. In some cases the lesion sits exclusively in the lower parietal region (the supramarginal gyrus also known as Brodmann's field 40), involving the underlying white matter extensively. In other cases the lesion involves a part of the auditory and insular cortices and the white matter underlying both, sparing the supramarginal gyrus. In such cases the lesion spares most of the auditory association cortex (Wernicke's area) while consistently involving the primary auditory cortex. In some instances the lesion encom-

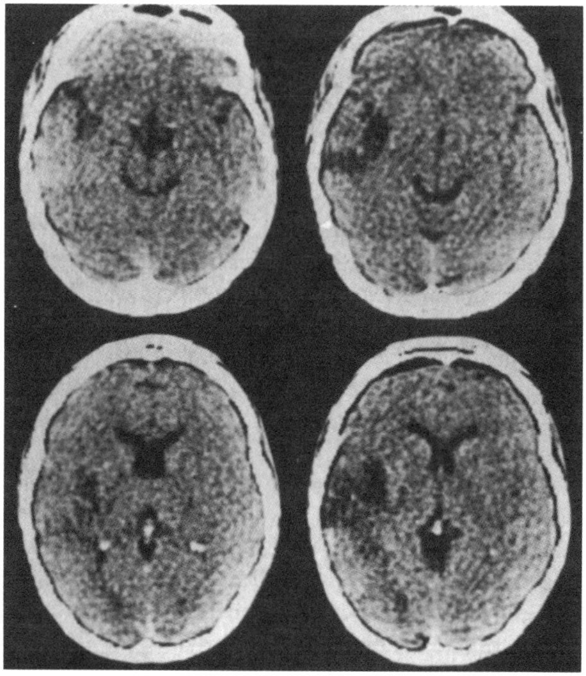

FIGURE 3. CT of a patient with conduction aphasia. The photos show a lesion involving the left primary auditory cortex and extending anteriorly into the insular region. It was caused by a nonhemorrhagic infarction.

passes all three loci: the supramarginal, auditory, and insular cortices (see Figure 3). Rarely, damage to the insular cortex and underlying white matter alone has been associated with this syndrome. Such findings, presented in studies by Naeser & Hayward (1978), Kertesz et al (1979), and Damasio & Damasio (1980), led to the inescapable conclusion that anatomically as well as behaviorally, conduction aphasia is an intermediate syndrome between Wernicke's and Broca's aphasias. The strategic placement of the lesion, with its complete or partial sparing of both Wernicke's and Broca's areas, results in remarkably preserved auditory comprehension and speech production. On the other hand, the lesion compromises structures capable of transferring auditory information into the motor system, a physiological step required for the act of repeating a verbal sentence verbatim.

## Global Aphasia

Patients with global aphasia have marked nonfluent speech, poor repetition, and poor comprehension. They have traditionally been thought to have extensive lesions involving, in contiguous fashion, all of the perisylvian territory of the left hemisphere. CT has largely confirmed that this is indeed the most common basis for that most devastating of the aphasias in which comprehension and expression of language, as well as repetition, are severely disturbed. In vascular cases, the lesion encompasses all the territories supplied by cortical branches of the middle cerebral artery and often involves the lenticulo-striate territory, too, damaging the basal ganglia and capsule. But CT has shown also that slightly different patterns can cause global aphasia. For instance, two noncontiguous lesions, one placed in Broca's area and another in Wernicke's area, can cause global aphasia with or without involvement of the underlying white matter and basal ganglia (Damasio 1981). Furthermore, the patients with basal ganglia components tend to have a more severe speech defect.

## Transcortical Motor Aphasia and Mutism

Transcortical aphasia is a curious term used to designate an aphasic disorder in which repetition is preserved. Patients with transcortical motor aphasia (TMA) have good repetition and good comprehension despite poor language output. The pathological basis of the transcortical aphasias had not been fully elucidated prior to the age of the CT scan. The original cases of transcortical aphasia had been identified clinically and related to a hypothesized anatomical basis long before the first postmortem cases became available. Traditionally, it had been accepted that lesions located anteriorly and superiorly to Broca's area could cause transcortical motor aphasia. Radioisotope scan data (Rubens 1975, Kertesz et al 1977) supported this association and extended the anatomical locus to include not only lateral frontal lesions but also mesial frontal lesions, the common anatomical denominator being that they spared Broca's area and were located in the left hemisphere. CT has changed this panorama remarkably. Most cases of true transcortical motor aphasia appear with lesions of the lateral frontal lobe that spare Broca's area totally or in part. In vascular cases damage is clearly the result of infarction in the prefrontal or vascular border zone territories (i.e. the border between the anterior and middle cerebral distributions). In a significant number of cases the lesions are exclusively subcortical, located deep in the frontal lobe, anteriorly and superiorly to the left frontal horn. Such lesions result from infarctions in the deep aspect of the border zone between the anterior and middle cerebral vascular territories. But the patients with lesions located in the mesial aspect of the frontal lobe, which involve the supplementary motor area, the cingulate gyrus, or both, do not have transcortical motor aphasia and present, rather, with a syndrome of mutism and akinesia. Although those patients share some characteristics with TMA, such as little spontaneous speech, comparatively good comprehension, and preserved repetition, their general behavior is entirely different in that they show no intent to communicate by word or gesture and have a marked disturbance of affect and emotion. In other words, their drive to communicate, not just to speak, is disturbed, while there is no conclusive evidence that their language processing is altered. In keeping with the fact that their lesions compromise the mesial limbic system cortices and not the lateral regions of neocortex, their disorder is motor and affective and not primarily linguistic.

### Transcortical Sensory Aphasia

In transcortical sensory aphasia (TSA), repetition is preserved despite poor comprehension. CT has not only shown that the most prominent lesion in Wernicke's aphasia is distinct from that in conduction aphasia but also that it is distinct from that of transcortical sensory aphasia. In TSA the lesion spares most of the auditory association cortex but involves either the nearby parietal or the nearby inferior temporal cortices, or both. Not uncommonly it involves visual association cortex, too, in the lateral aspect of the adjoining occipital lobe and in the white matter underneath (Damasio 1981). The lesions associated with transcortical sensory aphasia are generally the result of border zone infarcts, i.e. infarcts in the territory supplied by terminal branches of both the middle and posterior cerebral arteries.

CT clearly confirmed the notion that most cases of transcortical aphasia (motor or sensory) are related to lesions outside the immediate perisylvian circle. The reader is referred elsewhere for an appraisal of the physiopathologic significance of these "isolation of speech area" syndromes (Geschwind et al 1968). As for the clinical significance, it is obvious: The finding of transcortical aphasia is diagnostic of a specific cerebral location and, in vascular cases, is suggestive of a specific type of disease process.

### Atypical Aphasias

Systematic observation of CTs revealed that some syndromes of aphasia that could not be classified according to the Boston Diagnostic Aphasia Examination categories were associated with lesions that did not involve the cerebral cortex and that, instead, compromised structures of the basal ganglia and thalamus of the dominant hemisphere. Damasio et al (1982) and Naeser et al (1982) have noted that the head of the caudate, the anterior aspect of the putamen, and the anterior limb of the capsule are often involved in those aphasias. Some patients have fluent speech, others have nonfluent speech, but most have disturbed auditory comprehension and, invariably, have disturbances of articulation and right hemiparesis. It is too early to know the mechanisms that lead to these language disturbances and, in fact, whether those mechanisms are at all comparable to those which produce the cortical aphasias. It is also too early to decide whether or not more than one individual syndrome exists, or to comment on the relative severity of these aphasias in comparison with the more typical ones related to lesions involving cortical loci. Our current impression is that these are, in general, milder aphasias. Previously, Hier et al (1977) and Alexander & LoVerme (1980) had found atypical aphasias in association with hemorrhages of the basal ganglia in patients with hypertension. Those cases share some features with the ones described above but had, in addition, major disturbances of attention, which precluded a clear analysis of the linguistic deficits. Furthermore, those large hemorrhagic lesions, by virtue of their space-occupying nature, did not permit the same kind of anatomical correlation attempted in the studies by Damasio and by Naeser. Many of these reservations apply to the cases of atypical aphasias described with hemorrhages in the thalamus. A detailed anatomical localization is difficult on the basis of CT data. The clinical characteristics of those cases are highly variable, although they are generally suggestive of transcortical sensory aphasia. (Mohr et al (1975) and Cappa & Vignolo (1979) have described those clinical characteristics in detail.) A similar picture has been found recently in patients with nonhemorrhagic infarctions of the thalamus (Graff-Radford et al 1984).

## The Alexias

Some of the finest discoveries of classic aphasiology concern the anatomical underpinnings of reading disorders, the fundamentals of which were proposed by Dejerine based on the autopsy findings in two patients. One had lost the ability to read and write (acquired alexia-with-agraphia) (Dejerine 1891). The other had also lost the ability to read, but his ability to write remained intact (acquired alexia-without-agraphia, also known as "pure alexia") (Dejerine 1892). The reader is referred elsewhere for information on the physiological and clinical significance of these discoveries (Geschwind 1965). CT has confirmed beyond a shadow of a doubt that the two syndromes have markedly different pathological correlates. Alexia-with-agraphia, in its rare and pure form, is associated with lesions of the vast extent of association cortex that lies in the left parietal lobe, behind the auditory association cortex. Most commonly those lesions involve the angular gyrus or area 39 (quite often alexia and agraphia are associated with Wernicke's aphasia in patients in whom the underlying lesion extends from Wernicke's area to the angular gyrus). The syndrome of alexia-without-agraphia (pure alexia) is associated with a left occipital lobe lesion or lesions that compromise the flow of visual information from both the left visual cortex and the right visual cortex, in the direction of the left language cortex (information from the latter courses in the splenium of the corpus callosum). CT has been of help in demonstrating that more than one pattern of damage can accomplish such a complex pattern of disturbance (Damasio & Damasio 1983). For instance, patients can have an isolated lesion of the splenium of the corpus callosum interrupting leftward visual information outflow, combined with another lesion located more posteriorly in the occipital lobe and capable of disconnecting the left visual cortex from the left temporo-parietal language cortices. More commonly, patients have a continuous lesion that severs connections from both visual systems and thus cuts off both visual cortices from the left temporo-parietal region. It is interesting to note that, as might be predicted from the physiological mechanism, the lesion need not lie within the splenium of the corpus callosum itself, provided that the callosal fibers are indeed damaged in their intrahemispheric course after passing through the splenium. CT has also been crucial in clarifying the relation between pure alexia and a variety of possible accompanying manifestations, such as color "agnosia" (a condition in which the patient is unable to name colors shown to him or to identify colors given their names, but is capable of matching colors), achromatopsia (a condition in which the patient is unable to perceive color and reports the perception of shades of gray while he maintains normal form vision), and the visual agnosias. About half of all patients with pure alexia also have color "agnosia." A small percentage have achromatopsia but not color agnosia, and the remainder have alexia in the absence of either. The association between pure alexia and visual agnosia is uncommon. Its presence indicates that in addition to the left hemisphere lesion, a supplemental lesion of the right hemisphere has occurred in a fairly comparable location of the nondominant hemisphere's visual system (Damasio & Damasio 1982).

### Concluding Remarks

At a time in which autopsy studies have become much less common, the availability of accurate, in vivo, neuroimaging techniques is most welcome. When used proficiently, with an awareness of the many methodological limitations, CT has provided precious information concerning the neural basis of language. In addition to confirming cerebral localizations proposed on the basis of a handful of single case studies, CT has permitted experimental behavioral studies in relation to the lesions detected. Furthermore, it has made possible the discovery of several new, previously unsuspected, anatomo-clinical entities.

But, perhaps more importantly, by repeatedly revealing the consistency of brain/behavior correlations in aphasia, obtained in different research centers and with different technical equipment, CT has contributed to the acceptance and consolidation of a neuroanatomical way of conceptualizing behavior against which there was widespread resistance as late as a decade ago.

The introduction of PET scanning, tomographic regional cerebral blood flow (SPECT), and nuclear magnetic ressonance (NMR), all currently in their preliminary stages, will reinforce and amplify the results obtained with CT, by adding a dynamic component to the images now available.

## Anatomy of Human Cerebral Dominance

As late as the mid 1960s the standard view regarding cerebral dominance for language stated that it had no anatomical correlates, that it did not exist in other species, and that its evolution in humans could not be studied. Such a position (exemplified by Von Bonin 1962) implied the neglect or active rejection of the older anatomical studies on dominance (Pfeiffer 1936). But the discoveries of the past 15 years have proven that each of these standard views was false and have opened entirely new avenues of study. We present some data on human asymmetries as well as a brief discussion of findings in other species.

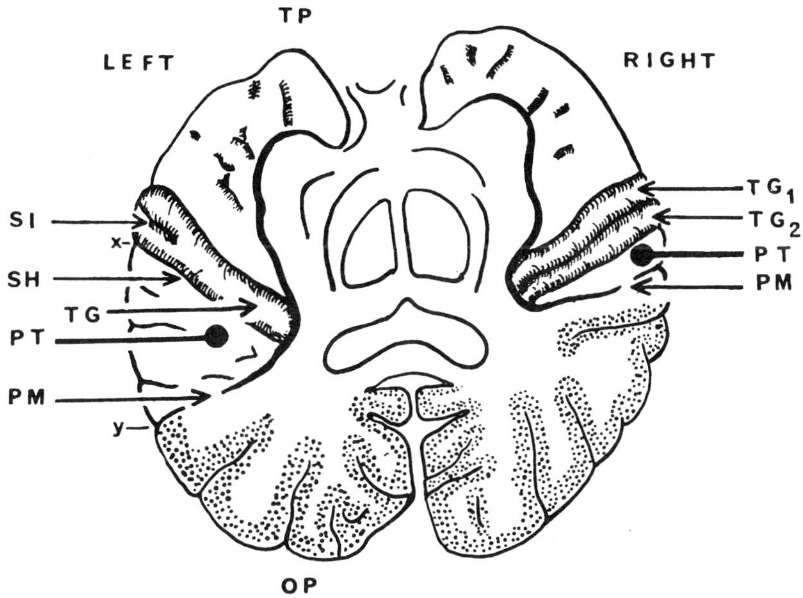


FIGURE 4. Upper surfaces of human temporal lobes exposed by a cut in the plane of the Sylvian fissure. Anatomical landmarks and typical left-right differences are shown. The posterior margin (PM) of the planum temporale (PT) slopes backward more sharply on the left than on the right, so that end y of the left Sylvian fissure lies posterior to the corresponding point on the right. The anterior margin of the planum formed by the sulcus of Heschl (SH) slopes forward more sharply on the left. In this brain there is a single transverse gyrus of Heschl (TG) on the left, but two on the right ($TG_1$, $TG_2$). TP = temporal pole; OP = occipital pole; SI = sulcus intermedius. Reproduced from Geschwind & Levitsky (1968).

Geschwind & Levitsky (1968) showed not only that anatomical asymmetry was present in the human brain but also that it was readily visible even to the naked eye. They studied the planum temporale, i.e. the area lying between the posterior margin of the first transverse gyrus of Heschl and the posterior end of the sylvian fossa, in the brains of 100 normal individuals. This area was larger on the left in 65%, larger on the right in 12%, and approximately equal in 23%—results that were highly significant statistically, and have since been replicated repeatedly. The area at issue is the portion of Wernicke's area contained within the sylvian fissure, on the upper surface of the temporal lobe. Most of Brodmann's cytoarchitectural field/22 is contained in the planum temporale (see Figure 4).

This asymmetry is present in the fetus and newborn infant (Wada et al 1975, Witelson & Pallie 1973) and appears by the thirty-first week of gestation (Chi et al 1977). The right side develops about a week earlier than the left. Galaburda et al (1978) showed that this gross asymmetry corresponded to asymmetry of the cytoarchitectonic area Tpt (in the nomenclature of Sanides). The left planum temporale is on the average one-third larger than the right planum, and is often many times as large. The magnitude of the microscopic asymmetry is even more striking. In the first brain studied, the left Tpt was more than 700% larger than the corresponding area on the right. Even when the right side is large, which Wada (1981) finds, interestingly, to be more frequent in females, it rarely attains this magnitude (see Figure 5).

Another human asymmetry described by LeMay & Culebras (1972) involves the sylvian fissures. The middle cerebral artery travels in the plane of this fissure and can be visualized by arteriography. In most people the right sylvian fissure turns up more sharply at its end than the left. This finding was of importance since it showed a marked asymmetry that could be visualized in the living human, thus creating the possibility of correlating asymmetries with functional characteristics, such as handedness. In right-handers, they found this pattern in 67%, with the reverse pattern in 8%, and fissures at equal levels in 25%. In left-handers the corresponding figures were 20%, 10%, and 70%.

Utilizing CT, LeMay (see Galaburda et al 1978) showed that in most individuals there is a wider occipital region on the left and a wider frontal region on the right, and she claimed that the distributions differed with handedness. There seems to be agreement that the left posterior region is generally wider but not that the distribution differs in left-handers (Chui & Damasio 1980). The reasons for the discrepancies are not entirely clear. In one study, one of the "normal" groups contained several patients with early brain disease, a group that might well have an anomalous pattern of asymmetry. There may also be variations in technique, e.g. different angles of the cut through the brain might give variable results. Another possibility now under investigation is that some computer programs may foreshorten the brain and thus obscure certain asymmetries. Further study is obviously needed in this area (see Figure 6).

Another of LeMay's findings replicated in the study by Chui & Damasio (1980) was that of predominant left occipital "petalia." Petalia is an anthropological term used to designate an impression in the inner table of the skull, produced by the bulging of the adjacent cerebral lobe.

## Evolution of Human Asymmetry

In many individuals, some major fissures and sulci may leave an imprint in the skull. Aware of this fact, LeMay & Culebras (1972) studied the endocranial casts of human fossils. It is apparent that in the cast of the Neanderthal man of LaChapelle-aux-Saints (dating back 30,000 to 50,000 years) the imprint of the right sylvian fissure is higher than that of the left, i.e. the same asymmetry seen in modern humans. It was also found in Peking man, probably dating back about 300,000 years. Because most of the cortical regions related to language processing lie near the sylvian fissure, these findings suggest an early evolution of language.

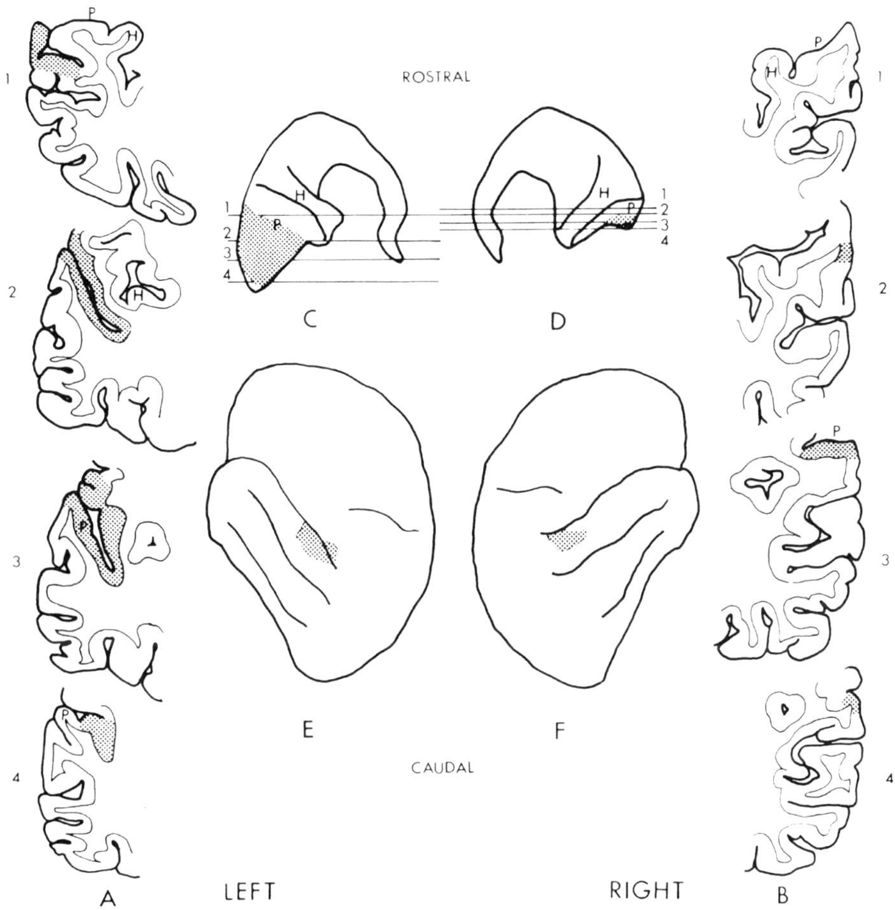


FIGURE 5. Coronal sections of a human brain are shown in A and B. The superior temporal planes are shown in C and D with planum temporale (P) and Heschl's gyrus (H). Lateral surfaces of brain show area Tpt (*shaded*) in E and F. *Arrowheads* point to Sylvian fissures. Note large planum asymmetry (C and D). Note buried temporal cortex on coronal sections (*arrows*). Reproduced from Galaburda et al (1978).

The significance of these data is increased by studies in nonhuman primates. LeMay & Geschwind (1978) found that there were patterns of asymmetry in the great apes identical to those of modern humans but that brains of rhesus monkeys showed no comparable asymmetry. Yeni-Komshian & Benson (1976) reported that in the chimpanzee the left planum temporale is typically larger than the right, as in humans. These results, showing for the first time a definite anatomical asymmetry in another mammal, raise an important question: Do the

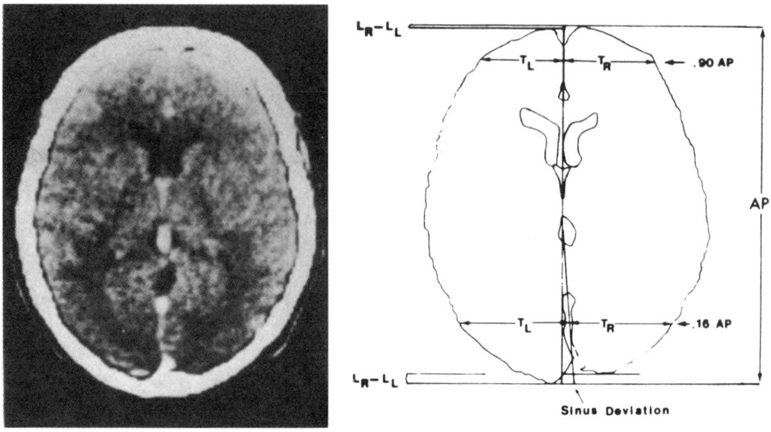


FIGURE 6. CT of a normal male with left occipital petalia and diagram of reference points used to measure petalia and other brain asymmetries with CT. AP—antero-posterior diameter. 0.16 AP and 0.90 AP—levels at 16% and 90% of AP length (measured from most posterior point) used to determine transverse diameter. $T_L$ and $T_R$ = left and right transverse diameters of cerebrum (occipital $T_L$ and $T_R$ are determined at 0.16 AP; frontal $T_L$ and $T_R$ at 0.90). $L_L$ and $L_R$ = length of left and right hemisphere, used to determine petalia.

great apes possess language abilities, or do their perisylvian regions contain structures destined for some still unspecified function that is a forerunner of language?

### Functional Asymmetry in Other Species

Nottebohm (1970) was responsible for overturning the standard belief that functional asymmetry existed in no other species. He has shown that in several species of singing birds, although not in all, cutting the left hypoglossal nerve will almost entirely abolish song, while cutting the right hypoglossal nerve will cause only minor alterations of song production. If the left nerve is cut in early life, compensation takes place and singing will occur in adult life. Since bird song (only present in males) is related to sex, the nucleus HVc, which contains testosterone receptors, is larger in males. It is of interest that there is no significant side asymmetry in this nucleus; this suggests that some forms of cerebral dominance might be based on biochemical differences. The hypoglossal nucleus is, however, significantly larger on the left side, which perhaps is important in determining asymmetrical function within the central nervous system.

Many examples of functional or anatomical asymmetry have been found in other species. We believe that both anatomical and functional asymmetry extend well back in the phylogenetic scale and that they are standard features of the animal world.

The most extensive experiments on functional asymmetry in a nonhuman mammalian species are those of Denenberg (1981) and his colleagues. He found that in the laboratory rat, lesions of the right or left hemispheres can have different effects. These studies provide evidence for right hemisphere advantage for spatial and emotional functions, a finding of special interest since the human right hemisphere has similar advantages for precisely the same functions. Studies on functional asymmetry in other species are summarized by Denenberg (1981), to which we refer the reader.

Anatomical asymmetry is not confined to primates. Diamond et al (1981) has shown greater cortical thickness in parts of the right posterior hemisphere in the rat and A. M. Galaburda (unpublished observations) has found larger cytoarchitectonic areas on the right side in the rat. Wada & Kolb have also found right-sided asymmetry in other species.

There are thus both anatomical and functional findings in other mammals that suggest the existence of right hemisphere dominance. Interestingly, in humans, right hemisphere dominance appears to be more consistent than language dominance. Thus, some adults develop crossed aphasias, i.e. aphasia with right hemisphere lesions. But it is not common to find visuospatial defects following left posterior lesions that are as severe as those seen after right posterior lesions. (The typical right hemisphere functions thus reverse sides less often than language.) We suspect that right hemisphere dominance appeared earlier in evolution than left hemisphere dominance, which only developed to its highest levels at a later period.

Anatomical asymmetry has been known for years in submammalian species. For instance, the pineal eye of lizards is asymmetrically placed. The right habenular nucleus of the lamprey is much larger than the left (Kappers et al 1936) and there is asymmetry of the same nuclei in the frog (Kemali & Braitenberg 1969). Such subcortical asymmetries may well be the forerunners of the cortical asymmetries.

## Chemical Asymmetries in the Nervous System

After studying epileptic patients undergoing surgery, Serafetinides (1965) suggested that LSD acted primarily on the right temporal lobe, thus raising the issue of neurochemical asymmetry. The work of Glick and his co-workers (1977) has clearly documented chemical asymmetries. They found that unilateral injection of dopaminergic drugs will cause the rat to circle to one side consistently. The dopamine content of the caudate nucleus that is opposite the direction of circling is higher than the one on the other side. Circling tendencies differ in males and females, a fact of interest since human females tend to be somewhat more right-handed than males. Animals that are strongly consistent circlers learn mazes better than those who are not, presumably because they have an inborn marker for right and left. The predominance of chemical asymmetry on one side is correlated with a consistent anatomical pattern of other chemical asymmetries. Neurochemical asymmetry in the human thalamus has been found by Oke et al (1978), who have described higher norepinephrine content in the left pulvinar and right VPI. Eidelberg & Galaburda (1982) have now reported anatomical asymmetries in the human thalamus.

### Asymmetries in Human Disease

Among children with dyslexia, stuttering, autism, and other developmental disorders, all of which are predominantly seen in males, there is some evidence for an increased proportion of left-handedness or ambidexterity. Galaburda & Kemper (1979) studied the asymmetries of cellular architecture in the brain of a severe childhood dyslexic with a strong family history of dyslexia. They discovered many microscopic anomalies confined to the left hemisphere that involved, in particular, area Tpt (part of Wernicke's area). Groups of nerve cells were found in abnormal locations and normal cortical structure was disrupted. There was distinct polymicrogyria, i.e. islands of cortex in the white matter. These disturbances clearly resulted from disordered migration of neurons during development. Such left hemisphere anomalies could well have been the cause of the patient's left-handedness. A careful review of the literature suggests that similar findings had been present in other cases, although they were not specifically commented on as the cause of the learning disability. A second case now being examined by Galaburda & Kemper (1979) shows similar anomalies.

It is interesting to note that Galaburda & Kemper found that the abnormal left hemisphere was larger, not smaller, than the right hemisphere. This could have been the result of slowed neuronal migration in that hemisphere, and is comparable, in milder degree, to what is found in megalencephaly in which striking neuronal migration deficits lead to a very enlarged hemisphere. If that is the case, the study of CT asymmetries may be useful in the investigation of variants in normal populations, but may not be helpful in cases of developmental disturbance.

Another type of disease association with cerebral dominance has recently been reported. Geschwind & Behan (1982) have shown that immune diseases were two and one-half times as common in 500 strong left-handers as in 900 strong right-handers, and have advanced an experimentally testable theory regarding the neurobiological basis of the development of dominance and of its pathology.

## Concluding Remarks

For most biological traits it would be ideal to know the relevant anatomy, genetics, fetal and childhood development, evolution, physiology, chemistry, immunology, associations with other traits, and its forms in other species. This type of information has been notably lacking for the language systems even though language ranks among the most distinctive human traits. The recent neurological discoveries in cerebral dominance have opened up areas previously considered inaccessible.

Human biology and medicine always proceed more rapidly when an animal model is available, and this is now the case for cerebral dominance. Many people would still assert that we will learn little from other species that do not have language. We believe, however, that animal models will lead to experiments that will cast significant light on the evolution of language and other human functions, as well as to new approaches to the study of disordered dominance, either developmental or acquired.

## References


Alexander, M. P., Lo Verme, S. R. 1980. Aphasia after left hemispheric intracerebral hemorrhage. *Neurology* 30:1193–1202

Benson, D. F. 1967. Fluency in Aphasia: Correlation with radioactive scan localization. *Cortex* 3:373–94

Benson, D. F., Sheremata, W. A., Buchard, R., Segarra, J., Price, D., Geschwind, N. 1973. Conduction aphasia. *Arch. Neurol* 28:339–46

Cappa, S. F., Vignolo, L. A. 1979. "Transcortical" features of aphasia following left thalamic hemorrhage. *Cortex* 15:121–30

Castaigne, P. Lhermitte, F., Signoret, J. L., Abelanet, R. 1980. Description et étude scannographique du cerveau de Leborgne (la découverté de Broca). *Rev. Neurol.* 136(10):563–83

Chi, J. G., Dooling, E. C., Gilles, F. H. 1977. Gyral development of the human brain. *Ann. Neurol.* 1:86–93

Chui, H. C., Damasio, A. R. 1980. Human cerebral asymmetries evaluated by computerized tomography. *J. Neurol. Neurosurg. Psychiatry* 43:873–78

Damasio, A., Damasio, H. 1982. Cerebral localization of complex visual manifestations: Clinical and physiologic significance. *Neurology* 32(4):96

Damasio, A., Damasio, H. 1983. The anatomical basis of pure alexia and color "agnosia." *Neurology.* In press

Damasio, A., Damasio, H., Rizzo, M., Varney, N., Gersh, F. 1982. Aphasia with nonhemorrhagic lesions in the basal ganglia and internal capsule. *Arch. Neurol.* 39:15–20

Damasio, H. 1981. Cerebral localization of the aphasias. In *Acquired Aphasia,* ed M. Taylor Sarno, New York: Academic

Damasio, H., Damasio, A., Hamsher, K., Varney, N. 1979. CT scan correlates of aphasia and allied disorders. *Neurology* 29:572

Damasio, H., Damasio, A. 1980. The anatomical basis of conduction aphasia. *Brain* 103:337–50

Dejerine, J. 1891. Sur un cas de cecité verbale avec agraphie, suivi d' autopsie. *Mem. Soc. Biol.* 3:197–201

Dejerine, J. 1892. Contribution a l'étude anatomo-pathologique et clinique des differentes varietés de cecité verbale. *Mem. Soc. Biol.* 4:61–90

Denenberg, V. H. 1981. Hemispheric laterality in animals and the effects of early experience. *Behav. Brain Sci.* 4:1–49

Diamond, M. C., Dowling, G. A., Johnson, R. E. 1981. Morphologic asymmetry in male and female rats. *Exp. Neurol.* 71:261–68

Eidelberg, D., Galaburda, A. M. 1982. Symmetry and asymmetry in the human posterior thalamus. Part I: Cytoarchitectonic analysis in normal persons. *Arch. Neurol.* 39:325–32

Galaburda, A. M., Kemper, T. 1979. Cytoarchitectonic abnormalities in developmental dyslexia: A case study. *Ann. Neurol.* 6:94

Galaburda, A. M., Sanides, F., Geschwind, N. 1978. Human brain: Cytoarchitectonic left-right asymmetries in the temporal speech region. *Arch. Neurol.* 35:812–17

Geschwind, N. 1965. Disconnexion syndromes in animals and man. *Brain* 88:237–94, 585–644

Geschwind, N., Behan, P. 1982. Left-handedness: Association with immune disease, migraine, and developmental learning disorder. *Proc. Natl. Acad. Sci. USA* 79:5097–5100

Geschwind, N., Levitsky, W. 1968. Human brain: Left-right asymmetries in temporal speech region. *Science* 161:186–87

Geschwind, N., Quadfasel, P., Segarra, J. 1968. Isolation of the speech area. *Neuropsychologia* 6:327–40

Glick, S. D., Jerussi, T. P., Simmerberg, B. 1977. Behavioral and neuropharmacological correlates of nigrostriatal asymmetry in rats. In *Lateralization in the Nervous System,* ed. S. Hamad, R. W. Doty, L. Goldstein, J. Jaynes, G. Krauthamer, pp. 213–49. New York: Academic

Graff-Radford, N., Eslinger, P., Yamada, T., Damasio, A. 1984. Nonhemorrhagic infarction of the thalamus: Behavioral, anatomical and physiological correlates. *Neurology.* In press

Hier, D. B., Davis, K. R., Richardson, E. P., et al 1977. Hypertensive putaminal hemorrhage. *Dev. Neurol. Behav. Pediatr.* 1:54–57

Kappers, C. U. A., Huber, G. C., Crosby, E. C. 1936. *The Comparative Anatomy of the Nervous System of Vertebrates Including Man,* Vol. 1. New York: Macmillan

Kemali, M., Braitenberg, V. 1969. *Atlas of the Frog Brain,* Berlin/New York: Springer

Kertesz, A., Lesk, D., McCahe, P. 1977. Isotope location of infarcts in aphasia. *Arch. Neurol.* 34:590–601

Kertesz, A., Harlock, W., Coates, R. 1979. Computer tomographic localization, lesion size, and prognosis in aphasia and nonverbal impairment. *Brain Language* 8:34–50

Konorski, J., Kozniewska, H., Stepien, L. 1961. Analysis of symptoms and cerebral localization of audio-verbal aphasia. *Proc. 7th Int. Congr. Neurol.* 2:234–36

LeMay, M., Culebras, A. 1972. Human brain morphological differences in the hemispheres demonstrable by carotid angiography. *N. Engl. J. Med.* 287:168–70

LeMay, M., Geschwind, N. 1978. Asymmetries of the human cerebral hemispheres. In *Language Acquisition and Language Breakdown,* ed. A. Caramazza, E. B. Zurif, pp. 311–28. Baltimore: Johns Hopkins Univ. Press

Mohr, J. P. 1976. Broca's area and Broca's aphasia. In *Studies in Neurolinguistics,* ed. H. Whitaker, New York: Academic

Mohr, J. P., Walters, W. C., Duncan, G. W. 1975. Thalamic hemorrhage and aphasia. *Brain Language* 2:3–17

Naeser, M. A., Hayward, R. W. 1978. Lesion localization in aphasia with cranial computed tomography and the Boston diagnostic aphasia exam. *Neurology* 28(6):545–51

Naeser, M. A., Alexander, M. P., Helm-Estabrooks, N., Levine, H. L., Laughlin, S. A., Geschwind, N. 1982. Aphasia with predominantly subcortical lesion sites: Description of three capsular/putaminal aphasia syndromes. *Arch. Neurol.* 39:2–14

Nottebohm, F. 1970. Ontogeny of bird song. *Science* 167:950–56

Oke, A., Keller, R., Mefford, I., Adams, R. N. 1978. Lateralization of norepinephrine in human thalamus. *Science* 200:1411–13

Pfeiffer, R. A. 1936. Pathologie der Horstrahlung und der corticalen Horsphare. *Hand. Neurol.* 6:533–626

Rubens, A. B. 1975. Aphasia with infarction in the territory of the anterior cerebral artery. *Cortex* 11:239–50

Serafetinides, A. E. 1965. The significance of the temporal lobes and of hemispheric dominance in the production of LSD-25 symptomatology in man. *Neuropsychologia* 3:69–79

Von Bonin, G. 1962. In *Interhemispheric Relations and Cerebral Dominance*, ed. V. Mountcastle, p. 6. Baltimore: Johns Hopkins Univ. Press

Wada, J. A. 1981. Presentation at Epilepsy Int. Congr., Kyoto, Japan

Wada, J. A., Clarke, R., Hamm, A. 1975. Cerebral hemispheric asymmetry in humans. *Arch. Neurol.* 32:239–46

Witelson, S. F., Pallie, W. 1973. Left hemisphere specialization for language in the newborn: Neuroanatomical evidence of asymmetry. *Brain* 96:641–46

Yeni-Komshian, G. H., Benson, D. A. 1976. Anatomical study of cerebral asymmetry in the temporal lobe of humans, chimpanzees, and rhesus monkey. *Science* 192:387–89

# PART III

# Alexia and Apraxia

*Orrin Devinsky*

Alexia and apraxia were major interests of Norman Geschwind through his early neurological career in 1960s. His interests in aphasia alexia, and apraxia formed the nidus for his disconnection syndromes paper and for rekindling interest in relating behavior and brain structure. Both alexia and apraxia provided insights into the cortical machinery for executing specific coordinated higher functions—reading and skilled, learned movements. The role of the dominant parietal lobe in reading, writing, and praxis was further defined by these contributions, as well as the effects of disconnecting left parietal input (alexia without agraphia) or output (one form of ideomotor apraxia).

Dejerine described two patients with alexia, each exemplified a syndrome resulting from different mechanisms. The first patient (1891) had both alexia and agraphia resulting from a left angular gyrus lesion.[1] The second patient (1892) had pure alexia from a lesion disconnecting visual input to the left angular gyrus.[2] Dejerine correctly analyzed the anatomy and mechanism of these cases. In the second case, destruction of the left visual cortex caused a right hemianopsia and destruction of the splenium prevented intact visual input from the left half of space from reaching the angular gyrus, a critical processing center for reading and writing. Dejerine's 1892 description of the classic disconnection syndrome, alexia without agraphia, was lost to the English-speaking neurological community after World War I.

In 1961, Norman Geschwind first read Dejerine's papers on alexia. One week later, Edith Kaplan asked for Dr. Geschwind's input on the strange case of a 41-year-old policeman, who had a left frontal resection for a glioblastoma. Postoperatively, he developed a grasp reflex in the right but not left, hand. Kaplan was shocked to find that he wrote normally with his right hand but asphasically with his left. Dr. Geschwind's wheels were spinning with thoughts of callosal syndromes and disconnection, fresh from Dejerine's description of alexia without agraphia. The role of disconnection in producing left-hand agraphia in the policeman, and a new case of alexia without agraphia with revival of Dejerine's mechanism, were described by Geschwind and Kaplan anonymously in the New England Journal of Medicine in 1962. The case of agraphia was more extensively reported in Neurology in 1962.[3]

Geschwind rediscovered and carefully described the syndrome of alexia without agraphia in his disconnection syndrome papers[4] and subsequently described a patient, with Fusillo (reproduced here, Color-Naming Defects in Association with Alexia (1966) [5]), similar to Dejerine's both clinically and neuropathologically. This man had alexia associated with color-naming defects. In this man's brain, disconnection of visual input from the angular gyrus prevented the language cortex from receiving the data to be named. Geschwind's summary of "The Anatomy of Acquired Reading Disorders" in 1962[6] (reproduced here) provided him with the background to recognize this disconnection syndrome, and add his original observations regarding defective color naming. Geschwind later described, together with Judd and Gardner, alexia and agraphia in a composer.[7] Together with Benson, Geschwind provided an excellent review of the alexias for the *Handbook of Clinical Neurology* in 1969 (reproduced here).[8]

Apraxia, like aphasia, was lucidly identified through brilliant clinical-pathological correlations by early German neurologists. However, in post-WWI England and France, apraxia was rarely mentioned in its original forms, but instead, was incorrectly applied to a variety of other motor disorders such as constructional tasks, gait, speech, and clumsiness.[9] His review of apraxia for the *Handbook of Clinical Neuropsychology*, written with Damasio,[9] is reproduced here. In his disconnection syndromes papers[10-12] and later publications,[9,13-16] Geschwind helped non-German neurologists revisit apraxia. Geschwind emphasized that apraxias are common, especially in patients with acute dominant hemisphere frontal strokes, although considered rare by most neurologists. This is because most apraxic patients can correctly manipulate familiar objects in their environment, but fail with specific testing. In other patients, apraxia is missed because it is only present during the early stage of the disorder. Geschwind also stressed that apraxia should be used to describe disorders characterized by impairment in executing a learned movement in response to a stimulus which would normally elicit the movement in the setting of intact sensation, strength, attention, and cooperation.[9] He recognized four principal settings in which apraxia could be demonstrated:[9]

1. failure to produce a correct movement in response to a verbal command
2. failure to correctly imitate a movement performed by the examiner
3. failure to correctly perform a movement in response to seeing an object
4. failure to handle and use and object correctly.

Liepmann first used the term apraxia. Conceptually, it was a motor asymbolia (Meynert's term). Geschwind fully credited Liepmann, recognizing the brilliant analysis of Regierungsrat case, in the patient's inability to performed learned movements was explained by a series of disconnecting lesions;[17] neuropathology confirmed the predicted lesions sites.[18] Leipmann and Maas later reported apraxia from a callosal lesion.[18] Geschwind and Kaplan's subsequent description of a similar patient with apraxia from a callosal (and left frontal) lesion[10] was a major impetus behind Geschwind's "Disconnexion Syndromes in Animals and Man.[4] Geschwind critically examined Liepmann's classification and considered the limb-kinetic form—characterized by inability to make fine, precise, independent movements of the contratlateral hand—to result from corticospinal pathway (neurons or fibers) lesions; thus the limb-kinetic form was not a true apraxia.[19] Apraxia is a disorder of higher functions (learned skilled movements) resulting from lesions in association cortex or association/callosal pathways, not a primary motor disorder.

Geschwind's analysis and teaching about apraxia reveals his fundamentals of his style: (1) passion for history, even when it has been discarded; (2) looking at what others see and seeing something new; (3) appreciating the value of detailed clinical and pathological case study; (4) synthesis of observations from daily life* to novels to current science; (5) and a love of talking about his thoughts and soliciting comments and criticisms.

## References

1. Dejerine, J. Sur un Cas de Cecite Verbale avec Agraphie, Suivi d'Autopsie. Mem Soc Biolog, 1891; 3, 197-201.
2. Dejerine, J. Contribution a l'Etude Anatomo-Pathologique et Clinique des Differences Variete Verbale. Mem Soc Biolog, 1892; 4, 61-90.
3. Devinsky, O. Disconnexion Syndromes. In SC Schachter and O Devinsky (eds.) *Behavioral Neurology and the Legacy of Norman Geschwind.* New York: Lippincott-Raven Press, 1997, pp. 115-126.
4. Geschwind, N. Disconnexion Syndromes in Animals and Man, I and II. Brain, 1965; 88, 237-294(I); 585-644(II).
5. Geschwind, N, and Fusillo, M. Color-Naming Defects in Association with Alexia. Arch Neurol, 1966; 15, 137-146.
6. Geschwind, N. The Anatomy of Acquired Disorders of Reading. In J. Money (ed.), *Reading Disability*. Baltimore: Johns Hopkins Press, 1962, pp. 115-129.
7. Judd, T, Gardner, H, and Geschwind, N. Alexia Without Agraphia in a Composer. Brain, 1983; 106, 435-457.
8. Benson, DF, and Geschwind, N. The Alexias. In P.J. Vinken and G.W. Bruyn (eds.), *Handbook of Clinical Neurology.* Vol. 4. Amsterdam: North-Holland, 1969, pp. 112-140.

* He loved to cite the example of multiple motor pathways for facial expression—a volitional one arising in pyramidal pathways and a mesial/subcortical pathway arising in cingulate, supplementary motor, amygdala and subcortical sites that mediate smiling. A patient with a frontal motor cortex lesion, when asked to smile would do so quite asymmetrically but perfectly in response to a joke. In contrast, a patient with a limbic lesion might smile volitionally fairly well, but asymmetrically to a funny remark. "Only actors and politicians can fairly well reproduce a natural smile to common." (Geschwind, teaching rounds).

9. Geschwind, N, and Damasio, AR. Apraxia. In PJ Vinken, GW Brown, and HL Klawans (eds.) *Handbook of Clinical Neurology Vol. 1(45): Clinical Neuropsychology*. Amsterdam: Elsevier Science, 1985, pp. 423-432.
10. Geschwind, N, and Kaplan, EA. Human Cerebral Deconnection Syndrome: A Preliminary Report. Neurology, 1962; 12, 675-685.
11. Geschwind, N. Disconnexion Syndromes in Animals and Man. I. Brain, 1965; 88(2), 237-294.
12. Geschwind, N. Disconnexion Syndromes in Animals and Man. II. Brain, 1965; 88(3), 585-644.
13. Geschwind, N. The Apraxias: Neural Mechanisms of Disorders of Learned Movement. Am Sci, 1975; 63(2), 188-195
14. Heilman, KM, Coyle, JM, Gonyea, EF, and Geschwind, N. Apraxia and Agraphia in a Left-Hander. Brain, 1973; 96(1), 21-28.
15. Geschwind, N. The Apraxias and Agnosias. In GA Talland, and NC Waugh (eds.), *The Pathology of Memory*. New York: Academic Press, 1969, pp. 3-8.
16. Heilman, KM, Gonyea, EF, and Geschwind, N. Apraxia and Agraphia in a Right-Hander. Cortex. 1974; 10, 284-288.
17. Liepmann, H. *Das Krankheitsbild der Apraxie ("Motorischen Asymbolie")*, Berlin, 1900.
18. Liepmann H, Storch E. Mschr Psychiat Neurol, 1902;11:115.
19. Heilman, KM, Rothi, LJG, and Watson, RT. Apraxia. In SC Schachter and O Devinsky, *Behavioral Neurology and the Legacy of Norman Geschwind*. New York: Lippincott-Raven Press, 1997, pp. 171-182.

# CHAPTER 10

# The Anatomy of Acquired Disorders of Reading

*Norman Geschwind*

To most educators and pediatricians, the term *dyslexia* means the failure to acquire the ability to read; it is this disturbance which is the focus of interest of this volume. It is worth recalling that historically the first reading problems to have been investigated were cases of the *loss* of the ability to comprehend written language, and it is therefore common practice among neurologists to distinguish *acquired* dyslexia or alexia from their *congenital* counterparts.

The distinction between these acquired disturbances and the congenital dyslexias is not an academic one. Remarkably restricted lesions in the left cerebral hemisphere of the adult may cause permanent severe disabilities. By contrast, total destruction of the left hemisphere in early childhood ordinarily does not prevent acquisition of language. It seems clear that the distribution of pathology in the congenital disturbances of language must involve something other than what is involved in the aphasias of adults.

Very uncommonly, the acquired disabilities are of functional psychiatric origin (hysterical *blindness* is much more common). In nearly all cases the disability results from damage to the brain readily distinguished at post-mortem examination, and the study of such lesions has been the most important technique for studying the parts of the nervous system involved in the comprehension of visual language in adults. An acquaintance with them is indispensable to any investigation of the apparently more elusive mechanisms involved in the failure to learn to read.

---

In the ensuing discussion, a certain number of neuroanatomical terms will be used that may be unfamiliar to those without special training. Such readers are advised to begin by reading the Appendix to this paper, p. 139, where a brief outline of the necessary information is presented.

Reprinted with permission from J. Money (ed), *Reading Disability*. Baltimore: The Johns Hopkins University Press, 1962; 115-129.

Three situations stand out prominently in which patients may lose the ability to read.[1] The most common is Wernicke's aphasia, in which the patient shows a severe incomprehension of both spoken and written language, together with a characteristic speech pattern (fluent speech which is often totally incomprehensible as the result of use of many distorted or incorrect words and extensive circumlocutions), and an inability to write correctly. A more restricted and less common syndrome is that of "pure word blindness with agraphia." The most restricted syndrome and the one whose mechanism I will discuss at some length is that of "pure word blindness without agraphia."

Before discussing this syndrome, the first question, oddly enough, must be whether I have a topic for discussion. Distinguished authors have disputed the existence of this entity. On the opposite side one finds equally distinguished adherents, Dejerine (1892); Bastian (1898); Holmes (1950); Symonds (1953); Warrington and Zangwill (1957); Hécaen, Ajuriaguerra, and David (1952); Alajouanine, Lhermitte, and Ribaucourt-Ducarne (1960). Some time ago those of us in the Aphasia Unit of the Boston Veterans Administration Hospital decided to review carefully individual case reports of this condition in the attempt to decide for ourselves whether it was justifiable to isolate the condition of "pure word blindness without agraphia."

We did not have to look far. The first reported case with a post-mortem examination is that of Dejerine (1892). Inexplicably this is a neglected paper. It is not mentioned in several works on aphasia. Where cited, it is often misquoted or even dismissed. Its value can be stated briefly. The careful description of the clinical picture has been confirmed more than once, and it established an anatomical localization which has also been repeatedly confirmed. It is, in fact, a masterpiece of neurological clinicopathological correlation.

Dejerine's patient was an extremely intelligent 68-year-old man who, on October 25, 1887, suddenly observed that he could no longer read a single word. He was examined first by Landolt (a distinguished ophthalmologist and a pioneer in physiological optics) and the original findings were confirmed by Dejerine repeatedly over the next four years.

The patient had a visual acuity of 8/10, spoke fluently without error, and understood all spoken speech. Objects were named perfectly, including pictures of technical instruments in a catalogue. He could identify his own morning newspaper by its form but could not read its name. On presentation he could not identify a single letter by name. The only written material he could read was his own name. Writing was correct, both spontaneously and to dictation, but what was written could not be read back. As Dejerine commented, his writing was rather like that of a blind man, larger than normal and with poor orientation of the lines.

---

[1] Throughout this presentation the word *read* is used in the narrow sense of "ability to comprehend language presented visually" and not at all in the sense of "ability to read aloud." Even in the neurological literature the two meanings are often confused. Many patients who cannot read aloud comprehend the written word correctly.

Although the reading of isolated letters was impossible, the patient could identify them by name after tracing their contours with his finger; if the examiner formed letters by moving the patient's hand through the air, he could name the letters produced in this way. This phenomenon had been described earlier in similar patients and many patients since then have shown the same finding.

A rather surprising contrast was the fact that even at the beginning of the illness, he could recognize individual Arabic numerals, but had trouble in reading several numbers simultaneously and in doing arithmetic calculations. With the passage of time all his difficulties in reading Arabic numerals and in doing even the most complex written calculations disappeared while his difficulties in reading letters persisted unchanged. Roman numerals were not tested. (Later observers have frequently confirmed the superiority in reading Arabic numerals in these patients, while Roman numerals seem to show the same difficulties as other letters.)

Like the other examples of this syndrome, this case showed a right hemianopia. Another frequently observed finding is a difficulty in color vision in the retained left visual field, but this is not mentioned by Dejerine.

The remarkable discrepancy between the loss of letters and preservation of numbers arouses one's interest in other visual symbols. The patient who had been a skilled musician now showed a total inability to comprehend musical notation, but could write a scale or particular notes on command. The ability to sing and play instruments was unimpaired.

The patient was observed carefully over the next four years. During this time he continued actively and very successfully in business, kept on writing, played cards skillfully, and learned and performed new music by ear. He had no difficulty in orientation even when going to strange parts of Paris.

On January 5, 1892, another cerebral vascular accident left him with paraphasic speech and incapable of writing. He died at 10 a.m. on the sixteenth of January, and an autopsy was performed in the patient's home by Dejerine, twenty-four hours after his death.

Dejerine gave a careful description of the external appearance of the cerebral hemispheres and of the internal appearances as revealed by gross horizontal sections. There was no report of the microscopic findings in the lesions in this original publication, but these appeared in a later paper and in his monumental work on the anatomy of the brain. They fully confirmed the impressions he had drawn from observation of the gross specimen and supported his theoretical conclusions.

Two major lesions were found in the brain (Figures 1–4). There was the recent lesion (with which the patient had become paraphasic and agraphic) involving the angular gyrus and adjacent portions of parietal lobe and temporoparietal junction. It showed the characteristic features of a recent lesion: there were signs of both white and red infarction, in the absence of atrophy of the involved gyri, in growth of new vessels, yellowish coloration, and thickening or adherence of the meninges. The older lesion (which is the one that is of major interest here since it is the one causative of the clinical picture I have been discussing) had

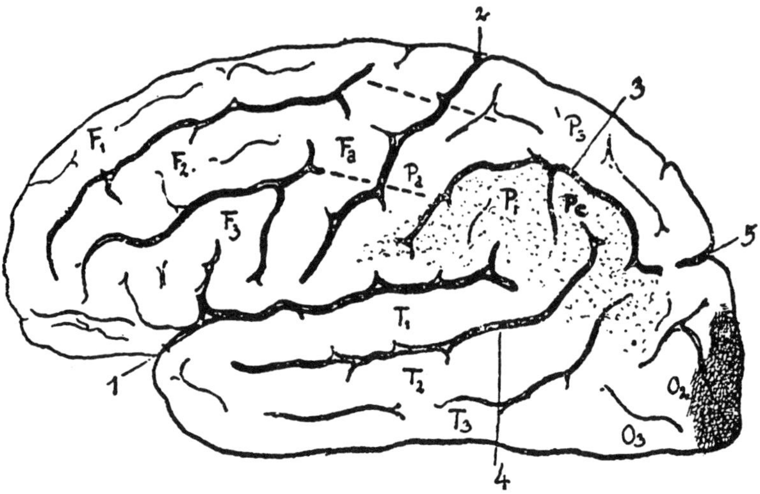


FIGURE 1. Left hemisphere of Dejerine's patient, lateral view. The dark area in the occipital lobe represents the old region of destruction, the stippled area the recent lesion. 1 = Sylvian fissure; 2 = Rolandic fissure; $F_3$ = third frontal gyrus; $T_1$ = first temporal gyrus; Pc = angular gyrus. Reproduced from Dejerine (1892).

caused destruction of the medial and inferior aspects of the occipital lobe. This showed the characteristic appearance of a lesion of considerable age with narrowing and atrophy of the gyri. The white matter of the occipital lobe was yellow and shrunken. In addition, there was a region of old destruction of white matter in the splenium of the corpus callosum.

In discussing the significance of the pathology, let us confine ourselves to the older lesion whose effects were apparent to Dejerine. He pointed out that for a word to be seen as language and not merely as an arbitrary design, there must be a connection between the visual centers in the occipital cortex and the language areas in the left hemisphere. But, in this patient, the destruction of the left occipital cortex and the resultant right hemianopia made it necessary for the patient to see only in his left visual field and hence, with his right occipital cortex. In this situation, for reading, it is necessary to have connections going from the right occipital cortex across the corpus callosum and to the left-sided language areas in the posterior temporal region. Dejerine argued that the extensive destruction of white matter in the left occipital lobe in this case would destroy the connecting fibers from the right occipital cortex. He thought that this destruction alone would suffice to disconnect the right visual area from the language areas without having to bring in the lesion of the splenium of the corpus callosum. There is good reason, however, to believe that the lesion of the corpus callosum did contribute significantly to the disconnection postulated by Dejerine. The anatomical

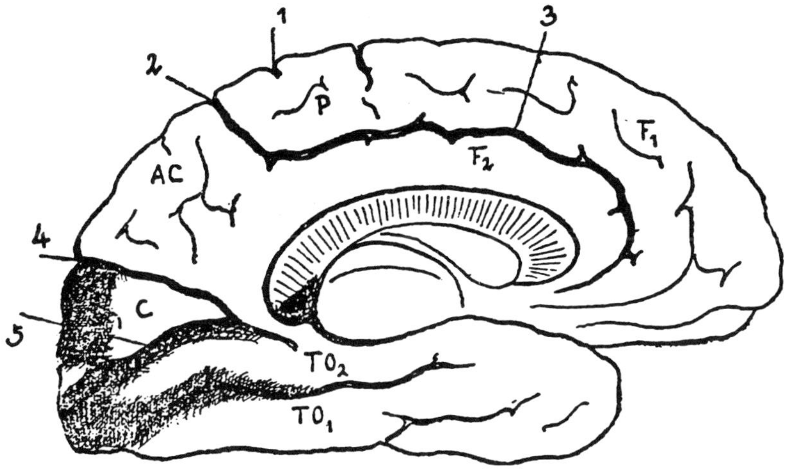


FIGURE 2. Left hemisphere, medial view. The structure marked by radiating lines is the corpus callosum, the posterior end of which (the splenium) is seen to contain an area of old destruction. 5 = calcarine fissure, along the lips of which lies the visual cortex, which is shown as involved in the area of old destruction. Reproduced from Dejerine (1892).

evidence supports strongly the view that fibers from the occipital lobes to the corpus callosum run in the splenium where they are rather tightly packed.

It is worth commenting here that Dejerine's anatomical conclusions from this case are frequently misquoted. A frequent statement is that he attributed this syndrome to a lesion of the angular gyrus. In fact, he carefully denied this. He had shown a year earlier that a lesion of the angular gyrus caused the syndrome of pure word blindness with agraphia and indeed, he thought that it was specifically disconnection of the right visual cortex from the left angular gyrus which led to pure word blindness without agraphia.

There is one feature of the clinical picture which is very compatible with the idea of a specialized disconnection. This is the fact that although letters could not be read by this patient when presented visually, they could be "read" when they were traced on his hand or when his hand was moved over the outline of a letter. This stimulation when presented to the right hand would go to the left sensory cortex and thence readily to the speech areas; when presented to the left hand, it would go across the corpus callosum (anteriorly to the splenium) from the right hemisphere and thus reach the speech areas. This preservation of tactile or kinesthetic "reading" in pure word blindness without agraphia contrasts to its loss in pure word blindness with agraphia. The latter syndrome is the result of a lesion of a cortical area which somehow functions in the operations done on visual language; once destroyed, it is obvious that comprehension of written language

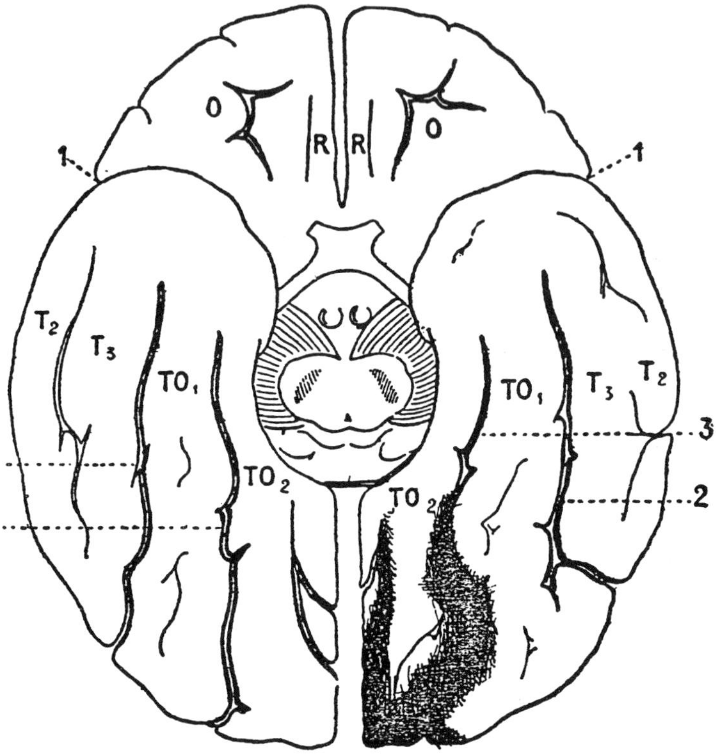


FIGURE 3. Cerebral hemispheres, seen from below. Reproduced from Dejerine (1892).

is lost regardless of its mode of presentation; but, by a suitably placed lesion one can specifically disconnect from this cortical area visually presented material alone, while preserving the transmission of somesthetically presented stimuli.

A few years later, Bastian (1898) reviewed two more cases (in addition to Dejerine's) which had come to post-mortem and had shown similar clinical and pathological findings and led him to defend essentially the same mechanism.

Foix and Hillemand (1925) advanced further evidence in support of a mechanism of disconnection and, in particular, of the importance of the lesion in the splenium. They had found that, in a case of destruction of the left occipital lobe with preservation of the splenium, there was no word blindness, despite the presence of the expected right hemianopia. By contrast, two cases which at post-mortem showed destruction of the splenium in addition to that of left visual cortex had manifested pure word blindness. The occurrence of this syndrome, dependent as it is on the concurrence of two lesions, is a result of the arrangement of the cerebral vessels. The posterior cerebral artery supplies not only the occipital cortex but the splenium of the corpus callosum. Hence, occlusions of this vessel are

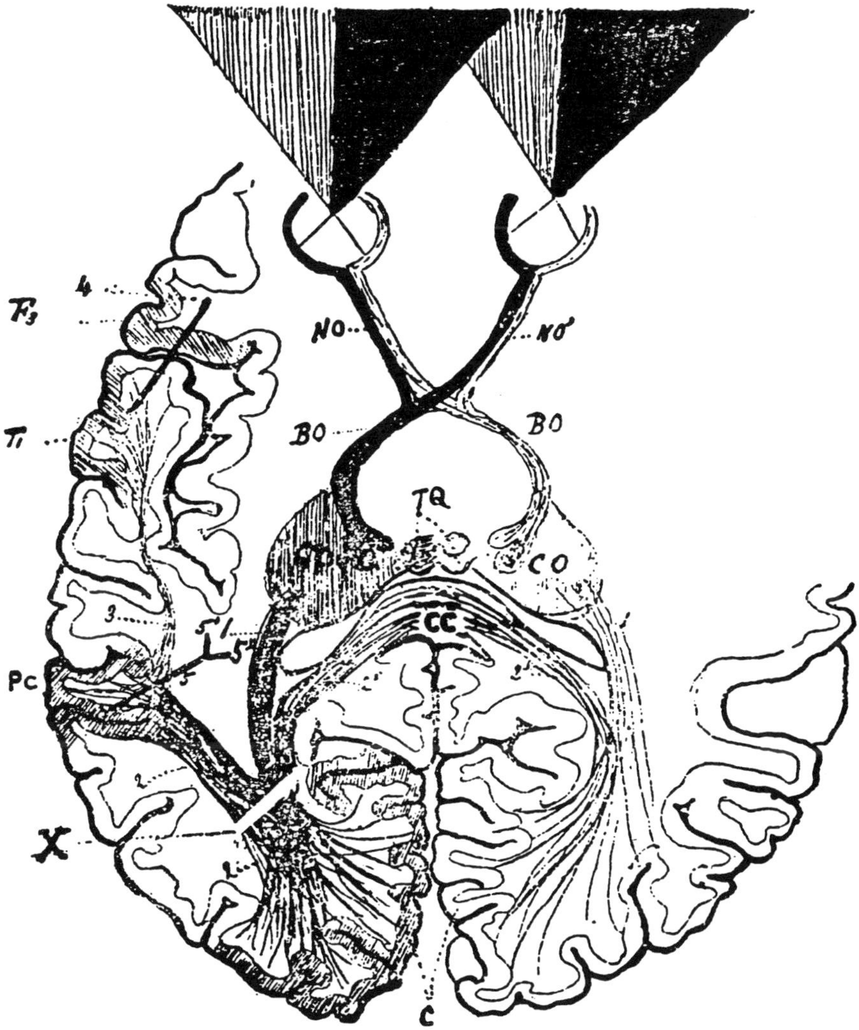


FIGURE 4. Diagrammatic horizontal cross section of cerebral hemispheres, illustrating the mechanism of pure word blindness without agraphia. NO = left optic nerve and NO– = right optic nerve. C = left and right calcarine cortex, shown destroyed on the left (oblique lines); Pc = left angular gyrus (when destroyed as shown here alexia with agraphia results; this region is intact in pure alexia without agraphia); X = large lesion in white matter of left occipital lobe destroying fibers from the right visual cortex going to the left angular gyrus; cc = corpus callosum (although no lesion is shown here, a lesion here will be easily as effective as the lesion at X in disconnecting the right visual cortex from the left angular gyrus). Reproduced from Dejerine (1892).

likely to lead to destruction of the two structures necessary for this syndrome. Had the posterior fifth of the corpus callosum been supplied like the anterior four-fifths by the anterior cerebral artery, I suspect that pure word blindness would be indeed an extremely rare syndrome.

The most recent confirmation both of the clinical picture and of pathology has been the work of Alajouanine, Lhermitte, and Ribaucourt-Ducarne (1960) who had six cases with the classical clinical syndrome, one of whom died showing the above distribution of pathology. They list several other workers who have also confirmed the pathological picture.

There is further evidence for the mechanism suggested by Dejerine and supported here. Cases of pure word blindness have been due most often to vascular disease and rarely to trauma. In the extensive studies of Teuber, Battersby, and Bender (1960) on 46 patients with war wounds of the occipital lobes, there was not a single case of word blindness. Furthermore, these authors point out that in World War I, no such cases were found by Marie and Chatelin or Wilbrand and Saenger. Professor Teuber has been kind enough to show me the notes on one patient seen after the completion of the above study who developed word blindness following trauma which, however, cleared in a few months.

The reason for the paucity of word blindness as a sequel of penetrating injury to the brain is, I believe, the fact that it would be extremely unusual to sustain injury simultaneously to the left visual cortex and the splenium of the corpus callosum. A missile penetrating the splenium would probably enter the upper brain stem and almost certainly lead to the patient's death.

The evidence from neurosurgical procedures lends further support to the argument. Hécaen, Ajuriaguerra, and David (1952) describe seven patients who underwent occipital lobe resection, all very extensive. Every one of these patients developed pure word-blindness, but in every case the disability cleared up within six months. (It is interesting, however, that all of these patients found reading unpleasant after their recovery.) If pure word blindness were the result of a lesion of some cortical region of the occipital lobe alone, permanent word blindness should have been seen in some of these cases. In contrast to the recovery of these patients is the fact that cases of this disorder that have a vascular origin have a very poor prognosis for recovery. The only difference between the vascular and surgical cases is the preservation of the splenium in the latter. Presumably the fibers from the right occipital lobe to the speech areas are so tightly packed in the splenium that they are more effectively destroyed here than they are by even a very extensive lesion of the white matter of the left occipital lobe.

The above suggested mechanism has further implications. If the splenium alone were destroyed, words presented in the *right* visual field should be read normally, but the patient should be word-blind for words presented in the *left* visual field. Two papers have presented such cases. Thus, Trescher and Ford (1937) found that a patient whose splenium had been sectioned for removal of a third ventricle tumor could not read letters in the left visual field although the standard visual field examinations were normal, nor could she name wooden letters placed into her left hand. On the other hand, objects placed in the left hand were named correctly and two-point discrimination was normal in this hand. Maspes (1948) presented two further cases in whom the splenium of the corpus callosum was cut for removal of colloid cysts of the third ventricle. Both these cases developed alexia in the left visual field alone.

For the past fifteen years attribution of clinical symptomatology to lesions of the corpus callosum has been unpopular because of the negative reports of physiologists on the effects of callosal section and particularly as a result of the studies of Akelaitis and his co-workers (1941, 1943, 1944) on interruption of the callosum in man. However, Sperry (1961) and his colleagues have recently conclusively shown that dividing the callosum leads to profound changes in animals, if they are examined properly. Sperry showed that if one hemisphere is trained, the learned material is transferred to the opposite hemisphere by way of the corpus callosum. After section of the callosum, new material presented to one hemisphere is not transferred to the opposite side. In man, the testing situation is simpler than in the animal, since language skills remain confined to the left hemisphere in normals. Hence, immediately following callosal destruction, appropriate testing should reveal defects if the right hemisphere is tested with language tasks. The effect of posterior section is to cut off the right occipital lobe from the language areas. Sections further forward should have more profound effect on the limbs. Elsewhere we have described the effects of more anterior involvement of the corpus callosum (Geschwind and Kaplan, 1962). I would like especially to express my debt to Dr. Sperry whose work alerted me to the possible importance of callosal disconnection in humans.

The most serious objection to the mechanism discussed here arises from the aforementioned work of Akelaitis and his co-workers. In particular, he described six patients in whom the splenium was cut; in none of them was there any subsequent alexia in the left visual field. These six cases stand in contradiction to the case of Trescher and Ford (1937) and the two cases of Maspes (1948). There is at present no obvious means of explaining the discrepancy, although some suggestions may be made. One possibility is that the sections performed on Akelaitis's cases were less complete than those done on the patients of the other authors, but since none of the patients has had a post-mortem examination, this cannot be verified. Maspes pointed out that in five of the six cases studied by Akelaitis, cerebral lesions had been present from early childhood. Language skills might not have been sharply localized in the left hemisphere in these cases, and callosal section would therefore have shown little effect. All of Akelaitis's cases were epileptics, while none of the contrasting group were. Could epilepsy favor the opening up of alternative pathways? This is a rather hazardous speculation which can only be mentioned here. Clearly, further observations are needed.

In this final section, I would like to turn to some more remote implications of the interpretation of pure word blindness without agraphia that have been defended here. First are its implications for the general problem of interpretation of the aphasias. Neurologists have frequently assumed that "mixed" aphasias were the result of mixtures of "pure" lesions. But, even the patient with pure word blindness with agraphia does not have the lesion of pure word blindness without agraphia "mixed" with another lesion. Very pure lesions may result only from disconnection from the language areas, and the possibility still remains that lesions directly in the speech areas can never produce a "pure" syndrome (in the sense of an aphasic disorder confined to a single modality). This view gains added support from the fact that many researches over the years have supported a similar mechanism for pure word deafness, i.e., a lesion of the left Heschl's gyrus, with destruction of callosal fibers from the right Heschl's gyrus, with no lesion in speech cortex. Hoff (1961) is the most recent investigator to have found pathological evidence for this mechanism.

The next point I would like to discuss is an apparent difficulty which arises from the mechanism for pure word blindness suggested above. Professor Davis Howes called my attention to the fact that none of the published cases of pure word blindness has had the symptom of so-called optic aphasia. By this term is meant the inability to *name* a seen object although the subject recognizes it (as proven, let us say, by his ability to select it afterwards from a group), with retained ability to name objects by feel, sound, smell, or taste. If indeed the right occipital lobe is disconnected from the language areas, how can the subject *name* seen objects? Let me sharpen this point by noting that in the patient mentioned earlier, studied by Mrs. Kaplan and myself, who shows evidence of anterior callosal disconnection, one finds an inability to name *letters* placed in the left hand, i.e., a "tactile alexia" of the left hand. He also shows an inability to name *objects* placed in the left hand although he can identify them nonverbally, i.e., he has the analogue to "optic aphasia" which has been called "tactile aphasia." Why does "optic aphasia" not accompany pure word blindness? One possible explanation is the straightforward anatomical one, i.e., that different pathways are used in naming an object, or more likely, that the sight of an object is much richer in associations than that of a letter and that eventually more anterior parts of the right hemisphere are stimulated whence pathways are found across the corpus callosum. Adolf Meyer (1950) supported essentially this latter version of the anatomical explanation.

There is another approach to the problem of the preservation of object-naming. Dr. Davis Howes and I have recently had the opportunity to study a patient with pure word blindness without agraphia who presented the classical clinical syndrome. In his paper in this symposium, Dr. Howes describes the studies that we have conducted, and in particular, he discusses the comparative data on object- and word-naming respectively. One possibility which emerges from these data is that while object- and word-naming may use the same pathways, object-naming may survive partial damage more effectively. The data do not clearly decide between the anatomic and functional explanations and this remains an interesting area for further investigation.

In closing, we can turn to the question of the possible relevance of what has been presented here to the problem of "congenital dyslexia." I think one can say with some assurance that the lesion described here is not the cause of congenital dyslexia. Children with this disturbance do not have hemianopias. Furthermore, even if such a lesion did rarely occur in a child under the age of six, I doubt that it would impair his ability to learn to read, or if he were already reading, I believe that the disability would be transient. The reason for this is the tremendous ability of the youthful nervous system to find alternative means of compensating for damage to localized areas, a faculty much attenuated in the adult. However, I suspect that I could guess the type of explanation that Dejerine *might* have given for congenital dyslexia. He would have argued that the angular gyrus acts in some specific way to process visual language, and that *bilateral* maldevelopment of this region would be the minimum substrate for difficulty in learning to read. Is this the true explanation? I do not believe that an answer is available. I would only suggest that we keep in mind the lesson to be learned from Dejerine of the importance of interweaving our functional with our anatomical knowledge.

## Appendix

This brief appendix is designed to aid the reader of this paper who lacks a technical background in neuroanatomy. The reader should refer to the illustrations given in the paper while reading this section.

The two halves of the brain (the *cerebral hemispheres*) are connected by a large bundle of nerve fibers called the *corpus callosum*, which can be seen on the inner surface of the divided brain. The posterior end of this structure is called the *splenium*. The cerebral hemispheres consist of an outer mantle of *gray matter*, which is called the *cortex*, which consists of *nerve cells*, and a central core of *white matter*, which consists of nerve fibers coming from or going to the cortex. The white matter carries to appropriate areas incoming sensations from the periphery, interconnects different parts of the cortex and carries impulses to muscles out of the cortex.

There are certain distinct specializations of the cortex. Visual impressions go to the posterior end of the cerebral hemisphere, the *occipital lobes*, with the right side of the visual field being represented in the left occipital cortex and the left side in the right occipital cortex. Language functions are carried out only on the left side of the brain in most people in the areas marked in Figure 1 as $F_3$ which is in the *frontal lobe*, in the area marked $T_1$ which is in the *temporal lobe*, and in the area marked $P_c$ (the *angular gyrus*) which is at the junction of the temporal, parietal, and occipital lobes.

The word *hemianopia* refers to a loss of vision in one half of the visual field. The *left* half of each retina receives the image from the *right* half of the visual field, since the incoming image from the visual field is inverted by the lens of each eye. The left half of each retina is connected to the left occipital lobe of the brain. Thus, a right hemianopia (for each eye) signifies impaired perception in the right visual field and results from destruction of the visual cortex in the left occipital lobe and vice versa for a left hemianopia.

## References

Akelaitis, AJ. Studies on the Corpus Callosum II. The Higher Visual Functions in Each Homonymous Field Following Complete Section of the Corpus Callosum. Arch Neurol Psychiat, 1941; 45,788-796.

Aklaitis, AJ. Studies on the Corpus Callosum VII. Study of Language Functions (Tactile and Visual, Lexia and Graphia) Unilaterally Following Section of the Corpus Callosum. J Neuropath Exp Neurol, 1943, 226-262.

Akelaitis, AJ. A Study of Gnosis, Praxia and Language Following Section of the Corpus Callosum and Anterior Commissure. J Neurosurg, l944;1,94-102.

Alajouanine, T, L'hermitte, F, and de Ribaucourt-Ducarne, B. Les Alexies Agnosiques et Aphasigues. In *Les Grandes Activites du Lobe Occipital.* Paris: Masson, 1960, p. 235.

Bastian, HC. A Treatise on Aphasia and Other Speech Defects. London: H. K. Lewis, 1898.

Dejerine, J. Contribution a l'Etude Anatomo-pathologique et Clinique des Differences Variete Verbale. Mem Soc Biolog, 1892; 4,61-90.

Foix, C, and Hillemand, P. Role Vraisembable du Spleniurn dans la Pathogenic de l'Alexie Pure par Lesion de la Cerebrale Posteriere. Bull Mem Soc Med Hop Paris, 1925; 49,393.

Geschwind, N, and Kaplan, E. A Human Cerebral Deconnection Syndrome. Neurology, 1962; 12,673-685.

Hecean, H, Ajuriaguerra, J, and, David, M. Les Deficits Fonctionnels Apres Lobectomie Oceipitale. Mschr Psychiat Neurol, 1952;123,239.

Hoff, H. Die Lokalisation der Aphasie. In: *Proceedings of the VII International Congress of Neurology*, Vol I. Soc Graf Rom, Rome, 1961, p. 555.

Holmes, G. Pure-Wood Blindness. Folia Psychiat Neurol Neurochir Neerlandica, 1950; 53,279.

Maspes, PK. Le Syndrome Experimental Chex 1'Homme de la Section du Splenium du Corps Calleux: Alexie Visuelle Pure Hemiansopsique. Rev Neurol 1948; 80,100.

Meyer, A. Writings on Aphasia. In *The Collected Papers of Adolf Meyer*. Vol I. Baltimore: John Hopkins Press, 1950.

Sperry, RW. Cerebral Organization and Behavior. Science 1961; 133,1749.

Symonds, CP. Aphasia. J Neurol Neurosurg Psychiat, 1953; 16,1.

Teuber, HL, Battersby, WS, and Bender, MB. Visual Field Defects After Penetrating Wounds of the Brain. Cambridge: Harvard University Press, 1960.

Trescher, JH, and Ford, FR. Colloid Cyst of the Third Venaicle. Arch Neuro Psychiat, 1937; 37,959.

Warrington, E, and Zangwill, O. A Study of Dyslexia. J Neurol Neurosurg Psychiat, 1957; 20,208.

The researches described here were supported in part by a grant (No. M-1802) to the Section of Psychology, Massachusetts Institute of Technology from the National Institute of Mental Health, United States Public Health Service.

# CHAPTER 11

# Color-Naming Defects in Association With Alexia

*Norman Geschwind and Michael Fusillo*

Disturbances of color identification in association with the syndrome of pure alexia without agraphia have been repeatedly recognized in the past. Lange[1] reviewed these extensively. More recently Critchley[2] has reviewed the literature on such disturbances of color identification. He expressed skepticism as to the existence of the syndrome of aphasia for color names and advanced the view that such cases probably represented the combination of a perceptual deficit with a minimal aphasia.

We have recently had the opportunity to clarify the problem of color-name aphasia by repeated study of a patient with the syndrome of pure alexia without agraphia over several months. On the basis of these studies, we believe that the evidence is now clear that a disturbance of color-naming, or more correctly, of matching the spoken name of the color to the seen color, can be shown to exist in the demonstrated absence of any perceptual disturbance. The patient to be described eventually came to postmortem examination and demonstrated, as will be pointed out, the classic pathology of the syndrome of pure alexia without agraphia as first described by Dejerine[3] and repeatedly confirmed since then. A preliminary description of this case has been published.[4]

## REPORT OF A CASE

H. C. (MMH 426-89), a 58-year-old machinist had been known to be diabetic for 17 years. He was transferred to the Massachusetts Memorial Hospital (where he was under the care of Dr. Charles Kane) from another hospital on Sept 24,

---

Reprinted with permission from *Archives of Neurology*. 1966; 15 (2): 137-146. 

1962, because of right-sided weakness, confusion, and difficulty expressing himself of several days' duration. These difficulties had come on abruptly during a hospitalization for reinvestigation of a long-standing severe sensorimotor polyneuropathy.

The past history was not contributory except for long-standing diabetes mellitus and episodes of postural hypotension in the few months preceding his admission. There was no history of hypertension or previous signs or symptoms of cerebral vascular disease.

Lumbar punctures performed at the other hospital on previous admissions had shown on one occasion a protein of 113 mg/100 cc, and on another 330 mg/100 cc. Pressure, cell count, and serology were normal on both occasions. On these admissions serum proteins were normal and a rectal biopsy for amyloidosis was negative. Except for the evidence of diabetes, the results of other laboratory studies were normal. Before admission to the Massachusetts Memorial Hospital the patient's medications had included protamine zinc insulin suspension (60 units per day), chlorpropamide (Diabinese) (25 mg three times per day), thiamine (100 mg daily), and liver extract and cyanocobalamin (Vitamin $B_{12}$) injections every other day.

General physical examination on admission to the Massachusetts Memorial Hospital revealed a well-developed, well-nourished white man in no acute distress who, although right-handed, showed lack of spontaneous use of the right arm. The vital signs were as follows: blood pressure, 128/78 mm Hg; pulse, 120 beats per minute and regular; respirations 24 breaths per minute and regular; and temperature, 98.6 F. If the patient remained erect for 15–20 minutes, his blood pressure would drop and he would develop a shock-like syndrome so that he had to be maintained almost continuously in bed. The skin revealed stasis dermatitis, dependent rubor, and trophic changes over both lower extremities. There was a trace of pretibial edema. The results of the remainder of the general physical examination were within normal limits.

On neurological examination the patient knew his name but did not recall his address. He stated his age incorrectly. He felt that he was still at the other hospital and that it was probably the fall of 1933. He realized, however, that his memory was poor and had insight into the fact that he had been having difficulty naming objects over the past several days prior to admission. He was able to perform simple one-digit calculations. He could recall none of four objects after one minute. There was mild difficulty in naming familiar objects or parts of objects. The patient could obey spoken commands reasonably well but had more difficulty with written commands. He had difficulty in writing, manifested by holding the pen clumsily and by misspelling words. His ability to write was clearly better than his comprehension of written material. There was minimal right-left confusion. The optic fundi revealed micro-aneurysms, deep punctate hemorrhages, and waxy exudates consistent with diabetic retinopathy. There was no papilledema. There was a dense right homonymous hemianopia. The right pupil was slightly larger than the left, but both reacted to light and on convergence. The rest of the cranial nerve functions were normal. There was a tendency for the right arm to drift downward and laterally when the patient's eyes were shut. There was severe wasting of all four extremities, especially distally. No fasciculations were observed. There was weakness of all four extremities in a distal distribution. Muscle tone was normal throughout. Fine movements were performed clumsily with the right hand. The deep tendon reflexes were absent throughout. The plantar responses were also absent. The patient showed an unsteady, wide-based gait. Sensory examination revealed that pin-prick, light touch, and vibratory appreciation were impaired in a fading stocking distribution over both feet to the level of the knees. In addition, position was impaired in the toes of the right foot and the fingers of the right hand. Two-point discrimination, tactile localization, and stereognosis were impaired in the right hand. The patient manifested extinction to touch over the right side of the body on double simultaneous stimulation.

During the first few days of his hospital stay, the patient developed congestive heart failure, pulmonary emboli, diabetic keto-acidosis, and gastro-intestinal bleeding, for all of which he was treated successfully. Serial electrocardiograms were consistent with a diagnosis of pulmonary emboli. A bilateral superficial femoral vein ligation was performed. A lumbar puncture showed normal pressures, clear cerebrospinal fluid with 2 red blood cells, a sugar of 133 mg/100 cc (with a corresponding blood sugar of 200 mg/100 cc), and a protein of 256 mg/100 cc. The colloidal gold curve was flat. The patient's serum proteins were 5.2 gm/100 cc, and there was a reversal of the albumin-globulin ratio. Serum electrophoresis was within normal limits. X-rays of the skull were also within normal limits. An electroencephalogram on the second hospital day was abnormal, with left postcentral preponderance due to the presence of theta waves at 4 to 7 per second. A repeat EEG about ten days later showed no essential change.

Because of the patient's condition, detailed examination of the higher functions was not possible until the fifth hospital day. At this time he was unable to name simple objects, written words, or letters. He was, however, able to name a circle, a triangle, and a square. There was no right-left confusion and no finger agnosia. The patient was able to follow verbal commands well. There was now some minimal weakness of the right lower extremity, above and beyond the weakness due to the patient's chronic sensorimotor polyneuropathy. On the 22nd hospital day the patient was still unable to name even simple letters, such as C or S. He could not read the words cat, dog, or his own first name. Using his left hand, he demonstrated that he could write much better than he could read. Although he could not read, he was able to copy letters as well as words without any difficulty. He was able to add simple 1 and 2 digit numbers in his head, but was unable to add the same numbers when they were written down on paper.

The patient was finally transferred to a nursing home on the 31st hospital day. The disability in reading was still present, although the medical problem had become well stabilized. During the next eight months, through the kindness of Dr. J. Litter, the patient's private physician, we were enabled to study the patient in detail, first at the nursing home, then at his own home, and finally (through the courtesy of Dr. William Timberlake) at the Lemuel Shattuck Hospital.

When the patient was first seen at the nursing home seven weeks after the acute episode, he demonstrated the following residual picture: The distal symmetrical sensorimotor polyneuritic signs were still present, as well as the right hemianopia. Speech production and comprehension were normal. The recent memory deficits had, however, cleared completely (except for the special difficulties in topography to be mentioned below). The right-sided sensory loss which had appeared at the time of his acute episode had cleared (leaving only the symmetrical distal loss due to the polyneuropathy). Right-left orientation and finger-naming were normal, and he could perform mental arithmetic well. There were no disturbances of consciousness or abstract thought. He could spell words correctly and write them with either hand separately. Handwriting was normal but he wrote slowly. There were no constructional difficulties. Optokinetic nystagmus was present and grossly equal to both the right and left sides. These aspects of his clinical picture remained stable over the next few months.

He showed severe disturbances in spatial orientation and topography. Thus, he could not tell us where the nursing home or his own home were located and incorrectly answered questions about how to get to various points in the Boston area with which he had had extensive experience in the past. It should be stressed, however, that these disturbances cleared to normal in the next few weeks.

In the last months of his life, he developed some new symptoms consisting of vague pains over the right side of the body, especially the thorax, which were diffuse and difficult to characterize. They were increased by repetitive sensory stimulation. Although these raised the suspicion of an incipient thalamic syndrome and were repeatedly complained of, they never became agonizing.

In addition to the findings listed earlier, he showed certain disabilities which remained essentially stable over the next eight months and which were the object of special study. He complained of distortions of his visual field which we failed to be able to characterize. These, however, did not in any way affect his ability to copy visual forms or words correctly. He could neither read words aloud nor comprehend their meaning but could copy them correctly. He could not match words to appropriate pictures. He could read only some single letters; two-digit numbers, by contrast, were usually read correctly. Only one error was made in several months in the naming of objects, photographs, or line drawings. He could spell words presented to him orally and could comprehend words spelled to him orally. He could write spontaneously and to dictation but could not read his own handwriting if it was shown to him later. Also, in striking contrast to his correct object identification was his difficulty in color identification, which was as persistent as his alexia. We will give in the next section a detailed account of the tests employed to study this color identification difficulty and the results obtained.

## Studies of Color Identification

*Naming of Seen Colors.* Colored sheets of paper were presented to the patient. He misnamed in almost all cases, and there was no consistency to his misnaming except that the response "gray" or "grayish" was the most common. His misnamings applied not only to colors in the narrow sense of the term but appeared also when he was presented with black, white, or gray.

Arbitrary Colored Objects: Colored pictures of objects which are not usually of a fixed shade, e.g., neckties, crayons, dresses, blankets, or curtains, were then presented to the patient. His errors were similar to those produced with colored pieces of paper.

Distinctively Colored Objects or Pictures: Objects or pictures of objects which are usually of a certain color or are conventionally regarded as being of a certain color, e.g., apple, banana, telephone, milk, or bricks, were presented to the patient. He failed in these as he had in the first two categories. These errors occurred although the patient could name the objects correctly and could, as shown below, tell what colors these objects normally were. Thus, the patient, shown a pad of writing paper, said it was tan; but when asked, said that writing paper was usually white. He insisted that this pad "looked tan" to him. He misnamed the color of the red bricks in the fireplace in his own living room.

*Verbal Memory for Colors of Objects.* The patient was asked to state the usual colors of specified objects, e.g., apples, bananas, the sky, etc. He performed without error on this task.

*Verbal Memory for Objects Having a Certain Color.* The patient was asked to name the usual colors of objects named by the examiner. He performed without error on this task.

*Comprehension of Names of Seen Colors (Matching of Seen Colors to a Name Given Verbally).* The patient was shown a group of colored objects or sheets of paper and was asked to select a specific color, e.g., "Show me the red sheet of paper." The patient failed in this task almost always. He would also fail in simpler form of this task: being shown an object and asked, "Is this red?" he would answer at random.

*Color-Matching.* Several versions of this test were carried out and all were performed correctly. Thus, the patient, when given two rows of colored papers, would successfully match each paper in one row to the same color in the other row. In order to rule out that the patient was doing this task by means of brightness differences, a more complex form of the test was set up whereby the colors differed markedly in brightness and saturation. The patient performed without error in this task.

A still more complex task was set up in which the patient was given a pile of colored chips of papers and permitted to sort them. He correctly collected all of the items of a particular kind. Thus, he correctly sorted a group of chips of two slightly different shades of green into two separate piles.

*Ordering Shades of One Color.* The patient could correctly arrange a series of reds in order from bright red at one end to pink at the other.

*Matching Seen Colors to Pictures of Objects.* The patient was given a group of colored papers or crayons and a group of line drawings of objects. He correctly matched the colors to the objects, e.g., a yellow crayon to a banana.

*Pseudo-Isochromatic Color Tests.* The patient was given both the American Optical Company and the Ishihara pseudo-isochromatic tests of color vision. He performed both without error. The American Optical test was performed readily because it uses geometrical forms which the patient could name readily. On the Ishihara test the patient either named the digits (as we have noted above the patient could read most two-digit numbers although he could not generally read two-letter pairs) or traced them out with his finger. On those parts of the Ishihara test using colored paths he traced these correctly. It should be noted that one of the examiners (NG), who is moderately red-green blind, performed very poorly on these tests, while the patient performed as well as the examiner (MF) with normal color vision. Despite this, the patient's descriptions of the color in which the correct answer was printed were grossly inaccurate. Thus, one of the cards which shows a bright red 7 on a gray background was described as having a gray 7.

In addition to these tests of the patient's color identification ability, certain features of his performance on these tasks deserve to be mentioned here. One of these was the fact that the patient never replied with a simple "I don't know" to the demand for naming a color. Furthermore, when offered the correct name from a group, he would not accept it. In fact, if the patient had replied "gray" and was told by the examiner that the correct answer was "red," he would often say, "It may look red to you, doctor, but it looks gray to me" or "Well, maybe it's a reddish-gray." When pressed, he would almost always insist that the color "looked" to him as he had named it. Sometimes he would explain his response by saying that his eyes weren't working well. On one occasion, shown a pad of writing paper, he said that it was tan. When we asked him what color writing paper normally was, he said, "It's usually white but this looks tan." When we told him that the paper was actually white, he suddenly said, "I don't understand what happened: it now looks white." We will return to this in the Comment section.

The patient only once made an error in sorting. Our usual technique for this task was to hand him a colored chip (without naming the color) and the patient was told to select all the chips which looked like the one demonstrated. This he did without error. His only faulty sorting occurred on a variant of the task. We showed him a chip and said, "This is red. Now pick out all the red chips." He proceeded to form a pile which contained all the red chips but also all the chips of one of the two shades of green that were in the group. When asked what his pile contained, he picked up a red chip and said, "This is red." He then picked

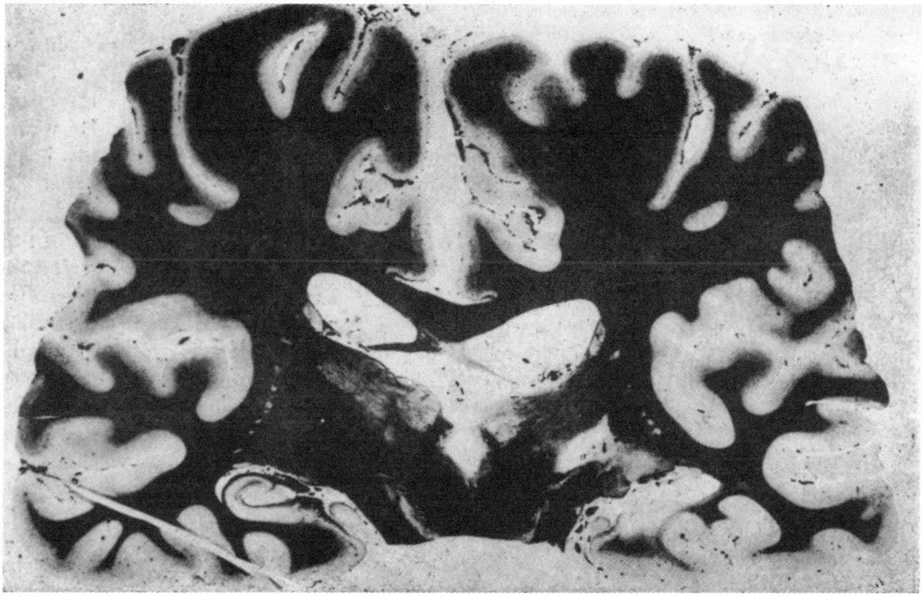

FIGURE 1. In this section (2200) the total degeneration of the left fornix is seen as well as the cystic lesion in the left posterolateral-ventral nucleus of the thalamus. Destruction of the left hippocampus and enlargement of the temporal horn of the left lateral ventricle is also evident.

up one of the chips of the particular shade of green that he had selected and said, "This is another shade of red." We then had him match the chips from his pile (without our mentioning any color names) to the green chips of the shade he had not chosen. He carefully matched all of the shade of green he had chosen to these but did not select out any of the red ones. We will return to this curious result in our Comment section.

## Pathological Examination

The patient died on Dec 21, 1963, 15 months after the onset of his original difficulty, at the Lemuel Shattuck Hospital. The brain after removal was fixed in formaldehyde solution (formalin).

On gross examination of the uncut brain fixed in formaldehyde solution, the only obvious finding was an old softening in the region of the left occipital pole.

The brain was embedded in celloidin, and sections were cut at 35μ intervals with alternate sections being stained for myelin and cells. Representative sections are shown in the figures.

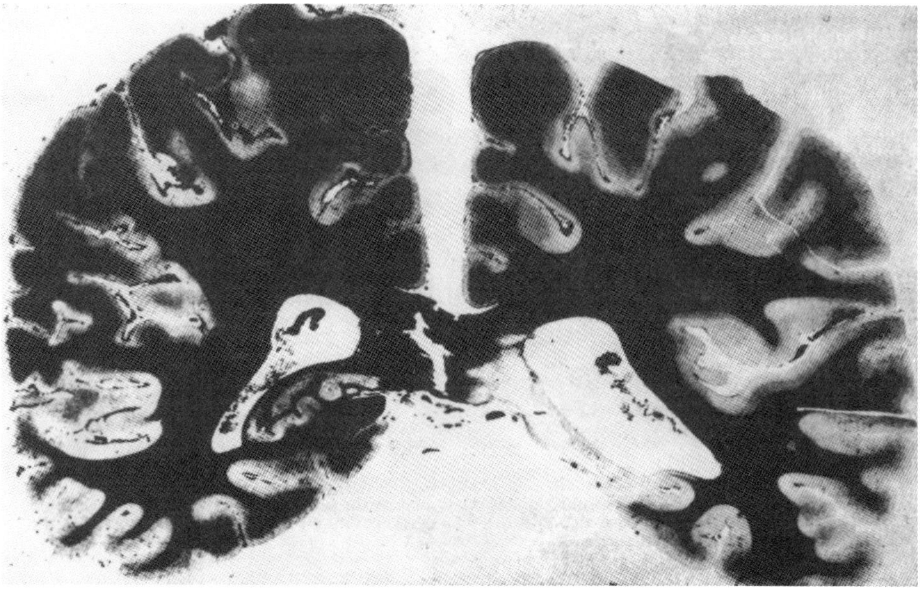

FIGURE 2. Total infarction and degeneration of the splenium of the corpus callosum is seen (section 2500). The cavity in the center of the splenium is a result of artifact and was not seen in adjacent serial sections of this region. The gross destruction of the hippocampus on the left is also evident.

The right hemisphere was normal except for secondary degenerations resulting from lesions in the left hemisphere. Figure 1 (section 2200) shows that the left hippocampus was infarcted with resulting complete degeneration of the left fornix. In addition, an infarct is seen in the posterolateral ventral nucleus of the thalamus. The corpus callosum is intact in this section. Figure 2 (section 2500) shows that the splenium is infarcted. Figure 3 (section 3200) shows the destruction of the left calcarine cortex by the infarct. No other lesions were found in the brain. It was concluded that the areas of infarction noted were all within the distribution of the left posterior cerebral artery.

## Comment

This 58-year-old man entered the hospital originally for investigation of a sensorimotor polyneuritis which was thought probably to be a complication of his diabetes. He exhibited severe postural hypotension which appeared after 15 to 20 minutes in the upright position and was thought to be a manifestation of the polyneuropathy. This may well have contributed to the acute episode of cerebral infarction from which the patient suffered. We will try to relate the lesions found

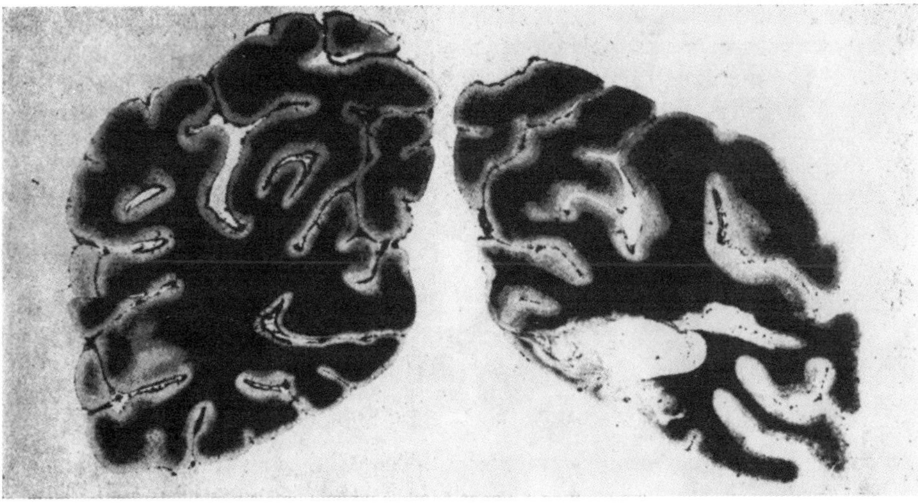

FIGURE 3. The visual cortex on the right is intact and on the left is completely destroyed (section 3200). The optic radiations are also affected. The cystic cavity on the left communicates with the posterior horn on the same side.

at postmortem to the clinical picture. In essence, we found a long-standing infarction in the distribution of the left posterior cerebral artery. The left calcarine cortex, the splenium, and the left hippocampal region were extensively involved, and there was also an infarct in the ventroposterolateral (VPL) of the left thalamus.

Certain aspects of this clinical picture cleared during our period of observation. The early general recent memory deficit and the later difficulty in topographic memory were in this category, as well as the right-sided sensory loss. It seems reasonable that the right-sided sensory loss was a neighborhood effect of the thalamic infarct seen at postmortem. We had conjectured that during his life the patient's complaint (appearing late in his course) of ill-defined vague pains over the right side of the body but sparing the face, and made worse by repeated stimulation, was an early thalamic syndrome, and this too may be attributable to the thalamic infarct which involved VPL but spared the trigeminal representation in ventroposteromedial nucleus (VPM). The early recent memory defect may have been only a nonspecific result of an acute episode or may have reflected bilateral ischemia of the medial temporal regions which produced transient but reversible damage on the right side, while leading to a permanent infarct on the left. The alternative possibility should, however, be kept in mind that an infarct of the medial temporal region on one side alone, particularly if that side is the dominant one, might itself be sufficient to cause transient recent memory disturbance despite complete normalcy of the nondominant side. The left medial temporal region might normally be most involved in verbal memory tasks since this is the side of the brain on which speech is localized. Thus, Meyer and Yates[5] and Milner[6] have shown that removal of the left temporal lobe back to 9 cm may produce a severe deficit in verbal memory, while a lesion of the right side does not have this effect. Both the findings of these earlier investigations and our own might be accounted for by assuming that the normal pathway for verbal memory is from left temporal speech areas to other areas of left temporal neocortex, lying more anteriorly which project in turn to the medial temporal region. A left medial temporal lesion would thus produce a recent memory disturbance at least for verbal material. The impairment would probably be transient since impulses from the left speech region could eventually follow an alternative route. Instead of the probable normal route, speech area to the left anterior temporal neocortex to the left medial temporal region, the following route could be taken: speech area to the left anterior temporal neocortex to the right anterior temporal neocortex (via the anterior commissure) to the right medial temporal region. We carefully checked the anterior commissure in the sections of our patient since, in its role as the major commissural connection between the temporal lobes (with the exception of the first temporal gyrus), it would play an essential role in such a compensatory mechanism. The anterior commissure was intact in our patient. Because we cannot rule out that the patient had more widespread ischemia during the acute stage, particularly of the medial temporal regions bilaterally, we can do no more than suggest the possibility of this alternative mechanism.

The difficulty in topographic memory was less transient, since it was still present more than six weeks after onset. It did, however, disappear subsequently. This might be attributable to transient damage to the posterior parietal regions which were not far from his permanent lesions. It is, however, of interest that he did not at this time show a full Gerstmann's syndrome. Another possibility is that the difficulty in topographic memory was simply a part of his more widespread recent memory deficit and had merely cleared more slowly.

The more stable deficits included the right hemianopia which is clearly the result of the infarct of the left optic radiation and calcarine cortex. The persistent complaint of distortion of the visual field was of interest and is similar to phenomena reported by other patients with posterior lesions. We did not investigate this in detail and can only comment briefly on its possible significance. Whitteridge,[7] confirming earlier suggestions by Hubel and Wiesel, and Myers, has recently brought evidence to show that the midline of the visual field is represented by a thin strip of cortex, area 18s (or juxtastriate 18). This region, unlike the primary cortical representation of the other parts of the visual field, has callosal connections; and Whitteridge has hypothesized that these fibers, running in the splenium of the corpus callosum, may serve to maintain continuity of the two visual fields and also to insure that direction of line is preserved across the vertical meridian. A lesion of the fibers of the splenium which interrupted these fibers might lead to a disruption of this mechanism so that lines crossing the vertical meridian might be distorted. For this to be operative in our patient, it would be necessary to assume that a small midline strip of the right visual field would have had to be intact. While our fields showed no gross sparing, we cannot in retrospect rule out a mild degree of such sparing. We can only mention his mechanism here with the hope that this possibility may be looked into more closely in the future.

The features which were the major objects of our interest were the reading disorder and the difficulty in color identification. The reading disorder cannot be attributed to any elementary visual disturbance, such as the distortion complained of above, since the patient correctly copied the words he could not read and because there was no difficulty in describing complex nonverbal visual arrays. The patient clearly showed the classic syndrome of pure alexia without agraphia,[3] many of whose aspects we have discussed elsewhere.[8,9] The postmortem findings of infarction of the left calcarine cortex and of the splenium coincide with the findings in Dejerine's case which have repeatedly been confirmed.

Our primary reason for presenting this patient is that he provided an especially rich opportunity for prolonged study of the difficulty in color identification, the results of repeated study of which over several months we have summarized above. Inspection of these results shows that the patient's pattern of disabilities can be summed up in one simple formula: The patient failed in all tasks in which he was required to match the seen color with its spoken name. Thus, the patient failed to give the names of colors and failed to choose a color in response to its name. By contrast, he succeeded on all tasks where the matching was either purely verbal or purely nonverbal. Thus, he could give verbally the names of colors corresponding to named objects and vice versa. He could match seen colors to each other and to pictures of objects and could sort colors without error.

By no nonverbal criterion could our patient be shown to have any deficit in color vision. In fact, a laboratory animal testable only by nonverbal means, who scored as well as our patient did on the nonverbal tasks, would clearly be accepted as having normal color vision. Our patient's perfect performance on pseudo-isochromatic tests of color vision reinforces this conclusion.

Our patient's one error on a special variant of the sorting test mentioned above is easily understood. We told the patient that a certain chip was red and to select all the other red ones. He picked up each chip and very slowly examined it. By specifying that we wanted "red" chips, we forced him to name every chip rather than simply to match to the sample chip. By misnaming a chip of one shade of green, he made an error. This error, because of the forced introduction of verbal mediation, may be called a secondary sorting error. Pick[10] referred to the possibility of this type of error. The importance of this type of error is that one must be very careful in testing for nonverbal matching or sorting not to introduce inadvertently forced verbal mediation which may lead to errors and confuse the examiner into believing that the patient had made a primary perceptual error. We suspect that some errors in sorting or matching described in the older literature may be on this basis.

One might describe the deficit as one of the naming of colors, but this might obscure the fact that the disturbance is a more widespread one since, in fact, the patient also fails to comprehend color-names under circumstances specified above. It is interesting that a similar defect occurs frequently in normal children. Thus, at the time of this study, the same tests applied to our patient were given to the four-year-old son of one of us. He also named colors incorrectly and showed incorrect comprehension of color names yet correctly sorted and matched colors and traced out the correct responses on the Ishihara test. This is not uncommon in children of this age and usually clears within a couple of years, as has indeed been the case for this child.

Color-name aphasia, as it was called, was well recognized by the classic German neurologists (as summarized by Lange[1]). There was, however, some reluctance to accept the defect as one of color-naming alone. Some of the patients made errors in matching or sorting tasks. We have already alluded to some of the difficulties in the interpretation of such tasks. Another problem was the fact that these patients commonly refuse to accept the correct name, as our patient did, or to insist as he did that the color really looks to them like the color they have mentioned and not like the correct color named by the examiner. These facts led to an assertion that these patients were manifesting an "agnosic" defect in addition to the naming defect. In order to consider this thesis, one must consider the anatomical lesions of these cases. Most typically the lesion, as first described by Dejerine[3] for his case of alexia without agraphia, destroys the left calcarine cortex and the fibers of the splenium which carry the callosal fibers of the visual regions. Thus, the left visual cortex is destroyed and the right visual region has lost its commissural connections, so that it is cut off from the speech area in the left hemisphere. This visual-verbal disconnection explains both the reading deficit and the inability to name colors or comprehend their names. It is also evident that the patient will not accept the correct name if offered to him since, if his lesion is extensive enough, he will not be able to compare the name heard in the left hemisphere with the color seen in the right hemisphere. Nor can he describe his color-vision experiences correctly since the part giving the description, i.e., the speech area, is disconnected from the part having the visual experience. It is of interest that in this situation the patient does not deny knowing the name but produces confabulatory responses. It has been pointed out elsewhere extensively that many of the so-called "agnosic" syndromes are actually produced by disconnections of primary sensory regions from speech area, with the resultant confabulatory responses.[9]

A final problem is presented by the discrepancy between color-naming and object-naming. Adolf Meyer[11] hinted at a possible mechanism. Thus, object-naming might be preserved despite the loss of reading in cases of pure alexia without agraphia because an object could arouse tactile associations further forward in the right hemisphere which could then get across the callosum over its intact portions anterior to the splenium. Written words lack tactile associations and, thus, would not reach the speech area via this roundabout route. Colors, like words, have verbal associations (their names)—but unlike objects, no tactile ones. The same explanation could account for the preserved readings of numbers[3,12] in many cases of pure alexia, since numbers have powerful tactile associations as a result of the strong tendency to count on the fingers in childhood.

The role of tactile associations in the syndrome of pure alexia without agraphia has been discussed more fully elsewhere.[9]

It is evident that our case effectively answers Critchley's[2] skepticism concerning the existence of amnestic color aphasia and would seem to go against his alternative suggestion that these cases might be accounted for on the basis of the combination of minimal dysphasia with minimal perceptual deficit. Our patient was exhaustively examined to rule out any defect in color perception, and his normal speech and the presence of only one error in object naming over months of repeated examination rules out the possibility of a general anomic aphasia. Furthermore, since the combination of a readily observable mild anomia with a visual field defect is not rare, such striking disturbances of color-naming and comprehension should be common. In fact, they are rare and are not commonly seen in such cases with mild anomias and visual field deficits, as would be demanded by Critchley's hypothesis. The close association of color-name aphasia to pure alexia without agraphia and to a highly specific anatomical lesion clearly runs against the highly nonspecific hypothesis suggested by Critchley.

We do not wish to suggest, however, that all disturbances of color identification are clinically identical with the type discussed here or result from the mechanisms we have outlined. Some of the cases with distortions of color vision (rather than with difficulties of color-naming) presented by Critchley may well be the result of complex alterations in color perception. It is clearly of great theoretical importance not to confuse such cases with the type of problem we have discussed here. Thus, Kinsbourne and Warrington[13] described a patient who had disturbances similar to those of our patient but also showed some difficulties in nonverbal matching, unlike our patient.

## Summary

A case history is presented of a patient exhibiting the syndrome of pure alexia without agraphia who also showed marked difficulties in color identification. The patient failed to name seen colors correctly and could not select a color from a group when given its name; in other words, he showed an isolated difficulty in uttering or comprehending the names of seen colors. By contrast, difficulties in color perception were ruled out by the following tests: the patient correctly matched colors by hue, despite great differences in saturation or brightness, correctly matched colored papers to uncolored pictures of objects, and performed without error on two pseudo-isochromatic tests of color vision. Verbal memory for color names was intact since he correctly named objects corresponding to named colors and named colors corresponding to named objects.

It was pointed out that the best characterization of his syndrome is "an inability to match seen colors to their spoken names."

At postmortem the patient showed the classic lesion of pure alexia without agraphia, i.e., infarction of the left calcarine cortex and of the splenium of the corpus callosum. The symptomatology is interpreted on the basis of these anatomical findings as a disconnection of the intact right visual cortex from the speech regions. Alternative interpretations are discussed. In particular, we show that the findings in our case cannot be interpreted as resulting from a minimal aphasia combined with a minimal perceptual disturbance.

## Generic and Trade Names of Drugs

Protamine Zinc Insulin Suspension—*Protamine Zinc Iletin.*
Chlorpropamide—*Diabinese.*
Cyanocobalamin—*Vitamin* $B_{12}$.

## References

1. Lange, J.: "Agnosien," in Bumke, O., and Foerster (eds.): *Handbuch der Neurologie,* Berlin: Springer Verlag OHG, 1936, vol 6, pp 807–885.
2. Critchley, M.: Acquired Anomalies of Colour Perception of Central Origin, *Brain* 88:711–724, 1965.
3. Dejerine, J.: Contribution à l'étude anatomopathologique et clinique des différentes variétés de cécité verbale, *Mem Soc Biol* 4:61–90, 1892.
4. Geschwind, N., and Fusillo, M.: Color-Naming Defects in Association With Alexia, *Trans Amer Neurol Assoc* 89:172–176, 1964.
5. Meyer, V., and Yates, H.J.: Intellectual Changes Following Temporal Lobectomy for Psychomotor Epilepsy, *J Neurol Neurosurg Psychiat* 18:44–52, 1955.
6. Milner, B.: "Laterality Effects in Audition," in Mountcastle, V. B. (ed.): *Interhemispheric Relations and Cerebral Dominance,* Baltimore: Johns Hopkins Press, 1962, pp 177–195.
7. Whitteridge, D.: "Area 18 and the Vertical Meridian of the Visual Field," in Ettlinger, G. (ed.): *Functions of the Corpus Callosum,* London: Churchill Co., 1965.
8. Geschwind, N.: "The Anatomy of Acquired Disorders of Reading," in Money, J. (ed.): *Reading Disability,* Baltimore: Johns Hopkins Press, 1962, pp 115–129.
9. Geschwind, N.: Disconnexion Syndromes in Animals and Man, *Brain* 88:237–294 and 585–644, 1965.
10. Pick, A.: "Aphasie," in Bethe, A., et al (eds.): *Handbuch der Normalen und Pathologischen Physiologie,* Berlin: Springer Verlag OHG, 1931, vol 15, pp 1416–1524.
11. Meyer, A.: Aphasia, *Psychol Bull* 2:261–277, 1905.
12. Symonds, C.P.: Aphasia, *J Neurol Neurosurg Psychiat* 16:1–6, 1953.
13. Kinsbourne, M., and Warrington, E.: Observations on Colour Agnosia, *J Neurol Neurosurg Psychiat* 27:296–299, 1964.

Dr. Julius Litter was the patient's private physician; Drs. Charles Kane and William Timberlake were in charge of the patient in different hospitalizations; Dr. Raymond D. Adams made the brain available for study; and Dr. Paul Yakovlev permitted the use of his laboratory for the preparation of the brain sections.

Some of the work reported was supported by NIH grants M-1802 and NB-6209 to Boston University.

# CHAPTER 12

# The Alexias

*D. Frank Benson and Norman Geschwind*

Alexia may be defined as an incapacity in the comprehension of written or printed words produced by a cerebral lesion. In current usage alexia refers only to acquired defects in contrast to dyslexia, a term designating an innate or constitutional inability to learn to read (Critchley 1967). This distinction has not gained universal acceptance but has become increasingly popular (Leischner 1957) and will be employed in the following discussion. The classical term "word blindness" is presently used by only a few investigators.

Many other terms have been employed to qualify the general term alexia. Most of these are best described in context with the particular symptom complex they denote, but several are used so extensively that they deserve mention here. Literal alexia indicates an inability to recognize letters while verbal alexia denotes a state in which letters are recognized but words are not. This division has been employed in many classifications such as those of Hinshelwood (1900), Brain (1961) and Hécaen (in press). The question as to whether these are truly separate entities or points on a continuum will be discussed later.

"Wortblindheit" (attributed to Kussmaul 1877) was the first widely used term describing acquired reading disturbances ("cécité verbale," commonly used by French authors and word blindness in English are exact translations). By analogy, various authors have spoken of letter blindness, mind blindness, "Seelenblindheit," "Notenblindheit," and "Zahlenblindheit." These terms are not frequently used at present, and the term word blindness has been replaced almost completely by the more general term alexia.

Early investigators stressed the presence or absence of agraphia in cases of alexia. Alexia without either agraphia or significant aphasia has often been called "pure" alexia ("reine Wortblindheit"). Several authors have asserted that there is no reported case of alexia without some other neurologic or neuropsy-

---

Reprinted with permission from P.J. Vinken and G.W. Bruyn (eds), *Handbook of Clinical Neurology. Volume 4*. Amsterdam: Elsevier Science B.V., 1969; 112-140.

chologic accompaniment (Beringer and Stein 1930; De Massary 1932) and question the use of the adjective "pure" in this disorder. For most authors, however, the word "pure" does not imply an absolutely isolated alexia but stresses that alexia dominates the clinical picture. The term "pure alexia" is thus still in use (Symonds 1953; Gloning et al. 1955) to describe alexia without significant agraphia or aphasia.

Many other terms have been used to differentiate varieties of alexia. Some are based on cortical localization (e.g. occipital or parietal alexia and even temporal and frontal alexia). Agnosia, as an explanation of alexia, has led to terms such as agnosic alexia, symbolic agnosia, and even to such combinations as subcortical visual verbal agnosia or occipital agnosic verbal alexia (Nielsen 1946). Goldstein (1948) suggested the more basic terms, primary and secondary alexia, to emphasize the absence or presence of associated aphasic disturbances. Some authors use total and partial as descriptive of the severity of alexia.

A difficulty in the assessment of the literature is the failure of some authors to differentiate the ability to read out loud from the comprehension of written material. By the definition offered in the first paragraph only failures of comprehension of written material may be designated by the term alexia. Those syndromes which may be confused with true alexia will be discussed in a later section of this chapter.

## History

Benton (1964), in his review of aphasia before the time of Broca, cites four early reports of alexia. The oldest is credited to Valerius Maximus, who, in 30 AD described a man who, after being struck on the head by an axe, lost his memory for letters but had no other defects. Mercuriale, in 1588, in describing a patient who had suffered a major seizure, noted "a truly astonishing thing; this man could write but could not read what he had written." In 1673 Johann Schmidt described two individuals with alexia, one who remained unchanged while the other responded to retraining. The last author quoted by Benton is Johann A. P. Gesner, who in 1770 described a patient with impaired reading who had more difficulty with his native German than he did with Latin. Genarin in 1838 and Trousseau in 1865 are credited by Charcot (1877) with early reports of reading disturbance in the French literature.

Despite the unique quality of these cases there was little interest in alexia until the time of Broca and the subsequent interest in the neuropathological basis of language disturbance. Even then cases of alexia were infrequently recorded, at least partially because illiteracy was still widely prevalent. Broadbent (1872) recorded a case of severe reading disability in an individual with only mild aphasic disturbances and minimal disturbance of writing. He also recorded the first postmortem findings but, since the patient had succumbed to a large intracerebral hematoma involving the left hemisphere, definitive study was impossible. Broadbent did, however, note evidence of an old infarction deep in the white matter of the parietal-occipital junction and suggested that this area was probably important for the association of visual and verbal material. Kussmaul (1877) described this same symptom complex and is credited with the first description of a right homonymous hemianopia in conjunction with alexia. Guéneau de Mussy (1879) described a patient able to read numbers, but not letters or words. Bertholle's (1881) patient suffered from asyllabia, an ability to read letters individually but not in combination. This patient read only a few words in isolation, but by spelling out each letter in the word was able to read a phrase or short sentence. Charcot (1877) reported a patient with a right visual-field defect who could read only by tracing the letter with his finger. This patient could read individual and grouped numbers but had a distinct calculation disturbance.

The study of alexia was advanced considerably by Dejerine (1891, 1892) with the publication of two clearly defined case reports including postmortem findings. The first report (1891) described a 63-year-old patient, who, eight months before death, suddenly discovered that he was no longer able to read. Examination revealed only minimal right-sided weakness and a "probable" right hemianopic visual-field defect. Verbal paraphasia was present in spontaneous speech and repetition, but there was no difficulty with object naming. The alexia was total, as was the agraphia, except for the retained ability of the patient to write his own name. One month after onset the paraphasia in speech had disappeared, but there was no improvement in reading or writing. When examined shortly before death the patient showed only slight change in the alexia (recognition of his own name and a few numbers) and no improvement in writing. The major finding at postmortem examination was an old, yellow infarct involving three quarters of the cortex of the angular gyrus and extending to the occipital horn of the lateral ventricle.

In the second paper Dejerine (1892) described an educated businessman who acutely lost the ability to read but had no evidence of aphasia, no disturbance of writing (spontaneously or to dictation), no difficulty in naming objects on visual confrontation, and no difficulty in number reading. There was a right homonymous hemianopia (he was originally seen by the ophthalmologist Landolt who published his findings in this and other cases, 1888) but no loss of ability to name colors. The patient was followed until a second vascular accident produced total agraphia in addition to the alexia, still without significant aphasic symptoms. Ten days later the patient expired and at autopsy two separate infarcts were demonstrated. One was a softening involving a major portion of the left angular gyrus, which by its pathological characteristics was of recent origin. The second was a yellowed, scarred lesion affecting the medial and inferior aspects of the left occipital lobe with additional involvement of the splenium of the corpus callosum. This older lesion lay entirely in the area supplied by the left posterior cerebral artery. Dejerine concluded that the occipital infarct had destroyed the visual pathways of the left calcarine area and the callosal lesion had severed the connections between the right hemisphere visual areas and the left hemisphere, thus isolating the left parietal cortex from its usual routes of visual stimulation. He further conjectured that the dominant angular gyrus acted as a center for the optic images necessary for written language; if this area remained intact but isolated from the visual regions, the patient retained writing skills despite severe alexia, but if the angular gyrus was destroyed, both reading and writing would be lost. The agraphia occurring shortly before death in this case was considered a result of the recent angular gyrus lesion.

Bastian (1898) supported the findings of Dejerine with several case reports and by 1900 Hinshelwood reported a series of 28 cases of "word blindness" taken from the literature and including 6 from his own practice. Thus by the beginning of the 20th century the presence of reading disturbance, both as an isolated phenomenon and in relationship with agraphia or aphasia, was well recognized and documented. In the ensuing years many cases have been added to the literature, most often in single case reports without pathological data. A myriad of neighborhood signs differing in many instances from case to case have been presented, and quite often the prominence of one of these signs has led the investigator to suggest it as the primary cause of reading disturbance itself. Thus the 20th-century literature on alexia contains many suggested theoretical mechanisms for the production of alexia.

Several comprehensive reviews of alexia have appeared since the monograph of Hinshelwood. De Massary (1932) thoroughly reviewed the French contributions to the subject but was somewhat incomplete in reports of German and English articles. Lange (1936) reviewed the German contributions. Weisenburg and McBride (1935) and Holmes (1950) have reviews in English, again suffering from inadequate reporting of foreign contributions. More recently Leischner (1957) has published a monograph on disorders of written speech which includes a good review of alexia.

Disagreements as to the underlying mechanisms of alexia have been less marked in the eastern European than in the western literature. Many good reports concerning reading disorder have emanated from the eastern European countries, almost all of which reflect the powerful influence of pavlovian thinking. Thus alexia is discussed in terms of a defect in the primary or secondary visual analyzer (Davidenkov 1956; Luria 1966), the former referring to integrative activities in the region of the primary visual cortex, while the latter indicates a separate area involved in complex visual associations. The recent work of Konorski (1967) in Poland has stressed the anatomical connections of these areas.

There are only a few reports from the Orient discussing alexia but these are significant for their comparison of phonetic script and the "Chinese" character (ideographic) type of writing. Imura (quoted by Panse and Shimoyama), Asayama (1914), and Panse and Shimoyama (1955) discuss reading disturbance in Japan where both types of writing are used and understood by most of the population. Asayama described in detail a case of alexia produced by a dominant hemisphere luetic vascular lesion that produced almost total alexia and agraphia in Kana script (a phonetic syllabic script), while there was a negligible loss of ability to handle the "Chinese" type script. This finding is supported by the other authors who note this dichotomy as the prevalent form of reading disturbance among the Japanese. They conjecture that the Kana script depends on auditory-visual (phonetic) function, more susceptible to damage in cases of aphasia than the more strongly visual "Chinese" script. A single case (Lyman et al. 1938) of an educated Chinese financier, fluent in both Chinese and English, with a surgically treated left parietal-occipital tumor indirectly supports this view by manifesting the opposite dissociation. Their case suffered severe disability in both reading and writing of Chinese characters while suffering only minimal disturbance with English written material. Their case had practically no aphasic residual, and the authors conjecture that the posterior location of the lesion produced most severe interference with the more visually oriented Chinese character script. Further studies of alexia in oriental languages would certainly be useful for both anatomical and functional theorizing.

## Classifications

The presence of variations in the symptom picture of alexia was noted even in early observations. These variations involved both the reading disorder itself and the associated neurologic and psychologic signs. These differences led to classifications based upon individual opinion as to the importance of the various findings. Leischner's (1957) monograph includes a good survey of such classifications taken from the world literature and has been used as the basis for the following presentation. (An asterisk marks the classifications taken directly from Leischner's review.)

Wernicke* proposed the following three varieties of alexia:

(1) Cortical alexia—in which both reading and writing are severely disturbed.
(2) Subcortical alexia—in which reading is impossible but writing is preserved. These patients have a right homonymous hemianopia.
(3) Transcortical alexia—which produces errors in both reading and writing while copying is preserved.

In addition, Wernicke* suggested the following separation of alexic syndromes:

(1) Literal alexia—in which the patient finds it impossible to name even a single letter and rarely comprehends a letter.
(2) Verbal alexia—in which the patient can read and recognize single letters but has great difficulty in reading words.

Weissenberg* proposed the following classification:

(1) Alexia—a loss of the ability to read letters which could be total or partial (hesitant reading with many errors).

(2) Dyslexia—in which letters are read aloud and apparently understood but can not be combined for the comprehension of words. This too can be total or partial.

It has already been noted that the term dyslexia is no longer popularly used in this manner, and most authors have preferred the terms literal and verbal alexia for the entities mentioned by Weissenberg.

Dejerine,* in a series of presentations, carefully described several varieties of alexia and introduced the following classification:

(1) Word blindness with agraphia ("cécité verbale avec agraphie"). The patient can neither read nor write, even with help of somesthetic and kinesthetic aids.
(2) Pure word blindness with preservation of spontaneous and dictated writing ("cécité verbale pure avec intégrité de l'écriture spontanée et sous dictée"). The patient cannot read, but writes to dictation or spontaneously. He cannot, however, read what he has written.

Pick (1931)* introduced a new concept in the following classification:

(1) "Störungen der Wortformfassung" (word-form blindness, defect of recognizing the appearance of a word). This occurs when the patient can no longer distinguish the form of a letter. The patient can neither read aloud nor understand when reading silently.
(2) "Störungen der Wortsinnerfassung" (word-meaning blindness, defect of comprehension of the meaning of a word). Here the patient can read words and letters aloud, but fails to recognize the meaning of what he has read.

Goldstein* simply divided alexia into primary and secondary varieties:

(1) Primary alexia—this is a comparatively isolated disturbance of reading which the author considered to be either a variety of visual agnosia or a defect in the ability to handle abstract language material.
(2) Secondary alexia—by this was meant that the alexia was part of a more complex language disturbance with major aphasic difficulties.

Hermann and Pötzl (1926)* proposed a classification based on Dejerine's:

(1) Pure word blindness without agraphia.
(2) Alexia-agraphia of the parietal type.

Kleist* suggested three types of alexia which in essence conform to Dejerine's classification:

(1) Subcortical alexia.
(2) Corticocommissural alexia.
(3) Cortical alexia.

The first two varieties have right visual-field defect and produce alexia by separation of the intact right visual cortex from the portion of the left hemisphere necessary for understanding written material, while the third type develops after damage to this left cortical area itself.

Misch and Frankl* emphasized in their classification the presence or absence of visual agnosia:

(1) Alexia accompanying a severe visual agnosia—a state in which recognition of words was lost along with all other visual recognition.
(2) Alexia as the primary symptom of an otherwise mild visual agnosia.
(3) Alexia without recognizable visual agnosia. These patients can read, but only with difficulty.

Joy* also divided reading disturbances into three varieties but utilized clinical and psychological terminology:

(1) Aphasic alexia—in which the ability to understand words is lost.
(2) Semantic alexia—in which simple words are recognized, but not more complex words.
(3) Agnosic alexia—in which the graphic symbols are not recognized (visual agnosia).

Nielsen* also used aphasic, agnosic, and semantic divisions in classifying alexia but included anatomical localization in his classification:

(1) Agnosic alexia—in which the lesion is in the dominant occipital white matter, often accompanied by a lesion in the splenium of the corpus callosum.
(2) Aphasic alexia—in which the lesion involves the angular gyrus of the dominant hemisphere.
(3) Semantic alexia—in which the lesion involves Wernicke's area of the dominant posterior temporal cortex.

Luria (1966) divided alexia into two main groups:

(1) Visual alexia—in which he defines two further subclasses, literal and verbal alexia, the former considered a variety of visual agnosia while the latter is a variant of simultanagnosia.
(2) Reading disturbances secondary to aphasic disturbances.

Brain (1961) returned to the familiar varieties of Dejerine, although with new terminology:

(1) Agnosic alexia—a failure to recognize visual symbols of speech with retention of the ability to write.
(2) Visual asymbolia—the inability to read is accompanied by difficulty in writing.

Hécaen (in press) has proposed the following classification of alexia:

(1) Aphasic alexia—the reading disturbance that accompanies Wernicke's aphasia.
(2) Alexia with agraphia—the combination of severe reading and writing disturbance in a patient with little evidence of aphasia.
(3) Alexia without agraphia—the presence of significant reading disturbance without aphasia or defect in writing. This syndrome is further subdivided into three subgroups: (a) literal alexia, (b) verbal alexia, and (c) global alexia.

Despite variation in the terminology employed, most of these classifications are remarkably similar indicating the existence of clinically distinct entities. We will use the following, simple clinical classification, loosely based upon Dejerine's original clinical descriptions:

(1) Hemialexia,
(2) Alexia without agraphia,
(3) Alexia with agraphia,
(4) Aphasic alexia,
(5) Pseudoalexia.

## Clinical forms

### Hemialexia

The presence of a unilateral reading disturbance (alexia) following section of the posterior part (splenium) of the corpus callosum has been reported by a number of investigators. The earliest such case was reported by Trescher and Ford (1937) in a patient whose posterior corpus callosum was sectioned by Walter Dandy for removal of a colloid cyst of the 3rd ventricle. These authors demonstrated that the patient was unable to recognize and comprehend words or letters presented to the left visual field alone, despite the presence of fully normal visual fields. The authors conjectured that material presented to the left visual field reached the right visual cortex but that section of the splenium had effectively separated this area from the portion of the dominant hemisphere necessary for comprehension of written symbols.

Maspes (1948) reported on six cases with posterior callosal sectioning; because of pre-operative or operative cerebral damage to four of the cases, he restricted observations to two individuals with no recognizable cerebral pathology except that produced by the callosal section. Both of these patients read and comprehended material presented to the right visual field but were unable to recognize or comprehend either words or letters presented tachistoscopically in the left visual field. More recently Gazzaniga et al. (1965), reporting several patients who had undergone complete callosal section, confirmed the earlier findings that the nondominant visual field is alexic while reading is normal in the other field. Thus there appears to be a condition of hemialexia produced by surgical sectioning of the splenium of the corpus callosum. That the same syndrome may be produced on a vascular basis is suggested by the statement of Trescher and Ford (1937) that "one of us has observed several cases of alexia on the left in elderly patients having a vascular lesion in the distribution of the posterior cerebral artery but has not had the opportunity to determine the exact site of the lesion by post-mortem examination."

There is, however, a series of reports in the literature of individuals who did not develop hemialexia after callosal sectioning. Akelaitis (1941, 1944) reported 24 cases of callosal sectioning, nine of which included the splenium. In six of these, reading was tested pre- and post-operatively, and Akelaitis reported no significant change in reading ability, thus suggesting a bilateral cortical capacity for reading. Criticism of the Akelaitis findings (Maspes 1948; Geschwind 1965) has emphasized the special character of the patient population. With only a few exceptions this consisted of patients with severe cerebral pathology, present from birth or early infancy (four of the six reported cases were left-handed secondary to early severe left-hemisphere pathology). Geschwind also suggested that the presence of life-long seizure disorder might favor the use of cerebral pathways not normally employed. By contrast the cases of Trescher and Ford (1937) and of Maspes (1948) had 3rd ventricle tumors and had not developed seizures prior to surgery. A further criticism may be advanced that the testing of reading ability by Akelaitis (1941, 1944) was inadequate. Reading was tested only by the recognition of a large block letter (4.5 cm in height) placed in one visual field and left there until a response was given. The author states that for best results the letter was placed between 2 and 10 degrees lateral to the fixation point and he fails to report any means of detecting eye movement. Thus his results are not comparable to those authors who used tachistoscopic presentation and leave open the possibility that the Akelaitis patients would also have had hemialexia if tested in this manner.

In a recent report, however, Gazzaniga and Sperry (1967) give some support to the Akelaitis view. They tested two patients who had undergone callosal sectioning by presenting single object names tachistoscopically to the left visual field only. The patients were unable to verbalize the word but pointed to the appropriate object with the left hand, demonstrating comprehension of the *written* word by the right hemisphere. A third patient, however, failed consistently in this test. The differences between the patient who failed and those who succeeded may account for the apparent differences in performance of this task. The patient who failed was entirely normal until he sustained brain injury as an adult whereas, of the two successful subjects, one was twelve years of age and the other had probably sustained brain injury in early childhood. These findings suggest that the nondominant hemisphere is capable of limited "reading" in patients with early brain damage but not if damage occurs after dominance has been well established. This agrees with experiences in cases where hemispherectomy has been performed for infantile hemiplegia. Thus, while agreeing with the observations of Akelaitis, the work of Gazzaniga and Sperry also confirms the occurrence of hemialexia in the adult following sectioning of the corpus callosum if there is no history of early brain damage or childhood seizures.

There is further evidence that reading comprehension is not present to any significant extent in the nondominant hemisphere of most adults. As will be noted later most patients suffering from alexia without agraphia have a right hemianopia plus a lesion of the corpus callosum primarily involving the splenium. Testing the patients is simple since the right visual-field defect removes problems of fixation and the necessity for use of tachistoscopic presentation. These patients are not able to point to objects presented to them with either the right or the left hand when written names are presented to them.

In summary, there is a condition in which a failure of reading comprehension (alexia) in one visual field (nondominant) follows destruction of the splenium of the corpus callosum. This is an understandably rare condition and can be termed hemialexia.

## Alexia Without Agraphia

The entity of alexia without agraphia has been recognized for many years and many reports appear in the literature, most of which consist of a single case, too often without autopsy correlation. There is great variation in the neighborhood signs which accompany the major symptoms. The constant features of all cases are the loss of the ability to read printed material with retained ability to write both to dictation and spontaneously. While the onset of this disorder is usually sudden it most often appears without other dramatic disabilities. In eight cases reported by Alajouanine et al. (1960), alexia occurred suddenly and without any significant forewarning. Occasionally the onset was accompanied by giddiness, vertigo, visual scotomata, or other symptoms referable to the posterior circulation, but more often there was no significant symptomatology at the onset. Because of this, many patients do not seek medical advice immediately and often are not seen by physicians for many months. Hinshelwood (1900) noted that as the loss of reading was the only symptom recognized by the patient, the ophthalmologist was often the first physician consulted.

The etiology of most reported cases of this type of alexia has been vascular, specifically thrombosis involving the posterior cerebral artery. There are no well-documented cases of alexia without agraphia produced by trauma or gunshot wounds, probably because the exact combination of dominant occipital and callosal lesions necessary to produce this syndrome is highly unlikely in a patient who survives major penetrating wounds. Alexia without agraphia has been produced by dominant occipital lobectomy (David et al. 1955) but in most instances has been transient, probably because the surgeon does not section the splenium in performing this procedure. The occipital lobectomy must destroy many of the fibers coming through the splenium but probably not all. Obviously if all the fiber connections traversing the splenium were destroyed, a permanent syndrome of alexia without agraphia could be anticipated.

*Clinical symptoms*

Some symptoms are frequently found accompanying alexia without agraphia, and many other symptoms are recorded in a few cases. A right homonymous hemianopia is most common, and many authors state that this is an invariable accompaniment (De Massary 1932; De Ajuriaguerra and Hécaen 1949), but there are several cases recorded in which no field defect was detected (Adler 1944; Alajouanine et al. 1960). A defect in the ability to identify colors on confrontation has been recorded in most cases. Defective ability to read musical notes or to read numbers has been recorded in many, but not all. In addition, a calculation disorder is frequently seen, and difficulty in naming objects and defect in topographical orientation are reported in some cases. Because the associated symptoms have so often led to theories concerning the mechanism of the alexia, the theories will be discussed together with the individual clinical signs. It is significant to note that paralysis, sensory loss, paresthesiae, and significant aphasia are rarely recorded and are almost never noteworthy in cases of alexia without agraphia.

*Alexia.* The most striking symptom recorded is of course the inability to read printed material. Many authors (Dejerine 1892; Hinshelwood 1900; Hécaen 1957) have divided this into two varieties, literal and verbal alexia. In addition some patients are described who were able to read letters, but unable to join them together to make syllables (asyllabia). Many authors have noted that most "pure" alexics have difficulty with both letter and word reading and that none are completely intact in one performance while failing the other and consider literal and verbal alexia as points on a continuum. Alajouanine (1951) feels that almost all alexic patients have some limitation of the ability to recognize letters, many have difficulty in orienting the letters in space or in recognizing the letters as a graphic symbol, disturbances which interfere with the visual-auditory associations needed for recognition. Frequently used letters are recognized better than infrequently used letters, often the patient's own initials being best preserved. Simply designed letters such as "I" and "O" are recognized more readily than more complex letters. Errors also occur for letters such as "P" and "R," "b," "d," "M" and "W," etc. which are frequently substituted for each other. Dejerine (1912) reported an individual who could not "read" the letters "R" and "F" until they were inscribed in a medallion signifying the French Republic at which time they were immediately recognized.

Some patients will read individual letters, place them together in syllables which are pronounced audibly and from this will decipher the word. If given adequate time, some of these patients can comprehend small quantities of written material. Usually, however, this process leads to both paralexia and omission, so that comprehension of sentences and paragraphs is almost impossible. The alexic patient is often able to read some simple, high-frequency words more readily than he can identify the component letters. Hinshelwood (1900) considered this as a separate and specific disability which he termed "letter blindness without word blindness." This condition is rarely reported now, probably because most investigators note that in fact only a few words are actually identified by these patients who thus can be considered "word blind" as well as "letter blind." There may, however, be a notable discrepancy in the ease with which an alexic handles letters and words; one patient may "name" letters while unable to "read" words while another patient may be unable to distinguish the separate letters of a word he is able to read aloud. This discrepancy has been emphasized in the recent classification of Hécaen (1957) who calls the first variety verbal alexia, the second literal alexia, and uses the term global alexia to describe the patient unable to "read" either letters or words.

It should be noted, however, that what might be considered as the syndrome of "letter blindness without word blindness" is seen frequently in aphasic patients. Thus patients with classical anomic aphasia who manifest severe difficulty in confrontation naming may be able to read words (i.e. show comprehension of written words) but may be unable to name out loud individual letters, just as they have difficulty producing the names of objects, body parts, etc. An important test of this would be matching of capital and lower case written and printed letters, which should reveal normal performance, and of course the presence of clinical aphasia excludes these individuals from the category of alexia without agraphia. We believe that these are cases of letter-naming difficulty rather than cases of literal alexia without verbal alexia and that some of the cases described in the literature as isolated literal alexia would fall within this description.

*Writing.* Most authors agree that the writing seen in alexia without agraphia is not entirely normal, but are impressed by the retention of considerable writing capacity compared to minimal reading ability. A frequent observation is that patients will write better to dictation or when asked to write a spontaneously formulated paragraph than in copying. This does not mean that they cannot copy, but this performance is slavish and often without understanding. The behavior of such a patient is like that of normals attempting to copy a meaningless design. The fact that the patient can copy exactly, although slowly, words whose meaning remains unknown to him is important in ruling out a primary perceptual disturbance and favors a disturbance in an associative mechanism. The ability to transfer written script to printed letters or to block letters is extremely difficult or impossible for the alexic patient. Even spontaneously performed writing shows certain disturbances. Many authors have noted the inability of the alexic patient to continue writing after a brief distraction. Many of these patients have difficulty in moving from one line to the next, and often the writing is slanted abnormally with the writing directed downward and to the right. Dejerine (1891) commented that the correct writing associated with poor following of printed lines resembles the written performances of a patient with acquired blindness. Purdon Martin (1954) found similar writing characteristics in an alexic patient and in normal individuals writing with their eyes closed. There are some reports of defective spelling but most authors believe that the written spelling of alexics is actually within normal limits. Adler (1944, 1950) extensively studied a single patient shortly after the onset of alexia and again five years later. There was a distinct deterioration in writing which she considered due to an inability of the patient to benefit from practice. There are, however, many other reports in which there is no deterioration of writing.

*Musical note and number reading.* There is far less agreement concerning the loss of the ability to read musical notation or the ability to read numbers. Some patients have been reported who have retained both of these abilities while totally losing the ability to read, while other patients, equally well studied, have lost one or both of these faculties. Thus the patient of Dejerine (1892) retained the ability to read numbers but lost the ability to read music. It should be noted, however, that he was still able to perform musically, both vocally and instrumentally even though he no longer read music, a situation analogous to alexia without agraphia. De Ajuriaguerra and Hécaen (1949) state that musical blindness always accompanies verbal blindness, but Bastian (1898) and others report cases of retained ability to "read" musical notation despite inability to "read" letters. This problem is complicated by the comparatively high rate of musical illiteracy in the general population and by variable, usually inadequate, testing of musical notation comprehension. It would appear that musical note reading may be lost in cases of "pure" alexia, but whether this is universally true remains a debatable point.

The ability to "read" numbers has been studied and recorded adequately in many cases. Many patients with alexia without agraphia have difficulty in "reading" numbers (Hécaen et al. 1957) but most investigators (Alajouanine et al. 1960) feel that number reading is likely to be preserved, as in Dejerine's original case (1892), suggesting as explanations that: (a) the number vocabulary is smaller and more thoroughly overlearned, and (b) the phonemic qualities of numbers are less complex than those of letters. A third explanation points out that numbers are first learned by counting on the fingers, thus producing bilateral somesthetic associations to the written numerals and that therefore alternate association pathways may be available for number reading (Geschwind 1962).

Calculating ability is often disturbed in patients with alexia without agraphia, again the severity ranging from no disturbance to total incapacity. Most authors are agreed, however, that acalculia per se is not a part of the alexic syndrome and if present suggests either a severe number-reading disturbance (De Massary 1932), a spatial orientation disability, or a combination of these. Dejerine's classic case (1892) provides a dramatic example in that his ability to read numbers and to calculate was normal despite a severe and persistent alexia.

*"Reading" by nonvisual stimulation.* (1) Somesthetic "reading." As early as 1877 Charcot reported a patient who could read only by using his finger to trace the outline of each letter, a finding that was strongly emphasized in the work of Goldstein and Gelb (1928). That this capability is not universal in alexia without

agraphia is attested by other observers (Hécaen et al. 1957; Alajouanine et al. 1960). Nonetheless, the ability of many patients to "name" a letter traced somesthetically after failure on purely visual stimulation is well documented. Similarly most patients with pure alexia can "read" anagram letters held in the hand. Patients with alexia with agraphia are unable to make use of these somesthetic stimuli. (2) Auditory "reading." The patient with alexia without agraphia readily comprehends words spelled aloud to him by the examiner and also spells aloud correctly, while patients with other varieties of alexia fail on these tasks (see later sections for further discussion of this evaluation).

*Color identification.* A fascinating and frequent accompaniment of alexia without agraphia is difficulty or even total inability to identify a color upon confrontation or to point to the proper color when the color name is offered. This defect is additionally striking because most of these patients can name objects without difficulty.

A color identification disorder was reported by Broadbent (1872), and has subsequently been reported frequently. In fact, defective color identification ranks in frequency just after alexia and right visual-field defect as a persistent finding in this syndrome. Not all cases of "pure alexia," however, show defective color identification (Quensel 1927; Davidenkov 1956; Ajax 1964).

The source of this color-identification defect remains controversial. One frequent suggestion is that this is a form of agnosia (Holmes 1950; Hécaen et al. 1957; Kinsbourne and Warrington 1964), a theory that has been discounted by others (Bay 1953; Critchley 1953; Teuber 1955). In a recent review Critchley (1965) stated that there are only a few cases of *color agnosia* recorded in the literature and that he did not feel that any of these were well studied. After further subdivision of the color identification problem, he stated ". . . it seems likely that the syndrome of *amnestic color blindness* really represents not a specific entity, but rather a very mild disorder of visual perception coupled with a minimal aphasia." This theory was critisized recently by Geschwind and Fusillo (1966). These authors presented a case of alexia without agraphia who showed complete inability to name colors on presentation or to properly select colors when the name was given. This individual could, however, accurately match colors despite marked differences in brightness and saturation and had no difficulty in the Ishihara test. Similarly he had no difficulty handling color names in a strictly verbal level (i.e. he could state the color of familiar objects such as a rose, the sky, a banana, etc). He showed no evidence of anomic disturbance in other categories. These authors suggested that their patient's color-name disability was a loss of purely visual-verbal association, similar to the reading disability, and suggesting a specific disconnection as the cause (see later section on disconnection theory). Geschwind (1967) has pointed out the difference between this syndrome and the usual aphasic anomia. Because the patient fails both in naming a color and selecting a named color, he suggests that it is best described as a failure to match a seen color and its spoken name. Recent work of De Renzi and Spinnler (1967) suggests that individuals with right brain damage have greater difficulty with nonverbal color identification tasks (color matching, Ishihara test) while those with left brain damage, as anticipated, have more difficulty in color-naming tasks. They point out, however, that their patients do not have the unique syndrome described by Geschwind and Fusillo and the possibility exists that the color-identification difficulty seen frequently in alexia without agraphia differs fundamentally from other color-naming and color-matching defects of brain-damaged patients.

*Visual agnosia.* Just as agnosia is often advanced as an explanation for the difficulties of color identification seen in alexia, it is also offered as an explanation of the alexia itself (Adler 1944; Holmes 1950; Gloning et al. 1955; Ettlinger and Hurwitz 1962). The topic of visual agnosia is complex and beyond the scope of this chapter, but does deserve comment because it has been implicated as the cause of "pure" alexia.

Unfortunately the term agnosia has been used in many different ways in the literature. Some use the term in a broad clinical sense to describe any failure in recognition tasks with preservation of elementary sensation. In this broad sense alexia can be accepted as a form of agnosia. Many investigators, however, also use the term agnosia as an explanation or mechanism for a specific behavioral abnormality, defective symbol recognition. In some cases this is only circular thinking, i.e., alexia is a form of agnosia and is therefore caused by agnosia. Others use the term agnosia to designate a disturbance of higher-level perceptual functions, i.e., they use the term agnosia for the disability that Lissauer (1889) designated "apperceptive mind blindness" and suggest that alexia is based on this difficulty. This is open to question, however; most alexics can copy adequately (an act that would seem to demand perceptual integrity). Furthermore, there are reports of patients with severe object-identification difficulties who can read (Davidenkov 1956). Quite possibly there are alexics with an apperceptive form of agnosia (Gloning et al. 1955) but this does not appear to be a factor common to most cases. Finally, some investigators consider alexia to be an agnosia of the associative type (in the terminology of Lissauer), i.e., a loss of the usual associations of the seen name. Thus agnosia as presently used appears too vague for the explanation of alexia unless the process producing this state is well described.

Some authors describe alexia as an agnosic phenomenon in a different sense, arguing that the difficulty in reading is part of a more widespread difficulty in visual identification. There are some recorded cases of alexia which have been accompanied by additional findings of defective visual recognition. A good example is the case of Adler (1944) in which the patient had alexia with minimal writing disturbance plus inability to identify objects, pictures of objects, faces, and geometric shapes. In this situation the inability to "recognize" letters and/or words can be considered part of an overall defect in symbol recognition, although the precise mechanism of this defect remains obscure. It is well recognized, however, that many cases do not have this combination of findings; some patients are alexic without agnosia and others agnosic without alexia (Hécaen et al. 1957). In this respect two cases reported by Davidenkov (1956) are illustrative. The first patient, following a vascular accident, was able to read and write but could not recognize (name) common objects on visual presentation but readily named these objects when he was allowed to touch them. The second individual lost the ability to read, although he retained full capacity for writing and had only minimal difficulty in naming objects (or colors) visually presented. Davidenkov emphasized that the first case was one of visual agnosia and was quite distinct from the second, a case of pure alexia with minimal evidence of "visual agnosia." The opinion offered by Davidenkov is shared by many other investigators who have noted that recognition (naming) of visually presented objects is retained in most cases of alexia without agraphia. Thus, while pure alexia and visual agnosia (in the sense of difficulty in identification of nonverbal visual material) certainly can coexist, they may also occur separately.

In summary, we feel that the term agnosia is not useful as an explanation for the occurrence of alexia without agraphia and that its use should be restricted to those cases which show widespread difficulties in visual identification, including the comprehension of written material.

*Defective Gestalt formation.* Some authors argue that alexic patients suffer from a defect in Gestalt formation, an inability to combine the parts into a whole. With this disorder the patient is able to recognize parts of the written material but unable to combine them into a meaningful whole or, vice versa, reads words without being able to isolate (read) letters. This explanation was particularly stressed by Wolpert (1924, 1930), Goldstein and Gelb (1928), Brain (1941), and Adler (1944). Unfortunately the Gestalt theory neither defines nor explains the disturbances underlying alexia. Furthermore, many patients with right hemisphere lesions seem to have difficulty in uniting parts into a whole but reading is usually less markedly disturbed than other visual functions in these patients, suggesting that defective Gestalt formation is not a basic mechanism in the production of alexia.

*Simultanagnosia.* Several authors (Wolpert 1924; Davidenkov 1956; Luria 1959; Kinsbourne and Warrington 1962b) have reported patients manifesting reading disability ("spelling dyslexia") who are able to describe a single item from a complex picture but not other items in the picture, and thus cannot recognize the story portrayed by the entire picture. This has been called simultanagnosia or a disorder of simultaneous form perception. The patients described were able to "read" single letters and thus laboriously decipher simple words but were both slow and liable to erroneous guessing (paralexic substitutions). The obvious similarity between identification of a single portion of a complex picture and a single letter of a word was duly noted and the "spelling dyslexia" was considered a natural consequence of simultanagnosia. Through tachistoscopic presentation of both single and double forms, Kinsbourne and Warrington (1962b) demonstrated that their patients with this disorder were unable to identify more than a single stimulus. They also demonstrated a need for a minimum of one second between exposures of two different forms for these to be properly identified by such patients. These authors suggested that these two observations were sufficient to "explain" simultanagnosia and spelling dyslexia and suggested dominant anterior occipital localization. This inviting theory cannot be considered in most cases of alexia without agraphia, however, as most reports describe no such defect in the comprehension of complex pictures and do not show "spelling dyslexia." This latter point is best demonstrated by the ability of many alexic patients to copy an entire word without identifying either the letters or the word. Thus simultanagnosia can be considered a source of alexia without agraphia, but only in selected cases.

*Eye-movement disorder.* Several authors have noted disturbances of eye movements in patients with reading difficulty. Luria (1966) includes a careful study of eye movements in his tests of reading ability. Beringer and Stein (1930) reported an individual who would read one or two words, stop, blink his eyes, and then read several more words. In addition, this patient had extreme difficulty in changing from one line of print to the next. The authors suggested that the reading disturbance was due to a combination of visual defect (right hemianopia) producing a need for increased stimulation of remaining visual tissue and an increased refractory phase of the remaining retinal tissue. The authors believed that with visual stimulation there would be slow and uneven stimulation of the visual cortex, abnormal motor response (eye-movement disorder), and subsequent reading difficulty. Warrington and Zangwill (1957) present a single case, unable to read words, but capable of reading individual letters. This patient had a persistent right visual-field defect, distinct abnormalities of saccadic and searching eye movement,s plus a tendency to read correctly the left portion of a multisyllable word and to guess the remainder (e.g., "them" for "these," "manager" for "management"). They considered that eye-movement disorder could produce a disability in word reading, but did not explain difficulties in letter reading, which they considered a true agnosia (defect in symbolic recognition). This theory fails to explain the absence of alexia in patients with severe paralysis of ocular movement. Although disturbances of eye movements do occur in some cases of alexia, it would appear logical that alexia itself could produce abnormal eye movements just as visual scanning of an unfamiliar form is less regular than the visual movements used to scan a familiar object. Thus the possibility must be raised that the alexia produces eye-movement irregularities rather than vice versa.

*Asthenopic alexia.* Pötzl (1928) describes a specific type of alexia without agraphia seen in patients who have had vision restored surgically after prolonged blindness. He termed this asthenopic alexia and noted that this was always a transient state. These patients can read for only a brief period and then must rest before reading further.

*Geometric form agnosia. Spatial disorientation.* A number of patients with alexia without agraphia have shown abnormality of spatial perception. That this is not constantly seen was pointed out by Charcot (1887) and Dejerine (1892), but the role of spatial perception disturbance as an etiologic factor in reading disturbances must be considered. Purdon Martin (1954) suggested that many alexic patients have defective visual-spatial perception. These patients have difficulty in drawing a line between dots or in defining the relationship of two lines. This author noted the similarity in these performances to those of a patient with a refractive error who would be unable to read without his glasses and whose performance in spatially oriented drawing tasks would be grossly hampered. Gloning et al. (1955) described a right-handed individual who suffered a right occipital lesion and subsequently had "pure word blindness," visual-spatial agnosia, constructional apraxia, and inability to read a clock. They considered that the reading disturbance in their case was caused by the severe visual-spatial agnosia and was not, therefore, the same as the alexia noted with left occipital defect. Adler (1944) also reported a marked geometric visual difficulty in her patient, but concluded that this, as well as the alexia, was on the basis of a figure-ground disturbance. Geschwind and Fusillo (1966) reported a case of alexia without agraphia who originally showed disorientation in space but recovered from this completely while the alexia persisted.

### *Pathology*

Despite the large number of cases quoted in the previous paragraphs, alexia without agraphia remains an uncommon condition, although reported more frequently than pure word deafness or isolated agraphia. Most papers in the literature report only a single case. One of the authors (F.B.) has observed only a single case of "pure" alexia in somewhat over 1,000 consecutively evaluated cases of language disturbance. Thus most neurologists, even those with large clinical practices and specialized interest in higher cortical dysfunction, cannot anticipate seeing more than a few cases of alexia without agraphia in a lifetime of practice.

The rare occurrence of this syndrome is amply substantiated by the infrequent appearance of autopsied cases of alexia without agraphia. Table 1 lists 17 cases taken from the literature, each with a clinical diagnosis of alexia without agraphia and a description of the neuropathology. Unfortunately the completeness of both clinical and pathological reports varies widely; the omission of at least some pertinent information in one or both categories occurs in many of the cases. Nonetheless, the basic clinical picture appears solidly established in each case and sufficient pathological data are included to offer useful comparisons. The pathological findings will be discussed under three headings: occipital, corpus callosum, and other involvement.

*Occipital.* With only one exception the left occipital lobe was involved in all cases. In the exceptional case (Gloning et al. 1955) the right occipital lobe was involved, but the authors strongly suggest that the reading disturbance in this case was produced by visual-spatial distortion and is not the same as that seen in "pure word blindness" produced by left occipital pathology. The description of the area involved is somewhat variable but usually includes the inner and under

TABLE 1. Published cases of alexia without agraphia with autopsy findings.

| | | |
|---|---|---|
| 1. Landolt | 1888 | Old cystic lesion involving the inferior portion of the left occipital lobe. Recent hemorrhagic lesion in the corpus callosum. |
| 2. Dejerine | 1892 | Old lesion in left occipital lobe and splenium of corpus callosum. Fresh lesion in left angular gyrus. |
| 3. Redlich | 1895 | Lesion involving left calcarine, lingual, and fusiform cortex, splenium, and posterior thalamus. |
| 4. Lissauer<br>Brissaud | 1889<br>1900 | Degeneration in left medial occipital lobe and splenium. |
| 5. Hahn | 1895 | Softening in left calcarine region, splenium and right tapetum. |
| 6. Dide and Botcazo | 1902 | Bilateral lesions of lingual gyrus. |
| 7. Hinshelwood and MacPhail | 1904 | Old lesion, left calcarine fissure. |
| 8. Paterson and Bramwell | 1905 | Lesion in the distribution of the left posterior cerebral artery including connections of the right visual areas with left angular gyrus. |
| 9. Bonvicini and Pötzl | 1907 | Two lesions in the left occipital cortex which enclosed an apparently intact calcarine cortex. |
| 10. Pötzl | 1928 | Destruction of left lingual, fusiform and part of cuneus, some degeneration in left parietal and temporal lobes, destruction of part of corpus callosum. |
| 11. Ehrenwald | 1929–30 | Old lesion involving the left lingual gyrus. |
| 12. Kleist | 1934 | Inner and under surface of left occipital lobe, small right occipital lesion with callosal degeneration. |
| 13. Niessl Von Mayendorff | 1935 | Left lingual and fusiform gyri, cuneus, precuneus, and tapetum. |
| 14. Gloning et al. | 1955 | Right occipital (lingual, fusiform, and lower cuneus) splenium and posterior thalamus. Recent left frontal and minimal left occipital necrosis. |
| 15. Geschwind and Fusillo | 1966 | Left calcarine region, splenium of corpus callosum, VPL of left thalamus, and left hippocampal region. |
| 16. Gloning et al. | 1966, case 1 | Meningioma, deep into left medial occipital lobe with considerable surrounding degeneration. |
| 17. Gloning et al. | 1966, case 2 | Cystic lesions in left lingual and fusiform gyri and splenium. |

surface of the occipital lobe, essentially the area directly dependent upon the posterior cerebral artery for vascular supply. Most often the lingual and part or all of the fusiform lobe are infarcted along with varying portions of the cuneus and the calcarine cortex. One report (Bonvicini and Pötzl 1907) stated that the calcarine cortex appeared intact, although surrounded by infarcted cortex. Dide and Botcazo (1902) and Kleist (1934) describe bilateral occipital infarction, but the remainder describe unilateral involvement.

*Splenium of the corpus callosum.* Infarction or "involvement" of the corpus callosum or of the "connection of the right visual area" is described in nine of the fifteen brains. This does not mean, however, that actual infarction was not present in the other cases. Infarction in the tightly packed white matter of the splenium may not produce the grossly obvious degenerative changes that are seen after involvement of cortical and subcortical tissues. One of the present cases (Geschwind and Fusillo 1966) was sectioned by a highly experienced neuropathologist who reported no evidence of corpus callosum infarction on gross inspection. Sections stained for myelin demonstrated, however, a pronounced destruction of the splenium. This does not mean, however, that an infarct of the splenium is essential for production of the syndrome of alexia. Several authors (Kleist 1917; De Ajuriaguerra and Hécaen 1949) have suggested that deep white-matter destruction in the left medial occipital region could just as readily disconnect the left-hemisphere language areas from right-visual sensory stimuli.

*Additional involvement.* In addition to the universal presence of occipital pathology and frequent splenium involvement in cases of alexia without agraphia, several areas of inconstant involvement are mentioned. Most of these structures fall within the area of distribution of the posterior cerebral artery. Thus some cases showed posterior thalamic or hippocampal infarction (producing thalamic pain or disturbance of recent memory). Three had parietal softening although in two of these the parietal lesion occurred later than the occipital involvement. Most authors report that the remainder of the brain and brainstem were free of significant pathology. Thus the only consistently demonstrated pathology involves the dominant occipital lobe and the connections of the nondominant visual association area with the dominant speech areas.

All of the reports listed in the table describe medial-inferior occipital involvement but a number of postsurgical cases of alexia without agraphia secondary to lateral parieto-occipital pathology have been recorded (Warrington and Zangwill 1957; Kinsbourne and Warrington 1964; Ajax 1967). The pathology in these cases was diverse including tumor, A-V malformation, and intracerebral hematoma. The exact depth of occipital involvement remains unknown as no postmortem follow up is available. As could be expected this type of case has a greater number of demonstrable neurologic side effects (mild aphasia, mild agraphia) but does show a distinct reading disturbance. Clinically these cases more closely resemble the cases of alexia without agraphia following dominant occipital lobectomy reported by David et al. (1955). The surgical cases, however, have either been transient or when persistent the reading disturbance has been mild. It is worth noting, however, that even following recovery of reading ability the surgical patients usually dislike the reading process. It would be possible to suggest that the fundamental pathology in these cases is also in the medial-inferior occipital region but this can not be confirmed by the available material. The possibility of a second anatomical localization for the production of reading disturbance without agraphia can be raised but at best must remain conjectural until better clinical and pathological proof is presented.

*Theoretical considerations*

Many of the symptoms associated with alexia without agraphia discussed above have also been suggested as possible causes of the alexia. These include visual agnosia, simultanagnosia, defective Gestalt formation, eye-movement disorder, and visual-spatial disorientation; inasmuch as these have already been discussed, they need not be reiterated, but one theory, that of *disconnection,* has not been brought forward and deserves additional attention.

Several authors have suggested that alexia without agraphia is produced by separation of two essential cortical areas (Dejerine 1892; Hinshelwood 1900; Nielsen 1946; and more recently Geschwind 1962, 1965). These investigators have suggested that alexia seen without other major language disturbances represents an inability to transfer visually perceived language stimuli to an area in the left hemisphere involved in interpretation of visual language (angular gyrus). This theory was advanced by Dejerine (1892) who pointed out that the primary visual area in the left hemisphere is damaged (thus causing the right visual-field defect) and that in addition there was destruction of connections from the right visual region (either by a lesion in the corpus callosum or in the white matter deep to the left parietal-occipital region) which effectively disconnects the dominant angular gyrus from the visual association areas of both sides. This theory proposes that the area for written language interpretation is intact, thus the patient can recognize spelled words and can spell accurately both orally and in writing. The separation of this area from visual stimuli not only produces alexia but also can cause a color-identification disturbance which is also dependent on pure visual-verbal associations. Most of these patients, however, retain object-naming ability and many can correctly "read" numbers, possibly through other pathways available for these visual associations.

## Alexia With Agraphia

The clinical syndrome and pathology of alexia with agraphia were presented by Dejerine (1891) whose case manifested almost total inability to read, limited writing ability, but only minimal aphasia and calculation disturbance. At postmortem examination Dejerine found a yellowed plaque confined to the angular gyrus on the left side with penetration into the white matter. Dejerine stressed that this syndrome must be carefully distinguished from "pure word blindness" (i.e., alexia with no difficulty in writing). The clinical picture of alexia with agraphia has been described many times since the work of Dejerine and most investigators have agreed that the angular gyrus is essential for the functions of reading and writing (Wolpert 1930; Nielsen and Raney 1938; Alajouanine et al. 1960).

This entity was also seen frequently before the time of Dejerine's lucid clinical description. For example, Starr (1889) collected 50 cases of "sensory aphasia" from the world's literature, 21 of which had proved angular gyrus lesions at autopsy. All of these had demonstrable alexia. Unfortunately many of the examiners had not recorded or tested writing, but whenever tested, writing was also noted to be abnormal, and the occurrence of both reading and writing disturbance following damage to the dominant angular gyrus was well accepted by that early date.

Alexia with agraphia has been designated by many other terms. Some authors speak of this symptom complex as "parietal alexia" (Quensel 1927; Pötzl 1927; Hoff et al. 1954); in the classification of Kleist (1934) mentioned previously, this entity was called "cortical alexia." Other authors (Nielsen 1946; Alajouanine et al. 1960) have considered this syndrome as one of a group called "aphasic alexia." A number of authors have pointed out that alexia with agraphia is a total defect in the use of written or printed symbols and have claimed that this suggests a "language defect" rather than a perceptual defect.

*Clinical symptoms*

There is greater variation in the clinical picture of this syndrome than in alexia without agraphia. Many cases begin acutely with sudden loss of the ability to read and write as a result of an acute infarction. This disorder has also been reported with neoplastic disease and following trauma; there are several fairly large series secondary to war wounds (Marie and Foix 1917; Poppelreuter 1917). Alexia with agraphia has been described on the basis of an A-V malformation (Casey and Ettlinger 1960) and tumors with left parieto-occipital localizations. While a variety of etiologies may produce this syndrome, most authors agree that involvement of the dominant angular gyrus is a constant finding. The wide variation in pathological causation contrasts significantly with alexia without agraphia (the permanent cases of which are nearly all of vascular origin) and helps make alexia with agraphia a far more common entity.

The clinical onset of alexia with agraphia may be insidious or quite acute. Almost invariably there are neighborhood clinical signs of significance. If the onset is acute, the patient will usually show a mild paresis and some degree of sensory loss. The paresis clears, either completely, or at least to the point where only minimal weakness is demonstrable, but in many cases a significant sensory disturbance involving the right side of the body remains. Almost all patients suffering alexia with agraphia have some degree of aphasia which ranges from a minimal degree of word-finding difficulty to a more marked sensory aphasia with paraphasia and comprehension disturbance. It should be emphasized, however, that the term alexia with agraphia, can be used only when the reading and writing disturbances are distinctly more severe than any other aphasic difficulties. In addition, the findings of the Gerstmann syndrome are often present. A right homonymous visual-field defect may be present, but there are many reports (De Massary 1932) where this sign is absent and it is clearly a less constant finding than in alexia without agraphia.

*Alexia.* The loss of the ability to read is almost invariably severe in cases of alexia with agraphia. The reading disturbance usually includes words, letters, numbers and musical notes, although there are some exceptions to the latter two categories (e.g., Casey and Ettlinger 1960). Not only is number reading frequently disturbed, but very often there is a severe calculation defect so that the patient cannot handle numerical computation even when the problem is given verbally and a verbal response is requested, a notable contrast with the usual situation in alexia without agraphia. Dejerine (1892) and De Ajuriaguerra and Hécaen (1949) point out that patients with this type of alexia are unable to trace letters or numbers with their finger and understand the symbol. While this capacity is not consistently preserved in "pure alexia," these authors emphasize that the recognition of letters or numbers as meaningful symbols regardless of modality of presentation is invariably disturbed in cases of alexia with agraphia. The difficulty in somesthetic "reading" is parallelled by difficulty in auditory "reading" (i.e., the inability to understand spelled words).

*Agraphia.* As the name suggests, writing disturbance is a distinct part of alexia with agraphia, but there is considerable disagreement as to the severity of the writing disturbance. Dejerine and many subsequent French investigators have stated that writing is less disturbed than reading. Other authors, however, find that reading and writing disturbances are approximately equivalent so that the individual who is able to read a few letters or a few words will also write a few letters or a few words. The writing disturbance is usually not so severe that the patient is unable to produce letters, but the writing is always paragraphic, consisting of recognizable letters combined into unrecognizable words. While these patients spontaneously produce correct letters, they are most often unable to produce letters upon dictation or will be paragraphic in this situation. These patients often show significant disturbances in copying printed material, in contrast to patients with alexia without agraphia who copy slowly and slavishly but correctly, while the alexic with agraphia will often reproduce the actual forms of the letters incorrectly.

*Gerstmann syndrome.* In addition to a calculation defect which appears on verbal testing and thus goes beyond the inability to read and write numbers, these patients often show the other findings making up the Gerstmann syndrome (Gerstmann 1930). Thus many patients with alexia with agraphia have difficulty in right-left orientation and difficulty in naming fingers or recognizing them by name, along with agraphia and acalculia. These symptoms are not invariably present and are, in fact, rarely mentioned in the literature. Our own experience has been that most patients showing the syndrome of alexia with agraphia will have an associated Gerstmann syndrome.

*Related symptomatology.* Many of these patients show other symptoms which are seen frequently in conjunction with the Gerstmann syndrome. Thus most of these patients have some form of constructional disturbance, showing distinct difficulty in copying drawings, performing match stick designs or Koh's Block Designs. Topographic memory disturbance (Critchley 1953) is not infrequent even when evaluated in a purely visual (nonverbal) manner. Many cases have been reported showing inability to recognize or locate an area on an outline map. It has been our experience, however, that most of these patients are oriented in their own and even new environments, and severe spatial disorientation is not a frequent accompaniment of this type of alexia.

*Aphasia.* Some form of aphasia is almost constant with this syndrome and, as noted above, is most pronounced if the onset is acute. The aphasia is fluent and in most cases the aphasic disturbance is mild, consisting primarily of somewhat empty speech with word finding pauses, difficulties in naming, usually in association with good repetition, and auditory comprehension. In other words, these patients often manifest a mild anomic type of aphasia. In the classification of alexia proposed in this chapter, individuals with severe aphasic disorders are considered as suffering from aphasic alexia rather than alexia with agraphia. Thus for a patient to be included under the term alexia with agraphia he must show much greater disturbance in reading and writing capacities than in spoken language functions. Some authors (De Ajuriaguerra and Hécaen 1949) believe that alexia with agraphia is always accompanied by a distinct disturbance of inner speech mechanisms. We have seen, however, many patients with severe reading and writing disturbance who are not functionally disabled in spoken language capability, despite the presence of mild aphasic symptoms.

*Spelling.* Geschwind (1962) and Howes (1962) have laid great stress on the inability of these patients to comprehend words spelled aloud by the examiner despite the presence of otherwise excellent auditory comprehension. The reverse task, the spelling of words out loud is also severely defective. This is in sharp contrast to the patients with alexia without agraphia who generally have little difficulty in either of these functions. Thus we believe that an excellent ancillary test for this particular variety of alexia is to ask the patient to spell aloud or to identify a series of words spelled aloud by the examiner. Of course cases with more significant aphasic defects, particularly of the sensory aphasia variety, will also fail this test, but in this situation the spoken language disturbance is sufficiently prominent to explain the failure in the spelling tasks.

Some investigators regard this difficulty in comprehending words spelled aloud as evidence of a mild degree of auditory comprehension difficulty, but this view is difficult to maintain in the face of evidence that patients with this disorder may show absolutely normal comprehension for long and complex sentences. Other authors (Symonds 1953) regard this as a specialized auditory comprehension defect which they call "letter-name deafness." We believe that a simpler explanation is available. As noted earlier, the alexic without agraphia is able to "read" when letters are presented tactilely or auditorily, while the alexic with agraphia fails in both these situations. The alexic with agraphia is in fact much like a patient returned to a state of illiteracy. One might almost say, by analogy to discussions of "inner speech," that "inner reading" is preserved in alexia without agraphia but lost in alexia with agraphia. The ability to comprehend orally spelled words requires ability to turn the heard letters into their visual form, an ability never acquired by the illiterate and lost in alexia with agraphia.

*Paralexia.* In some patients with long-standing alexia with agraphia an unusual form of paralexia may be noted. These patients are unable to comprehend most written material. Occasionally, however, when attempting to read aloud, they will produce responses which show comprehension of the word. These responses are often paraphasic substitutions. Thus one of our patients read the word "kitten" as "a small cat." When asked to read the word "livingroom" she said, "Oh, I know what that is, it is the place we go after dinner to watch TV." It should be stressed that this patient had a significant defect of naming (word finding) on visual confrontation. It appears possible that certain written words aroused visual images which were then named paraphasically. Obviously this type of "reading" is possible only for picturable words and she was unable to respond to written prepositions, most verbs, and abstract nouns (e.g., liberty, truth, etc.). Also, the stock of correct responses was limited and had taken many years to develop so that this individual, while comprehending a few written words, would still be considered alexic.

### *Pathology*

Dejerine (1891) reported postmortem findings of an old, yellowed infarct involving about three quarters of the left angular gyrus as the only significant pathological finding. From this base the author surmised that the angular gyrus was essential for the optic recall of written letters and that damage to this structure produced both alexia and agraphia. This pathological localization has been almost universally confirmed, and it is generally accepted that destruction of the dominant angular gyrus will cause significant disturbance in both reading and writing (Wolpert 1930; De Massary 1932).

### *Theoretical considerations*

Several interpretations have been placed on this syndrome. It is difficult to accept the notion that this is simply a more severe degree of alexia without agraphia, since the differences in clinical picture and pathology militate against the notion that these are disturbances distributed on a continuum. It is also not possible to accept the idea that this is simply a portion of a more widespread aphasic syndrome, since the reading and writing disturbances may clearly dominate the clinical picture. Dejerine (1891) felt that this syndrome resulted from an actual lesion of the cortical center for written words. The effect of the lesion may be roughly considered as reducing the patient to a state of illiteracy. In what way does the angular gyrus subserve this function? Although it is clear that it is a vital link in the process of reading, this does not clarify the fundamental activity of this region. The suggestion has been made recently (Geschwind 1965) that the angular gyrus plays a major role in the formation of associations between vision, somesthesis, and audition and thus is basic to the visual-auditory associations involved in reading. While the theoretical problems remain unsettled clinical experience clearly demonstrates the important status of the dominant angular gyrus in written language function in that significant angular gyrus damage can produce both alexia and agraphia with comparative sparing of spoken language function.

## Aphasic Alexia

Most investigators of aphasic syndromes have described reading disturbance associated with aphasia. Many agree with De Massary (1932) who stated that significant aphasic symptoms may produce so much disturbance of language that reading is secondarily involved. He concluded that such cases belong properly in a classification of aphasia and not in an outline of alexia. Nonetheless, certain characteristic reading disturbances are present in some forms of aphasia and will be outlined briefly. It should be noted that one of the greatest difficulties in outlining the aphasic alexias stems from the diverse classifications of aphasia. Most of these classifications actually describe the same or significantly similar symptom complexes but use different terminologies. We have elected to use the terminology presently in use in our unit, modified from the classic outlines of the early continental investigators.

### *Wernicke's aphasia*

In this type of aphasia the patient does not understand spoken language or shows severe defect in comprehension of spoken words. His speech is usually fluent, but filled with paraphasia. Repetition of spoken language is severely disturbed, and most patients with this type of aphasia have extreme difficulty in producing names of objects on confrontation. These patients have an alexia accompanied by agraphia of a variety similar to that described under the category of alexia with agraphia, in other words a sprawling paragraphic output made up of real letters combined in an incorrect manner. The defects in reading and writing are generally of the same order of magnitude as those seen in producing and comprehending spoken language.

It is generally accepted that the pathology producing Wernicke's aphasia is located in the posterior superior temporal lobe of the dominant hemisphere. This area lies directly adjacent to the angular gyrus and shares at least some of the same vascular supply. Thus it would be easy to conjecture that the alexia and agraphia seen with Wernicke's aphasia is secondary to involvement of the angular gyrus by the same pathological process. It is true that such pathological involvement is present in many cases. There is, however, reasonable evidence that angular gyrus involvement is not essential and that posterior superior temporal pathology alone can produce severe alexia. Nielsen (1939) presented 16 cases, primarily collected from the literature, with clinically significant alexia who at postmortem had dominant temporal lobe infarction without involvement of the angular gyrus. Each of these individuals, of course, demonstrated the other features of Wernicke's aphasia.

There is a further argument against the theory that the alexia and agraphia of Wernicke's aphasia are secondary to extension of the lesion to the angular gyrus.

This theory would carry the implication that the full syndrome of Wernicke's aphasia actually consisted of separate components. It is, however, a commonplace of clinical experience that while alexia with agraphia may be seen in relative isolation, rarely or never does one see severely fluent and paraphasic speech together with auditory comprehension disturbance in the absence of alexia and agraphia.

The lesion producing Wernicke's aphasia lies in a region of auditory association cortex. Wernicke (1874) felt that the syndrome was not a mixture of separable components but that all the elements resulted from a lesion of the area subsequently given his name. It should be noted that the area described by Wernicke was confined to the posterior superior temporal region. Some recent authors (e.g., Penfield and Roberts 1959) have tended to enlarge Wernicke's area to include all the retrorolandic speech regions. This nomenclature is, however, not justified historically, and appears not to coincide with either anatomical or clinical data. Wernicke argued that language is initially acquired auditorily in the great majority of mankind and that subsequent acquisition of visual language is by reference to this initial auditory acquisition. This would correspond with the clinical data that visual language may be disturbed in isolation by a lesion which prevents visual-auditory associations to be made, while lesions in the cortical areas involved in this auditory learning will affect all modalities of language.

*Pure word deafness*

By definition the patient with this disorder is able to read with little or no difficulty, whereas he does not understand spoken language. Similarly the patient with pure word deafness has at most mild difficulty in speech or writing, although at times he may have slightly paraphasic speech, and some paragraphic errors may be present in his writing. The classically accepted lesion for this entity lies deep in the dominant posterior temporal lobe separating the auditory association cortex from Heschl's gyrus but not involving the cortex itself or bilateral lesions in the middle of the superior temporal gyrus (Gloning et al. 1963).

*Broca's aphasia*

Loss of the ability to read is not anticipated in this type of aphasia, one in which the patient has no apparent difficulties with comprehension of spoken language. Many investigators, however, have noted reading disturbance in cases of Broca's aphasia (Nielsen 1938; Goldstein 1948; Leischner 1957). Nielsen labeled this as "one of the unsolved problems of aphasia" when describing ten cases taken from the literature, each with Broca's aphasia secondary to a purely frontal lobe lesion, as demonstrated by autopsy and each said to be alexic. Review of the cases quoted by Nielsen is disappointing, however, as the evidence documenting loss of reading ability was poor. Several of the cases lacked evidence of premorbid ability to read (an important factor in the 19th century when illiteracy was common), and in others the ability to read aloud was not distinguished from reading comprehension. Certainly none of the cases quoted had the extensive clinical evaluation given to the patients with alexia mentioned thus far.

We would surmise that most cases reported as alexic with Broca's aphasia are explained in one of the following ways: (a) the patient was illiterate, (b) the patient was unable to read aloud, or (c) the patient suffered multiple lesions, one of which was posterior. We cannot exclude that true alexia may exist with a purely anterior lesion but evidence for this occurrence is not convincing. The possibility exists that a transient alexia may be present after frontal damage as a secondary effect of transient visual inattention such as described by Kennard (1939) and Welch and Stuteville (1958) in animals. Another possibility was raised by Charcot (1887) who thought that the poorly literate would be more likely to read aloud and could thus be expected to become alexic with onset of a Broca's aphasia. This theory has not, however, been subjected to careful investigation and remains unconfirmed.

We have had a limited experience with reading difficulties in patients with Broca's aphasia. Some of these patients had evidence for additional posterior lesions. In others the disturbance of reading was not entirely similar to that seen in the other forms of alexia. It was found that these patients could, in fact, comprehend written material but did so with tremendous difficulty, often needing several minutes to "read" a ten or twelve word sentence. These patients disliked reading, considering it very hard work, but most of them, if directly questioned, stated that they were able to read, a view confirmed by formal testing. It would thus appear that the clinical evaluation of such patients demonstrates preserved reading comprehension. At present there is no adequate explanation for the slowness and dislike of reading in some patients with Broca's aphasia.

*Transcortical aphasia (isolation of the speech area)*

This rare entity is characterized by the presence of normal or near normal ability to repeat spoken language coupled with severe auditory comprehension defect and grossly abnormal expressive speech. Of the few patients described in the literature with this disorder (Goldstein 1917; Geschwind et al. in press) all have been totally alexic and agraphic. It was theorized by Goldstein that in the isolation syndrome, the auditory area of the posterior superior temporal region, the motor speech area in the posterior inferior frontal region and fibers connecting these two areas are intact but are, in essence, isolated from the remainder of the cortex, a view confirmed by the pathological findings of Geschwind et al. Thus while the patient is able to repeat words and phrases that he hears, he does not comprehend them as words and is totally unable to recognize or comprehend printed material.

*Conduction aphasia*

This type of aphasia, originally, although incompletely, defined by Wernicke (1874), is not rare. The patient is able to comprehend spoken language, but unable to repeat correctly what he hears. In our own experience we note that these patients have a haltingly fluent speech, many literal paraphasias, good comprehension of spoken language, poor ability to name on confrontation, and marked disturbance of repetition. In addition they cannot read aloud, but the great majority comprehend written material readily. Thus we have seen patients who cannot read a simple four- or five-word newspaper headline out loud but are able to read novels or even textbooks of medicine with apparently normal comprehension. They have difficulties in writing which parallel those of speaking. The written material produced by patients with conduction aphasia consists of real letters and even real words but is contaminated with misspellings (literal paragraphias) and omissions. In a small minority of patients who otherwise manifest the syndrome of conduction aphasia, there is significant difficulty in reading comprehension despite good auditory comprehension. We have hypothesized that these patients have a posterior extension of their lesion from the parietal operculum (the usual site of the lesion of conduction aphasia) to the angular gyrus.

## Pseudoalexia

In the discussion of the ability to read printed material there are several varieties of difficulty which are not truly alexias but may present clinically as a severe difficulty in reading. Since they must be considered in the differential diagnosis of alexia they deserve comment here.

*Reading aloud.* The differentiation between the ability to read out loud and to comprehend written material is essential in any discussion of aphasic alexia. This has been emphasized by Goldstein (1948) and recently by Luria (1966) who note that many patients with aphasia in spoken language will have great difficulty in reading out loud and yet may have normal or near normal comprehension of written language. This will be true in particular of cases of conduction aphasia and Broca's aphasia. The opposite situation, i.e., the preservation of reading aloud in the face of inability to comprehend printed material is also seen but is much less common (Dejerine 1880). Incomplete examination of the patient, using the ability to read aloud as the sole test of reading, may lead to incorrect labelling of these patients as alexic. By the definition offered at the beginning of this paper it is the comprehension of printed material that is significant so that the patient who comprehends printed material but does not read out loud should not be regarded as alexic while the rare patient who reads aloud without comprehension may be accepted as alexic.

*Unilateral paralexia.* Incorrect reading of part of a word or part of a sentence is known as paralexia. This may occur in any alexic patient but of particular interest is the patient who makes paralexic errors only for material falling in one visual field, a unilateral paralexia. The error is either one of omission or substitution, these errors consistently occurring in the part of the word or sentence falling in the hemianopic field when the visual focus centers on the mid portion of the word or sentence. Thus a patient with a right homonymous field defect may read the word "northwest" as "north" or "northern" and the sentence "He went out to dinner" simply as "He went out." The individual with a left field cut may read these as "west" and "out to dinner" respectively. As would be anticipated, unilateral paralexia is far more common in patients with left visual-field defects but is also seen occasionally with right hemianopic disturbances. Kinsbourne and Warrington (1962a) reported a detailed study of this disorder, using six cases with right posterior hemisphere damage secondary to either vascular or neoplastic disease. Each case had presented with distinct left visual neglect and all demonstrated the phenomenon of unilateral paralexia. Each patient could correctly identify individually presented letters and none exhibited any form of aphasia. The reading errors that they made, either omissions or substitutions, occurred exclusively in the left half of space. If, however, the words were presented in a vertical column instead of the traditional horizontal row, the full phrase could be correctly and easily read out loud and comprehended. It should be noted that this disturbance does not occur in all patients with a left hemianopia and probably requires inattention in addition to the hemianopia.

This form of misreading may be extremely disabling since the confabulatory responses and omissions of material in the left field may lead to gross distortions of comprehension. These patients are not, however, truly alexic since they do read correctly, both in their good visual field and with vertical presentation. This must then be considered only as a reading disturbance, a pseudoalexia. It may well be similar in basic mechanism to the hemialexia described earlier as resulting from lesions of the splenium of the corpus callosum. It is clear that a necessary component of this disorder is that the patient is unaware of or inattentive to his hemianopia and may either confabulate to complete stimuli not seen in the hemianopic field or omit this area entirely.

*Unrecognized developmental dyslexia.* It has been our experience on one occasion to examine a patient with a typical Broca's aphasia who had a severe reading disorder. This was not a reading disturbance of the type mentioned earlier during the description of Broca's aphasia, but a true disability in reading. It was only after considerable testing of the patient and questioning of the family that information was obtained revealing that the patient had never been able to read in a normal manner, had attended special schools because of his reading problem, and that his reading performance since the onset of aphasia was unchanged from premorbid performance. By the definitions stated in the opening part of this paper, this patient would not be considered alexic, but rather a case of developmental dyslexia. It is worth stress since such cases may occasionally present clinically and may be confusing unless this possibility is appreciated.

*Mental retardation.* Many individuals with significantly limited mental capacity never gain the ability to read. This can be considered as similar to developmental dyslexia but in no sense should be considered as alexia, the individual never having acquired reading ability. Nevertheless, generalized mental retardation is not always obvious to the examiner, especially when dealing with an adult who presents with signs of acute cerebral disorder, and must be considered in the differential diagnosis of reading disturbance. Usually a good history of premorbid intellectual capability will distinguish this disorder.

*Confusional state.* Inability to read coupled with many other "mental" symptoms such as disorientation, depressed attention span, hallucinations, apathy, agitation, loss of accepted social manners, agraphia, acalculia, disturbed visual and spatial orientation, etc., is seen not infrequently in both neurologic and psychiatric practice. While the reading disturbance may be profound, it is obviously part of the widespread cerebral dysfunction generally known as a confusional state. This state presents a diagnostic problem only when the patient is quietly confused and the other components are overlooked by the examiner. When the confusion clears, the reading disturbance will generally disappear along with the other findings. Defective attention (inability to attend to stimuli) is probably the basic factor underlying this reading disturbance which is not a true alexia. It may be difficult in some cases to rule out that confusional disorder and alexia are both present. It should be stressed that isolated alexia is never the result of a confusional state.

*Psychogenic disorders.* Only on rare occasions will the patient with purely psychogenic dysfunction be considered as alexic. Certainly both severely depressed patients and active or deteriorated schizophrenics may refuse to read upon request, just as they may refuse to carry out other requests, but when considered in the context of the entire disease picture the reading disturbance does not stand out. Reports of alexia as a significant hysterical symptom are rare (Teitelbaum 1941). It would appear that this symptom is too subtle, subjective, and lacking in drama for use by the hysterical patient. Thus reading disturbance (pseudoalexia) may well be part of a psychogenic syndrome but it is rarely sufficiently prominent to warrant confusion with true alexia.

## Additional Theoretical Considerations

*Hemispheric dominance.* In the great majority of cases the pathology of the alexic syndrome is compatible with left-hemisphere dominance, although a few cases have been recorded in left handers in whom the pattern of lesions was reversed (Gloning et al. 1966). There is very little evidence which even suggests bilateral representation of reading comprehension. Akelaitis (1941) and Gazzaniga and Sperry (1967) suggested that some of their cases of callosal section showed evidence of bilateral reading ability as discussed earlier in the section on hemialexia. Our experience in a small number of cases of alexia without agraphia has not demonstrated preservation of comprehension in the apparently intact right hemisphere. Thus these patients with right hemianopia and involvement of the splenium but with an intact left visual field not only fail to read aloud but cannot match written words with pictures or objects and fail to carry out written commands with either hand. This problem, in common with other issues of right-hemisphere substitution, deserves further study. It can be stated with some confidence however, that the ability to comprehend written language is dependent upon intactness of the dominant (usually left) hemisphere in the majority of adults and conversely, that the presence of clinical alexia is a strong indication of dominant-hemisphere pathology.

*Childhood lesions.* We know of no reports of acquired alexia in childhood except in cases demonstrating considerable language loss. Whether this is due to paucity of cases, inadequate examination, or because lesions adequate to produce alexia in adult life do not do so in childhood (or would be rapidly compensated) is not known. Descriptions of the clinical pictures, course, and pathology of acquired alexia in childhood would be most welcome.

*Alexia in the deaf or blind.* We do not know whether lesions which produce alexia alone or in combination with other clinical features in the normally hearing and seeing would have the same effects in the congenitally deaf or blind. Thus, if Wernicke's interpretation of alexia as a part of Wernicke's aphasia (cited earlier) is correct, one would expect that a lesion of Wernicke's area in a congenitally deaf patient who knew only manual language and lip reading might produce no alexia for written material or indeed, for the manual language, since the patient would never have learned these by reference to auditory language and hence would not use the auditory association cortex.

Similarly, it would be reasonable to assume that the patient with either acquired or congenital blindness who "read" Braille would not lose this ability after the usual lesion of alexia without agraphia. What would happen to this patient after the usual lesion for alexia with agraphia? One such case has been observed (Gloning 1967) and did demonstrate loss of the ability to understand the Braille language as would be anticipated from our earlier discussion of alexia with agraphia.

*Relationship to developmental dyslexia.* In recent years there has been a resurgence of interest in the problem of the child with exceptional difficulties in learning to read and write. Such individuals have at least a superficial resemblance to the patient with alexia with agraphia in that they may have normal use of spoken language and normal intelligence but are unable to master the written form of language. By our original definition these cases are not considered with the alexias as they have never gained the function of reading, but the obvious similarity of symptomatology is at least suggestive of a common factor. To date there are no pathological data available in the developmental dyslexias and any relationship must remain conjectural. It is conceivable that bilateral defective maturation of the angular gyrus could lead to this syndrome, but this too is purely speculative. The developmental dyslexias are discussed in Chapter 19.

## Test of Reading

In earlier sections, the ability to read aloud and the ability to comprehend written material have been presented as separable functions. It is therefore obvious that they are to be evaluated separately. At the same time, however, it must be recognized that many of the factors which disturb reading capability, may interfere with both types of reading function simultaneously. The following brief outline of test procedures will aid in differentiating varieties of alexia but must always be considered within the entire context of neurologic and aphasic defects.

*Reading aloud.* In testing this ability the examiner requests that the patient read aloud letters, numbers, words and sentences. In addition to omissions, the examiner watches for substitutions, verbal paralexias, and omissions or errors restricted to one visual field.

*Comprehension of letters.* This is tested by having the patient match lower case to capital letters and print to script. If there is failure at this level, the patient should be asked to trace the letter with his finger, or the letter should be moved slowly in front of the patient (Botez et al. 1964). This test may be made more difficult by cross hatching or other mild disguise of the letter or by tachistoscopic presentation. Number comprehension may be tested by having the patient match a written number with the proper number of objects or fingers.

*Comprehension of written words.* This is tested by requesting that the patient match a written word with the proper object or body part. Tachistoscopic presentation may be used.

*Comprehension of phrases and sentences.* This testing can be carried out in several ways. Matching of a short descriptive phrase or sentence with an object or simple yes-no questions can be used. With longer sentences, conditional clauses, unstressed prepositions, and absurd statements may be used to probe the quality of comprehension.

*Paragraph comprehension.* This is tested by offering a factual paragraph followed by questions based on the information in the paragraph. This can challenge both the grasp of specific information and the understanding of the basic ideas put forth in the reading material.

*Visual function.* Special attention should be given to visual function as it influences reading. This includes tests of visual acuity, visual field determinations of both confrontation and extinction varieties, optokinetic nystagmus, color vision, and the ability to identify objects presented visually. Eye movements should be observed and special note taken of the ability to scan a line of print and move to the next line. Complex machinery for recording eye movements during visual scanning has been described (Garron and Cheifetz 1967) but is too complicated for use except in research.

*Speed of reading.* The rapidity with which a patient is able to read silently a passage is obviously of interest but is of limited use in clinical evaluation. There is great individual variation in the speed of reading and a given patient's premorbid ability is rarely known by the examiner. In addition, there are some patients who read painfully slowly but if allowed sufficient time can demonstrate that they have comprehended the material. This may be the only residual of a previous alexia.

*Spelling aloud and comprehension of spelled words.* One additional evaluation, not truly a test of reading, has proved of distinct value in the study of alexia. This is the determination of the patient's ability to spell aloud and to recognize words spelled aloud by the examiner. Both of these acts will be failed by the patient with alexia with agraphia or with the alexia associated with Wernicke's aphasia. In cases of alexia without agraphia, however, the response to both tests will be at a normal level, and individuals with Broca's or conduction types of aphasia will usually recognize spelled words even if they cannot produce the letters to spell a requested word. Failure in both of these tests is suggestive of pathology affecting the dominant temporoparietal area.

The simple test procedures outlined above offer considerable information for differentiation of the varieties of alexia. The ability to read aloud *and* to comprehend letters, words, phrases, and longer written language is readily determined and the presence of alexia can be demonstrated. The ability to handle spelled words will aid in differentiating the so-called "pure" alexia from that produced by dominant temporoparietal disorder. Observation may reveal sources of nonalexic reading disturbances. In the final assessment, however, the exact variety of alexia or nonalexic reading disturbance must be determined by a complete clinical evaluation of which the above-mentioned tests are only one portion.

## Therapy

In the face of the extensive literature available on the alexias including discussions of the clinical state, pathology, physiology, development of reading skills, and breakdown with cerebral disease, there has been surprisingly little specific information concerning therapy for alexia. Most authors are quick to point out that the techniques of remedial reading cannot be employed in alexia without considerable alteration, since the alexic has lost this skill because of cerebral damage, whereas the "slow reader" has yet to accomplish reading. Thus, while remedial reading techniques can be utilized, treatment must be individualized for the alexic patient.

Kinesthetic aid to reading has been emphasized by Goldstein (1948) and many other authors. In essence, this consists of having the patient run his finger over the outline of a given letter while teaching him to say the letter name aloud. With continued practice this may become easier for the patient, and eventually some patients may develop a kinesthetic sense for eye movements to replace the clumsier and slower use of the hand. This technique, however, has proved unsuccessful in most cases of alexia and at best appears to have limited therapeutic value.

Wepman (1951) emphasizes five steps in therapy for alexia which he admits are borrowed from remedial reading experience. These five steps are:

(1) The determination of residual reading level to provide a starting level for therapy.
(2) The building of sight vocabulary of simple words, primarily accomplished by intensive drilling.
(3) The phonetic sounding of letters and phrases, again done by intense drilling.
(4) The comprehension of connected written material (sentences and phrases) which is built up by repeated drill on material of interest to the patient.
(5) The continued practice of reading under supervision with occasional testing to ascertain the accuracy of comprehension.

The author points out that the third step may be impossible for individuals with aphasic disorders producing expressive abnormalities and may be deleted. While admitting that alexia may prove difficult to treat, Wepman (1951) suggests that with patience and considerable therapy many patients "can be started on the road to recovery of reading."

For retraining of reading skills Goldstein (1948) suggests starting at a somewhat more elementary level and warns that progress beyond this level may be difficult or even impossible. He strongly recommends the use of pictures of familiar objects printed together with the first letter of the name of the object (e.g., "*A*" and a picture of an *Apple*). This printed material is combined with verbalization by the therapist until the patient associates the letter and the object and can produce the sound of the letter by saying the known name of the object. Goldstein notes that this technique is frequently used in initiating reading skills in children, but is rapidly dropped as it is both inefficient and unnecessary. In alexia, however, this technique may be necessary for a long period. Another technique advised by Goldstein concerns learning of the alphabet. He advocates dividing the alphabet into groups of five, equating each letter with one of the fingers and drilling sequentially until the alphabet can be recited. Similar drill is then used to equate the spoken letter name with the written letter name. Both Goldstein and Brain (1961) emphasize that some alexic patients perform better when taught immediately to read words without attempting to spell or pronounce letters. This relieves the patient of the arduous task of reaccomplishing phonetic skills, quite impossible for some aphasic patients, but places additional pressure upon the therapist who must beware of paralexic errors.

In summary, the therapy of alexia must be individualized, demands arduous labor on the part of both the patient and the therapist, plus considerable ingenuity on the part of the therapist, and in many cases an end result far below normal levels must be accepted.

## References


Adler, A.: Disintegration and restoration of optic recognition in visual agnosia. Arch. Neurol. Psychiat. (Chicago) 51 (1944) 243–259.

Adler, A.: Course and outcome of visual agnosia. J. Nerv. Ment. Dis. 3 (1950) 41–51.

Ajax, E. T.: Acquired dyslexia. Arch. Neurol. (Chic.) 2 (1964) 66–72.

Ajax, E. T.: Dyslexia without agraphia. Arch. Neurol. (Chic.) 6 (1967) 645–652.

Akelaitis, A. J.: Studies of the corpus callosum. II. Arch. Neurol. Psychiat. (Chicago) 45 (1941) 788–796.

Akelaitis, A. J.: A study of gnosis, praxis and language following section of the corpus callosum. J. Neurosurg. 1 (1944) 94–102.

Alajouanine, Th., F. Lhermitte and B. de Ribaucourt-Ducarne: Les alexies agnosiques et aphasiques. In: Les grandes activités du lobe occipital. Paris, Masson & Cie. (1960).

Asayama, T.: Über die Aphasie bei Japanern. Dtsch. Arch. klin. Med. 113 (1914) 523–529.

Bastian, H. C.: A treatise on aphasia and other speech defects. London, H. K. Lewis & Company (1898).

Bay, E.: Disturbances of visual perception and their examination. Brain 76 (1953) 515–550.

Benton, A. L.: Contributions to aphasia before Broca. Cortex (Milano) 1 (1964) 314–327.

Beringer, K. and J. Stein: Analyse eines Falles von reiner Alexie. Z. ges. Neurol. Psychiat. 123 (1930) 472–478.

Bertholle: Asyllabie ou amnésie partielle et isolée de la lecture. Gaz. hebd. Méd. Chir. 6 mai (1881).

Bonvicini, G. and O. Pötzl: Alexie. Wien. klin. Wschr. 29 (1907).

Botez, M. I., T. Serbancescu and I. Vernea: Visual static agnosia with special reference to literal agnosic alexia. Neurology (Minneap.) 14 (1964) 1101–1111.

Brain, W. R.: Visual-object-agnosia with special reference to the Gestalt theory. Brain 64 (1941) 43–62.

Brain, W. R.: Speech disorders. London, Butterworths (1961).

Brissaud, E.: Cécité verbale sans aphasie ni agraphie. Rev. neurol. 8 (1900) 757.

Broadbent, W. H.: Cerebral mechanism of speech and thought. Med. Chir. Trans. 55 (1872) 145–194.

Casey, T. and G. Ettlinger: The occasional 'independence' of dyslexia and dysgraphia from dysphasia. J. Neurol. Neurosurg. Psychiat. 23 (1960) 228–236.

Charcot, J. M.: Sur un cas de cécité verbale. In: Leçons sur les maladies du système nerveux, Vol. III of Œuvres complètes de J. M. Charcot. Paris, Delahaye & Lecrosnier (1877).

Critchley, M.: The parietal lobes. London, Edward Arnold (1953).

Critchley, M.: Acquired anomalies of colour perception of central origin. Brain 88 (1965) 711–724.

Critchley, M.: Aphasiological nomenclature and definitions. Cortex (Milano) 3 (1967) 3–25.

David, M., H. Hécaen, R. Angelergues and C. Magis: Les tumeurs occipitales. Neurochirurgie I (1955) 85–108.

Davidenkov, S. N.: Visual agnosias—lecture 8. State Publishing House of Medical Literature 2 (1956a).

Davidenkov, S. N.: Visual agnosias—lecture 9. State Publishing House of Medical Literature 2 (1956b).

Dejerine, J.: Aphasie et cécité des mots. Progr. méd. 8 (1880) 629.

Dejerine, J.: Sur un cas de cécité verbale avec agraphie, suivi d'autopsie. Mém. Soc. Biol. 3 (1891) 197–201.
Dejerine, J.: Des différentes variétés de cécité verbale. Mém. Soc. Biol. (1892) 1–30.
Dejerine, J. and André-thomas: Contribution à l'étude de l'aphasie chez les gauchers. Rev. neurol. 24 (1912) 214–226.
De Ajuriaguerra, J. and H. Hécaen: Le cortex cérébral. Paris, Masson & Cie. (1949).
De Massary, J.: L'alexie. Encéphale 27 (1932) 134–164.
De Renzi, E. and H. Spinnler: Impaired performance on color tasks in patients with hemispheric damage. Cortex (Milano) 3 (1967) 194–217.
Dide, M. and Botcazo: Amnésie continue, cécité verbale pure, perte du sens topographique, ramollissement double du lobe lingual. Rev. neurol. 10 (1902) 676–680.
Ehrenwald, H.: Über das Lesen mit Umgehung des optischen Wahrnehmungsapparates. Z. ges. Neurol. Psychiat. 123 (1929–30) 204–223.
Ettlinger, G. and L. Hurwitz: Dyslexia and its associated disturbances. Neurology (Minneap.) 12 (1962) 477–480.
Garron, D. C. and D. L. Cheifetz: Stimulus rotation and visual scanning in subjects with copying disability. Percept. mot. Skills 24 (1967) 1015–1024.
Gazzaniga, M. S., J. E. Bogen and R. W. Sperry: Observations on visual perception after disconnection of the cerebral hemisphere in man. Brain 88 (1965) 221–236.
Gazzaniga, M. S. and R. W. Sperry: Language after section of the cerebral commissures. Brain 90 (1967) 131–148.
Gerstmann, J.: Zur Symptomatologie der Hirnläsionen im Übergangsgebiet der unteren parietal- und mittleren Occipitalwindung. Nervenarzt 3 (1930) 691–695.
Geschwind, N.: The anatomy of acquired disorders of reading. In: John Money, ed.: Reading disability. Baltimore, Johns Hopkins Press (1962).
Geschwind, N.: Disconnexion syndromes in animals and man. Brain 88 (1965) 237–294.
Geschwind, N.: The varieties of naming errors. Cortex (Milano) 3 (1967) 97–112.
Geschwind, N. and M. Fusillo: Color naming defects in association with alexia. Arch. Neurol. (Chic.) 15 (1966) 137–146.
Geschwind, N., J. Segarra and F. Quadfasel: Isolation of the speech area. Neuropsychologia (Oxford) in press.
Gloning, I., K. Gloning and H. Hoff: Aphasia—a clinical syndrome. In: L. Halpern, ed.: Problems of dynamic neurology. Jerusalem, Jerusalem Post Press (1963).
Gloning, I., K. Gloning, K. Jellinger and H. Tschabitscher: Zur Dominanzfrage bei reiner Wortblindheit-Farbagnosie. Neuropsychologia (Oxford) 4 (1966) 27–40.
Gloning, I., K. Gloning, F. Seitelberger and H. Tschabitscher: Ein Fall von reiner Wortblindheit mit Obduktionsbefund. Wien. Z. Nervenheilk. 12 (1955) 194–215.
Gloning, K.: Personal communication (1967).
Goldstein, K.: Die transkorticalen Aphasien. Jena, Gustav Fischer (1917).
Goldstein, K.: Language and language disturbance. New York, Grune and Stratton (1948).
Goldstein, K. and A. Gelb: Psychologische Analysen hirnpathologischer Fälle auf Grund von Untersuchungen Hirnverletzter. Z. ges. Neurol. Psychiat. 41 (1928) 1–142.
Gueneau de Mussy, N.: Contribution à l'étude pathologique et physiologique de l'amblyopie aphasique. Rec. Ophtal. (Paris) 3 (1879) 129–142.
Hahn, E.: Pathologisch-anatomische Untersuchung des lissauerschen Falles von Seelenblindheit. In: Arbeiten aus der psychiatrischen Klinik in Breslau, 3. Leipzig, Georg Thieme (1895) pp. 109–119.
Hécaen, H.: Aspects des troubles de la lecture (alexie) au cours des lésions cérébrales en foyer. In press.

Hécaen, H., J. de Ajuriaguerra and M. David: les déficits fonctionnels après lobectomie occipitale. Mschr. Psychiat. Neurol. 123 (1952) 239–290.

Hécaen, H., J. de Ajuriaguerra and R. Angelergues: Les troubles de la lecture dans le cadre des modifications des fonctions symboliques. Psychiat. Neurol. (Basel) 134 (1957) 97–129.

Hécaen, H. and R. Angelergues: Pathologie du langage. Paris, Larousse (1965).

Hermann, G. and O. Pötzl: Über die Agraphie. Abh. Neurol. Psychiat. Psychol. 35. Berlin, Karger (1926).

Hinshelwood, J.: Letter, word and mind-blindness. London, H. K. Lewis (1900).

Hinshelwood, J. and A. MacPhail: A case of word blindness with right homonymous hemianopsia. Brit. med. J. 2 (1904) 1304–1307.

Hoff, H., I. Gloning and K. Gloning: Über Alexie. Wien. Z. Nervenheilk. 10 (1954) 149–162.

Holmes, G.: Pure word blindness. Folia Psychiat. Neerl. 53 (1950) 279–288.

Howes, D.: An approach to the quantitative analysis of word blindness. In: John Money, ed.: Reading disability. Baltimore, Johns Hopkins Press (1962).

Kennard, M.: Alterations in response to visual stimuli following lesions of the frontal lobe in monkeys. Arch. Neurol. Psychiat. (Chicago) 41 (1939) 1153–1165.

Kinsbourne, M. and E. K. Warrington: A variety of reading disabilities associated with right hemisphere lesions. J. Neurol. Neurosurg. Psychiat. 25 (1962a) 339–344.

Kinsbourne, M. and E. K. Warrington: A disorder of simultaneous form perception. Brain 85 (1962b) 461–486.

Kinsbourne, M. and E. K. Warrington: Observations on colour agnosia. J. Neurol. Neurosurg. Psychiat. 27 (1964) 296–299.

Kleist, K.: In: K. Bonhoeffer, ed.: Handbuch der ärtzliche Erfahrungen im Weltkriege 1914–1918. Vol. 4. Leipzig, Barth (1934).

Konorski, J.: Integrative activity of the brain. Chicago, University of Chicago Press (1967).

Kussmaul, A.: Die Störungen der Sprache. Leipzig, Vogel (1877).

Landolt, E.: In: Feestbundel aan Franciscus Cornelis Donders. Amsterdam, F. Van Rossen (1888a).

Landolt, E.: Alexia or word blindness. Neurol. Cbl. 7 (1888b) 605–606.

Lange, J.: Alexie. In: O. Bumke and O. Foerster, eds.: Handbuch der Neurologie. Berlin, Springer (1936).

Leischner, A.: Die Störungen der Schriftsprache. Stuttgart, Georg Thieme (1957).

Lissauer, H.: Ein fall von Seelenblindheit nebst einem Beiträge zur Theorie derselben. Arch. Psychiat. Nervenkr. 21 (1889) 2–50.

Luria, A. R.: Disorders of 'simultaneous perception' in a case of bilateral occipital-parietal brain injury. Brain 82 (1959) 437–449.

Luria, A. R.: Higher cortical functions in man. New York, Basic Books (1966).

Lyman, R. S., S. T. Kwan and W. H. Chao: Left occipito-parietal brain tumor with observations on alexia and agraphia in Chinese and English. Chin. Med. J. 54 (1938) 491–516.

Marie, P. and Ch. Foix: Les aphasies de guerre. Rev. neurol. 1 (1917) 3–18.

Martin, J. Purdon: Pure word blindness considered as a disturbance of visual space perception. Proc. roy. Soc. Med. 47 (1954) 293–295.

Maspes, P. E.: Le syndrome expérimental chez l'homme de la section du splénium du corps calleux. Rev. neurol. 2 (1948) 101–113.

Misch, W. and K. Frankl: Beitrag zur Alexielehre. Mschr. Psychiat. Neurol. 71 (1929) 1–47.

Nielsen, J. M.: The unsolved problems in aphasia. I. Bull. Los Angeles neurol. Soc. 4 (1938) 144–122.
Nielsen, J. M.: The unsolved problems in aphasia. II. Bull. Los Angeles neurol. Soc. 4 (1939) 168–183.
Nielsen, J. M.: Agnosia, apraxia, aphasia: their value in cerebral localization. New York, Hoeber (1946).
Nielsen, J. M. and R. B. Raney: Symptoms following surgical removal of major (left) angular gyrus. Bull. Los Angeles neurol. Soc. 3 (1938) 42–46.
Niesl von Mayendorf, E.: Zur Lehre von der Seelenblindheit. Z. ges. Neurol. Psychiat. 152 (1935) 345–382.
Panse, F. and T. Shimoyama: Zur Auswirkung aphasischer Störungen im Japanischen. Arch. Psychiat. Nervenkr. 193 (1955) 131–138.
Paterson, J. and E. Bramwell: Two cases of word blindness. Med. Press (1905) 507–508.
Penfield, W. and L. Roberts: Speech and brain mechanisms. Princeton, Princeton University Press (1959).
Pick, A.: In: W. Bethe, ed.: Handbuch der normalen und pathologischen Physiologie. Berlin, Springer (1931).
Poppelreuter, W.: Die Störungen des Lesens und Schreibens bei zerebral Sehgestörten. In: Die psychische Schädigungen durch Kopfschuss im Kriege, 1 (1917) 256–270.
Pötzl, O.: Zur Kasuistik der Wortblindheit-Notenblindheit. Mschr. Psychiat. Neurol. 66 (1927) 1–12.
Pötzl, O.: Die optisch-agnostischen Störungen. Leipzig, Deuticke (1928).
Quensel, F.: Ein fall von rechtsseitiger Hemianopsie mit Alexie and zentral bedingtem monokulärem Doppeltsehen. Mschr. Psychiat. Neurol. 65 (1927) 173–207.
Redlich, E.: Ueber die sogenannte subcorticale Alexie. Jb. Psychiat. Neurol. 13 (1895) 1–60.
Starr, A.: The pathology of sensory aphasia. Brain 12 (1889) 82–99.
Symonds, C.: Aphasia. J. Neurol. Neurosurg. Psychiat. 16 (1953) 1–6.
Teitelbaum, H. A.: Psychogenic body image disturbances associated with psychogenic aphasia and agnosia. J. Nerv. Ment. Dis. 93 (1941) 581–612.
Teuber, H. L.: Physiological psychology. Ann. Rev. Psych. 6 (1955) 267–296.
Trescher, J. H. and F. R. Ford: Colloid cyst of the third ventricle. Arch. Neurol. Psychiat. (Chicago) 37 (1937) 959–973.
Warrington, E. K. and O. L. Zangwill: A study of dyslexia. J. Neurol. Neurosurg. Psychiat. 20 (1957) 208–215.
Welch, K. and P. Stuteville: Experimental production of unilateral neglect in monkeys. Brain 81 (1958) 341–347.
Weisenburg, T. S. and K. McBride: Aphasia: a clinical and psychological study. New York, The Commonwealth Fund (1935).
Wepman, J. W.: Recovery from aphasia. New York, Ronald Press (1951).
Wernicke, K.: Der aphasische Symptomencomplex. Breslau, Franck and Weigert (1874).
Wolpert, I.: Die Simultanagnosie. Z. ges. Neurol. Psychiat. 93 (1924) 397–415.
Wolpert, I.: Über das Wesen der literalen Alexie. Mschr. Psychiat. Neurol. 75 (1930) 207–266.

Part of the work reported here was supported by Grant NB-06209 from the National Institutes of Health to the Boston University School of Medicine.

# CHAPTER 13

# Apraxia

*Norman Geschwind and Antonio R. Damasio*

Apraxia is an impairment of the execution of a learned movement in response to a stimulus which would normally elicit the movement, subject to the condition that the afferent and efferent systems involved are intact, and in the absence of inattentiveness or lack of cooperation. This is a very broad definition applicable to many different types of stimulus, including some highly specialized ones. For the overwhelming majority of clinical situations, however, one can use the following operational definition: apraxia is (a) failure to produce the correct movement in response to a verbal command, or (b) failure to imitate correctly a movement performed by the examiner, or (c) failure to perform a movement correctly in response to a seen object, or (d) failure to handle an object correctly. The incorrect performance cannot be explained by weakness, incoordination, akinesia, abnormal reflexes, impaired auditory comprehension, or impaired visual or tactile perception. Furthermore, the patient must be attentive and cooperative.

The exclusionary criteria of our operational definition indicate that apraxia is not a disorder of the effector apparatus of the motor system, which controls the initiation, direction, stability, and strength of a movement, nor is it a disorder of the somatosensory system, which provides crucial information to the motor system. The definition also excludes the possibility that apraxia is a consequence of defective comprehension, be it auditory or visual, of the command given by the examiner in the process of testing for the phenomenon. Finally, it implies that the movements are learned. Thus defined, apraxia is a disorder of the high level control of the execution of some classes of movement, as requested by an observer in the verbal or visual mode. The movements fail to be carried out entirely or are performed defectively.

---

Reprinted with permission from P.J. Vinken, G.W. Bruyn, and H.L. Klawans (eds), *Handbook of Clinical Neurology. Volume 1 (45): Clinical Neuropsychology.* Amsterdam: Elsevier Science Publishers B.V., 1985; 423-432.

The use of the term apraxia for the types of difficulty described above was originated by Hugo Liepmann in the first years of the twentieth century. Although it continued, in the years between the wars, to be employed in this sense in the German-language literature, there was almost no discussion of this type of disorder in English or French publications. As a result, the word apraxia came to designate a wide variety of other types of incorrect motor performance. It has commonly been used for disorders in constructional tasks, for certain disorders of gait, for certain difficulties in speech, and often for unexplained clumsiness. In this chapter none of these other disorders are considered.

In spite of its frequency, apraxia often fails to be recognized. Thus it is usually the case that one patient who is apraxic on testing will, in a natural setting, perform learned movements normally, especially when he can see and manipulate objects he has previously known in their proper environment. Unless specifically tested for, apraxia will almost never be evident to the examiner and is not likely to be a complaint of either the patient or the family. Another reason why apraxia may fail to be recognized is that, in some patients, the phenomenon tends to be especially marked during the acute stage of the causative lesion but to recover fairly rapidly, so that in later stages the patient may fail to exhibit apraxia. Furthermore, apraxia is often wrongly diagnosed. The clumsy movements that result from weakness, ataxia or dystonia, the difficult initiation of movements due to akinesia, or the slow movements consequent to bradykinesia, are not apraxia.

## Testing for Apraxia

The appropriate testing of apraxia comprises assessment of the ability to carry out *limb*, *buccofacial*, and *axial* movements. Apraxia is usually easier to demonstrate in the upper limbs, i.e,. with movements of arm and hand, than in the lower limbs. Each side should be tested separately. Some movements should be *transitive*, i.e., movements that normally involve the manipulation of an implement, and others intransitive, i.e., movements such as saluting that do not utilize an implement. In both cases the patient should be tested first with a *verbal command* to pantomime the movement. It is important to note that in the testing of responses to verbal command, the patient should not be given the implement in the case of transitive movements. He is thus asked to pretend that he is using a comb, or shaving, or eating soup with a spoon in the absence of the object. It is essential that the examiner should not himself pantomime the movement as he gives the command. Should the patient fail the execution on verbal command, with one or the other hand, arm, leg, or foot, or in some cases both, the ability of the patient to imitate is then tested with a *visual command*, i.e., the examiner pantomimes the movement and the patient is asked to imitate.

The same rules of testing used apply to buccofacial movements, i.e., movements of the cranial musculature other than movements of the eyes, the lids and the sternomastoids, which should be first requested by verbal command and then by visual command (imitation). The examiner should test movements that normally do not require an object, e.g., showing the teeth or sticking out the tongue. It should be noted that failure to demonstrate emotional expressions, e.g., surprise or anger, may reflect a special mechanism for which the right hemisphere is thought to be important and which is discussed elsewhere. In the patient with facial apraxia on verbal command and/or imitation, the emotional movements will not be impaired selectively. The patient is also asked to pantomime (and later to imitate) movements which normally require an object, e.g., pretending to blow out a match.

Another type of task relates to axial movements, i.e., movements which involve midline structures other than the face, jaws, larynx, pharynx, or tongue. They include movements of the eyes and eyelids, the head and neck, the trunk, and also movements which simultaneously involve the trunk and limbs synergistically. Examples are 'look up and open the eyes,' 'bend the head down,' 'stand up and walk backwards,' or 'show me the position of a boxer.' On the other hand, commands such as 'kick,' 'stamp out a cigarette,' 'make a fist,' or 'punch,' involve specific movements of the arm-hand or leg-foot and therefore fall under the category of limb movements.

In further testing, the patients should be asked to demonstrate a movement in response to a specific object which is seen or handled. It is also useful to observe such movements in a natural setting with the patient unaware of the observer. Finally, patients should be asked to pantomime serial actions both in the absence of objects and in their presence, to use several objects in a given sequence, e.g., remove a cigarette from a packet, light it, and use the ashtray. This tests for *ideational apraxia.*

It is obviously important in the testing of apraxia to any particular type of stimulus, to be certain that the requirements listed in the definition are met. Thus one must show that the patient can comprehend the command. When the patient is not aphasic in spoken speech one can easily document this by having the patient describe verbally what is demanded of him. If aphasia is present in spoken speech, the patient can be asked to respond to questions. Because Broca's and conduction aphasics can often respond 'yes' or 'no' correctly, this is easily done. Thus the patient who has been asked to show, in the absence of the object, how a hammer is used, can be asked: 'Did I ask how to cut wood?' 'Is a hammer used for eating?' Or, if the examiner himself performs the movement: 'Did I show the use of a hammer?' The latter type of question also helps to be sure that a failure or imitation is not the result of failure of visual recognition.

The simplest method of demonstrating that a failure is not the result of weakness, incoordination, akinesia, or some other motor disorder is the performance, by the patient, of the demanded movement in response to another stimulus. Thus when a patient who fails to pantomime the use of a hammer to verbal command or on imitation, then handles an actual hammer correctly, one can be certain that there is no motor impairment. If the patient fails with the actual object, one must use information obtained from motor examination and from observation of the patient obtained in a natural setting.

A protocol for the testing of apraxia is available in Goodglass and Kaplan's Manual for the Assessment of Aphasia and Related Disorders (1983).

## Types of Apraxic Errors

The simplest type of error is total failure to perform the movement. More commonly one observes an incorrect movement. Thus, a patient asked to salute with the left arm may simply raise the arm in the air, or may posture the hand correctly yet fail to carry it to the correct position. In many cases the nature of the parapraxic error may provide clear evidence that a verbal command has been comprehended.

In limb movements, certain types of error are commonly seen. In particular, one should note the *use of the body part as the object* (BPO). Thus the patient asked to show the use of a hammer may strike the surface with the closed fist rather than manipulate an imaginary hammer. Asked to show how the hair is combed he may smooth the scalp with the hand.

In testing of bucco-facial praxis one may observe several types of errors: (a) *incomplete gestures*, i.e., failure to round the lips when blowing; (b) *'onomatopoetic' responses*, e.g., responding to 'show me how you blow out a match' with the forcefully uttered words 'blow out a match,' 'blow,' or 'puff.' This type of error is almost never seen with limb or axial commands; (c) *achieving the purpose of the movement with the hand*, e.g. pretending to shake a match in the air rather than blowing it out, or wiping the lips with the hand rather than licking them; (d) *self-cuing*, e.g., the patient, when asked how he would blow out a match, first pantomimes the movement of striking a match with the hand, and then the imaginary match is carried to the lips. This is then followed by either a correct or an incorrect movement. If the blowing movement is correct, the examiner should repeat the command while holding the patient's hand.

## Classification

The classification and terminology used in the literature on apraxia is often confusing. In terms of the principal region of involvement, the terms *limb apraxia* and *buccofacial (or oral) apraxia* should be retained. They are self-explanatory. Both terms were first introduced by Liepmann in his early papers. The terms *ideomotor* and *ideational*, also used by Liepmann, are sometimes used with varying meanings. *Ideomotor apraxia* applies to the failure to carry out a requested movement properly. The term *ideational apraxia* applies only to impairments of limb movement, and generally denotes an impairment in the ability to carry out a sequence of movements. Since such a sequence normally deals with movements that require the use of one or more objects, some authors have used this term for any failure with objects. Liepmann, however, used the term ideomotor for failure of a single movement with an object, and *ideational apraxia* applies to any failure to produce a sequence. In ideational apraxia, therefore, the patients may actually carry out individual verbal or visual commands correctly, often using the same implements they fail to use properly in serial action, provided they involve only one step. Even when the series is executed, the individual movements may be correct but may occur at the wrong time.

The physiopathologic mechanism behind ideational apraxia is probably different from the one responsible for the much more frequent ideomotor apraxias. In many instances of ideational apraxia, the control of attention is impaired and the full grasp of the instruction is questionable. In some especially severe cases, we suspect a component of agnosia may actually be responsible for the failures. At any rate the phenomenon is seen often in patients with advanced Alzheimer's disease or in other patients with bilateral parietal lobe dysfunction. Some very well defined cases appear to have left posterior lesions.

## The Presentation of Apraxia

Apraxia is most commonly seen in patients with left hemisphere lesions who often have aphasia as well, and in patients with lesions of interhemispheric pathways crossing in the corpus callosum, especially the anterior portions. The apraxias seen in patients with callosal lesions were the first ones described by Liepmann and provide the most clear illustration of the definition given above and will be discussed first.

### Apraxia following callosal lesions

The patient described by Geschwind and Kaplan (1962) is a standard example of this form of apraxia. The patient had undergone excision of a glioblastoma in the left hemisphere at which time the left anterior cerebral artery had been sacrificed. (At post-mortem the right hemisphere was fully intact and there was an infarction of the anterior 4/5 of the corpus callosum). All elementary motor functions of the left arm and leg were intact. There was weakness of the right shoulder and in the right leg as well as a grasp reflex confined to the right arm. Despite the elementary difficulties in the right arm, the patient, when asked to carry out a verbal command with that limb, would do so immediately and correctly, e.g., 'show me how you would use a hammer,' or 'show me how you salute.' Buccofacial movements were also done correctly. But, when he was asked to carry out a command with his left arm, e.g., 'show me how you would use a hammer with your left hand,' he would either not respond or else perform an incorrect movement. On visual command, e.g., if the examiner pantomimed the correct response, the patient could perform normally with his left arm. Similarly, if he were handed the hammer in the left hand, he could then handle it correctly. Furthermore, in a natural setting, he could be seen to use his left arm normally to manipulate objects. Such correct operations performed by the left arm clearly showed that the failure to respond to the verbal command could not be due to a basic defect in the operation of the motor system, such as weakness or ataxia. In other words, this patient failed both transitive and intransitive verbal commands related to his *left* limbs, but he could perform verbal commands related to the oral musculature. Furthermore, he could carry out left limb movements to *visual* command, or spontaneously, or when the implement was available rather than imaginary, and axial movements were carried out correctly. In particular, he would fail to carry out a single movement with the left leg, e.g., 'kick,' yet would use this limb correctly in response to commands for walking, turning, etc., i.e., when it was used as part of a synergism with trunk movements. Eye movements were also done correctly.

The correct responses to right arm commands showed that this patient could comprehend language properly and was attentive and cooperative enough to carry out motor tasks. The impaired movements respected certain criteria: (a) they were learned, (b) they represented a real action, object, or concept, and (c) they involved a single limb. Using the traditional classification, this patient had limb apraxia of the ideomotor type involving the left limbs in response to verbal command but not on imitation or object handling.

From an anatomical and functional point of view, this means that spoken commands arrived normally in the auditory cortices of this patient and were appropriately decoded in the left posterior language regions necessary for auditory comprehension. The neural code of the movement requested by the examiner was properly evoked in the left posterior cortices, i.e., parietal and occipital, where we believe both visual and somatosensory traces of the experience of representational movements are stored. From this left posterior region the appropriate information could be transmitted to the left premotor region, and from there, movements of both the right hand and mouth region could be activated in the precentral motor cortex (either by direct projections or by using the ipsilateral basal ganglia and thalamic reentrant relays). But the ability to move the left-sided extremities was dependent on *right* premotor structures and it is apparent that the transmission of crucial control information to those right premotor structures was precluded by the callosal lesion. Geschwind and Kaplan interpreted the left arm apraxia precisely in this way, as a result of an interruption of information flow from the motor structures in the left frontal regions to the equivalent structures in the right frontal lobe, from which the operation of the left arm is controlled. They predicted that the patient had suffered destruction of the anterior portion of the corpus callosum, a hypothesis later confirmed at autopsy. This finding replicated and validated Liepmann's observations in comparable patients (Liepmann and Maas 1907). We will return to a comparison between these patients and to an intriguing difference between them: Liepmann's patient could *not* perform on visual command.

It is of importance to note that since the posterior one-fifth of the corpus callosum was intact, it appears that potential transmission of information from the left visual region to the analogous regions of the right hemisphere could not substitute for the circuitry interrupted by damage in the anterior corpus callosum. That the control of the left hand in the right premotor region was intact could be ascertained because when visual information reached the right hemisphere, i.e., when the examiner carried out a movement for the patient to imitate, the patient executed the appropriate motions of the left limbs. Buccofacial movements could be carried out on both sides from the left hemisphere because of the extensive bilateral representation of these movements from each side.

Just as was the case with movements of the right limbs and of the facial musculature, movements of the axial musculature could be directly elicited from the language hemisphere of this patient without any need for controlling information to traverse the corpus callosum. This happens because, just as with buccofacial movements, the control of the axial musculature can be operated from one hemisphere only for both sides of the body. Movements of this type are often preserved in other apraxic patients with lesions of the left hemisphere, indicating that their control is of a special nature. In all probability, after the verbal command has been translated into the appropriate neural code, activation can proceed through non-pyramidal motor cortices which deal primarily with axial movements. Such cortices are located in many sites, including the posterior superior temporal region and the sensory association cortices in the posterior sensory regions of the left hemisphere. There is even evidence that the right hemisphere may be capable of controlling these movements by itself. Some patients with major lesions of the left hemisphere which destroy most or all language cortices, motor cortex, and parietal cortex, perform axial movements to command without difficulty. It is thus possible that both Wernicke's areas can respond to such movements.*

Patients with surgical section of the corpus callosum also develop this form of apraxia. It is interesting to note that most of these patients can perform correct left limb movements on visual command, i.e., using the right hemisphere to transfer information from the right visual cortex to the right premotor region. This is similar to what was seen in the patient of Geschwind and Kaplan (1962). And yet the patient of Liepmann and Maas (1907) was not able to carry out visual commands with the right hemisphere (in spite of the fact that the right hemisphere was intact and the left limbs could be moved normally). We think this disparity underscores the varied individual endowment of the right hemisphere for the learning and performance of skilled limb movements. This apparent disparity further emphasizes Liepmann's notion that, in most individuals, the storehouse for learning and performance of skilled movement is located in the left hemisphere.

---

*It has recently been claimed that axial movements are not spared relative to limb and buccofacial movement in apraxic patients (Poeck et al. 1982). Howes has, however, reanalyzed the data of this paper and has shown that in fact axial movements were carried out to verbal command at much higher rate than limb and buccofacial movements in all the different aphasic populations studied. It is of interest that on imitation axial movements were not significantly different from the other categories (Howes, in press).

## Apraxia with left hemisphere lesions

Apraxia is most often seen with left hemisphere lesions and is thus often associated with aphasia, although, as we shall note later, the relation is not causal. One of the most frequent forms of apraxia occurs in patients with Broca's aphasia who commonly also have a paralysis of the right arm and hand and a right-sided central facial paralysis. Although these patients usually move the left limbs spontaneously in an entirely appropriate manner, they typically fail to perform correctly with them when asked to carry out a verbal command (this phenomenon is also known as *sympathetic apraxia,* a term that denotes the pairing of left apraxia with right paralysis; it is, of course, simply a limb apraxia to verbal command of the ideomotor type). They may show as much puzzlement in their sudden inability to move the left hand as patients with callosal lesions demonstrate in similar circumstances. It is also typical for them not to carry out correctly verbal commands for movements with the lips, jaw and tongue, e.g., 'pretend that you are blowing out a match.' On the other hand, if the natural context for the movement is recreated, the patient often performs well, i.e., he will blow out a real lit candle when minutes before he may have failed to pantomime the blowing of an imaginary candle. *Buccofacial apraxia,* as this type of apraxia is generally called, is seen in most patients with Broca's aphasia. De Renzi et al. (1966) found it in at least half of their Broca's patients and further noted that the apraxia and aphasia were not causally related, as there were instances of both aphasia without apraxia and the reverse. More recently, Tognola and Vignolo (1980) have noted the strong association between buccofacial apraxia and lesions of the left frontal operculum, lower precentral gyrus, and insula. Furthermore, when the command to move the left limbs or both sides of the facial musculature comes in a visual form, some patients succeed in the movement, i.e., if the patient who has just failed to show how to eat soup with his left hand is asked to copy the pantomime of the examiner eating soup with his left hand, some patients may be able to carry out the command. As noted above, however, the majority of these patients will also fail on imitation (Goodglass and Kaplan 1983). We believe this is especially so in patients with the most standard cerebral organization of left language dominance and right-handedness.

The lesion responsible for the aphasia and the apraxia in these patients damages not only the same type of connections which are affected in the patients with callosal lesions, i.e., connections linking the left premotor region to the right premotor region, but also damages the motor area of the left hemisphere. The callosal connections are damaged in their origin in the cortex or in their course through the subcortical white matter on the left. The parsimonious explanation for the failure to carry out verbal commands with the left hand is thus similar to the one invoked for the patients with callosal damage, that is, crucial control information is prevented from crossing the corpus callosum into the right premotor region. As far as the facial movements are concerned, it is apparent that the destruction of the left primary motor cortex prevents the activation of any facial movement from the left side. Thus, the bilateral movements of facial and pharyngo-laryngeal musculature become entirely dependent on the right premotor and precentral cortices, which cannot be properly controlled from the left because of the lesion of the callosal connections. Such right-sided cortices can often be directly activated through the visual mode in a situation in which the examiner asks for the imitation of an action he pantomimes, or in which the subject is presented with the actual objects on which he is supposed to act, e.g., the sight of a lit candle may arouse right hemisphere visual imagery sufficient to drive the right motor apparatus into action.

Patients present with apraxia in association with other types of aphasia, for instance, conduction aphasia. As is well known most patients with conduction aphasia have mild or absent right facial paralysis and typically have no right upper limb paralysis at all. It is of special interest, then, that they have difficulty carrying out movements with *either* superior limb as well as with the face. The most parsimonious account of this intriguing defect is that the lesion in the left hemisphere prevents the crucial control of information from reaching the left premotor region. Thus, the command cannot reach the right premotor region because it can not get to the origin of the callosal fibers. Apraxia can also be seen in transcortical types of aphasia, both motor and sensory, and even in Wernicke's aphasia. Although the presence of auditory comprehension defects clearly may raise questions regarding the full understanding of the instructions, there is little doubt in many cases that the apraxic symptomatology of many of these patients cannot be explained by a defect of auditory comprehension. This problem does, however, require further study.

Many other patients with parietal lobe damage but without aphasia can have apraxia. The apraxia commonly involves both limbs but movements of the face may be preserved. Axial movements are, as a rule, intact. The parietal lesions associated with apraxia must encompass the lower parietal region in the angular and supramarginal gyri. We have noted that in patients with lesions located exclusively in the higher parietal lobe, i.e., areas 5 and 7, no apraxia ensues, although the patients show optic ataxia, a visuo-motor impairment of the guidance of arm and hand movements towards a visual target (Damasio and Benton 1980). Defects of that type have been reproduced in experimental animals following damage to white matter connections between the superior parietal lobule and the premotor region (Haaxma and Kuypers 1975), and have generally been interpreted as a disconnection of important visual and somatosensory information from the premotor region which, directly or indirectly, controls the pyramidal cortex responsible for fine finger movements (Lawrence and Kuypers 1968).

The finding of such pervasive apraxia in patients with lower left parietal lesions is of the highest importance. It indicates that, in most individuals, this region of the brain probably contains the master control for the kind of representational limb movements impaired in apraxia. The flow from this controlling area is interrupted by lesions that cause conduction aphasia, or Broca aphasia, or that block anterior callosal transfer. The master control itself is impaired if the lesion is in the appropriate posterior location. This master control is likely to depend on the integration of somatosensory and visual information and can be activated by verbal or visual commands but is independent from the language system.

**Apraxia in non-right-handers**

Most of what is written above and in fact most of the literature on apraxia, applies to patients with standard cerebral organization, i.e., those patients that have left hemisphere dominance for language and also left hemisphere dominance for skilled movements of the hands and phonatory apparatus. Those patients are, almost invariably, right-handed. But there is little doubt that dominance for language and dominance for skilled movements are functionally dissociated, and in some cases, related to different hemispheres. The case of Heilman et al. (1973) provides a powerful indication that this is so. Their patient was left-handed, and he sustained paralysis in the left limbs as the result of a right middle cerebral infarction. Placed in the left hemisphere of most individuals, this lesion would have caused a Broca's aphasia and right hemiparesis. But in this patient no aphasia appeared, indicating that cerebral dominance for language was in the left hemisphere. What the patient showed, however, was a severe apraxia of the *right* limbs only, i.e., an inverted sympathetic apraxia. The likely explanation for this finding is that dominance for learned, representational movement of the limbs was in the right hemisphere, as indicated by the patient's left-handedness, and that in spite of normal language processing and of an intact left motor region, the proper control information from the right hemisphere was no longer available for transfer to the left premotor region. This case presents evidence against the view that disorders of oral language and praxis represent impairments of a common function.

**Apraxia in the deaf**

Bellugi et al. (1983) have studied four deaf patients who depended on American Sign Language (ASL) for communication and who sustained focal cerebral lesions caused by stroke. Three patients had left hemisphere lesions and one had right hemisphere damage. The right hemisphere patient had neither sign aphasia nor apraxia. The three left hemisphere patients had sign aphasia but only *one* of them had apraxia (limb apraxia for transitive and intransitive movements and buccofacial apraxia), and only one other patient was impaired in a set of non-representational movement tasks of the type designed by Kimura (see below). These findings also constitute evidence against the belief that communication defects—in oral language or praxis—are the result of a primary disorder of movement control. Two patients who passed the Kimura tasks were severely aphasic in ASL, i.e., they made numerous linguistic errors expressed in complex, sequential, spatially organized movements. Furthermore, the patient who had apraxia also passed the Kimura tasks, a strong indication that the presence of apraxia does not predict impairment in non-representational types of movement.

These findings lend support to the concept that not only are the control of language and movement separate, but even that the control of language and that of *representational* movement are distinct.

### Disturbances of the control of non-learned, non-representational movement

Some investigators have attempted to study the relation between focal brain lesions and the execution of different types of movement. For instance, Kimura (1982) used non-representational meaningless gestures, both isolated and in sequence, involving the oral musculature or the hand. Her subjects included patients with cerebral vascular disease and brain tumors and the localization of the lesions was not based on neuroimaging methods or autopsy. Her general conclusion was that impairment of the execution of single meaningless movements of the oral musculature was associated with left anterior lesions and that impairment in meaningless single movements of the hand was more closely associated with lesions of the left posterior region. In both instances, she attributed the defect to a general difficulty in the selection of correct postures from a pre-programmed plan. Kolb and Milner (1981) also studied meaningless, complex arm movements in a population of epileptic patients without aphasia. They noted that the impairment in non-representational arm movements was especially associated with left parietal lobe excisions while impairment in meaningless facial movements was especially associated with lesions of the left or the right frontal lobe, which in turn had no influence on the arm movement. These studies add to our knowledge of the physiopathology of movement but do not really relate to the understanding of the phenomenon of apraxia. It is conceivable that the impairment of non-representational arm movements after left parietal damage reflects another aspect of the constructional disorder observed with lesions in this location.

## The Significance of Apraxia

Apraxia in the sense employed in this chapter was for many years almost entirely neglected, and even today some authors regard it as rare. The fact is that apraxia is a frequent phenomenon that can be identified in many patients with cerebral lesions, especially in those caused by stroke. It can be a useful sign for a clinical neurologist, but its greatest importance lies in what it tells us about cerebral organization in relation to movement. Perhaps the most important of these lesions was made clear by Hugo Liepmann, in his pioneering studies of this phenomenon: in most humans, the ability to learn how to execute skilled, representational movements depends on structures of the left hemisphere. Liepmann made this point clear after studying patients with lesions of both the premotor and parietal regions and of the corpus callosum. Modern lesion studies as well as study of patients with surgical split brain have confirmed the correctness of Liepmann's conclusions (Geschwind 1975; Heilman 1979). The strong association in most people between these types of skilled movement and the left hemisphere is made all the more clear when one appreciates the relatively poor abilities of the isolated right hemisphere for those same movements. This is especially evident in those apraxic patients with an intact right hemisphere who fail to improve on imitation of a visual command. We believe this reflects the fact that the learning of skilled, representational movements is so strongly rooted in the left hemisphere in most people, that the right hemisphere of most individuals has minimal ability to imitate a visual model, and even less ability to carry out movements of the limbs or buccofacial musculature to verbal command. It should be recalled that correct imitation of a movement depends on having the movement in one's learned repertoire. Thus most people cannot handle chopsticks correctly the first time, even when they can observe a demonstration. But, of course, the ability to imitate is variable, even in right-hand individuals with standard cerebral organization, because there are instances in which the intact right hemisphere is able to perform far better on imitation than on verbal command. This is an indication that the endowment of the right hemisphere for this particular task is varied and that in some individuals the right visual cortices are able to transfer information into the somato-sensory and motor system of the right side and thus drive certain muscular groups into motion. In many, if not most cases, this may well reflect that some motor learning has taken place in the right hemisphere.

Another important conclusion derived from the study of apraxia is that axial movements are organized and driven from brain different structures from those used for separate movements of small joints especially in the hand. This is evident from the fact that axial movements are commonly intact in patients with apraxia. This conclusion is strongly concordant with the known anatomical facts concerning the motor systems. Thus it has long been known that sensory association cortices, including the posteriorly located language areas, have direct connections to subcortical motor structures without the intervention of the precentral cortex, either directly or via the supplementary motor area. It is also conceivable that the right hemisphere may actually be more adroit at controlling this type of complex synergy than the left hemisphere, which appears far more specialized for fragmented, fine motions of the hand or buccofacial musculature. It is of interest to note that axial synergies are phylogenetically and ontogenetically older than the fine motions of fingers and phonatory apparatus. This might well explain the more widespread representation of their control and perhaps even a leading role for the right hemisphere, the specializations of which may well be phylogenetically older.

The dramatic dissociation between limb and buccofacial movements, on the one hand, and axial movement on the other, is in keeping with the knowledge that the cerebral cortex contains both a pyramidal system devoted primarily to the production of multiple nonstandard fine movement, and non-pyramidal systems that can be associated with innate although somewhat modifiable synergies. The non-pyramidal systems play a greater role in relatively automatized, 'spontaneous' movements. The natural smile which occurs with amusement is obviously emotionally driven from non-pyramidal motor structures, whereas the smile which we attempt to make for a photographer on command is likely to result from the engagement of the pyramidal motor cortex; it usually has only a poor resemblance to the naturally occurring emotional expression. There is ample proof that the control of these two types of movement is differently located in the brain. Patients with lesions in the lower tier of the precentral cortex have a contralateral, central, facial paralysis, which is marked in all voluntary motions; but when they smile or laugh in response to a joke, they often correct the asymmetry of the mouth and perform an entirely normal movement. Conversely, patients with lesions in the mesial cortices (for instance, anterior cingulate gyrus and supplementary motor area, as well as other mesial frontal lobe cortices), or in subcortical structures such as the amygdala, thalamus, and neostriatum, often have what is known as an 'emotional' type of facial paralysis in which poor innervation on one side appears during smiling, laughing, or crying, although in response to verbal command the facial musculature is moved symmetrically (Damasio and Maurer 1978). Such dissociations strongly indicate that the brain has multiple generators of movement and that those different generators are engaged according to the *type of movement* and to the *context* in which it is performed.

The motor systems, when activated either spontaneously or at the request of an examiner, through a verbal or a visual mode, make use of programs of movement, some of them innate, others learned. It is possible to say that apraxia reflects a loss of, or a failure to, evoke those programs in response to normally effective stimuli, or especially, a loss of the access of those programs to the motor generators which guide representational movements of the limbs and buccofacial apparatus.

## References

Bellugi, U., H. Poizner and E.S. Klima: Brain organization for language: clues from sign aphasia. Human Neurobiol. 2 (1983) 155–170.

Damasio, A. and A. Benton: Impairment of hand movements under visual guidance. Neurology 29 (1979) 170–178.

Damasio, A. and R. Maurer: A neurological model for childhood autism. Arch. Neurol. 35 (1978) 777–786.

De Renzi, E., A. Pieczuro and L.A. Vignolo: Oral apraxia and aphasia. Cortex 2 (1966) 50–73.

Gazzaniga, M., J. Bogen and R. Sperry: Dyspraxia following division of the cerebral commissures. Arch. Neurol. (Chicago) 16 (1967) 606–612.

Geschwind, N.: Disconnecxion syndromes in animals and man. Brain 88 (1965) 237–294, 585–644.

Geschwind, N.: The apraxias: Neural mechanisms of disorders of learned movements. Am. Scientist 63 (1975) 188–195.

Geschwind, N. and F. Kaplan: A human cerebral disconnection syndrome. Neurology 12 (1962) 675–685.

Goodglass, H. and E. Kaplan: The Assessment of Aphasia and Related Disorders. Philadelphia: Lea and Febiger, 2nd Ed. (1983).

Haaxma, R. and H.G.J.M. Kuypers: Intrahemispheric cortical connexions and visual guidance of hand and finger movements in the rhesus monkey. Brain 98 (1975) 239 260.
Heilman, K. M.: Apraxia. In: K. M. Heilman and E. Valenstein (Eds), Clinical Neuropsychology. London & New York: Oxford University Press (1979).
Heilman, K. M., J. M. Coyle, E.F. Gonyea and N. Geschwind: Apraxia and agraphia in a left-hander. Brain 96 (1973) 21–28.
Kimura, D.: Left-hemisphere control of oral and brachial movements and their relation to communication. Philosoph. Trans. R. Soc. London, Series B 298 (1982) 135–149.
Kolb, B. and B. Milner: Performance of complex arm and facial movements after focal brain lesions. Neuropsychologia 19 (1981) 491–503.
Lawrence, D. G. and H. G. J. M. Kuypers: The functional organization of the motor systems in the monkey. Brain 91 (1968) 1–36.
Lepmann, H.: Drei Aufsatze aus dem Apraxie-Gebiet. Berlin: Karger (1908).
Liepman, H. and O. Maas: Fall von linksseiter Agraphie und Apraxie bei rechtsseitiger Lahmung. Z. Psychol. Neurol. (Lpz.) 10 (1907) 214–227.
Moll, L. and H. G. J. M. Kuypers: Premotor cortical ablations in monkeys: Contralateral changes in visually guided reaching behavior. Science 198 (1977) 317–319.
Mountcastle, V. B., J. C. Lynch and A. Georgopoulos: Posterior parietal association cortex of the monkey: Command functions for operations within extrapersonal space. J. Neurophysiol. 38 (1975) 871–908.
Poeck, K., G. Lehmkuhl and K. Willmes: Axial movements in ideomotor apraxia. J. Neurol. Neurosurg. Psychiatr. 45 (1982) 1125–1129.
Tognola, G. and L. A. Vignolo: Brain lesions associated with oral apraxia in stroke patients: A clinico-neuroradiological investigation with the CT scan. Neuropsychologia, 18 (1980) 257–272.

The work presented in this chapter was supported in part by grants from the NIH (NS-06209), the Orton Research Fund, and the Essel Foundation, to the Department of Neurology and Dana Research Laboratories, Beth Israel Hospital, Boston; Department of Neurology, Harvard Medical School; and Boston University Aphasia Research Center, VA Hospital, Boston (N.G.) and supported by NINCDS Grant PO1 NS 19632-01 (A.R.D.).

# PART IV

# Hemispheric Asymmetries, Cerebral Dominance, and Handedness

*Steven C. Schachter*

Geschwind's interests in hemispheric asymmetries, cerebral dominance, and handedness were natural extensions of his work in aphasia and apraxia, and grew out of his desire to "explore the possibility that the human brain was endowed with anatomical asymmetries that could account for the various aspects of cerebral dominance."[1]

Not surprisingly, Geschwind began his study of asymmetries and cerebral dominance with the temporal lobe. Temporal lobe asymmetries had received only minor attention in the literature over the preceding century and had never been correlated with handedness.[2] Geschwind and his colleague, Walter Levitsky, were particularly influenced by the anatomic findings of Pfeifer and by Von Economo and Horn.[3,4] and using only a ruler and a camera, cut 100 adult brains postmortem in the planes of the Sylvian fissures and compared the appearance of the left and right plana temporale. In this landmark study, they found a larger left planum temporale in 65 of 100 brains and a larger right planum in 11.[5] This approximate 2:1 ratio of left-right asymmetry was central to Geschwind's later concept of "standard structural dominance."[6]

Juhn Wada was greatly influenced by a lecture Geschwind gave in 1966, during which he described his as-yet-unpublished study with Levitsky.[7] Subsequently, Wada and others repeatedly confirmed the findings of Geschwind and Levitsky in adult, infant, and fetal brains.[8,9] Many other investigators were also personally inspired and motivated by Geschwind to study human cerebral asymmetries. One notable member of this group was the radiologist Marjorie LeMay, who together with several colleagues, performed a number of radiographic studies which documented cerebral asymmetries and their relationships to handedness.[10–13]

The intermediate step between Geschwind's interest in cerebral dominance and handedness, and his complete theory of cerebral lateralization,[14–16] was his work on the correlation between autoimmune disease and handedness, done largely in collaboration with Peter Behan. As Behan recalls,

> My wife and I spent some time in late 1980 working at Massachusetts General Hospital with Dr. E. P. Richardson. At that time Norman had already begun his major work on cerebral dominance. While we were having dinner at his home one evening, the question arose whether any of us had observed an association between any diseases and left-handedness. Curiously, I had just treated two cases of progressive dementia in patients who had premature white hair and who were strongly left-handed. These patients were also interesting for another reason: they each had thyroiditis and had responded to thyroid replacement therapy. Norman stated that he had seen a patient with a similar case that week. He also immediately recalled a professor and his daughter whom he knew intimately and both of whom were left-handed and had premature gray hair and possible early dementia.[17]

Based on this dinner conversation, Geschwind and Behan set out to investigate the relationship of left-handedness with autoimmune disease and carried out a study in Glasgow. The results, published in the *Proceedings of the National Academy of Sciences* in 1982,[18] received widespread attention because of the implied linkage of the development of the nervous and immune systems.

During the early 1980s, additional studies were performed and published[19] and Geschwind, in conjunction with his colleague Albert Galaburda, formulated a far-ranging hypothesis which integrated handedness, cerebral dominance, and autoimmune disease. The publication of this hypothesis,[14–16] often called the Geschwind-Behan-Galaburda (GBG) hypothesis, stimulated innumerable additional investigations and papers, and generated considerable support and skepticism.[20–22] Bryden et al.,[20] for example, recognized the GBG hypothesis as "a major scientific phenomenon of sudden onset and immediate influence," yet concluded that "psychologists and physicians have more useful things to do than to carry out further assessments of the model." At an Academy of Neurology meeting several years ago, the winner of the McHenry award for an outstanding paper on a topic in the history of neurology lauded Geschwind for his brilliant contributions to the field of aphasia, yet rejected the significance of the GBG hypothesis, which drew a sharp reaction from Geschwind's long-time friend and colleague Frank Benson, who was in the audience.

The publication of the hypothesis was nearly circumvented because of similar reactions from journal reviewers. Robert J. Joynt became chief editor of the *Archives of Neurology* in 1982 and invited Geschwind to become one of the associate editors. Shortly after, following many conversations with Joynt, Geschwind submitted the manuscript to the *Archives*. Joynt[23] recalls that responses by the reviewers "ran the gamut from great enthusiasm to outright rejection." Joynt, too, was skeptical, but he was eventually swayed by the manner in which "Norman traced the evolution of his theoretical construct, buttressed by facts and observations from a broad range of fields: biology, physiology, endocrinology, genetics, etc." Joynt decided to accept the article because "it offered a whole new view of the role of the nervous system in controlling noncognitive function."

The resistance to widespread acceptance of the GBG hypothesis derives from three sources. First, the study of the fetal origins of cerebral dominance is at odds with the work of Marian Annett, an influential handedness researcher and theorist, who purports that the genetic theory of cerebral development is a more powerful determinant of cerebral development than the "pathology model" of Geschwind. She has argued that intrauterine factors are less important than genetic factors in determining brain structure.[21] However, her theory and the GBG hypothesis actually complement one another. The latter approach may be able to shed light on the mechanisms by which genes control cerebral development. For instance, identifying the fetal insults or factors (e.g., testosterone) that modify brain structure and cerebral dominance from what would otherwise be predicted on strictly genetic grounds may provide clues to the mechanisms by which genes control normal brain development. Further, distinguishing the biologic associations of cerebral dominance and handedness may shed light on other genes that may be tightly linked with the "right shift" gene, which according to Annett controls the development of handedness.[21] For example, if autoimmune illness is associated with left-handedness, as was thought by Geschwind, then the search for the right shift gene could be directed toward those genes that are associated with autoimmune illness.

Second, the lack of consistency in handedness studies has resulted in a number of "negative" studies of handedness and biological associations, casting further doubt on the GBG hypothesis.[24] Yet review of this handedness literature reveals that many studies do not include enough subjects to demonstrate statistical significance, or use measuring instruments that do not produce a handedness score that is proportional to the degree and direction of handedness. Further, investigators often do not test the distribution of handedness scores for normality and yet use statistics for normally-distributed data.

Third, and most importantly, the interpretation of the hypothesis has often been too narrow.[25] As originally put forward by Geschwind and Galaburda,[14] the hypothesis states that "the most powerful factors [in determining the patterns of cerebral asymmetry] are variations in the chemical environment in fetal life and to a lesser extent in infancy and early childhood. The factors that modify cerebral dominance also influence the development of many other systems, e.g., the organs involved in immune response." Restatements of this hypothesis by other authors and critics often focus exclusively on the possible role of testosterone, though it is only one of many possible fetal factors. For example, Bryden et al.[20] wrote: "To simplify [the GBG hypothesis], alterations in the level of fetal testosterone are seen as having many effects." True, Geschwind went on to propose that testosterone was one of the major influences on brain development, but this was not the *essence* of the hypothesis.

The GBG hypothesis gives special importance to handedness correlation studies by seeking to increase our understanding of the interrelationships between structural and functional cerebral dominance. Consistent with Geschwind's other contributions, it was based on his insightful recognition of a *connection*—in this case between fetal factors, brain development, and human behavior. The assertion that intrauterine factors influence fetal brain development is a profound concept that further revises the nature-nurture argument. Conceptually, this was one of Geschwind's most insightful contributions. How tragic, as pointed out by Joynt,[23] that he died suddenly before this opus was ever published in its complete form.

## References

1. Geschwind, N. Anatomical asymmetry as the basis for cerebral dominance. Fed Proc, 1978;37,2263-2266.
2. Eberstaller, O. Zur Oberflachen-Anatomie der Grosshirn-Hemispharen. Wien Med Blatter, 1884;7,644.
3. Pfeifer, RA. Pathologie der Horstrahlung und der corticalen Horsphare. In O Bumke and O Foerster (eds.), *Handbuch der Neurologie.* Berlin: Springer, 1936, pp. 534-626.
4. Von Economo, C, and Horn, L. Uber windungsrelief, masze und rindenarchitektonik der supratemporalflache. Z Gesamte Neurol Psychiat, 1930;130,678-757.
5. Geschwind, N, and Levitsky, W. Human brain: left-right asymmetries in temporal speech region. Science, 1968;161,186-7.
6. Schachter, SC, and Galaburda, AM. Development and biological associations of cerebral dominance: review and possible mechanisms. J Am Acad Child Psychiatry, 1986;25,741-750.
7. Wada, JA. Pre-language and fundamental asymmetry of the infant brain. Ann N Y Acad Sci, 1977;299,370-9.
8. Wada, JA. Interhemispheric sharing and shift of cerebral speech function. Excerpta Medica International Congress Series, 1969;193,296-297.
9. LeMay, M, and Schachter, SC. Cerebral Asymmetries. In SC Schachter and O Devinsky (eds.), *Behavioral Neurology and the Legacy of Norman Geschwind.* Philadelphia: Lippincott-Raven, 1997, pp. 243-256.
10. LeMay, M, and Culebras, A. Human brain—morphologic differences in the hemispheres demonstrable by carotid arteriography. N Engl J Med, 1972;287,168-170.
11. Hochberg, FH, and LeMay, M. Arteriographic correlates of handedness. Neurology, 1975;25,218-222.
12. LeMay, M, and Kido, DK. Asymmetries of the cerebral hemispheres on computed tomograms. J Comput Assist Tomogr, 1978;2,471-476.
13. LeMay, M. Asymmetries of the skull and handedness. Phrenology revisited. J Neurol Sci, 1977;32,243-253.
14. Geschwind, N, and Galaburda, AM. Cerebral lateralization. Biological mechanisms, associations, and pathology: I. A hypothesis and a program for research. Arch Neurol, 1985;42,428-59.

15. Geschwind, N, and Galaburda, AM. Cerebral lateralization. Biological mechanisms, associations, and pathology: II. A hypothesis and a program for research. Arch Neurol, 1985;42,521-552.
16. Geschwind, N, and Galaburda, AM. Cerebral lateralization. Biological mechanisms, associations, and pathology: III. A hypothesis and a program for research. Arch Neurol, 1985;42,634-654.
17. Behan, PO. Handedness and Autoimmune Disease. In SC Schachter and O Devinsky (eds.), *Behavioral Neurology and the Legacy of Norman Geschwind*. Philadelphia: Lippincott-Raven, 1997, pp. 287-292.
18. Geschwind, N, and Behan, P. Left-handedness: association with immune disease, migraine, and developmental learning disorder. Proc Natl Acad Sci USA, 1982; 79,5097-5100.
19. Geschwind, N, and Behan, PO. Laterality, hormones, and immunity. In N Geschwind and AM Galaburda (eds.), *Cerebral dominance: the biological foundations*. Cambridge, MA: Harvard University Press, 1984, pp. 211-224.
20. Bryden, MP, McManus, IC, and Bulman-Fleming, MB. Evaluating the empirical support for the Geschwind-Behan-Galaburda model of cerebral lateralization. Brain Cogn, 1994;26,103-167.
21. Annett, M. The right shift theory of a genetic balanced polymorphism for cerebral dominance and cognitive processing. Current Psychology of Cognition, 1995; 14,427-480.
22. Dellatolas, G, Annesi, I, Jallon, P, Chavance, M, and Lellouch, J. An epidemiological reconsideration of the Geschwind-Galaburda theory of cerebral lateralization. Arch Neurol, 1990;47,778-782.
23. Joynt, RJ. A Darlin' Man. In SC Schachter and O Devinsky (eds.), *Behavioral Neurology and the Legacy of Norman Geschwind*. Philadelphia: Lippincott-Raven, 1997, pp. 3-4.
24. Schachter, SC. Studies of handedness and anomalous dominance: problems and progress. In AM Galaburda (ed.), *Dyslexia and Development: Neurobiological Aspects of Extra-Ordinary Brains*. Cambridge: Harvard University Press, 1993, pp. 269-96, 358-65.
25. Schachter, SC. Evaluating the Bryden-McManus-Bulman/Fleming critique of the Geschwind-Behan-Galaburda model of cerebral lateralization. Brain and Cognition, 1994;26,199-205.

## CHAPTER 14

# Cytoarchitectonic Left-Right Asymmetries in the Temporal Speech Region

*Albert M. Galaburda, Friedrich Sanides, Norman Geschwind*

The concept of cerebral dominance, the asymmetric control by the hemispheres of certain cerebral functions, is firmly established in man.[1] Each hemisphere appears to play a predominant role in the performance of certain functions such as language, fine motor activities, visuomotor tasks, and music, to name a few. Likewise, the brain clearly shows gross morphological asymmetries between the hemispheres,[2] of which one of the most striking is the difference in size between the left and the right planum temporale, the region on the superior temporal plane lying posterior to the transverse gyrus of Heschl (first transverse gyrus) and extending back to the end of the Sylvian fossa. It has been shown in large numbers of brains that the left planum is usually larger than its mate.[3–8]

The importance of the gross anatomic asymmetries is not yet clearly established. Laboratory data on behavioral auditory asymmetries,[1] in addition to clinical data obtained from aphasia-producing lesions on the planum,[9] when taken together with the planum asymmetries, make it tempting to presume that the larger left planum may represent the anatomic substrate for language lateralization to the left hemisphere. One cannot, however, argue purely from the gross asymmetries. It is conceivable that areas of specific cytoarchitectonic structure might be equally large on both sides, and that the gross asymmetries result from differences in the pattern of folding of the two hemispheres. This might suggest that the gross asymmetries have no relationship to function. Furthermore, even if cytoarchitectonic asymmetries were present, it would be important to deter-

---

Reprinted with permission from *Archives of Neurology*. 1978; 35 (12): 812-817. 

mine whether they involve regions likely to be implicated in language function. Thus, asymmetries in the planum might be secondary to asymmetries in nearby parietal cortex or subcortical structures that might also be responsible for the asymmetries of the Sylvian fissures found by LeMay and Culebras.[10] Indeed, our evidence that the asymmetries of the planum temporale represent cytoarchitectonic asymmetries in language-related regions is very limited.

Von Economo and Horn[11] published data supporting the view that the difference between the plana was the result of a larger extent of the auditory association cortex on the left side. Their study, however, presents certain difficulties. These authors measured the extent of the auditory-related cytoarchitectonic areas on the planum alone; they did not measure the full extent of these areas, which in addition to lying on the planum, also extend beyond its borders, e.g, onto the temporal convexity. Furthermore, they did not include the cortex that lies in the depths of the sulci on the planum, nor did they consider variations in cortical thickness but instead restricted their measurements to the two-dimensional representations of the areas on the surface. Such a study could not exclude the possibility that sufficient quantities of association cortex existed on the right side either beyond the planum or in the depths of sulci, which could counterbalance any differences on the plana themselves. On the other hand, their study might have easily erred in the opposite direction, i.e., they could have underestimated the left-sided preponderance by measuring only the portions of cytoarchitectonic areas on the planum alone.

To test more adequately the hypothesis that the planum asymmetries truly reflect cytoarchitectonic asymmetries in auditory-related cortex, we have made measurement of the full extent of the distinctive cellular areas of the auditory regions.

## Materials and Methods

### The Specimens

Four human brains were randomly selected from the Yakovlev Collection at the Armed Forces Institute of Pathology and the Harvard Medical School. This collection consists of normal specimens that have been embedded whole in celloidin and cut in gapless serial sections at a thickness of 35μ. Every 20th section has been stained for nerve cell bodies with Nissl stain and the adjacent section by the Loyez method for myelinated fibers. The methods of fixation, embedding, cutting, staining, and mounting assure that artifacts of distortion affect both hemispheres equally. Photographs of each brain prior to processing exist in the collection and have been used to reproduce the lateral views in the figures.

### Planum Reconstructions

The planum temporale of each hemisphere (Figures 1–4, C and D) was reconstructed from the coronal sections by the use of a specially designed projection

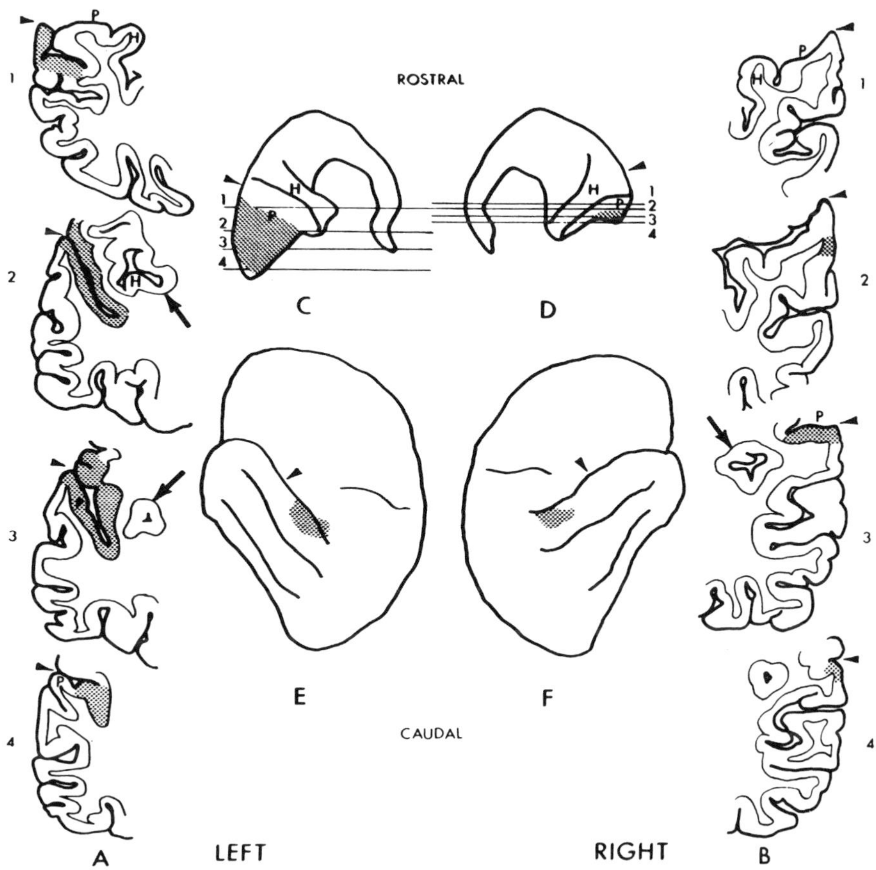


FIGURE 1. Case 1. In this figure, as with figures 2, 3, and 4, coronal sections are shown in A and B, superior temporal planes in C and D, showing planum temporale (P) and Heschl's gyrus (H), and lateral surfaces of brain showing area Tpt (shaded) in E and F. Arrowheads point to Sylvian fissures. Note large planum asymmetry (C and D). Also note buried temporal cortex on coronal sections (arrows). (Also see text.)

apparatus. The serial sections were projected on a flat surface without distortion and the limits of the plana were marked on graph paper. Since the projected magnification was known, as was the distance between sections, it was possible to reconstruct the plana to scale. The plane of section varied slightly from one specimen to the other; therefore, it is not possible to make direct comparisons for the shape and size of the plana among the different specimens; comparisons, however, are possible between the right and left plana in each specimen. For ease of identification, only Heschl's gyri are shown in the planum reconstructions,

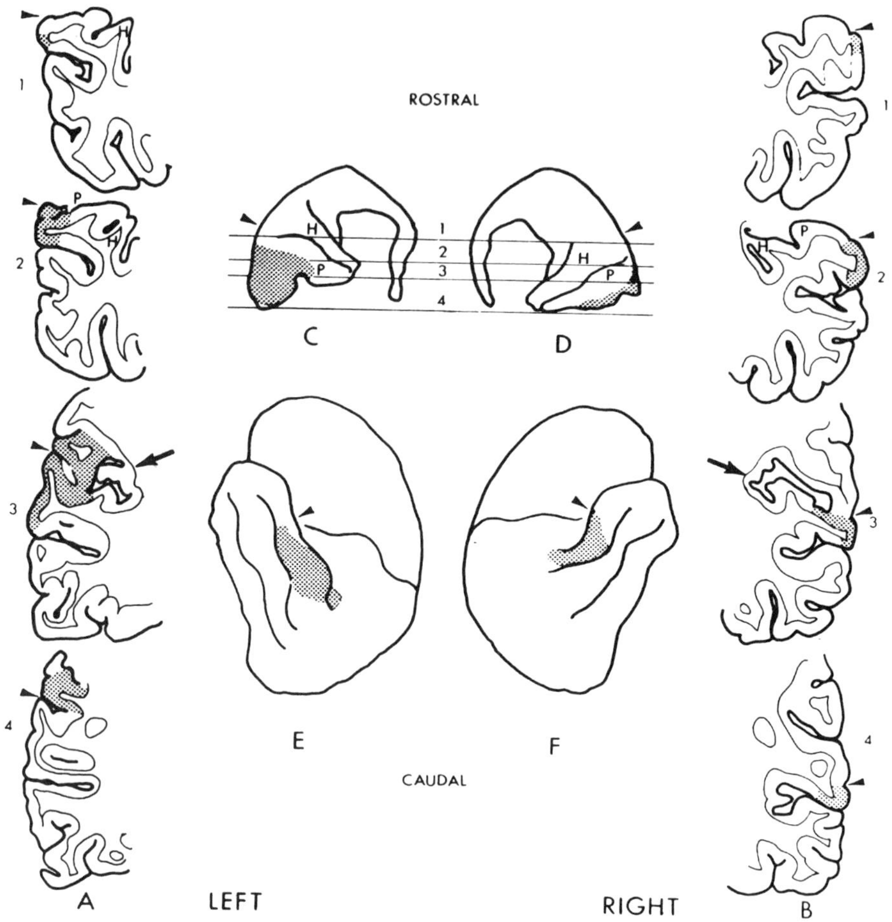


FIGURE 2. Case 2. Note extension of Tpt onto parietal lobe by way of cortical bridges (A3 and E). This case also shows buried temporal cortex (arrows). (See legend for Figure 1 for explanation of letters arrows, etc, and see text.)

leaving out other convolutions on the upper surface of the temporal lobe. The areas of the plana were measured directly on the graph paper reconstructions.

## Cytoarchitectonic Parcellation and Measurement

The cytoarchitectonic areas were identified by the use of a stereomicroscope under low-power magnification. The borders of each area were found on the Nissl-stained sections and then checked against the borders found on the myelin preparations. Photographic templates at fixed magnification were made of

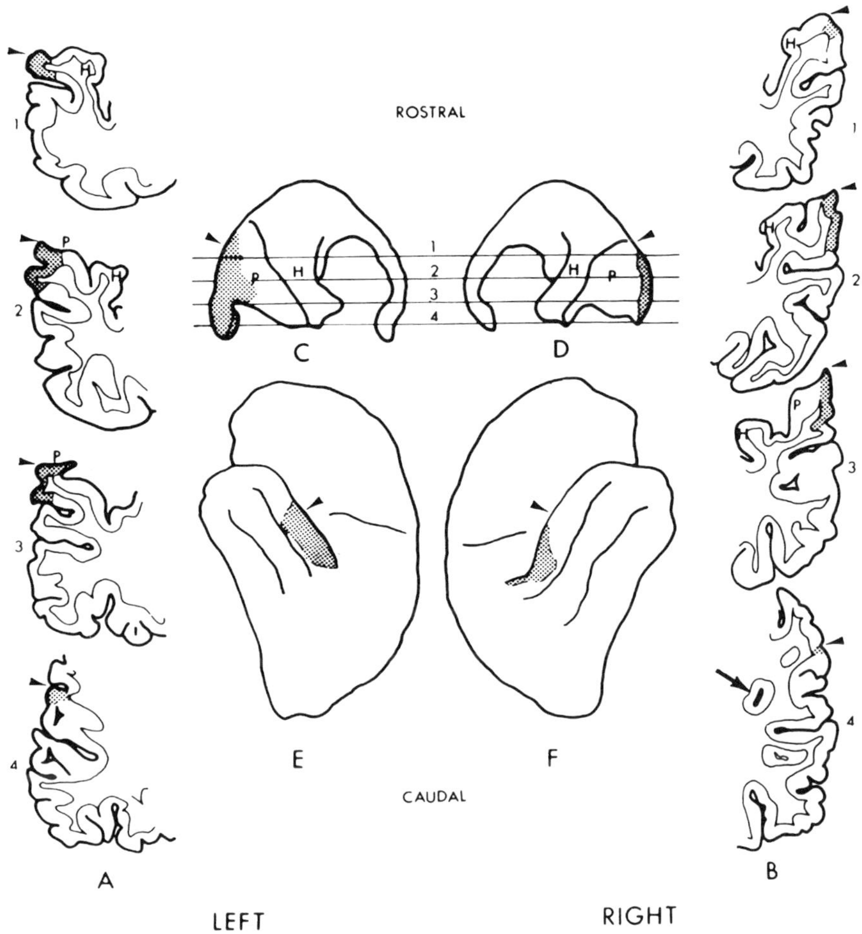


FIGURE 3. Case 3. Note buried temporal cortex (arrow). On the right, more Tpt is present on convexity than on planum. (See legend for Figure 1 for explanation of letters, arrows, etc.)

each section and the borders of the areas marked on them. The criteria used for area identification and the detailed maps of each auditory region have been given elsewhere;[12,13] for the purpose of this study, only the results of mapping temporoparietal area Tpt[2,12,13] will be presented. Area Tpt corresponds on architectonic grounds to the posterior portion of Brodmann's area 22[14] and von Economo's and Koskinas' area $TA_1$.[15] In this area, lamina IV cannot be easily separated from adjacent laminae III and V because pyramids from the latter two layers encroach on the former, thus obliterating the borders (Figure 5). Tpt can easily be distinguished from the neighboring association area Pa Ae[16] which

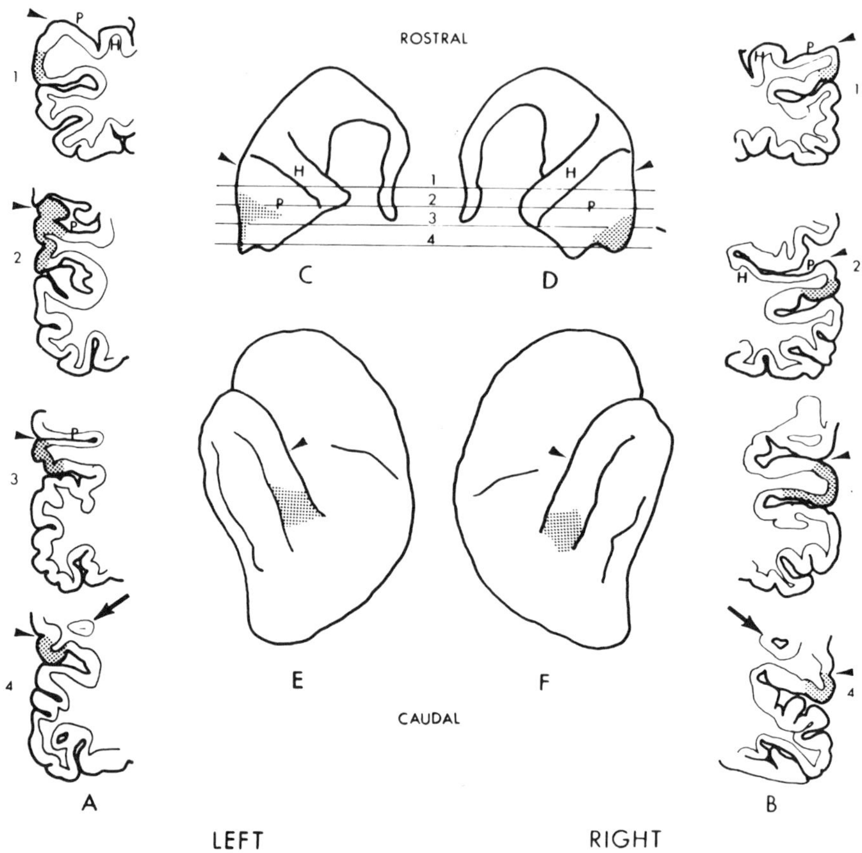


FIGURE 4. Case 4. Note slight predominance of right planum temporale (see text). Note also that left planum temporale is somewhat more folded, which may explain slight left-sided Tpt predominance. There is also buried temporal cortex (arrows). (See legend for Figure 1 for explanation of letters, arrows, etc.)

has a less dense lamina V and a lamina III containing slender pyramids disposed in columns (Figure 5). The area occupies the posterior portion of the planum and extends onto the temporal convexity to make up a major part of the posterior half of the superior temporal gyrus (Figures 1–4). In some specimens, it also extends around the posterior end of the Sylvian fissure and onto the parietal lobe (Figures 1E and 2E). It is likely that most lesions in the region of the posterior Sylvian fissure that cause Wernicke's aphasia involve substantial portions of area Tpt.[9]

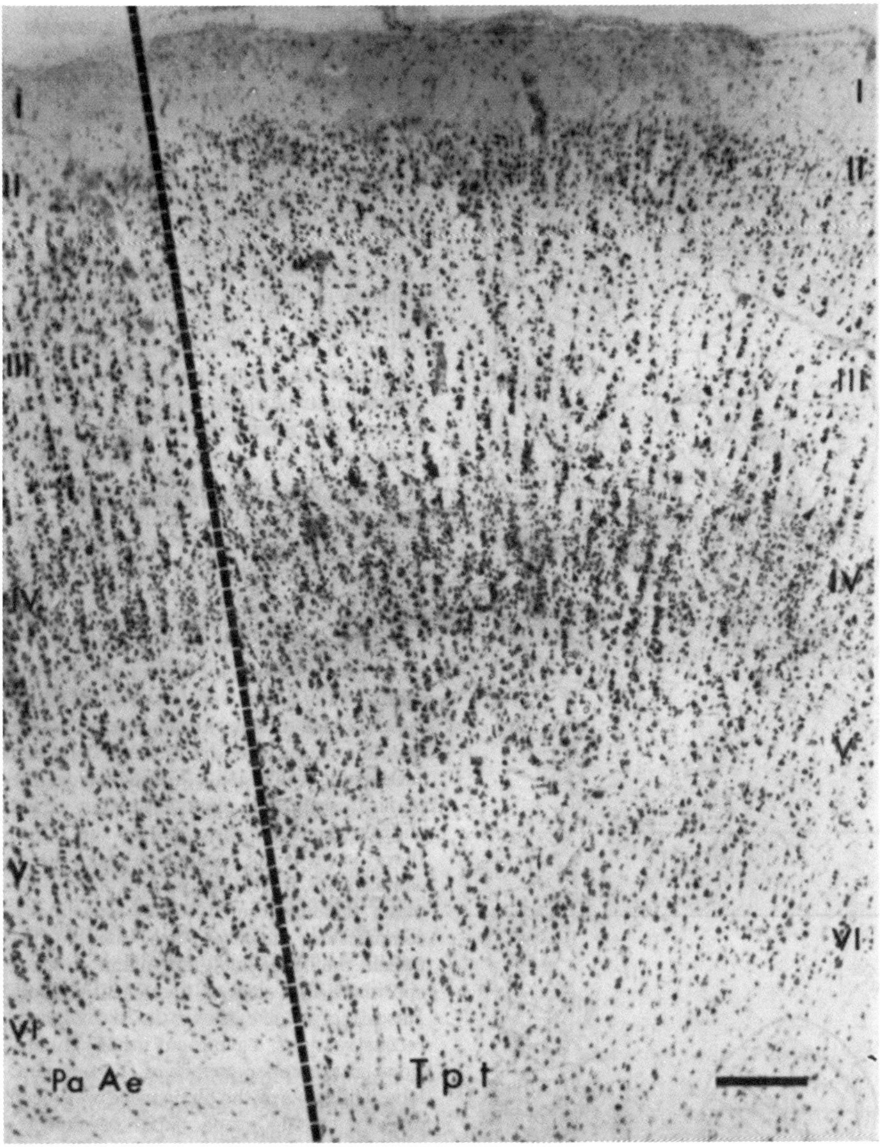


FIGURE 5. Areas Tpt and Pa Ae (see text). Note differences in sizes of pyramids in lamina III and difference in coarseness of pyramids in lamina V. Area Tpt represents a transition between auditory association cortex (cf Pa Ae) and cortex of the inferior parietal lobule. Bar = 200 .

Measurements of surface extent were made on the graph paper reconstructions of the plana and directly on the photographic templates showing cytoarchitectonic areas by the use of a compensating polar planimeter. The figures given in the tables are in relative units of area for the plana and in relative units of volume for area Tpt. The volumes of Tpt were calculated from the relative area measurements on the templates and the known data of section thickness and distance between sections.

## Results

### General Observations

The serially sectioned material affords the possibility of making several general observations concerning the auditory region that would otherwise escape the eye in other types of preparations. The plana reconstructed from these sections illustrate several features (Figures 1–4, C and D). The shapes of the plana vary from one specimen to the other but generally assume that of a triangle bound laterally by the Sylvian fissure (Figures 1 and 4, arrowheads), medially by Heschl's gyrus (Figures 1–4, H), and posteriorly by the posterior wall of the Sylvian fossa. The curvilinear appearance of the posterior border is produced by the uneven fusion of the posterior parietal operculum with the posterior planum temporale, allowing for the formation of deep pockets of cortex in the depths of the hemispheres. Some of these pockets can be seen in the coronal sections as concentric rings (Figures 1 and 4, arrows). Substantial amounts of the cortex can be buried in this manner. Plana that are visualized by drawing a knife blade in a posterior direction from the end of the Sylvian fissure,[3] thus unroofing the superior temporal plane, would not uncover this feature of the posterior planum. The plana, furthermore, can be extremely folded, so that large amounts of cortex are buried in long sulci. The sulci may be of the simple, unbranched type, or they can assume complex configurations (Figure 1A, section 1).

On the planum area, Tpt occupies the posterolateral aspect and appears to constitute most of the excess area in the cases where the right and left plana are different in size. This finding is particularly noticeable in case 1 (Figure 1, C and D) where the huge excess of the planum on the left side is covered by the Tpt cortex. In such cases, it can be seen that if Tpt were to be removed from both sides, the plana would be much more symmetrical in size and shape. Thus, Tpt seems to contribute substantially to the planum asymmetry. Also, in the cases showing Tpt asymmetry, the excess occurs mostly in a posterolateral location; this produces asymmetries in the lengths of the Sylvian fissures on both sides. Asymmetries in the lengths of the Sylvian fissures have been previously reported;[10] the findings of this study suggest that they may reflect, at least in part, asymmetries in the extent of area Tpt on the planum temporale.

Area Tpt extends outside of the planum onto the cerebral convexity. In some cases, more of Tpt is present on the superior temporal gyrus than on the planum itself (cf. Figure 2, D and F). In addition, at times Tpt extends onto the parietal

TABLE 1. Right-Left Measurements

| | *Planum Temporale Planimetric Units* | | *Area Tpt Volumetric Units* | |
|---|---|---|---|---|
| *Case* | *Right* | *Left* | *Right* | *Left* |
| 1 | 55 | 171 | 35 | 254 |
| 2 | 68 | 153 | 69 | 151 |
| 3 | 114 | 156 | 73 | 101 |
| 4 | 136 | 118 | 95 | 108 |

TABLE 2. Left-Right Ratios Based on Table 1

| *Case* | *Planum Temporale* | *Rank* | *Area Tpt* | *Rank* |
|---|---|---|---|---|
| 1 | 3.11 | 1 | 7.26 | 1 |
| 2 | 2.25 | 2 | 2.19 | 2 |
| 3 | 1.37 | 3 | 1.38 | 3 |
| 4 | 0.87 | 4 | 1.14 | 4 |

convexity (Figures 1E and 2E). This is probably accomplished through the extension of this type of cortex onto the parietal operculum along the posterior wall of the Sylvian fossa (Figures 1A, section 2, and 2A, section 3).

## Planum Asymmetries

The results of measuring the extent of the planum on the two sides are given in Table 1. In three of the four specimens, the left planum is larger than the right. In case 1, the left planum exceeds the right by more than 200%, and in case 3 by 37%. In the remaining case, the difference is only 13% (the right planum being larger), which may be within the error of measurement. Therefore, in this series of four brains three plana are greater on the left and is approximately equal on the two sides. In a much larger series, Geschwind and Levitsky[3] found a larger left planum in 65%, equal plana in 24%, and a larger right planum in 11%,[3] a roughly similar distribution of asymmetries. One is of course unlikely to encounter a case with a distinctly larger right planum in a small series.

## Cytoarchitectonic Asymmetries

The results in one brain (case 1) have been given elsewhere.[2] The volumes of Tpt are given in Table 2. Tpt is larger on the left side in the three cases in which the left planum is larger. The difference between the sides varies from greater than 626% in case 1 to 38% in case 3. Case 4 has Tpts that are only 14% different in size, a difference that is probably within the range of the error of the method. The data also show that in the case in which Tpt is very asymmetric in size (case 1), the volume on the right side is quite small, while that on the other side is very large. On the other hand, in the case that shows little asymmetry (case 4), the volumes of the two Tpts lie approximately halfway between the largest and the smallest in the series.

A pattern begins to arise from the data. The specimens studied show a distribution of asymmetries of the planum similar to that found in larger series. They also show a distribution of asymmetries in cytoarchitectonic area Tpt. In three cases, area Tpt is larger on the left; in one case, both Tpts are equal. The distribution of Tpt asymmetries seems to match that of planum asymmetries. Furthermore, the same cases that show planum asymmetries also show Tpt asymmetries, and the extent of the asymmetries also seem to match. Thus, in case 1 where the planum asymmetry is the largest, the asymmetry in the volumes of Tpt is also the largest, while in case 4, where there is no substantial planum asymmetry, the sizes of the Tpts area do not differ. Table 3 gives the ratios of the left over the right planum areas and the ratios of the left over right Tpt volumes. In all but case 1, the ratios are in agreement. In case 1, the ratio of Tpts is very large, reflecting the high degree of folding of the planum in that specimen. Still, when the ratios of the plana and the ratios of the Tpts are ranked and correlated, the coefficient of correlation is +1. In a series of four brains, such a perfect positive correlation is significant at the .05 level.[16]

## Comment

The findings of this study indicate that asymmetry in the size of the planum temporale of both hemispheres in man possibly reflects asymmetry in the size of a cytoarchitectonic area, which on morphological grounds belongs to the auditory region. This cytoarchitectonic auditory asymmetry, furthermore, may well represent the anatomic substrate of language function. Although much information on verbal lateralization to the left hemisphere exists in the literature,[1] and gross anatomic asymmetries have been described in the temporal lobe,[3–8] no previous report has shown unambiguously cytoarchitectonic asymmetries in the auditory region that could explain the functional differences. Although von Economo and Horn[11] attempted to demonstrate such cytoarchitectonic asymmetries, their study was incomplete and did not exclude other possibilities. It is clear from this study that an attempt to measure cytoarchitectonic areas just on the planum would miss portions lying on the convexities. Furthermore, as our study shows, large amounts of cortex can be buried in sulci, thus making measurements restricted to the brain surface incomplete. However, despite the limitations of previous studies, our results support the earlier notions of cytoarchitectonic asymmetry and suggest that the auditory cytoarchitectonic areas on the planum reflect, at least in part, the full asymmetry. This realization is important since, with the introduction of computerized tomography of the brain, it is now possible to visualize in many cases the planum asymmetries in living patients.[2] Knowledge about the relationship between cytoarchitectonic and planum asymmetries might allow one to infer the presence of cytoarchitectonic asymmetry after examination of the computerized scans.

The degree of dominance for language function by one or the other hemisphere may be a function of the degree of asymmetry in cytoarchitectonic areas such as Tpt. Thus, in brains where the asymmetry of Tpt is striking, dominance for language may be greatly lateralized, whereas in those in which Tpt is nearly equal on the two sides, the degree of functional lateralization may be much less. Similarly, asymmetries in Tpt may form part of a continuum extending from cases with a much larger area on the left side, through cases with nearly equal Tpts, to cases in which Tpt on the right side is larger. This anatomic continuum may underlie a similar distribution of dominance for language function.

The anatomic asymmetries might help to explain the variability in degree of recovery from lesions that produce language deficits. For instance, in brains where one of the sides has a much larger Tpt, a lesion on that side could produce more severe and long lasting aphasic disturbances, whereas in brains where Tpt is distributed more equally on the two sides, a unilateral lesion might not produce aphasia, or the deficit might be mild and short lived. This possibility is particularly tempting in view of the results of this study showing that in the case with extensive Tpt asymmetry the left area is very large, while the right is much smaller than average, and in the case in which Tpt is more symmetrical on the two sides, both areas are relatively large. The latter situation may be the case in some left-handed persons who tend to have more symmetrical brains[2] and also seem to acquire less severe aphasic disorders from unilateral lesions on either side.[17] Sex differences in certain neuropsychological processes[18,19] may also reflect the possibility that planum asymmetries are less striking in women.[8]

Absence of asymmetry may help to explain some developmental disorders of language function. Children with some forms of developmental dyslexia have been shown to be less lateralized on testing for verbal function.[19] It has even been suggested that these children possess two right hemispheres.[20] It is conceivable that the same children have brains with Tpts that are small on both sides, showing the probably typical right hemisphere size for Tpt bilaterally.

Finally, cytoarchitectonic asymmetries may shed some light on the language capabilities of nonhuman primates. Asymmetries in the lengths of the Sylvian fissures similar to those found in man have been reported in some great apes.[10] As demonstrated by the findings of this study, the Sylvian asymmetries seem to reflect planum asymmetries (which in turn might reflect Tpt asymmetries), which would support claims of language capability in these animals.[21]

## Abstract

The auditory regions in four normal brains were mapped and the full extent of the cytoarchitectonic subdivisions was measured for the presence of right-left asymmetries. It was found that asymmetries similar to those found in the planum temporale (left commonly larger than right) are also seen in auditory cytoarchitectonic area Tpt, an area of probable importance for language function. There is a strong positive correlation between the planum asymmetry and the asymmetry of Tpt. It is concluded that the previously described planum asymmetries probably reflect asymmetries in an auditory cytoarchitectonic area and therefore may represent, at least in part, the anatomic substrate for language lateralization.

## References

1. Milner B: Hemispheric specialization: Scope and limits, in Schmitt FO, Worden FG (eds): *The Neurosciences: Third Study Program.* Boston, MIT Press, 1974, pp 75-89.
2. Galaburda AM, LeMay M, Kemper TL, et al: Right-left asymmetries in the brain. *Science* 199:852-856, 1978.
3. Geschwind N, Levitsky W: Human brain: Left-right asymmetries in temporal speech region. *Science* 161:186-189, 1968.
4. Teszner D, Tzavaras A, Gruner J, et al: L'asymmetrie droite-gauche du planum temporale: A propos de l'étude anatomique de 100 cerveaux. *Rev Neurol* (Paris) 126:444-449, 1972.
5. Witelson SF, Pallie W: Left hemisphere specialization for language in the newborn: Neuroanatomical evidence of asymmetry. *Brain* 96:641-646, 1973.
6. Wada JA: Interhemispheric sharing and shift of cerebral speech function. *Excerpta Medica Int Congress Series* 193:296-297, 1969.
7. Wada JA, Clarke R, Hamm A: Cerebral hemispheric asymmetry in humans. *Arch Neurol* 32:239-246, 1975.
8. Chi JG, Dooling EC, Gilles FH: Gyral development of the human brain. *Ann Neurol* 1:86-93, 1977.
9. Meyer A: *The Collected Papers of Adolf Meyer.* Baltimore, The Johns Hopkins Press, 1950, pp 358-373.
10. LeMay M, Culebras A: Human brain, Morphologic differences in the hemispheres demonstrable by carotid arteriography. *N Engl J Med* 287:168-170, 1972.
11. Von Economo C, Horn L: Über Windungs-relief, Masse und Rindenarchitektonik der Supratemporalfläche, ihre individuellen und ihre Seitenunterschiede. *Z Neurol Psychiat* 130:678-757, 1930.
12. Pandya DN, Sanides F: Architectonic parcellation of the temporal operculum in rhesus monkey and its projection pattern. *Z Anat Entwickl-Gesch* 139:127-161, 1973.
13. Galaburda AM, Sanides F: The human auditory cortex: A new cytoarchitectonic map. *Neuroscience Abstr* 3:67, 1977.

14. Brodmann K: *Vergleichende Lokalisations lehre der Grosshirnrinde.* Leipzig, Barth, 1909, pp 144-145.
15. Von Economo C: *The Cytoarchitectonics of the Human Cerebral Cortex,* London, Oxford University Press, 1929, pp 111-114.
16. Ferguson G: *Statistical Analysis in Psychology and Education.* New York, McGraw-Hill Book Co, Inc, 1966, p 414.
17. Gloning I, Gloning K, Haub G, et al: Comparison of verbal behavior in right handed and nonright handed patients with anatomically verified lesion of one hemisphere. *Cortex* 5:41-52, 1969.
18. McGlone J, Davidson W: The relation between cerebral speech laterality and spatial ability with special reference to sex and hand preference. *Neuropsychologia* 11:105-113, 1973.
19. Marcel T, Katz L, Smith M: Laterality and reading proficiency. *Neuropsychologia* 12:131-139, 1974.
20. Witelson SF: Developmental dyslexia: Two right hemispheres and none left. *Science* 195:309-311, 1977.
21. Premack D: Mechanisms of intelligence: Preconditions for language, in Harnad SR, Steklis HD, Lancaster J (eds): *Origins and Evolution of Language and Speech.* New York, The New York Academy of Sciences, 1976, vol 280, pp 544-561.Accepted for publication March 4, 1978.

This investigation was supported in part by grant NINCDSS06209 to the Boston University Aphasia Research Center from the National Institute of Health, grant NSF-BNS 77-05674 to the Beth Israel Hospital, Boston from the National Science Foundation, and a biomedical support research grant from the Beth Israel Hospital, Boston.

Thomas L. Kemper made the specimens from the Yakovlev Collection available for this study.

# CHAPTER 15

# Left-Handedness: Association with Immune Disease, Migraine, and Developmental Learning Disorder

*Norman Geschwind and Peter Behan*

Cerebral dominance—i.e., greater proficiency of each cerebral hemisphere in acquisition and performance of certain specific functions—has been recognized as a biological characteristic of humans for over 100 years. In most people there is dominance of the left hemisphere for language and of the right side for certain spatial functions. The older literature dealt predominantly with humans, with major stress on the laterality of lesions producing certain cognitive deficits. Since World War II there have been many studies that demonstrate dominance in normals.

By contrast, few studies on laterality deal with the kinds of data that are often found in studies of other biological traits, such as eye color. Examples of such data include the anatomical structures involved, biochemical and immunological properties, genetics, ontogeny, evolution, and comparative features in other species. In older publications one finds a few discussions of associations of handedness, such as asymmetries in fingerprints.[1] More recent studies deal with anatomical asymmetries in the human brain, especially in language areas,[2–6] asymmetries of function and structure in other species,[7–11] the genetics of handedness,[10,12,13] and the relationship of sinistrality to learning disabilities and to artistic, athletic, and other talents.[12,14] Anatomical maldevelopment has been

---

Abbreviation: LQ, laterality quotient.

Reprinted with permission of the author from the *Proc. National Academy of Sciences*. 1982; 79: 5097–5100.

demonstrated in the left side of the cortex[15] and in the thalamus[16] of a left-handed childhood dyslexic. These studies reflect growing interest in the biological associations of dominance.

Since the autumn of 1980, one of us (N.G.) has been impressed by observations on both patients and normals with an apparently elevated frequency of certain disorders in left-handers and in their families, including immune disorders (e.g., ulcerative colitis, celiac disease, and Hashimoto's thyroiditis) and migraine. Developmental learning disorders (e.g., dyslexia and stuttering) were also present in elevated frequency, as described by others.[12,17] Several family trees of left-handers included, over several generations, many left-handers and individuals with immune disorders, migraine, or learning disorders, either alone or in combination. The decision was made to test these clinical impressions in studies on left-handers and controls. We also studied the frequency of left-handedness in groups of patients with migraine and immune disorders.

## FIRST STUDY

*Methods.* For use in our investigation, we developed a questionnaire containing a series of questions concerning personal and family history as well as a modification of the Oldfield Handedness Inventory.[18] The score on this inventory is expressed as a laterality quotient (LQ) which ranges in value from +100 (right-handedness in all tasks) to –100 (complete left-handedness). The $\chi^2$ test was used in all statistical comparisons.

The first study consisted of two separate investigations. In the first, we distributed 500 questionnaires in a shop in London that supplies items for use by left-handers, and we received 253 responses from individuals who had a LQ of –100, Questionnaires were also filled out by unselected individuals from the general population of Glasgow, including civil service applicants, attendants at conferences of teachers and nurses and their spouses, and individuals coming to a shop in Glasgow in which one of our assistants was employed. We selected from this group the questionnaires of 253 individuals, all of whom had a LQ of +100 and who were matched for age and sex to the 253 left-handers.

In the second part of the first study we administered questionnaires to additional individuals gathered in the same manner as the general population group described in the preceding paragraph. Of this group we selected 247 individuals with a LQ of –100 and 647 individuals with a LQ of +100. In the first part of the study we had calculated the frequencies of immune disease entirely on the basis of the subjects' responses to the questionnaire. In the second part we scored a subject as suffering from immune disease only if the diagnosis had been made in a hospital.

*Results.* In part 1 of this study, the frequency of immune disease reported by the left-handed subjects was 2.7 times greater than in the control right-handers ($P < 0.005$). The left-handers also reported significantly larger numbers of first- and

TABLE 1. First study, part 1

| | *Immune disorders* | | | *Learning disorders* | | |
|---|---|---|---|---|---|---|
| | LH | RH | *P* | LH | RH | *P* |
| Subjects* | 27(10.7) | 10(4.0) | 0.005 | 24(9.5) | 2(0.8) | 0.005 |
| First-degree relatives† | 48 | 25 | 0.01 | 21 | 7 | 0.01 |
| Second-degree relatives† | 45 | 23 | 0.01 | 11 | 1 | 0.001 |

LH, left-handers ($n = 253$); RH, right-handers, ($n = 253$).

*The number and percentage (in parentheses) of subjects suffering from one of the indicated disorders.

†The number of relatives suffering from these disorders.

second-degree relatives with immune disease (Table 1). Although several types of immune disorders were reported, the frequency of thyroid and bowel disorders was notable. (The following immune disorders were reported: celiac disease, dermatomyositis, diabetes, Hashimoto's thyroiditis, myxedema, regional ileitis (Crohn's disease), rheumatoid arthritis, thyrotoxicosis, ulcerative colitis, and uveitis.)

We also found a much higher frequency of developmental learning disorders (dyslexia and stuttering) reported by the left-handers than by the right-handers ($P < 0.005$). The left-handers also reported significantly larger numbers of relatives with learning disorders (Table 1).

In part 2 of the first study, the absolute rates of immune disorder in both the left- and right-handers were lower than those in part I because we accepted only those with diagnoses established in a hospital. However, the relative rates were comparable to those found in part 1, with the rate for left-handers 2.3 times as high as that in the right-handers ($P < 0.025$) (Table 2). Again the left-handers reported significantly higher rates of immune disorders in relatives. The left-handers reported a much higher rate of learning disorders than the right-handers ($P < 0.001$), as well as higher rates in their relatives (Table 2).

We could not study the frequency of migraine in the two groups because we found that the answers to questions concerning headache were too vague for proper distinction between migraine and other forms of headache.

## SECOND STUDY

In the second study we compared the frequency of left-handedness among patients with migraine or immune disorders seen in the neurological clinics in Glasgow and in a group of general population controls.

TABLE 2. First study, part 2

| | *Immune disorders* | | | *Learning disorders* | | |
|---|---|---|---|---|---|---|
| | LH | RH | *P* | LH | RH | *P* |
| Subjects* | 13(5.3) | 15(2.3) | 0.025 | 27(10.9) | 8(1.2) | 0.001 |
| First-degree relatives† | 58 | 102 | 0.025 | 19 | 24 | 0.025 |
| Second-degree relatives† | 19 | 18 | 0.005 | 2 | 4 | ‡ |

LH, left-handers (*n* = 247); RH, right-handers (*n* = 647). Footnotes (*, †) as in Table 1.

‡Numbers too small for calculation of *P*.

TABLE 3. Left-handedness in patient and control groups

| LQ | C | M | *P** | MG | *P** |
|---|---|---|---|---|---|
| <0 | 82 (7.2) | 17 (11.6) | 0.1 | 13 (13.3) | 0.05 |
| <–30 | 71 (6.2) | 17 (11.6) | 0.02 | 9 (9.2) | 0.3 |
| <–50 | 59 (5.2) | 15 (10.3) | 0.02 | 7 (7.1) | 0.5 |

C, controls (*n* = 1,142); M, migraine patients (*n* = 146); MG, myasthenia gravis patients (*n* = 98). Each entry indicates the number and percentage (in parentheses) of controls or patients with a LQ below the level indicated on the left.

**P*, probability of difference between the patient group and the controls.

We expected the study of the patient groups to give results less clearcut than those of the first study. We did not have available groups of patients with those immune disorders (i.e., involving thyroid or bowel) that our first study had found most often in the left-handers. Second, even the patient groups available to us were much smaller than those of the groups in the two parts of the first study.

*Methods.* The patient groups consisted of carefully diagnosed patients with severe migraine or with immune disorders. The control group consisted of 1,142 individuals from the general population of Glasgow, selected by the same methods as those described in the first study. The questionnaire and statistical methods were the same as those used in the first study. We compared the frequencies of individuals with different degrees of left-handedness among the patients and the controls. In the 1,142 controls there were 82 individuals with a LQ < 0 (i.e., with all degrees of left-handedness)—i.e., 7.2%, a figure comparable to that found by Oldfield[18] in a Scottish population.

*Results.* Table 3 summarizes the findings from the comparisons of patient groups and controls. There was a higher percentage of left-handedness among the severe migraine patients. The difference in the frequency of left-handedness was marginally significant ($P < 0.1$) at LQ < 0 and significant at LQ < –30 ($P < 0.02$) and –50 ($P < 0.02$).

In 98 patients with myasthenia gravis there was an elevated frequency of left-handedness at all three cutoff points, although the difference was significant only at LQ < 0 ($P < 0.05$).

The differences in the frequency of left-handedness found in comparisons of other patient groups (102 patients with rheumatoid arthritis, 168 with mixed-collagen vascular diseases, and 118 with multiple sclerosis) and the general population controls were not statistically significant.

## Discussion

The findings of the first study were in conformity with the hypothesis that immune disorders would be present more often in left-handers and their families than in right-handers. However, the data from this study suggest that the elevated rate is the result of preferential increases in certain forms of immune disorder, especially those involving bowel and gut. The first study is also concordant with the hypothesis of a higher rate of learning disabilities in left-handers and their relatives—a result in conformity with many, although not all, earlier studies.[12,17]

Although we believe that the data on immune disorders and learning disabilities reflect large differences between left-handers and right-handers, the reported frequency differences in relatives may be less reliable. An individual with a learning disability or an immune disorder may be more aware of the presence of these conditions in relatives than would individuals free of these disorders.

As we have already pointed out, we could not carry out an adequate study of the frequency of migraine in sinistrals because the answers to the questionnaire did not permit reliable distinction between migraine and other forms of headache. However, in the second study, we did find a significantly higher number of left-handers among carefully diagnosed patients with migraine.

We found an elevated frequency of left-handedness among patients with myasthenia gravis that was statistically significant only at LQ < 0, although it was of the same order of magnitude as the elevation in migraine. We did not find significantly elevated frequencies of left-handedness in the other immune disease groups studied. However, we did not have available large groups of cases with the forms of immune disorder found in greatest numbers in the first study. Furthermore, because the frequency of left-handedness in any one form of immune disease is probably lower than is the frequency of all such diseases among left-handers, much larger patient groups will be required than those which were available to us.

The increased rate of learning disorders among left-handers is not difficult to understand because impairments of the left hemisphere that disturb language functions may also cause a shift of handedness to the right hemisphere.[19]

The association of sinistrality, learning disorders, and immune disorders suggests the possibility of a common origin that may help in accounting for certain findings in childhood autism, one of the forms of developmental cognitive disorder. Coleman et al.[20] report that 10% of a group of autistic children suffered from well-diagnosed celiac disease, confirming other studies. A common interpretation is that celiac disease may be one cause of autism. An alternative hypothesis is that celiac disease, linked to HLA-B8,[21] is another manifestation of immune disorder in a group with elevated left-handedness. This interpretation is consistent with an elevated rate of hypothyroidism in parents of autistic children and with an elevated number of relatives with Down's syndrome,[22] another condition often accompanied by immune alterations in both the patients and their relatives.[23]

The most surprising finding in this study is the markedly elevated frequency of immune disorders in left-handers and in their relatives as compared to the rates in right-handers and their families. One possible explanation is that immune disorders are the result of stress in patients with learning disorders. This explanation is difficult to accept because immune disorders may be found in elevated frequency among relatives without learning disorders.

Another possible explanation for the association of immune disorders and sinistrality is that of separate genes on the same chromosome, with incomplete penetrance, for left-handedness and immune disease. The association would only indicate joint chromosomal localization and not causal connection. However, there is an alternative explanation based on a hypothesis formulated by one of us (N.G.) on the biological foundations of laterality, of which only a very brief summary can now be given.

The neurons that will occupy the cerebral cortex are formed before 20 weeks of gestation in the central core of the developing brain and then migrate to their future locations.[24] The study of fetal brains shows that the hemispheres are asymmetrical during gestation.[3,25] We have found that the gyri and sulci of the cortical convexity usually appear earlier on the right side. Chi et al.[4] have found a larger left planum temporale, part of the language area of Wernicke,[2] at 31 weeks of gestation, but the homologous region on the right side develops earlier. Ounsted and Taylor[26] hypothesized that the left hemisphere matures later—especially in males—on the basis of the finding that febrile convulsions were most likely to damage the left temporal lobe in boys in the first year of life.

It is proposed that a major influence that slows growth of the convexity of the left hemisphere in utero is testosterone. This effect will usually be greater in males because the fetal testes secrete testosterone. The effect of testosterone on neuronal development has been documented in such structures as the preoptic nucleus in which it has been shown to cause dimorphism in male and female rats.[27–29] Diamond et al.[11] have found the right posterior cortex to be thicker in male rats, and it has been found in our laboratory that the cytoarchitectonic areas in the same region are larger in male rats (unpublished observation). The findings of Goldman and Brown[30] are also consistent with differential cortical maturation in males and females.

Delayed growth in the left hemisphere as a result of testosterone would account for the greater frequency of left-handedness in males. When testosterone effects are more marked and neuronal migration is interfered with to a greater extent, abnormalities in the formation of the left hemisphere will result—especially in males—such as those described by Galaburda and Kemper[15] in the left temporal speech area of a severe childhood dyslexic. This type of effect would account for the much greater incidence of learning disorders in boys.

During fetal life the immune system is also maturing. Testosterone has important suppressive effects on the thymus both in utero and after birth.[31,32] Thus, during periods of increased testosterone effects on left brain development, maturation of the immune system is also likely to be affected. There are studies that support the hypothesis that the fetal thymus controls development of lymphocytes which are responsible for recognition of self-antigens and thus for prevention of autoimmunity.[33,34] Suppression of thymic growth during fetal life might therefore favor the development of autoimmunity in later life.

One might expect that this hypothesis would imply earlier development and higher frequency of immune disease in males. However, testosterone continues in postnatal life to exert a suppressive effect on the thymus. Thus, certain immune disorders such as myasthenia gravis and lupus erythematosus have a higher incidence in young women and older men[35]—i.e., groups in which testosterone effects are lowest. In the genetically autoimmune New Zealand black mouse[36] the disease develops later in the male. Castration accelerates autoimmunity in the male and testosterone administration slows it in the female.

The hypothesis that testosterone has a major role in the development of immunity is in conformity with several experimental studies. Iványi[37] has shown that several loci on the major histocompatibility complex in the mouse control not only the immune system but also various aspects of male differentiation, including mass of testis and thymus, blood testosterone and testosterone-binding globulin levels, sensitivity to testosterone, and expression of H-Y antigen on thymus. Androgens also control the serum level of the fourth component of complement in mice.[38] The minor histocompatibility complex controls β-2-microglobulin which is essential for immune responses; Ohno[39] has proposed that it also controls expression of H-Y antigen which is necessary for development of testes. There is thus an intimate bond between the control of male development and many aspects of the immune system.

One must raise the question as to participation of genetic factors in thc familial clustering of left-handedness, immune disorders, and learning disabilities. The hereditary patterns can be explained at least in part by the gene complexes mentioned in the preceding paragraph. We presume that other genes also participate in the joint control of anatomical asymmetry and immunity.

The hypothesis summarized here thus proposes that testosterone slows neuronal development in the left hemisphere, while simultaneously affecting immune development, and thus favoring later immune disorder. Conversely, genes controlling immune responsiveness also regulate testosterone effects.

## Abstract

We report an experimental study designed to test the following hypothesis derived from clinical observations: There is an elevated frequency in left-handed individuals and in their families of immune disease, migraine, and developmental learning disorders. In two separate investigations the frequency of these conditions was compared in strongly left-handed subjects and in strongly right-handed controls. In each of the investigations we found markedly higher frequencies of immune disease in the left-handers than in the right-handers. The rate of learning disabilities was also much higher in the left-handers than in the right-handers in both investigations. In a second study the frequency of left-handedness was compared in patients with migraine or immune disease and in general population control subjects free of these disorders. There was a higher frequency of left-handedness in patients with migraine and myasthenia gravis than in controls. We present a brief outline of a hypothesis that may account for an increased frequency of immune disease in left-handers and in their families.

## References

1. Cummins, H. & Midlo, C. (1943) *Fingerprints, Palms and Soles: An Introduction to Dermatoglyphics* (Blakiston, Phildelphia).
2. Geschwind, N. & Levitsky, W. (1968) *Science* 161, 186–187.
3. LeMay, M. & Culebras, A. (1972) *N. Engl. J. Med.* 286, 168–170.
4. Chi, J. G., Dooling, E. C. & Gilles, F. H. (1977) *Ann. Neurol.* 1, 86–93.
5. Galaburda, A. M., LeMay, M., Kemper, T. L. & Geschwind, N. (1978) *Science* 199, 852–856.
6. Eidelberg, D. & Galaburda, A. M. (1982) *Arch. Neurol.* 39, 325–332.
7. Glick, S. D., Jerussi, T. P. & Fleisher, L. N. (1976) *Life Sci.* 18, 889–896.
8. Nottebohm, F. & Nottebohm, M. E. (1976) *J. Comp. Physiol.* 108, 171–192.
9. Denenberg, V. H., Garbanati, J., Sherman, G., Hutzey, D. A. & Kaplan, R. (1978) *Science* 201, 1150–1152.
10. Corballis, M. C. & Morgan, M. J. (1978) *Behav. Brain Sci.* 2, 261–336.
11. Diamond, M. C., Dowling, G. A. & Johnson, R. E. (1981) *Exp. Neurol.* 71, 261–268.
12. Annett, M. (1979) *Behav. Genet.* 8, 227–249.
13. Porac, C. & Coren, S. (1981) *Lateral Preferences and Human Behavior* (Springer, New York), pp. 69–92.
14. Porac, C. & Coren, S. (1981) *Lateral Preferences and Human Behavior* (Springer, New York), pp. 181–191.
15. Galaburda, A. M. & Kemper, T. M. (1979) *Ann. Neurol.* 6, 94–100.
16. Galaburda, A. M. & Eidelberg, D. (1982) *Arch. Neurol.* 39, 333–336.
17. Porac, C. & Coren, S. (1981) *Lateral Preferences and Human Behavior* (Springer, New York), pp. 147–156.
18. Oldfield, R. C. (1971) *Neuropsychologia* 9, 97–113.
19. Porac, C. & Coren, S. (1981) *Lateral Preferences and Human Behavior* (Springer, New York), pp. 116–123.

20. Coleman, M., Landgrebe, M. A. & Landgrebe, A. R. (1976) in *The Autistic Syndromes,* ed. Coleman, M. (Elsevier/North-Holland, New York), pp. 197–205.
21. Dohan, F. C. (1981) *Biol. Psychiatry* 16, 1115–1117.
22. Wiedel, L. & Coleman, M. (1976) in *The Autistic Syndromes,* ed. Coleman, M. (Elsevier/North-Holland, New York), pp. 11–20.
23. Fialkow, P. J. (1967) *Transplantation* 5, 989–995.
24. Rakic, P. (1972) *J. Comp. Neurol.* 145, 61–84.
25. Wada, J. A., Clarke, R. & Hamm, A. (1975) *Arch. Neurol.* 32, 239–246.
26. Ounsted, C. M. & Taylor, D. C. (1972) *Gender Differences: Their Ontogeny and Significance* (Churchill-Livingstone, Edinburgh, Scotland), pp. 220–223.
27. Dörner, G. & Staudt, J. (1969) *Neuroendocrinology* 5, 103–106.
28. Raisman, G. & Field, P. M. (1973) *Brain Res.* 54, 1–29.
29. Gorski, P. A., Harlan, R. E., Jacobson, C. D., Shryne, J. E. & Southam, A. M. (1980) *J. Comp. Neurol.* 193, 529–539.
30. Goldman, P. & Brown, R. M. (1975) *Neurosci. Abstr.* 1, 494 (abstr.).
31. Dougherty, T. F. (1952) *Physiol. Rev.* 32, 379–401.
32. Frey-Wettstein, M. & Craddock, C. B. (1970) *Blood* 25, 257–271.
33. Littman, B. H. (1980) *Triangle* (*Engl. Ed.*) 19, 53–60.
34. Rocklin, R. E., Kitzmiller, J. L. & Kaye, M. D. (1979) *Annu. Rev. Med.* 30, 375–404.
35. Ounsted, C. M. & Taylor, D. C. (1972) *Gender Differences: Their Ontogeny and Significance* (Churchill-Livingstone, Edinburgh, Scotland), pp. 235–236.
36. Talal, N. (1976) *Transplantation Rev.* 31, 240–263.
37. Iványi, P. (1978) *Proc. R. Soc. London Ser. B* 202, 117–158.
38. Michaelson, J., Ferreira, A. & Nussenzweig, V. (1981) *Nature* (*London*) 289, 306–308.
39. Ohno, S. (1977) *Immunol. Rev.* 33, 59–69.

We express our special thanks to Colin Howat and Nicola Hanna, medical students at the University of Glasgow, not only for their help in the collection and analysis of data but also for invaluable suggestions concerning the project. We thank Mr. Bloom, proprietor of Anything Left-handed Limited, for his help. This research was supported in part by grants from the National Institutes of Health (NINCDS 06209 and NS17018), the National Science Foundation (BNS 77-05674), the William B. Underwood Company through the Orton Research Fund, and from the Essel Foundation.

# CHAPTER 16 (I)

# Cerebral Lateralization
## Biological Mechanisms, Associations, and Pathology: I. A Hypothesis and a Program for Research

*Norman Geschwind and Albert M. Galaburda*

We present a set of hypotheses about the biologic mechanisms of lateralization, i.e., the processes which lead to an asymmetrical nervous system. It would have been difficult even 20 years ago to formulate such a theory in the face of the prevalent belief that cerebral dominance lacked an anatomic correlate. It is proposed that cerebral dominance is based in most instances on asymmetries of structure. Although genetic factors are important we will lay stress on several factors that, in the course of development, both prenatal and postnatal, modify the direction and extent of these structural differences. Special attention will be directed to the intrauterine environment as a determinant of the pattern of asymmetries, and in particular sex hormones, e.g., testosterone or related factors. We will discuss the associations of anomalous cerebral dominance which include not only developmental disorders such as dyslexia and certain talents but also alterations in many bodily systems, including the immune system, the skin, and the skeleton. It is proposed that the same influences that modify structural asymmetry in the brain also modify other systems.

Although we have worked closely we have each taken special responsibility for certain sections, A.M.G. for sections dealing with normal development of the brain, asymmetry of the human brain, asymmetries in other species, and pathology of asymmetry in developmental disorders, and N.G. for the remaining sections.

---

Reprinted with permission from *Archives of Neurology*. 1985;42(6):428-459. 

## Background of the Theory

We briefly summarize the major findings that have stimulated our studies and theoretical considerations. Each of these subjects will be presented in greater detail in later sections.

*Anatomic Asymmetry of the Brain* It was demonstrated[1] and later confirmed in several studies that there was an easily detectable asymmetry in the human brain that involved the upper surface of the posterior portion of the left temporal lobe. Because this region, the *planum temporale,* constitutes a large portion of the temporal speech region of Wernicke, asymmetry of this zone may account for the predominant localization of speech to the left hemisphere in the majority of humans. Other asymmetries in the human brain have been described.[2,3] The larger size of the left planum temporale reflects the greater extent of a particular temporoparietal cytoarchitectonic area (TPT) on the left.

*Asymmetry of the Fetal Brain* Asymmetry is found in the brain of the human fetus and newborn infant, thus establishing the importance of genetic and/or intrauterine influences.[5–7]

*Male-Female Differences in the Brain* A higher frequency of left-handedness (LH) in men has been reported in many studies[8] although not in all. Recent studies support the view that men and women differ on the average in their patterns of abilities.[9–11] There is a predominance of men among cases of autism, dyslexia, stuttering, and other developmental disorders.[12]

*Laterality in Developmental Disorders* Many studies have reported elevated rates of LH in autism, stuttering, dyslexia, and other developmental disorders, although this has been denied in others.[13] We have found a markedly higher rate of dyslexia and stuttering in strong sinistrals than in strong dextrals.[14,15]

*Abnormal Cytoarchitecture in Childhood Dyslexia* The cortex of a severe childhood dyslexic contained an abnormal pattern of cytoarchitecture virtually confined to the left hemisphere, in particular the temporal speech region. These anomalies were the result of disordered neuronal migration and/or assembly.[16] The brain of a second dyslexic patient studied in our laboratory has abnormalities of neuronal architecture in the same regions,[17,18] and we have evidence for similar anomalies in living patients, with arteriovenous malformations in the left temporal region. Postmortem brains from two other dyslexics have similar anomalies. In the brains so far studied, the anomalies are exclusively or predominantly on the left.

*Patterns of Maturation of the Brain* On the basis of studies of patients with early febrile convulsions and later temporal lobe epilepsy, it was concluded that the male brain matures later than that of the female and that the left hemisphere matures later than the right.[19] The left planum temporale appears at the 31st week of gestation while the corresponding structure on the right develops a week to ten days earlier.[7] In fetal brains, there is generally earlier gyral and sulcal maturation on the right side.[20] Even in infancy dendritic development on the left side in the vicinity of Broca's area lags behind its homolog on the right, catching up only later.[21]

*Cell Death in the Developing Brain* In all species studied, neurons are formed in excess and many die when they fail in the competition to form connections.[22]

*Reorganization of Brain After Intrauterine Lesions* After surgical ablation of a region of cortex in the fetal monkey, the corresponding cortex of the other side develops a more extensive pattern of bilateral connections than is usually seen.[23] Other cortical regions both in the same and in the opposite hemisphere increase in size as the result of such lesions.[24]

*Hormonal Influences on Brain Structures* The formation of sexually dimorphic nuclei in the hypothalamus and other structures is dependent on hormonal influences and especially on variations in testosterone level during development.[25–30] Several authors[31,32] have proposed a relationship between either sex chromosomes or hormones and patterns of cerebral dominance.

*Genetic Studies of Handedness* Annett[33] has brought evidence that there is a population in whom cerebral lateralization for speech and handedness is random. Corballis and Morgan[34] have postulated that asymmetry is an inherent characteristic of the ovum. In twins and their first-degree relatives the rate of LH is higher than that in second-degree relatives.[35] This result is consistent with older findings of higher rates of LH in twins and their singleton relatives than in the general population. Anatomic and functional asymmetries in other species have been demonstrated by several investigators.[2,36–38]

*Chemical Asymmetry of the Brain* Serafetinides[39] found that hemispheric responses of humans to LSD were asymmetrical. Glick and co-workers[40] established the presence of an asymmetry of dopamine content in the rat caudate nucleus, differing in distribution in males and females, and have gone on to establish many other chemical asymmetries.

*Evolution of Asymmetry* LeMay and Culebras[2] demonstrated asymmetry of the sylvian fissures in fossil human skulls. Other asymmetries present in modern humans have been found in fossil primate skulls.[41]

*Associations of LH* We have observed a large group of associations with LH. Controlled studies[14] demonstrated a markedly higher frequency of immune disease in strong left-handers than in strong right-handers, and this has been confirmed in later studies[15,42] (and M. Kinsbourne, MD, and B. Bemporad, MA, written communication, July 13, 1983). Elevated rates of sinistrality have been found in patients with childhood allergies, certain adult immune disorders, and migraine. Older studies documented other associations, e.g., an elevated rate of LH among patients with harelip.[43] These observations (as well as others under investigation) have led us to postulate that some of the processes that influence lateralization also affect the development of the immune system, and are in turn influenced by it, and that processes which disturb cerebral lateralization will frequently have widespread effects on other bodily systems.

*Relationships of Laterality to Special Talents* Dyslexics and their families tend to have superior right hemisphere talents.[44,45] Left-handedness is much more common in certain groups, e.g., architects[46] and mathematically gifted children,[42] who also have a very high rate of allergies.

The lateralization of the nervous system which has interested clinical neurologists for 120 years has assumed increasing importance in developmental studies, genetics, linguistics, and psychology. We believe that its significance extends well beyond these disciplines into anthropology, evolution, and comparative zoology, and even into apparently more remote biological fields. As we hope to show, it is relevant to nearly every branch of clinical medicine and to most preclinical disciplines. Lateralization is a central theme in biology and medicine and not simply the esoteric concern of a small number of investigators.

## Cerebral Dominance: A Brief History of Some Concepts

The concept of lateralization grew out of the discovery in the last century of cerebral dominance, i.e., the superior capacity of each side of the brain to acquire particular skills. The major emphasis over the past 120 years has been on *functional asymmetry,* i.e., on the differences in function of the two sides of the brain and of specific regions within them. This section will review the major changes that have taken place in ideas concerning functional lateralization. Later sections will deal with the *biologic mechanisms or associations* of cerebral dominance. As we shall see, concepts of cerebral dominance have undergone major changes, and beliefs that were at one time widely accepted have been shown to be incorrect or to require extensive revision.

Broca[47] was the first to attract widespread attention to cerebral dominance. Although predominant use of the right hand had long been recognized, the possibility that manual preference had its origin in the organization of the brain had been considered little or not at all. Broca found that the lesions of his first group of aphasics all lay in delimited regions on the left side. It thus became clear that dominance existed within the human brain, i.e., the acquisition of certain abilities appeared to depend on structures located on one side. The special role of the left hemisphere in language seemed to fit in naturally with the preferential use of the right hand by the majority of humans.

The belief that verbal and manual dominance were two aspects of the same function dominated thinking for many years; it was assumed that right-handers had left cerebral dominance for language and that the reverse held for left-handers. It was soon found, however, that left-handers sometimes developed aphasia with left-hemisphere lesions and that some right-handers became aphasic after right-hemisphere lesions. This phenomenon, called *cross aphasia,* was regarded as a curious exception to the general rule that language and manual dominance shared the same substrate. It was not until after World War II that several investigators demonstrated the inaccuracy of the rule that language dominance and hand dominance were in the same hemisphere.[48,49] A new formulation stated that, with rare exceptions, right-handers had left cerebral dominance for language while 60% of left-handers had left dominance and 40% had right dominance. This formulation, still widely accepted, has also been challenged. It has been claimed that left-handers are likely to develop aphasia regardless of the side of the lesion.[50,51] This suggests that strong right cerebral dominance for language either does not exist, or is rare (except after early gross left hemisphere damage), and that in left-handers cerebral dominance for language is either leftsided or bilateral. Since even in right-handers extensive left-hemisphere damage still leaves some residual language, one might argue that bilateral representation is the rule, ranging, at one extreme, from almost total left dominance, through varying degrees of left superiority, to equal dominance, or, at the other extreme, moderate right-sided dominance (with only rare cases of strong right dominance). Annett[33] argues that aphasics with right-hemisphere lesions, although still a distinct minority, are far more common than was previously thought. It is clear that any simple assertion of equivalence between dominance for language and handedness cannot be correct.

Another aspect of the conventional theory, the belief that there was a single dominant hemisphere, grew out of the concept of unitary dominance for language and handedness. The minor (or nondominant) hemisphere was thought to subserve only elementary motor and sensory functions. Those who had dominance divided between the two hemispheres were often regarded as abnormal.

Investigations since the second World War have upset the notion of an active, dominant hemisphere and a minor, passive one. Many studies have shown that each hemisphere is usually superior in certain functions.[13,52–54] The left hemisphere is usually dominant for language and manual skills while the right hemisphere is more involved in certain spatial and musical abilities, attention, and many aspects of emotion.

The standard theory taught that cerebral dominance was a distinctive feature of humans and of no other species. Only within the past 20 years has this teaching been definitively disproved. Nottebohm and Nottebohm[36] demonstrated cerebral dominance for song in certain species of birds. Some skeptics believed that avian and human dominance were examples of convergent, i.e., independent, evolutionary trends, but the more recent demonstration by Sherman and co-workers[37] of right-hemisphere dominance for spatial function and emotion in a mammalian species, the rat, has made it likely that functional dominance is widespread in the animal kingdom. Older descriptions of anatomic asymmetries in other species[55,56] were generally overlooked, but more recently, structural asymmetry has been found in several other species[57–59] as well as chemical and pharmacologic asymmetry.[60]

The classic theory also taught that dominance was a property of the cerebral cortex, the latest stage in neurologic evolution, which had achieved its greatest complexity in humans. Penfield and Roberts[61] argued for language dominance in the left thalamus, but this view did not command wide agreement. Milner[52] demonstrated that left hippocampal removal led to predominantly verbal memory disorders while right-sided ablations led to nonverbal memory difficulties. The participation of subcortical structures in language function has been demonstrated by thalamic stimulation[62] and by the finding of aphasias after subcortical lesions.[63–65] Asymmetries of function are found even in the brainstem and spinal cord. Several years ago, David Cohen pointed out to one of us that the cardiac autonomic pathways descended predominantly on one side of the brain stem; more recently, Faden et al[66] found evidence for lateralization of cardiomotor function in the spinal cord.

The classic and contemporary views agree to a great extent on the effects of early and late lesions on dominance. Function often shifts to the opposite hemisphere after unilateral lesions in the first decade of life. Even in adults, transfers of this type occur, although much less often. Adult left-handers and those right-handers with LH first-degree relatives show, on the average, better recovery from aphasia than unequivocal right-handers.[67]

One aspect of the older ideas concerning early and late lesions, does, however, require revision. The term *early* lesions is usually applied not only to those occurring in about the first decade of life, but also to prenatal lesions. Yet as we will discuss later, unilateral lesions and maldevelopments in fetal life, and perhaps even in early postnatal life, will affect lateralization differently from childhood lesions. One must distinguish the effect of disturbances in at least three different stages, i.e., fetal (and perhaps early postnatal) life, childhood and adolescence, and adult life.

Despite the vast literature on dominance, few articles have dealt with its neural substrate, its nonbehavioral associations, or its comparative and evolutionary aspects. A few older articles that attempted to account for dominance in terms of anatomic asymmetry aroused little interest, but the genetics of dominance received greater attention. There were some publications on possible structural associations, e.g., asymmetries of limb length, of fingerprints and other dermatoglyphics, and of other structures, such as hair whorls. Since the existence of dominance in other species was almost universally denied, little consideration was given to the evolution of lateralization. Although developmental disorders such as dyslexia appeared to have a relationship with anomalous dominance, the possible biologic mechanisms of these conditions received only occasional comment.

Since the late 1960s there has been a surge of interest in the biology or dominance, reflected in articles on anatomic and chemical asymmetry structural and functional asymmetries in other species, and biological associations and mechanisms. Many of these studies were reviewed at a meeting in Boston in April 1983.[68] Another recent publication deals extensively with studies in nonhuman species.[69]

It has been shown repeatedly that knowledge of biological mechanism is likely to suggest new approaches for prevention and treatment of disease. The attempted specification of the processes of development opens the way to use of animal models, although the typical immediate reaction is that it must be impossible to gain useful information about language or developmental dyslexia from experiments in nonhuman species. The brains of all cases of childhood dyslexia so far studied contain cortical regions whose structure is anomalous as a result of disturbances in utero.[16,70,71] If dyslexia itself does not occur in the rat or mouse, one can still study neuronal organization and the influences that modify it and thus gain information of potential importance for the prevention and treatment of this disorder. In fact, we have already found two mouse strains in which prenatal unilateral developmental brain lesions are found (while they are absent in the other strains studied), comparable to those of the dyslexics. It is also likely, although the reasons will not be presented in detail, that the study of brain mechanisms of dominance in other species will lead to a deeper understanding of the underlying principles of language and cognition.

## Theory of Lateralization

This section summarizes the essentials of our hypothesis, and supporting data will be presented in detail in subsequent sections. The simplest theory of lateralization, which is widely accepted, is that patterns of asymmetry are strongly determined genetically. As we will try to demonstrate, this theory has serious shortcomings. Our thesis is that while genes contribute importantly many influences that lie outside of the gene pool of the fetus can alter lateralization patterns. The most powerful factors are variations in the chemical environment in fetal life and to a lesser extent in infancy and early childhood. The factors that modify cerebral dominance also influence the development of many other systems, e.g., the organs involved in immune response.

It is the intent of this hypothesis to account for the following: (1) left-handedness is usually found to be more common in men than women.[8] (2) The developmental disorders of language, speech, cognition, and emotion, e.g., stuttering, dyslexia, and autism are strongly male predominant.[12] (3) Women are on the average superior in verbal talents, while men tend on the average to be better at spatial functions.[9,10] (4) Left-handers of both sexes and those with learning disabilities often exhibit superior right-hemisphere functions.[44–46] (5) Left-handedness and ambidexterity are more frequent in the developmental disorders of childhood.[13,72,73] (6) Certain diseases are more common in non-right-handers, e.g., immune disorders.[14,15]

### Factors That Influence Lateralization

The human brain is asymmetrical even in fetal life with a pattern resembling that seen in adult life, e.g., a right sylvian fissure angled up more at its posterior end than the left[2] and a larger left planum temporale.[5–7,74] In the course of development the gyral and sulcal patterns develop earlier on the right side.[20] These findings are compatible with the concept that the fundamental pattern of the brain usually includes strong asymmetries favoring the structures around the left sylvian fissure. There is probably some influence that slows the growth of parts of the left hemisphere so that, for reasons to be given shortly, the corresponding regions on the right side develop relatively more rapidly. It is postulated, on the basis of the higher frequency of sinistrality and of learning disorders in men, that this influence is related to male sex, e.g., testosterone or some factor related to it. Histocompatibility-Y (H-Y) antigen, to be discussed later, is normally present only in male fetuses, but this cannot be the exclusive male-related factor, since, if it were, one could not account for similar, although less marked effects in women. Both the male and female fetus are exposed to maternal and placental hormones. Once the male testes develop, the titer of testosterone rises to high levels. The formation of the testes and the secretion of testosterone are essential to the development of most of the features that differentiate males from females in most species. The female fetus is also exposed to testosterone although in lower quantities. Factors that determine sensitivity to testosterone or other male-related influences will be important in both sexes. Both sexes are exposed to high levels of progesterone, which may have masculinizing effects on female fetuses at certain stages of development.[75]

The male-related influence thus acts to alter the expression of certain genes that play an important role in neural development. Many other influences could, of course, act on these genes, but some male-related factor must be of special importance.

Major effects of testosterone on neuronal development have been demonstrated in many studies, mostly in the rat, on the factors determining gender-specific sexual characteristics (such as the cyclic release of gonadotropins in the female) and behavior. Testosterone induces a change in the structure of specific nuclei in the hypothalamus and limbic system. Sex hormone receptors are widely distributed in many neural and nonneural tissues[76] and are found in the cortex of the newborn rat (gestationally equivalent to the human fetus in late pregnancy). Sex hormone receptors have recently been found in the cortex of the infant monkey, especially in association areas.[77]

If some factor delays the growth of portions of the left hemisphere, changes must take place in other regions (particularly the homologous ones in the opposite hemisphere, and unaffected areas in the same hemisphere) as a result of mechanisms which have been studied in recent years. Many neurons in the fetal nervous system die in utero and, in the rat, also in the early postnatal period. Recent data suggest that postnatal cell death also occurs in the human.[78] Although all the factors involved in cell death have not been specified, it is known that a neuron is more likely to die if it fails to establish connections. Goldman[23] has studied the changes in the pattern of connections that follow intrauterine lesions of one frontal cortex in the monkey. Normally each frontal cortex projects primarily to the ipsilateral thalamus and caudate nucleus. After an intrauterine lesion of one frontal cortex, the intact homologous cortex on the opposite side not only forms the usual ipsilateral connections, but also develops a large number of connections with the caudate nucleus and thalamus on the side of the lesioned cortex. It has also been shown that after ablation of a cortical area in intrauterine life, other cortical regions are found in later life to be larger than normal.[24] The homologous area on the side opposite the lesion and areas adjacent to the one lesioned are likely to show such an increase in size. This enlargement is presumably the result of death of fewer neurons and possibly of greater size of neurons in the intact regions of cortex because neurons in the lesioned area have been taken out of the competition competing for targets. A delay in development of some cortical regions on the left side should lead to the same effects, i.e., it should favor growth of cortical regions on the opposite side, and in unaffected regions of the same side. The larger of two areas will probably have not only more surviving cells but also more extensive bilateral connections, a feature which may well be characteristic of dominant regions.

The hypothesis suggests that growth retardation will generally be more marked in certain left-hemisphere regions in men, who will therefore show on the average a greater degree of shift to right-hemisphere participation in handedness and language and will therefore more likely have augmented right-hemisphere skills. In addition they may have elevated skills related to unaffected regions on the left. Excessive delays caused by male-related factors will be more common in men. In some cases there will be markedly delayed neuronal migration and/or abnormal neuronal assembly especially in left-hemisphere language regions, e.g., there will be disrupted cortical architecture and neurons in abnormal locations. Regions of disordered cytoarchitecture or disturbed neuronal migration confined to the left hemisphere have been found in the brains of several childhood dyslexics. The higher rate of such disruptions of cortical architecture in the left speech regions in men accounts for the greater rate of developmental learning disorders in boys.

The effect of testosterone may depend either on the level of the free hormone (i.e., not bound to sex hormone binding globulin) or on tissue sensitivity. Thus some female fetuses in whom sensitivity is high will also manifest excessive testosterone effects. Progesterone effects that are not the result of exogenously administered hormone may also reflect individual differences in sensitivity.

Testosterone also affects the growth of many other tissues. In particular it retards the growth of structures involved in immunity, i.e., the bursa of Fabricius in the fetal chick[79] and the thymus gland in the rat postnatally.[80] Recent experiments in the rabbit by Behan are consistent with similar retarding effects on the fetal thymus. Thus when testosterone effects on the brain are most marked, altered development of the immune system may occur, heightening susceptibility to later immune disorders. It might be argued that this mechanism would lead to a higher rate of immune disorders in men. There is, however, another effect that protects men especially in the postpubertal period. Testosterone suppresses the thymus even in adult life[80,81] so that thymic involution after puberty is more pronounced in men. In the New Zealand black/white (NZBW) autoimmune mouse model, the milder course of disease in the male depends on the presence of testosterone.[82] This hypothesis is compatible with the fact that certain autoimmune disorders, e.g., lupus erythematosus and myasthenia gravis, are most frequent in young women, i.e., when testosterone effects are at a minimum, and that the proportion of male cases rises with age, as testosterone effects decline. We have also found that atopic disorders (e.g., asthma, eczema, and hay fever) are more frequent in left-handers. The fact that atopic disorders in childhood are more common in males (before the pubertal rise in testosterone), but after puberty more common in females,[83] is also compatible with this hypothesis.

The relationship between testosterone and immunity is probably a very close one. Ivanyi[84] has shown that several loci in the major histocompatibility complex of the mouse, whose importance in immune mechanisms is established, also code for various aspects of the production and metabolism of testosterone and for expression of the H-Y antigen on the thymus gland. These and other relationships between sex hormones and immunity will be detailed later. Whether or not the specific hypothesis proposed here is the correct one (and, even if basically correct, it will certainly undergo major modification) it appears clear that there is an intimate interrelationship of sex hormones, immunity, and laterality.

Asymmetric development is a property not only of the cortex but of many other parts of the nervous system and of other organs. The factors that influence cortical asymmetry and the structures of the immune system will also modify development and, in particular, asymmetric development, in other systems. We will discuss in particular the evidence for asymmetry in neural crest migrations and will raise the possibility that some changes in neural structures are secondary to effects on the neural crest. It has been shown that influences acting in utero or in very early postnatal life may permanently alter certain metabolic systems; the possibility will be raised that such alterations may accompany shifts in dominance. We will also suggest that such intrauterine influences may modify susceptibility to certain diseases in later life, even in old age. In particular, regions whose development is disturbed in fetal life may be especially susceptible to later immune or infectious attack.

It should be stressed that frank left-handers constitute only one easily identifiable group with an anomalous (i.e., nonstandard) pattern of dominance. We postulate that the basic pattern of the brain is one with strong left-hemisphere asymmetry for the substrates of language and handedness. Influences that delay left-hemisphere growth thus tend to create brains in which the normal asymmetry of these regions is diminished, so that the corresponding areas on the two sides are more symmetrical. The group with symmetric brains should manifest a phenomenon postulated by Annett,[33] i.e., random dominance. Many individuals subjected to left-hemisphere delays will have random handedness, and thus roughly as many will be right-handed as left-handed. Left-handers will thus constitute only a fraction of the anomalous dominance group (our guess is about one third), which in total includes perhaps 30% of the population.

There is another reason why LH will not be present in many cases in which there is slowed growth of the cortex. There is no reason to assume that the delaying effect will be present all through gestation. It is likely that the observed patterns of dominance of cortical regions will differ depending on the exact period or periods in pregnancy in which the effects of testosterone or related factors are elevated. In some cases the as yet unknown substratum of handedness may have developed during a period in which there is no significant retarding effect. A delaying influence appearing later, e.g., a subsequent rise in testosterone levels or sensitivity may slow the formation of later-developing regions, e.g., the temporal speech area. If this type of pattern occurred frequently, one might find anomalous dominance for language more often than for handedness.

The earlier development of the right hemisphere mentioned above implies that it will be less subject to disrupting influences. As a result we expect that disturbances in cytoarchitectonic structure will be less frequent on the right than on the left. In addition early influences that disturb the development of the right hemisphere will often persist through later periods and thus have more widespread effects. Right-hemisphere retardation may thus often be accompanied by left-hemisphere delay, but in many cases retardation of left-sided development will follow normal development of the right side. In the latter case the right-sided areas may, after the period of cell death, be larger than normal.

Certain implications of these findings will be discussed. We will suggest that while genetic influences must play a large role, nongenetic factors will have a large influence on the development of dominance. Implications for giftedness will also be presented. Since the influences that produce delays in the left hemisphere will lead to final greater extent of other cortical regions, this process may be a mechanism of giftedness. This accounts for the elevated level of non-right-handedness (RH) in architecture and certain other occupations. Frank neuronal migration disorders may thus be not only a pathology of defect, but also a "pathology of superiority," which explains the presence of very high talents in many cases of autism, dyslexia, and stuttering and the common occurrence of superior right-hemisphere functions in dyslexics and their families.

In the final section, we will address the question of the fundamental mechanisms by which asymmetric structures are formed and will deal with the possibility that certain common mechanisms may be at play in both the plant and the animal kingdoms.

The following sections will contain more detailed data and discussions of the points presented in this summary of our hypothesis.

## Normal Development of the Brain

Cerebral asymmetry is found even during early fetal life. A review of the stages of normal cortical development will be helpful in later consideration of the processes that lead to lateralization. No neuron is formed in the cortex itself. All cortical neurons are generated in the neural tube, from which they migrate to their future locations.

Although many earlier descriptions of brain development were derived from observations on the human fetus, recent research has been carried out primarily on experimental animals. Thus while the general outlines of the schedules and patterns of human cerebral development are known, certain details can be drawn only by inference from studies in other species.

The development of neural structures proceeds in an orderly sequence as follows: (a) *neural induction,*[85] i.e., formation of the primitive neural elements; (b) *differentiation of the neural plate;*[86] (c) *formation of the neural tube*[87] which will give rise to the central nervous system; (d) *formation of the neural crest*[88,89] dorsal to the neural tube, from which cells will migrate to form peripheral sensory and autonomic ganglia and other derivatives, e.g., certain endocrine glands, some components of the thymus, thyroid, and parathyroid glands, some elements of the musculoskeletal system, nearly all pigmented cells of the skin, and other structures, and the skin and bones of the face; (e) *formation of germinal zones*[90] which generate neuronal and glial precursors; (f) *cell migration*[91] during which neuronal and glial elements will travel to their permanent locations; (g) *cellular differentiation and maturation*[90] during which neurons in their final locations grow and establish connections; and (h) *massive neuronal death and axonal attrition*[92] (although cell death probably occurs to some extent during each stage and continues even into the postnatal period).

In the first weeks of fetal development there is rapid replication of DNA. After the later phase of DNA replication, cells move toward the lumen of the neural tube to form the *ventricular germinal zone* (also known as the *subependymal zone,* the *subependymal cell plate,* or the *ependymal cell layer*) in which cells proliferate. The neural tube is thus differentiated into a *germinal* zone and a cell-free *marginal* zone. It is possible later to distinguish an *intermediate* zone, lying between the ventricular and the marginal zones, that contains postmitotic cells moving toward the pial surface. The *subventricular zone* appears as an additional germinal zone between the ventricular and intermediate zones, and contains proliferating glia and some special classes of neurons. Mitosis takes place only in the germinal zones, and cells migrate only after the completion of mitosis. Every neuron found in the cortex of a mature animal migrated in fetal life from the neural tube to its final location.

During the period of proliferation the generation of cells obeys the following rules: (a) there are spatial and temporal gradients; (b) cells destined to populate separate architectonic zones have separate origins; (c) cells are produced in a specific sequence of sizes, i.e., first large neurons, then intermediate-sized neurons, and finally, small neurons; (d) glia destined for a given region of the brain tend to originate after neurons; and (e) phylogenetically older parts of the brain tend to arise earlier in ontogeny.

The cellular migration that follows proliferation occurs in waves. During this stage the cortical mantle begins to form at the junction of the intermediate and marginal zones, and it increases in thickness with each successive wave of arriving neurons and glia. The cortical plate is soon differentiated into a deeper layer containing more mature cells that have arrived at an earlier period, and a more superficial layer containing later arriving, more immature neurons. Those cells that arrive later must thus move through the layers already formed in order to reach the outer surface. The process is even more complex; nerve cells seem to be in constant movement so that they may pass through their eventual permanent sites and then return to them. The ventricular zone becomes thinner as it continues to lose cells during the course of migration, and the two-layer cortical plate thickens.

The production of neurons and the consolidation of the ventricular zone begin at around six weeks of gestation. The first wave of migration to the cortical plate and its first differentiation take place between the sixth and eighth weeks. The subventricular zone is formed between the eighth and tenth weeks. From the 11th to the 13th weeks, the cortical plate differentiates into two layers, thickening of which continues through the end of the 15th week. Cellular migration to the cortex is completed between the sixth and eighth fetal months.

The stage of *cell differentiation,* especially in the deeper layers, begins roughly during the 16th week, i.e., before cell migration to the superficial layers is completed, and continues well into the postnatal period. During cell differentiation, neurons grow, develop their dendrites and axons, and establish synaptic contacts. Cortical maturation also involves *myelogenesis,* which takes place in an orderly, regionalized fashion; it begins in the cortex before birth, and continues well into adult life, the myelination of the tangential intracortical layers taking place very late. The great postnatal increase in brain weight is largely the result of accumulation of myelin. Myelination, like cellular proliferation and migration, generally occurs earlier in phylogenetically older regions; large neurons with long axons (present mostly in the deeper layers) myelinate before small neurons with short axons.

As will be discussed in greater detail later, the neuronal migration and assembly may be modified by circulating sex hormones. Estrogens enhance cortical maturation and myelogenesis in the rat,[93,94] whereas androgens interfere with this estrogen effect[95] in vitro and in vivo. Sexual dimorphism in neural organization can result from the differential effects of gonadal hormones during the stage of cell maturation,[95] but sex hormones may also affect the proliferation and migration of neurons. At the time in the early postnatal period in which one finds the maximum number of estradiol receptors in the rodent brain and peak estradiol levels, there is also intense sprouting of neurites and myelination of axons. It is important to stress that these hormonal effects are limited to brain areas having the appropriate hormone receptors and enzymes and to critical periods during which the receptors are sensitive to the effects of the particular hormone.

A crucial factor in cortical development, which helps to match the number of presynaptic neurons with available synaptic sites, is the process of cell death, which reduces the great excess of neurons produced in fetal life. Cell death can be enhanced experimentally, e.g., a focal lesion placed at a critical time decreases the number of postsynaptic sites and thus leads to increased death of neurons projecting to that structure. The process is graded; reduction of the number of appropriate synaptic sites results in an increased rate of cell death, while the experimental addition of postsynaptic sites can diminish it. The absolute number of available postsynaptic sites only partly determines which cells will die; there appear to be specific recognition properties that place some cells at an advantage in establishing connections. It is likely, however, that of two presynaptic axons having equal affinity for the postsynaptic site, the one arriving first has a greater chance of surviving. Thus, a neuronal system that develops quickly, or whose axons grow more rapidly comes to predominate over slower competing systems. When differences in developmental rate are affected by the numbers of receptors for hormones or other substances the relative extent of cell death in competing presynaptic systems may come under hormonal regulation during critical periods.

The lack of a given postsynaptic site need not lead to the loss of the presynaptic cell if that cell can establish connections elsewhere.[96,97] The reshaping of neuronal circuits because of availability of alternative postsynaptic sites has been shown by the placement of lesions during development. These experiments reveal the patterns of cell death resulting from the removal of postsynaptic sites, the rerouting of presynaptic axons to other available postsynaptic sites, and the invasion by other axons of postsynaptic sites left vacant by the loss of neurons destroyed by the lesion. When a cortical-visual area in the cat which normally receives transcallosal axons is lesioned in early life, there is a marked loss of neurons in the appropriate contralateral cortex[97]; some of the contralateral neurons do, however, survive because their axons change their trajectories and establish ipsilateral connections. Reorganization of connections may occur across the midline. Thus, unilateral collicular lesions in hamsters increase projections to the contralateral colliculus,[98] and contralateral projections from frontal cortex to thalamus are enhanced when the ipsilateral frontal cortex is lesioned.[99] It is likely that the striking findings in these experiments reflect mechanisms of adaptation to normal variations in the environment of the growing brain, which can alter the availability and location of postsynaptic sites in the developing nervous system.

## Asymmetry of the Human Brain

In this section, we will discuss the advantages of an asymmetric nervous system, summarize some of the known anatomic asymmetries found in the human at a gross and cytoarchitectonic level, and present the available data on their development. Studies in nonhuman species will be cited when relevant, but a fuller discussion of animal asymmetries will be left to a later section.

### The Advantages of a Lateralized Brain

The common belief that most animals are symmetrical is far from true. An axis of external symmetry is usually present, but internal asymmetry is probably the rule. It was believed for a long time that the brain was symmetric in both humans and other species. It is likely, however, that every vertebrate species will be shown to have an asymmetric nervous system, and, as will be pointed out later, the same is probably true for invertebrates, and, surprisingly, even single-celled organisms are commonly asymmetric. It is possible, however, that the most complex nervous systems show the most elaborate patterns of asymmetric function. Humans are not unique in the possession of lateralized functions, but they may well be endowed with the most extensively asymmetric brains.

The ability to learn and to adapt to changing environments has played a major role in the survival of higher animals: The human who survives in almost any ecologic niche owes his biological success primarily to his brain, and the cerebral dominance must have contributed heavily to human adaptive capacities.

It may appear strange that dominance has increasingly won out over duplication, but the advantages of redundancy are not as great as at first appears. The cat's superior recovery from hemiplegia is of little advantage in the wild since a few days or even a few hours of disability mean almost certain death. By contrast, lateral specialization makes possible a larger complement of talents that may be useful in survival. Furthermore, the more functions represented in the brain the greater will be the diversity of endowment within the species so that some members will survive almost any new threat. The modification of dominance by intrauterine environmental changes increases diversity to a far greater extent than a rigid genetic mechanism would allow.

It might be argued that dominance could be present even in the absence of structural asymmetry. An example may be the hyperstriatum ventrale, pars caudalis (HVc) nucleus of the singing bird,[100] which does not differ in size on the two sides, despite unilateral dominance for song. Even in the singing bird there is a small but significant difference in the size of the 12th nerve nucleus (which is about 15% larger on the left dominant side in the chaffinch). We suspect, however, that at least in mammals anatomic asymmetry will be the rule. At the very least one would expect an asymmetric pattern of connections so that each side could control different functions. A pattern that may well be common will be that of a unilaterally larger area with more extensive bilateral outputs and inputs than the opposite region.

In the last section of the article, we will discuss some of the known causes of anatomic asymmetry and will also present some hypotheses as to other possible mechanisms. Several different types of process may contribute to the neural asymmetries of higher animals.

## Gross Anatomic Asymmetries

Ever since Broca discovered the functional lateralization of the human brain, structural asymmetries have been sought to explain left-hemisphere specialization for language. Some early articles described asymmetries of hemispheric length, weight, or total surface area, but these were often very small or inconsistent.[101] Later authors did, however, find reproducible asymmetries,[102–105] but their publications were generally neglected. In 1962, von Bonin[106] dismissed the earlier work as uncontrolled or lacking in adequate statistical support and concluded that there were minor anatomic asymmetries in the brain that could not account for the dramatic functional asymmetries. Geschwind and Levitsky[1] reinvestigated this question and found a striking asymmetry of the portion of the upper surface of the temporal lobe behind the gyrus of Heschl. Their findings have been confirmed repeatedly, and other human brain asymmetries have been described. A summary of these lateral differences is presented in Table 1.

The first consistently found asymmetry in the human brain was described almost simultaneously by Cunningham[107] in Ireland and by Eberstaller[108] in Germany. They found the sylvian fissures to be asymmetric at the posterior end, i.e., the sylvian point at which the middle cerebral artery exists from the sylvian fossa. The right fissure curls upward posteriorly and thus ends in a higher position than the left, an asymmetry that can be seen in cerebral arteriograms and in postmortem specimens.[2] The pattern of this asymmetry varies with handedness.[109] As can be seen in Table 1, a bias toward a higher right sylvian fissure is much stronger among self-described right-handers than among left-handers.

It was also demonstrated quite early that the left sylvian fissure is usually longer than the right, a result which suggests that the temporal and parietal opercula, which make up the floor and the roof of the sylvian fossa, are larger on the left than on the right. The fact that the posterior temporal operculum is larger on the left side was originally shown by Pfeifer,[102] who pointed out that the planum temporale, a triangular region lying caudal to the transverse gyrus of Heschl on the superior surface of the temporal lobe, was larger on the left side. Subsequently, Geschwind and Levitsky[1] showed in 100 adult human brains that the left planum was usually larger, a result since confirmed by several other investigators.[5,6,74,110] Adolf Meyer[111] showed that the planum temporale is involved in language functions; it is, in fact, the extension on the upper surface of the temporal lobe of the speech area of Wernicke.

We would like to indicate some of the potentially important features of these data. In the first place, asymmetry is the rule in the planum, being evident in at least three quarters of the brains studied in all series. Second, the asymmetry is often dramatic in magnitude so that the left planum is sometimes ten times larger than the right. Although asymmetries of this magnitude may be seen in *subcortical* structures of other species, e.g., the habenular nucleus of the lamprey,[56] no nonhuman species yet studied has shown such a degree of lateral disparity in the cortex.

Pfeifer also pointed out that a second transverse gyrus was more likely to be found on the right than the left side, a result confirmed by later authors.[112,113] Even in fetal life the right planum, which develops earlier than the left is more likely to have two transverse gyri.[7]

Broca[114] was the first to give a detailed description of the anterior horizontal and ascending limbs of the sylvian fissure, located in the opercular portion of the frontal lobe. The horizontal limb makes up the rostral border of the pars triangularis, and the ascending limb makes up the caudal boundary. Eberstaller[108]

TABLE 1. Anatomic Asymmetries in Human Brain*

| Structure | RH N | RH L> | RH L = R | RH R> | LH N | LH L> | LH L = R | LH R> | Comments |
|---|---|---|---|---|---|---|---|---|---|
| Frontal lobe[118] | 297 | 28 | 23 | 49 | | | | | Petalia in East African skulls; no handedness; percentages |
| Frontal lobe[144] | 174 | 9 | 21 | 70 | 49 | 21 | 40 | 39 | Width by CT scan; adults and children; percentages |
| | 206 | 7 | 63 | 30 | 58 | 21 | 60 | 19 | Petalia by CT scan; adults and children; percentages |
| Frontal lobe[117] | | | | | 39 | 18 | 29 | 53 | CT width in nonfamilial left-handers; percentages |
| | | | | | 39 | 28 | 21 | 51 | CT petalia in nonfamilial left-handers; percentages |
| | | | | | 41 | 25 | 40 | 35 | CT width in familial left-handers; percentages |
| | | | | | 41 | 41 | 25 | 34 | CT petalia in familial left-handers; percentages |
| Frontal lobe[245] | 50 | 8 | 56 | 36 | 25 | 16 | 56 | 28 | CT petalia; percentages; LH includes ambidextrous |
| Frontal lobe[246] | 5 | 1 | 0 | 4 | | | | | Petalia in endocasts of Solo Man; no handedness |
| Frontal lobe[247] | 40 | | | 80 | | | | | Volume of frontal lobe from Yakovlev Collection; adults, children, and infants; no handedness; percentages |
| Inferior frontal gyrus[5] | 100 | 21.5 | | 26.7 | | | | | Mean convexity area of opercular portion; adults; no handedness |
| | 85 | 21.7 | | 25.8 | | | | | Mean convexity area of opercular portion; infants and fetuses; no handedness |
| Inferior frontal gyrus[125] | 102 | 26 | 61 | 13 | | | | | Brains with extra sulcus in pars opercularis; adults and children; no handedness; percentages |
| Inferior frontal gyrus[248] | 54 | 44 | 39 | 17 | | | | | Convexity area of pars opercularis and pars triangularis; no handedness; adults |
| | 10 | 66 | 17 | 17 | | | | | Childen |
| | 4 | 0 | 100 | 0 | | | | | Infants |
| Inferior frontal gyrus[115] | 12 | 8 | 1 | 3 | | | | | Total area of frontal operculum |
| Inferior frontal gyrus[125] | 10 | 6 | 3 | 1 | | | | | Total volume of opercular architectonic area 44; no handedness; adults and children |
| Temporal lobe[104] | 75 | 75 | 12 | 13 | | | | | Area of PT; no handedness; percentages |

TABLE 1. Anatomic Asymmetries in Human Brain* (continued)

| | RH | | | | LH | | | | |
|---|---|---|---|---|---|---|---|---|---|
| *Structure* | *N* | *L>* | *L = R* | *R>* | *N* | *L>* | *L = R* | *R>* | *Comments* |
| Temporal lobe[1] | 100 | 65 | 24 | 11 | | | | | Length of lateral edge of PT; adults; no handedness; percentages |
| Temporal lobe[74] | 100 | 75 | 12.5 | 12.5 | | | | | Area of PT; adults; no handedness; percentages |
| Temporal lobe[6] | 16 | 81 | | | | | | | Length of PT; no handedness; percentages; adults |
| | 14 | 86 | | | | | | | Infants |
| | 16 | 69 | 0 | 31 | | | | | Area of PT; no handedness; percentages; adults |
| | 14 | 79 | | | | | | | Infants |
| Temporal lobe[5] | 100 | 82 | 8 | 10 | | | | | Area of PT; no handedness; percentages; adults |
| | 100 | 56 | 32 | 12 | | | | | Infants |
| Temporal lobe[249] | 21 | 67 | | | | | | | Length of PT; no handedness; adults; percentages |
| Temporal lobe[113] | 30 | 3 | 47 | 50 | | | | | Percentages with more than 1 Heschl's gyrus; adults and children; no handedness |
| Temporal lobe[110] | 103 | 77 | 1 | 22 | | | | | Area of PT; no handedness; percentages |
| Temporal lobe[248] | 54 | 83 | 9 | 7 | | | | | Area of PT; no handedness; percentages; adults |
| | 10 | 70 | 20 | 10 | | | | | Children |
| | 4 | 50 | 50 | 0 | | | | | Infants |
| Temporal lobe[115] | 12 | 10 | | 2 | | | | | Area of PT |
| Temporal lobe[4] | 4 | 3 | 1 | | | | | | Volume of architectonic area TPT; children and adults; no handedness |
| Occipital lobe[118] | 297 | 52 | 24 | 24 | | | | | Petalia in East African skulls; no handedness; percentages |
| Occipital lobe[144] | 150 | 64 | 20 | 16 | 50 | 22 | 32 | 16 | Width by CT scan; adults and children; percentages |
| | 269 | 69 | 22 | 9 | 62 | 56 | 24 | 20 | Petalia by CT scan; adults and children; percentages |
| | | | | | 40 | 37 | 39 | 24 | Width by CT scan; adults and children; percentages; familial LH |
| | | | | | 37 | 59 | 22 | 19 | No familial LH |
| | | | | | 41 | 29 | 32 | 39 | Petalia by CT scan; adults and children; percentages; familial LH |
| | | | | | 39 | 59 | 15 | 26 | No familial LH |

TABLE 1. Anatomic Asymmetries in Human Brain* (continued)

| | RH | | | | LH | | | | |
|---|---|---|---|---|---|---|---|---|---|
| *Structure* | *N* | *L>* | *L = R* | *R>* | *N* | *L>* | *L = R* | *R>* | *Comments* |
| Occipital lobe[245] | 50 | 60 | 20 | 20 | 25 | 44 | 36 | 20 | CT petalia; percentages; LH includes ambidextrous |
| Occipital lobe[246] | 5 | 4 | 1 | 0 | | | | | Petalia in endocasts of Solo Man; no handedness |
| Occipital lobe[247] | 40 | | | 80 | | | | | Volume of occipital lobe from Yakovlev Collection; adults, children, infants; no handedness; percentages. |
| Occipital horn[116] | 87 | 60 | 30 | 10 | 13 | 38 | 31 | 31 | Length by PEG; percentages |
| Occipital horn[145] | 75 | 39 | 44 | 17 | | | | | Length by PEG; children, some with neurologic abnormalities; no handedness; percentages |
| Parietal lobe[126] | 8 | 5 | 1 | 2 | | | | | Volume of architectonic area PG; direct correlation with asymmetry in PT; adults and children; no handedness |
| Sylvian fissure[2] | 44 | 5 | 9 | 86 | 18 | 11 | 72 | 17 | Height of posterior end of sylvian fissure on carotid A-grams; adults and children; percentages |
| Sylvian fissure[109] | 100 | 7 | 26 | 67 | 28 | 7 | 71 | 22 | Height of posterior end of sylvian fissure on carotid A-grams; adult and children; percentages |
| Sylvian fissure[249] | 36 | 75 | | | | | | | Length of sylvian fissure; adults; no handedness; percentages |
| Sylvian fissure[158] | 25 | 84 | 0 | 16 | | | | | Length of sylvian fissure; no handedness; percentages |
| Sylvian fissure[250] | 38 | 21 | 21 | 58 | 20 | 15 | 35 | 50 | Height of posterior end of sylvian fissure on carotid A-grams; percentages |
| Thalamus[131] | 9 | 8 | 0 | 1 | | | | | Volume of nucleus lateralia posterior; adults and children; no handedness |
| Bulbar pyramids[122] | 123 | 73 | 10 | 17 | 7 | 86 | 0 | 14 | Side from which decussation is higher in the brain stem; adults and children; percentages |

*RH indicates right-handed; LH, left-handed; CT, computed tomography; PT, planum temporale; TPT, temporoparietal cytoarchitectonic area; A-gram, cerebral arteriogram; PEG and PG represent two cytoarchitectonic areas lying in the inferior parietal lobule (modified from Eidelberg and Galaburda[126]).

noted that the ascending sylvian limb was more often branched on the left than on the right. This suggested that the left frontal opercular region, which makes up part of Broca's speech area, was more infolded, and thus contained more cortex than the corresponding region on the right. Falzi et al,[115] in a recent study of brains of right-handers, have found an average of 22% more infolded cortex in the left than in the right frontal operculum.

McRae et al[116] showed that in pneumoencephalograms of right-handers the occipital horn of the left lateral ventricle is usually longer than the one on the right, while in left-handers the occipital horn asymmetry is nearly equally distributed between the right and left sides. Similar asymmetries in the occipital horns have been demonstrated by the use of computed tomography (CT).

The petalias are another group of anatomic asymmetries which can be seen in modern and fossil skulls and in CT. A petalia is a more marked indentation in the inner table of the skull on one side that results from the greater protrusion of the adjacent cerebral lobe on that side than on the other. LeMay[117] has shown in RH individuals a predominance of left occipital petalia, i.e., a wider and/or longer occipital lobe is found nearly four times more often on the left than on the right; a wider and/or longer frontal lobe is almost nine times more frequent on the right than on the left. In LH subjects, the distribution is much more symmetrical. All investigators agree that the left occipital lobe is usually wider or longer, but there is disagreement as to the exact statistics and as to whether the distribution varies with handedness. There is also disagreement on the part of some investigators as to whether the right frontal lobe is usually the larger one. Thus the one lobar asymmetry whose existence is agreed to generally is that of the left occipital region. The reasons for the disagreements are still unclear. They may reflect differences in radiologic technique or methods of measurement, in selection of subjects (e.g., one study used children with epilepsy as normal controls, which is probably not justified), or in criteria for handedness.

Another problem is that of how many independent petalias exist. Gundara and Zivanovic[118] in a study of East African skulls found not only predominance of right frontal and left occipital petalias but also a predominance of left parietal petalias which appears to be independent of the occipital petalia. We cannot go further into these issues at this point. We believe that these questions will be resolved only by further studies and by further anatomic investigations of brains obtained at post mortem.

These studies raise, however, an issue of theoretical importance, i.e., are certain asymmetries linked, or are they independent? Assume, for example, that one particular asymmetry in favor of the left side occurs in 80% of brains, while another asymmetry in favor of the right side is found in 80%. If the two asymmetries were linked, we might expect as many as 80% of brains to show both. If they are independent, both should occur together in 64%. If they are negatively related, there would still be co-occurrence in not less than 60% of cases. Very large samples would be needed to distinguish the three cases. In the study of Gundara and Zivanovic,[118] the frequencies of the eight possible combinations of occipital, frontal, and parietal petalia are in accordance with independent occurrence of the various asymmetries.

The larger the number of independent asymmetries, the greater the possible diversity of the population. In any case the data should be ascertained since they will place important constraints on any theory.

There is a spectrum of degrees of human cerebral asymmetry. While the left planum may be many times larger than the right, equally dramatic examples of right-sided planum superiority are uncommon. Furthermore, in about a quarter of cases there is little difference between the sides. Finally, the distribution observed for the planum, i.e., about 65% favoring the left, with 36% roughly equal or favoring the right, reappears in relation to other asymmetries. It is conceivable that the figure of 35% may represent the proportion of the population with anomalous dominance for language, i.e., without strong left preponderance. All or most of the clearly LH people probably belong to this group. Thus Gloning et al[50] and Satz et al[119] have argued that left-handers are likely to become aphasic regardless of lesion side, and that pure right-sided dominance is unusual. The anomalous language dominance group probably includes many individuals in addition to obvious left-handers. Luria[67] found that while almost all patients with penetrating wounds in the primary speech areas on the left were aphasic at onset, at a year about 30% had made good or excellent recoveries. Left-handers and right-handers with LH first-degree relatives were most likely to be in this group, but they did not constitute the entire good recovery group. We offer the speculation that the 35% without a larger left planum make up this group. Our guess is that this group will include most non-RH (a term which we will define more precisely later), as well as most of those with childhood learning disorders, and a large proportion of those with first-degree relatives in either of these categories. Gordon[44] found superior performance on right-hemisphere tasks in all members of a group of childhood dyslexics and in nearly all their first-degree relatives. A more recent article by Gordon[45] adds further evidence. Much more study will, however, be needed before this can be accepted.

There is, however, at least one important limitation on the use of CT scan asymmetries in the determination of anomalous dominance. As will be pointed out later, the childhood dyslexic, the maldevelopment of whose left hemisphere was described by Galaburda and Kemper,[16] had a larger temporal lobe on the left side. Since the publication of that article, the brains of three other childhood dyslexics have been studied, all of whom have shown similar lesions, predominantly on the left. In all three cases the left temporal lobe was larger than the right. This is probably explained by the presence of neuronal migration defects on the left, i.e., the larger size of the left hemisphere was the reflection of abnormality, just as the greater size of the brain in megalencephaly reflects delayed neuronal migration. Some individuals with anomalous dominance, especially those with learning disorders, may thus have an apparently normal pattern of radiologic brain asymmetry. If anomalies of this type are common, radiologic studies in life may be unreliable indicators of the pattern of lateralization. It is important to realize that imaging techniques are not adequate substitutes for direct anatomic studies.

## Asymmetry of Pathways

Flechsig[120] pointed out an asymmetry in the number of pyramidal fibers crossing from one side to the other in the medullary decussations in about 40% of post-mortem human brains. Yakovlev and Rakic[121] reported asymmetry in the pyramidal decussations of newborn and fetal human brains. Kertesz and Geschwind,[122] in a study of 158 adult brains, found that the decussation of the left pyramidal tract occurred more rostrally than that of the right in 82% of cases. Yakovlev and Rakic[121] noted that a complete decussation was more common for the pyramid arising from the left hemisphere than for that from the right, which they considered compatible with greater control by the left hemisphere than by the right over the opposite upper limb. Because of the apparently small number of non-RH in the study of Kertesz and Geschwind, the pyramidal asymmetry could not be correlated with handedness. The relative lack of non-RH was most likely an artifact since the handedness information obtained from the surviving relatives was probably unreliable.

Another asymmetry is found in the lower medulla:[123] an aberrant circum-olivary bundle deriving from the pyramidal tract is present on the left side much more commonly than on the right. It is believed by some that the aberrant bundle is destined to innervate the facial nucleus of the opposite side. This asymmetry would thus provide an anatomic substrate for the control of some of the speech-related muscles on the dominant side. The literature also contains data on asymmetries at lower levels of the central nervous system in other species, which will be discussed in a later section.

Certain asymmetries in the peripheral nervous system have been well known for many years, e.g., those in the sympathetic and parasympathetic systems which reflect the distribution of autonomic fibers to grossly asymmetric structures such as the heart, the gut, and the solid abdominal organs. In view of the asymmetries in the intrathoracic and intra-abdominal organs, it is likely that there are marked differences in the pattern of visceral sensory innervation from the two sides.

## Cytoarchitectonic Asymmetry

Cytoarchitectonics refers to the characteristic arrangement of neurons in different structures which render them distinguishable from their neighbors. Among the features studied are cell size and packing density, the presence of particular cell types (e.g., giant pyramids and Meynert stellates) and, as in the case of the cortex, the arrangement of neurons into layers and columns of specific widths and densities. Although gross anatomic features such as gyri and sulci may mirror to a great extent the boundaries of cytoarchitectonic areas, they probably also reflect the actions of physical forces exerted by the brain and skull. Since individual architectonic areas differ in connections and physiology, they are probably functional units.

Asymmetries in the volumes of specific architectonic areas have been demonstrated for several regions involved in language function. Thus area TPT is usually larger on the left. This area, part of the extended cortical auditory representation, is located predominantly on the planum temporale and posterior third of the lateral surface of the superior temporal gyrus.[124] Galaburda et al[4] have shown that the magnitude of the asymmetry in TPT correlates positively with gross asymmetry in the planum temporale; because of its location TPT is a major contributor to the asymmetry of the planum. This region makes up a portion of the classic Wernicke's area, so that TPT is probably an important part of the anatomic substrate of language lateralization.

Another asymmetric architectonic area is located in the pars opercularis of the frontal lobe. In eight of ten brains this opercular area was larger on the left side, with six brains showing a volume asymmetry in excess of 30%.[125] The specific frontal area that is larger on the left is found at the center of a region, lesions of which tend to lead to Broca's aphasia.

The left inferior parietal lobule also participates in language function, but the architectonic parcellation of this region did not receive detailed attention in the past. In a recent study, Eidelberg and Galaburda[126] have parcellated the parietal lobes of nine normal human brains and found asymmetry in parietal cytoarchitectonic area-G (PG), which lies on the angular gyrus. These investigators also found a significant positive correlation between planum asymmetry and asymmetry in the volume of PG. Furthermore, they postulated that size asymmetries in the cortex may be linked so that several areas involved in similar functions will be larger on one side. They suggested that the planum temporale, the inferior frontal gyrus, and the inferior parietal lobule would contain certain areas that are usually all larger on the same side of a given brain. Since the number of cases so far studied is small, the existence of discordant cases cannot be ruled out. It, however, remains possible that there are occasional discordant cases (also see section under gross anatomic asymmetries). Eidelberg and Galaburda[126] demonstrated asymmetry which favors the right side of parietal area-EG (PEG), located on the dorsal lip of the inferior parietal lobule. Because of the architectonic and connectional characteristics of area PEG, these authors postulated a role for it in visuospatial function.

Asymmetries in sizes of neurons have also been shown. L. Seldon, PhD, (oral communication, Dec 1, 1983) found that Golgi-impregnated neurons were on the average larger in the left than in the right primary auditory cortex. As a result there were thicker columns and broader intercolumn intervals on the left side in Nissl's-stained sections. Dendritic contacts were greater in number in the right auditory temporal association cortex area-A (TA).

Lesion and stimulation data have shown that certain subcortical regions, especially in the posterior thalamus, and usually on the left side, are also involved in language function.[127–130] Although the left pulvinar is most often involved in language disorders resulting from thalamic damage, no consistent asymmetry has yet been demonstrated for this nucleus. Eidelberg and Galaburda[131] have, however, recently shown that in eight of nine brains studied, the lateralis posterior nucleus was larger on the left. This nucleus, part of the posterior thalamic complex, closely abuts the pulvinar and is also likely to be involved in language functions.

## Chemical and Pharmacologic Asymmetry

Lateral asymmetries in the content of several transmitter substances have been demonstrated in animal and human brains. The most extensive studies are those of Glick and co-workers in the rat,[132,133] which have established the existence of chemical and pharmacologic asymmetry beyond any doubt. We will deal with this pioneering work later, and will, in this section, confine ourselves to studies in the human.

Oke et al[134] have shown an asymmetry in content of norepinephrine in the human thalamus. The left pulvinar contains more norepinephrine than the right, while the ventrobasal complex of the right side is richer in this neurotransmitter. A chemical asymmetry has been reported recently in the human cerebral cortex. Amaducci et al[135] showed that the left Brodmann area 22 (part of which corresponds to area TPT) contained greater cholineacetyltransferase (CAT) activity than the same region on the right. The asymmetry becomes more striking posteriorly in the region of area TPT. Glick et al[136] have found a linked pattern of chemical asymmetries in the human brain.

The first demonstrations of pharmacologic asymmetry in any species were, to our knowledge, the studies of Szara[137] and Sai-Halasz et al[138] who found that dimethyltryptamine, a psychotogenic serotonin derivative, produced both subjective and objective left-body findings in human volunteers. Gentili and Tiberi[139] reported similar findings with diethyltryptamine. Serafetinides[39] administered LSD (another drug related to serotonin) both preoperatively and postoperatively to 12 patients who underwent right anterior temporal lobe removals and to 11 with left-sided ablations. The typical perceptual responses to LSD disappeared after right, but not left, temporal lobectomy. This finding, which has not to our knowledge been investigated by any other group, might, of course, have several explanations. One possibility of particular interest is that lateralized differences in the responses to a drug administered systemically might result from an asymmetric distribution of receptor sites. Mandell and Knapp[140] reported asymmetry in serotonin distribution in the rat. Other recent data are also compatible with asymmetric actions of transmitters in humans. Thus elementary left-sided neurologic signs that disappear after treatment, have been reported in depression[141] and our own experience is in conformity with these reports.[142] Drug-induced dyskinesias have also been reported to occur more often on one side,[143] but later studies question this result.

**Development of Asymmetry**

Since anatomic asymmetries have been found even during early brain development, they cannot be ascribed exclusively to postnatal influences, although a role for these cannot be excluded. A sylvian fossa is visible soon after the tenth week of gestation, and a higher right sylvian point is distinguishable at least by the 16th week.[2]

Wada et al[5] were the first to show that the planum asymmetry described in adult brain was present in the fetus and newborn, and Chi et al[7] have shown that it can be observed as early as the 31st week of gestation.

Petalias are also seen in the brains of fetuses and children. LeMay[144] studied photographs of 49 fetal and newborn brains from the Yakovlev collection at the Armed Forces Institute of Pathology, Washington, DC, and from the Eunice Shriver Kennedy Center, Waltham, Mass. The left hemisphere was longer in 24, the right longer in only eight, and there was equal length in 17. Asymmetries have also been reported in the lengths of the lateral ventricles in brains of children from 5 months to 18 years of age. McRae et al[116] reported that in 100 consecutive pneumoencephalograms (87 in right-handed individuals), the occipital horn was longer on the left in 60%, and longer on the right in 10%, with symmetry in 30%. The 75 young patients of Strauss and Fitz[145] had a longer left occipital horn in 29 cases (39%), a longer right horn in 13 (17%), with symmetry in 44%. If, however, cases with probable damage before the first year of life were excluded, the left horn was longer in 54% and the right was longer in 8%, with symmetry in 38%. These data are compatible with the following interpretation. Assume that the probability of unilateral brain damage was equal on the two sides. When the damage was on the left it would in the majority of cases affect a left occipital horn that was already longer. By contrast, damage on the right would usually increase the size of a horn that was smaller. The net effect would be to produce a proportionally greater increase in right-longer cases.

It was observed early in the 19th century that the gyri and sulci often appear at different times in the two sides of the brain. Herve[146] called attention to the earlier gross anatomic development of the inferior frontal region of the right side, as compared with the left, and disagreed with other authors who had claimed the reverse without adequate data. Fontes[20] showed a similar delay in the appearance of cortical markings surrounding the sylvian fissure of the left side. Chi et al[7] demonstrated that the sulci of the sylvian region appear later on the left side; in the case of the superior temporal region, some of the cortical landmarks on the left trail those on the right by one to two weeks. Scheibel[21] has reported that development of higher order dendritic branches in the anterior language area occurs later on the left than on the right. It thus appears to be the case that regions on the left side that will be larger in the mature brain develop more slowly than the corresponding areas on the right.

An interesting related observation was made recently by Wada and Davies.[147] They reported that in a series of infant brains approximately the same proportion of male and female subjects have a larger right planum (14% males, 17.7% females). By contrast, in adult specimens there is a much lower proportion of male brains with a larger right planum (6% males, 16% females). The authors suggested that the left planum may enlarge more than the right after birth, especially in male infants. The right planum may, in fact, lose cells, thus increasing the asymmetry. An alternative explanation not considered by the authors, one which will be brought up again later, is that there may be a greater demise of men with a larger right planum during the early years of life. A third explanation will be discussed in the final section.

As already mentioned, Amaducci et al[135] found a higher level of CAT in the left superior temporal region of the adult human. A later study from these investigators deals with fetal human brains from 20 to 39 weeks gestational age.[148] The CAT level in the right temporal region was already at its adult level in this period, and was higher than that of the left temporal region even in the oldest fetuses. These data suggest that the delay in maturation of this region on the left persists into the postnatal period. This pioneering study also suggests that neurochemical as well as structural asymmetry must be taken into account if one is to understand lateral differences in function. A larger area has a potentially greater capacity than a smaller one, but the full realization of this capacity can be limited by a lack of full neurochemical development.

In later sections we will present further evidence for the earlier development of the human right hemisphere.

The exact developmental mechanism underlying the asymmetric rate of development of the cortical markings is not known. We believe that asymmetries may date back even to the period of neural induction when the first primitive neural elements form, and to subsequent early stages of development, so that there may be lateral differences in rates of DNA replication, cell division, neuronal migration, neuropil growth, and cell death. Preliminary evidence from a study performed in the rat suggests that asymmetries in growth rates are present during the period of active neuronal migration. DeBassio et al[149] have shown that the stream of neurons migrating to the olfactory bulb of the rat grows at different rates on the two sides. The stream on the right leads that on the left. It is interesting to observe that in the rat strain used in these studies, the left hemisphere develops more slowly, as appears to be the case in the human. In the rabbit, the right optic nerve myelinates in most cases before the left.[150]

It is important to stress that not every asymmetry in the adult brain is the result of normal development. Some instances of cerebral asymmetry shown both in post mortem specimens and in radiologic studies may be the result of disorders of hemispheric development. Enlargement of a lateral ventricle, for instance, may reflect an atrophic lesion of the ipsilateral hemisphere. Likewise, reversal of normal petalias seen on CT scans may reflect excessive delays in growth of a hemisphere, most often the left. Unilateral megalencephaly associated with mental retardation has also been described, and the enlarged hemisphere was distinctly the abnormal one.[151] A left hemisphere that was larger than the right and which contained cortex with evidence of abnormal neuronal migration was seen in the case of childhood dyslexia described by Galaburda and Kemper.[16] One must, therefore, be wary, as we have already noted, especially in clinical populations, of simple interpretations of lateral asymmetries observed by means of radiologic methods.

## Evolution of Human Asymmetry

It was thought only a few years ago that it was impossible to retrace the evolution of human cerebral dominance, since neither the brains of our ancestors nor any records of their linguistic capacities are available. The presence of lateral differences in the sylvian fissures led LeMay and Culebras[2] to the unexpected discovery that the asymmetry of brains of ancient humans could be reflected in the impressions on the inner surfaces of their skulls.

Several of the gross anatomic asymmetries present in the fetal and mature human brain have been demonstrated in the fossil skulls of our ancestors. The sylvian fissures often leave their impression on the inner table of the skull. The endocast of the skull of the Neanderthal man of La Chapelle-aux-Saints who lived 30,000 to 50,000 years ago exhibits the typical sylvian asymmetry of a longer, straighter left fissure and a fissure on the right which turns up at the end. A similar pattern is seen in the endocast of *Sinanthropus pekinensis* (Peking man). The cast of Pithecanthropus I shows a right occipital petalia, while the more common left occipital petalia is seen in Pithecanthropus II. Neanderthal skulls often show a left occipital petalia and a right frontal petalia. Holloway and de la Coste[41] have shown that skulls of hominoids show the same pattern of asymmetries found in modern humans. While the skulls of fossil nonhuman primates manifest asymmetry less often than those of humans, when asymmetries are present they show the same patterns as those found in modern humans.

## Right-Hemisphere Conservatism

The precocious development of the right hemisphere compared with that of the left deserves some consideration at this point, since it plays a major role in our hypothesis about the influences controlling dominance. Since the right hemisphere develops earlier, those influences during fetal life and in early postnatal life which act on the brain are more likely to affect development in the left hemisphere, which is at risk over a longer period. Woo[152] found greater variability in the left side of the human skull than in the right. Since growth of the skull closely reflects brain growth, these data provide further evidence for the greater modifiability of the left hemisphere in development. The earlier development of the right hemisphere is probably not a new phenomenon in humans, but rather one with a long evolutionary history. The development of the individual seems, in this case, to recapitulate the course of evolution, a parallel for which there are good reasons in this particular case. The advantage of earlier development of the right hemisphere derives from its specializations which will be discussed briefly.

Among the functions for which the human right hemisphere is dominant are certain types of spatial function, particularly the analysis of external space, and the orientation of the body within this space. It also plays a major role in emotion, both in the subjective experience and the external expression of emotion, as well as in the appreciation of emotion manifested by others. It is also of predominant importance in attention, a not unexpected finding since attentional systems rely heavily on the emotional systems and on spatial orientation. The role of attentional systems in shifting the focus of concentration to external stimuli is of major importance for survival; this is dealt with in detail in the review of Mesulam.[153]

There are also important controls by the right hemisphere over certain autonomic activities, e.g., as demonstrated by Heilman et al.[154] The right hemisphere thus has a special role in a group of activities essential for survival. It is not surprising that right-hemisphere dominance might have appeared early both in the course of evolution and in individual development.

The earlier development of the right hemisphere is probably relevant to what we refer to as the greater "conservatism of right hemisphere function." Although speech and handedness usually depend predominantly on the left hemisphere, there are individuals in whom right-hemisphere regions contribute significantly to these functions. There are also those who are especially skillful in use of the left arm, who make up from 6% to 14% of different populations. Aphasia sometimes follows right-hemisphere lesions. On the other hand, the appearance, after left-sided lesions, of syndromes typically observed after right posterior hemisphere lesions is less common, e.g., severe persistent right unilateral inattention is uncommon even in left-handers.[155] Furthermore, even lesions of the right hemisphere which lead to aphasia are likely to be accompanied by the typical right hemisphere spatial and emotional alterations.

Since the right hemisphere develops earlier, it is subject to interfering influences over a shorter period of time and its development is, therefore, less likely to be impaired. In other words, enlargement of left-sided regions in response to disturbance of the developmental pattern of the right will be less common than the reverse situation, i.e., larger size on the right as a result of left-sided delay and subsequent diminished cell death on the right. This probably accounts for the conservatism of the posterior right-hemisphere syndromes.

## Mechanisms of Development of Anatomic Asymmetry in the Human Brain

A fundamental question in any discussion of asymmetry is that of its ultimate origins. The system may at its beginnings be symmetrical, and some mechanism may later induce asymmetry. An alternative possibility is that asymmetry is present even at the earliest stages, i.e., in the ovum itself, as suggested by Corballis and Morgan.[34] It is possible to conceive of mechanisms that could induce asymmetry in a previously symmetric system, e.g., the effect of light on the chick embryo, as shown by Rogers.[156] The discussion of basic mechanisms of asymmetry will be left to the last section of the article.

Asymmetry, as already pointed out, is found in the fetal brain. In the photographs of brains of fetuses of 16 weeks in the monograph of Fontes[20] one sees the typical asymmetry of the adult, i.e., a left sylvian fissure that is longer than the right, while the sylvian point, i.e., the termination of the right sylvian fissure, is higher than that on the left. The fundamental pattern of the brain thus appears to be asymmetric with the same pattern of asymmetries found in most adults. Metabolic influences on the fetus do not usually alter the direction of this fundamental pattern which is thus retained by most adults. There are, however, influences in pregnancy that tend to diminish the extent of left-sided predominance, at least in the regions involved in handedness and language and thus secondarily to result in larger regions on the right side. As already stated earlier, our hypothesis is that some factor related to male sex, perhaps testosterone or some closely related factor, is the most likely candidate. The net effect of these intrauterine influences is to produce a shift from left predominance to symmetry and in a smaller number of cases to modest right predominance.

There are several mechanisms that could lead to greater relative size on the right. One might speculate that the modifying factor leads to more rapid growth on the right. Conversely, one might postulate that the effect of this modifying factor is to retard growth on the left. The right side then increases in size because it is more successful in the competition for synapses and therefore undergoes diminished cell death. We believe that the latter mechanism is the correct one, i.e., that the male-related factor retards growth at least in the language areas of the left side, as evidenced by the impaired neuronal migration and/or assembly on the left side in our cases of developmental dyslexia, which will be described more fully in a later section.

One cannot exclude the possibility that while the most common effect of this factor is to delay growth in the left superior temporal gyrus, it may have other effects in other regions and at other periods in gestation. Migration defects can, of course, be found on the right side, although we suspect less commonly than on the left, on the basis of evidence to be presented in later sections. The presence of right-sided migration defects clearly indicates that some influences can cause delayed growth on that side. The predominance of effects in the left superior temporal region may reflect the fact that this area might be at risk over a longer period. It is well known that most teratogens have a "window," i.e., a limited period in gestation before and after which they cannot alter some given system. The length of this window may be greater in some regions on the left side. The earlier formation of the right side probably places it at risk over a shorter period. It is likely that there will be variations from individual to individual in the sensitivity of particular regions to the delaying factor. The fact that neuronal migration is slowed preferentially on one side probably implies lateral differences in the chemistry of the system, i.e., either in receptor structure or density or even in immune properties, a point to which we will return later. It is also possible that there are factors which are operative only at certain periods in development.

The pattern of asymmetry is probably magnified when cell death occurs, since the larger area will be at an advantage in the competition for targets and will attain a more extensive set of bilateral connections. The same influences that delay growth on the left may also slow the growth of axons from cortical regions on the left, thus putting these neurons at a further disadvantage since they may find many targets now occupied by axons from the right side.

## Asymmetries in Other Species: Structure, Chemistry, and Function

We have already discussed data derived from the study of asymmetries in other species. In this section we review some of the findings concerning these asymmetries and their implications. As was pointed out earlier, the standard teachings concerning cerebral dominance held that this was a characteristic of humans alone, so that until the 1960s it was almost universally assumed that functional asymmetry simply did not exist in other species. In tests of handedness individual animals typically showed a consistent preference, but the distribution in the population was evenly divided. In the past 20 years there has been a major revolution in our thinking. Although there were suggestions in the work of such authors as Dewson[157] that functional asymmetry might be found in monkeys tested appropriately, it was Nottebohm and Nottebohm[36] who clearly demonstrated left cerebral dominance in a nonhuman species, i.e., song birds. Another advance came from the work of LeMay and colleagues[2,57] who showed that the anatomic asymmetries found in human sylvian fissure were also present in the brains of great apes. Sherman and co-workers[37] demonstrated the presence of functional asymmetry in a mammalian species, the rat.

It is curious, however, that knowledge of anatomic asymmetry in the brains of other species goes back many years, e.g., Larrabee[55] demonstrated early in the century the striking asymmetry of the decussation of the optic chiasm in the trout and in the cod and Kappers et al[56] reported the presence of a consistently much larger right habenular nucleus in the lamprey. It is intriguing to consider why these findings fail to excite the interest of students of human cerebral dominance and why researchers in animal behavior did not explore the possible functional implications. The belief that animals could not possess functional asymmetries, and the rejection of anatomic asymmetry as the basis for human dominance, probably account for the neglect of these data.

### Asymmetries in Animals

Differences between the hemispheres—anatomic, functional, and chemical—have recently been found in the brains of some nonhuman species (Table 2).

LeMay and Geschwind[57] have shown asymmetries in the sylvian fissures of great apes similar to those found in the human brain. Yeni-Komshian and Benson[158] have shown a larger left planum temporale in the chimpanzee. Cain and Wada[159] have documented a larger right frontal lobe in the baboon.

Asymmetries in structure have been noted in the brains of cats,[160,161] although these are inconsistent. On the other hand, regular anatomic asymmetries have been demonstrated in the rat. Diamond et al[162] found that the cortex was significantly thicker in several areas on the right than on the left in male rats, while in the female the left-sided areas were thicker. In females ovariectomized at birth, the male pattern was seen, which suggested that ovarian hormones modified morphologic asymmetries in the female cortex. In a later study, Diamond[59] found that removing the testes in newborn male rats also led to a reversal of the asymmetry pattern in several cortical regions. We have shown that the total neocortex, the primary visual area, and the sensory-motor cortex may be larger on the right side in the rat.[163] The motor zone is symmetrical, but definitive conclusions must await the examination of additional cases. Asymmetries have been reported in the hippocampus by Diamond et al[59,164] and we have also found similar lateral differences.

In nonmammalian species, several anatomic asymmetries have been reported. Braitenberg and Kemali[165] reported consistent asymmetries in the size and shape of the habenula in amphibians and fishes. A recent study, moreover, reports that the parietal eye of the lizard, a photosensitive structure, has asymmetric connections with the habenula.[166] The functional significance of these architectonic and connectional asymmetries remains to be studied.

Developmental asymmetry has been found in the rabbit. Narang[150] described the usually earlier myelination of the right optic nerve as compared with the left, and this correlates with asymmetry in functional maturation. Again precociousness of a right-sided neural structure is observed.

Functional asymmetries have been demonstrated in nonhuman primates, the rat and other rodents, and in birds. Petersen et al[167] described ear asymmetries for the perception of conspecific calls in Japanese macaques, and Dewson[157] reported functional asymmetries in auditory discrimination tasks in macaques in studies with temporal lobe lesions.

Asymmetries have been found in rats in open field activity, in mazes, and in swimming, as well as in tail position. In addition, studies have been made of the effects of lateralized lesions in a variety of rearing conditions. Thus it has been shown that, as in the human, the right hemisphere of the rat subjected to early handling mediates certain aspects of emotional behavior.[168]

In nonmammalian species, the most striking demonstrations of lateralization of function are those of Nottebohm[169] in singing birds. In finches and canaries song is abolished by lesions of the left but not the right side of the brain. Nottebohm has shown striking size differences in the song control nuclei between singing male and nonsinging female birds, but has failed to reveal consistent right-left anatomic asymmetries. Asymmetries in visual discrimination and auditory inhibition have also been demonstrated in chicks.[170]

TABLE 2 Anatomic Asymmetries in Brains of Nonhuman Species

| *Structure* | *N* | *L>* | *L = R* | *R>* | *Comments* |
|---|---|---|---|---|---|
| *Nonhuman primates* | | | | | |
| Skull[251] | 6 | 6 | | | Left occipital skull prominence found in old male gorillas |
| Skull[252] | 11 | 4 | | 1 | Difference in length of two sides of skull in gorillas |
| Sylvian fissure[107] | | X* | | | Length of fissure in mangabee chimpanzee, orangutan, baboon, but not macaque monkey; no figures |
| Sylvian fissure[253] | 24 | 50 | 33 | 17 | Percentage with longer sylvian fissure; chimpanzees |
| Sylvian fissure[57] | 12 | 0 | 2 | 10 | Height of sylvian point in orangutan |
| Sylvian fissure[57] | 9 | 1 | 4 | 4 | Height of sylvian point in chimpanzee |
| Sylvian fissure[67] | 7 | 0 | 5 | 2 | Height of sylvian point in gorilla |
| Sylvian fissure group with other sylvian fissure[158] | 25 | 80 | 12 | 8 | Percentages with asymmetries in sylvian fissure length; chimpanzees |
| Frontal lobe[159] | 7 | 0 | 1 | 6 | Frontal petalia in baboons |
| Temporal lobe[254] | 30 | 5 | 25 | | Difference between posterior ends of sylvian fissure and superior temporal sulcus in old world monkeys |
| *Other mammals* | | | | | |
| Total hemisphere[161] | 25 | 7 | 0 | 18 | Weight differences in cat |
| Total hemisphere[161] | 30 | 7.8 | 51.1 | 41.1 | Width of hemispheres in cat; percentages |
| Total hemisphere[161] | 30 | 11.1 | 41.1 | 47.8 | Height of hemispheres in cat; percentages |
| Total hemisphere[161] | 27 | 13.6 | 55.6 | 30.8 | Hemisphere width in rabbit; percentages |
| Total hemisphere[161] | 27 | 13.6 | 55.6 | 30.8 | Hemisphere height in rabbit |
| Total hemisphere[161] | 14 | 4 | 0 | 10 | Hemisphere weight in mouse |
| Neocortex[162] | 225 | | | 94 | Percentage of measures showing asymmetry in cortical thickness; rats and rat pups |
| Neocortex[38] | 20 | | | 18 | Male rats with thicker cortex in area 17 |
| Neocortex[38] | | | | 15 | Male rats with thicker cortex in area 39 |
| Neocortex[38] | 9 | 8 | | | Female rats with thicker cortex; difference not significant |
| Neocortex[255] | 42 | | | 71 | Percentage of male brains with thicker cortex; rats |
| Neocortex[255] | 54 | 9 | | | Percentage of female brains with thicker cortex; rats |
| Neocortex[256] | 11 | 1 | 2 | 8 | Volume of neocortex in male rats |
| Neocortex[256] | 9 | 5 | 3 | 1 | Volume of neocortex in females; not significant |
| Neocortical sulci[160] | 39 | | 55 | | Percentage with symmetric fissure patterns; in 45%, patterns were asymmetric; cats and kittens |

TABLE 2 Anatomic Asymmetries in Brains of Nonhuman Species (continued)

| *Structure* | *N* | *L* | *L = R* | *R* | *Comments* |
|---|---|---|---|---|---|
| Central region[257] | 10 | | | 10 | Cross-sectional neocortical area in rats |
| Hippocampus[258] | 18 | | | | Mean weight of left hippocampus 64 ±6 mg; mean weight of right hippocampus 58 ± 11 ($P \leq .001$); in rats |
| Hippocampus[163] | 17 | 1 | 3 | 13 | Hippocampal volume in handled, environmentally enriched rats; male and female |
| Hippocampus[163] | 15 | 11 | 1 | 3 | Hippocampal volume in nonhandled; standard environment female rats |
| Hippocampus[259] | 24 | | | 14 | Weight in male rats; not significant |
| Hippocampus[259] | 23 | | | 14 | Weight in female rats; significant |
| Optic nerve[150] | 24 | 5 | | 19 | Earlier opening of eye in rabbit during postnatal development |

* X indicates only category where examples were found, although no numbers were provided.

Chemical and pharmacologic asymmetries are also demonstrable in animals. In the last several years, research in normal rats has established asymmetries in striatal dopamine content,[171] striatal dopamine receptors,[172] striatal dopamine metabolism and dopamine-stimulated adenyl cyclase activity,[173,174] striatal deoxyglucose uptake,[40] and striatal γ-aminobutyric acid (GABA) turnover.[175] These biochemical asymmetries have been correlated with the preferred direction of rotation after administration of amphetamines and the direction of spontaneous nocturnal circling. Additional asymmetries have been demonstrated in nucleus accumbens, thalamus, hippocampus, neocortex, and others. In several of these studies, sex differences in asymmetry of structure and function have been found.

## Implications of Animal Asymmetries

The demonstrations of asymmetry in animals appear to confirm the belief that biologically determined asymmetry has existed throughout vertebrate evolution, and that human asymmetries are not a recent development nor an example of convergent evolution, but rather only the most recent example of a fundamental feature of neuroanatomy and behavior.

Biological, psychological, and medical research always sustains an important impetus from animal models which permit experimental manipulations that cannot be carried out in humans. Data from such models have led repeatedly to revisions of theories based only on studies in normal humans and those with brain lesions.

It should be possible to breed strains for marked asymmetry of specific structures, or for marked functional asymmetry, and thus to carry out studies on highly uniform animals, in contrast to the necessarily high variability of human groups. It should also render possible experimental study of different mechanisms of asymmetry, and in particular of the effects of manipulations during pregnancy and early postnatal life. It will also be easy to study the effects of pregnancy during different seasons and under differing conditions of light, temperature, and other variables.

Experimental animal studies may be particularly useful for investigation of functions that have long been thought to be confined to the human, e.g., language. The common response that such study is not possible in view of the lack of convincing evidence of language function in any other species, is, we believe, based on a narrow view of language. Human language depends on specific brain regions, which must have evolved and which probably share common activities with homologous areas in other species.

In the recent heated discussions as to whether apes could acquire language, there was complete neglect of the implications of the finding of asymmetries in the brain of the chimpanzees in areas homologous to the language regions of humans. If destruction of such a homologous cortical area on the left side had abolished the asserted linguistic capacities of the animal, this would have supported the belief that the animals had learned some activity related to human language. If on the other hand the animal's acquired abilities had been abolished only by bilateral ablations of nonhomologous regions, the argument against the possession of linguistic capacities would have been supported.

One of the major stumbling blocks to a study of language forerunners in other species is the assumption that language is primarily a means of communication between humans. This has led investigators to stress the training of animals to *produce* language. Yet language is clearly used as an internal processing mechanism by humans. The fact that this is usually perceived as inner speech has strengthened the assumption that this must reflect the internal use of learned language. The interconnected language areas must, however, possess a method of neural coding. We suggest that such internal codes exist in other species and are used for internal cognitive processing. The external communicative aspect of language may have been a late development in the human, but the fundamental features of an internal language system may have existed at a far earlier period.

If such systems are present in lower species one may be guided to them by the presence of anatomic asymmetries similar to those found in the human. It should be possible to breed animals for increased size of these regions. One could also use the technique devised by Goldman,[23] i.e., placement of lesions during fetal life in one area so as to increase the size of the corresponding contralateral area or of adjacent areas. The development of animals with superior functions of these regions might permit cognitive studies that could illuminate as yet unexpected features of language. Such studies should be guided by information concerning the possible homologues of human language regions. The chimpanzee has asymmetry in the planum temporale like that of the human[158] and the great apes have asymmetries similar to those of humans in the sylvian fissures.[57]

Similarly the lack of animal models has held up the study of psychiatric illness. The described relationships of some of these to handedness suggests an important role of dominance. As the study of disorders of lateralized brain disorder in psychosis advances, it should be possible to carry out studies on the functions of homologous unilaterally asymmetric regions in other species. Data from such models will perhaps make it possible to restate the concept of psychosis in new—and perhaps unexpected—terms that are more susceptible of neurologic and cognitive analysis than those now available.

The study of animal models has already uncovered some intriguing findings, e.g., the poorer maze performance of rats who do not show strong turning tendencies to either side,[176] the importance of early experience in establishing dominance in male rats,[37] altered callosal projection patterns in animals with early visual system lesions,[97,177] and the higher rate of left-turning in females who have been in utero with many males.[178] Animal studies have already cast important light on mechanisms of asymmetry in the claws of crustaceans[179,180] and in the chick brain.[156] Since animal models will probably be available in very large numbers, the possibilities for important additions to and modifications of ideas concerning dominance are almost without limit.

## Pathology of Asymmetry in Developmental Learning Disorder

Just as asymmetries in the structure of the hemispheres may begin to appear at least as early as the period of neuronal migration, changes in the pattern of cerebral lateralization may result from factors operating at different stages of the normal developmental process. Gross alterations of symmetric structures have been produced experimentally. The formation of paired optic vesicles may be altered by a lesion during the time of neural induction.[181] Damage to the chordal plate portion of the mesoderm at that period produces an amphibian embryo with a single midline eye. Kallen[182] has suggested that drugs such as thalidomide might act at this early stage by producing errors in the induction of ectodermal structures in the limbs. As we will note later, many influences which lead to abnormal limb formation act primarily on one side.

Evidence from the study of brains of individuals with developmental dyslexia suggests another mechanism, occurring later in fetal development, which may lead to disorders of lateralization. Because of its relevance to the hypothesis presented in this article, the evidence from the brain in dyslexia will be presented here in greater detail.

### Neuropathology of Developmental Dyslexia

Neuropathologic findings in the brain in developmental dyslexia have been described in three cases, and preliminary observations are available in two additional cases. In the first case, Drake[70] reported excessive numbers of neurons in the subcortical white matter especially in the parietal region, which suggested a disorder of neuronal migration. He did not, however, mention any significant lateral differences. Anomalies were also found at other levels, e.g., an arteriovenous malformation in the cerebellum.

A second case, reported by Galaburda and Kemper,[16] was studied with particular attention to lateralization of abnormalities and to cytoarchitectonic structure. The findings in that case may be summarized as follows: (a) a large area of micropolygyria (a malformation of cortex consisting of abnormal folding, fewer layers, and primitive orientation of neurons, thought to result from an alteration in neuronal migration) in the left planum temporale and posterior third of the superior temporal gyrus; (b) clusters of subcortical neurons especially in perisylvian areas; (c) clusters of neurons in layer one of the cortex, especially in the superior temporal gyrus; and (d) abnormal, primitive layering and primitive neurons in numerous perisylvian and pericingulate areas. These findings were present only in some parts of the left cortex, and none were found on the right. Later review disclosed five small extopias involving right frontal cortex.

The findings in another case included primitive left-hemisphere cortical differentiation and frank cortical dysplasias, especially in perisylvian cortex, and clusters of ectopic neurons in layer one, some associated with brain wart formation. In this case again the right-hemisphere cortex was more normal.[17]

Preliminary findings in a third case[183] have included bilateral cortical dysplasias and ectopias in the temporal lobes, both more striking on the left side. A fourth case, recently studied, has revealed similar findings.

Additional architectonic abnormalities in the thalamus of the Galaburda and Kemper case[16] have been reported by Galaburda and Eidelberg.[184] The medial geniculate nucleus and the lateralis posterior nucleus were distorted in shape and showed clusters of primitive cells and abnormal myelination. In contrast to the findings in the cortex the thalamic abnormalities were present more symmetrically. This brain was also abnormal on gross examination. The left hemisphere was large and contained an excessive volume of subcortical white matter. Asymmetric enlargement of a single hemisphere has been reported in unilateral megalencephaly,[151] which involved the right hemisphere of a 13-month-old infant with intractable seizures. The cortex was simple in gyral pattern, and abnormal in cytoarchitecture, with clusters of primitive neurons and indistinct cortical layering. The subcortex contained cells arrested in migration.

It has been noted often that malformed cortex frequently contains abnormal blood vessels. Arteriovenous malformations (AVMs), which are more common in men than women, are often found in the posterior perisylvian regions. Levine et al[185] recently reported a case of learning disability in a young patient who had undergone a left temporal lobectomy following a hemorrhage probably originating in an AVM. The authors suggested that the developmental reading disorder in this case was the result of the acquired lesion. It is, however, quite possible that the AVM was embedded in abnormally developed temporal cortex so that the patient would probably have been dyslexic even if the malformation had not ruptured. We are aware of six patients with lifelong reading disability but no early history of bleeding or surgery, who were shown to have AVMs in the left temporoparietal region. Caron et al[186] reported a series of AVMs in the language areas of the left hemisphere. The population was overwhelmingly male, and although left superior temporal AVMs were common in the men none were found in the women. Persistent aphasia occurred infrequently after surgery, suggesting that speech representation was anomalous in most of these cases. In another series from Japan,[187] cortical AVMs were found predominantly in men on the left side.

In summary, the brain abnormalities in dyslexia are developmental in nature and can be attributed to alterations in the cortex and connectionally related subcortical structures resulting from disturbances in neuronal migration and assembly. It is likely that in some individuals the postulated slowing of the rate of migration of neurons to the left cortex is even more marked than in the normal state; this excessive delay can lead to lateralized developmental arrest and malformation, thus leading to childhood dyslexia and possibly other developmental disorders.

It is conceivable, furthermore, that delay of left cortical development results in more successful competition by right-hemisphere neurons for available synapses and thus leads to diminished rates of neuronal death on the right. This would explain the reported excess of reversed asymmetries in severe dyslexics[188–190] but these have not yet been confirmed. We wish to stress again that in the four dyslexics studied at postmortem in our laboratory we have not found reversal of the usual asymmetry but rather symmetry of the planum temporale. The potential for enhanced right-hemisphere development in the dyslexics helps to explain the apparent excess of LH and right-hemisphere skills[44,45] in dyslexics and their families.

## Are Minor Neuronal Migration Defects Normal?

Neurologists and neuropathologists have usually regarded extensive disorders of neuronal migration and assembly as dramatic abnormalities typically associated with mental defect and epilepsy, while the pathologic significance of less severe and more localized malformations of this kind has, in general, been neglected. There has existed a common tacit assumption that while the gross disorders produce rather crude neurologic defects, those of lesser degree are of little significance, with one important exception, i.e., even minor migrational defects are accepted as causes of epilepsy.

The common ascription of little importance to minor developmental defects is based on the belief that they are frequently found in normal brains. This standard teaching may, however, be erroneous. The assertion that these defects are not associated with neurologic impairment means only that they are found relatively frequently in the brains of patients who have died of nonneurologic illness and in whose records no mention is made of neurologic disorder. It is, however, clear that a wide variety of neurologic defects without relatively crude manifestations are overlooked by most physicians. Despite the high frequency of the many forms of learning disability, they are rarely mentioned in medical records, even on neurologic services, and histories of mental illness are often not sought after. Patients and families often fail to mention these conditions either because they do not regard them as medical illnesses, or through a desire for concealment. If facts about learning disability or psychiatric disorder are not obtained from the patients themselves, the errors in family histories are even greater. It is extremely rare to find a reference to dyslexia in a sibling, or to stuttering in an uncle. Furthermore, good personal histories of handedness are rarely obtained even on neurologic services, and are almost never recorded in other departments; familial histories of handedness are almost entirely lacking. Even when such data are obtained they are usually of low reliability.

It is by deliberate intent that allusion to the failure to obtain histories of learning disabilities, handedness, and psychiatric disorders is coupled to the discussion of the tendency to dismiss lesser degrees of anomalies of neural development as of little or no pathologic significance. We suspect that it is precisely this type of "minor" developmental pathology that is responsible for many of the learning disabilities and related disorders and psychiatric conditions. The study of Veith and Schwindt[191] is relevant. They found a much higher rate of minor anomalies in postmortems of social derelicts than from other individuals.

Another form of developmental anomaly that is probably even more widely overlooked than minor migrational disorders is failure of normal maturation of neuronal organization within a particular brain region. Neuropathologists who usually deal with adult material do not always have experience with developmental patterns and may thus overlook failures of full maturation of neuronal assemblies. A recent disagreement about the postmortem findings of a case of Tourette's syndrome illustrates this problem. Balthasar[192] concluded that the caudate nucleus of his patient with Tourette's showed a cytoarchitectonic pattern usually seen only in infancy. Eminent students of the pathology of the basal ganglia disagreed as to the validity of these conclusions.

These problems illustrate some standard conceptions concerning the teratology of the nervous system. Many congenital malformations, e.g., neural tube defects, are correctly regarded as causes of gross neurologic disorder, but the possibility that apparently minor degrees of these conditions may have important effects on function receives much less attention. In agenesis of the corpus callosum, the entire structure or major portions of it are absent. It is unlikely that the underlying causes of this condition will manifest themselves only in such gross deficits; there are probably many individuals in whom the corpus callosum contains a much smaller than normal complement of fibers in certain portions. Recent studies[23,97,177] confirm that the local pattern of callosal connections can be altered by intrauterine or postnatal interventions and thus make it likely that such cases exist. Such a condition should be reflected in accompanying functional changes, although of a different and less coarse nature than those seen in patients with total agenesis. The same may be true of neural tube defects.

**Pathology of Superiority**

There is another possible, although surprising, reason why lesser degrees of neural migration deficits or of other forms of teratology may be overlooked. It has already been suggested that in mild cases of this type certain types of disturbed function may occur commonly. We must consider another apparently paradoxical possibility, i.e., that minor malformations may often be associated, not with abnormal function, but rather with distinctly superior capacities in certain areas. The idea that a "pathologic" disorder could manifest itself primarily by superior abilities is alien to standard modes of thinking about neurologic disease. It may seem bizarre to speak of "the neuropathology of superior intellectual functions"; yet we suggest that a superior outcome, with or without accompanying problems in other areas, is not at all unusual. The reasons have already been advanced. If the growth of one portion of the hemisphere is delayed, then other regions will be larger than they normally would have been. When this increase in size is marked superior or even remarkable talents may develop.

A likely example of such reciprocal increased development is afforded by the case of Galaburda and Kemper[16] who despite lifelong difficulties in reading was a talented metalsmith. The superior right-hemisphere talents of dyslexics documented by Gordon[45] illustrate the same point. The case of Sano[193] manifested remarkable artistic talents in the face of very limited linguistic capacities. The author concluded, on the basis of careful comparison with control cerebra, that the brain of this individual showed poor development in both frontal and temporal lobes but markedly enlarged posterior regions. The remarkable talents of some autistic patients[194,195] possibly represent further examples of the operation of this mechanism.

The occurrence of high talents through this mechanism may also help to explain the high frequency of such disorders as childhood dyslexia. The high spatial talents of many of the affected individuals may counteract the evolutionary disadvantage of their disabilities. This would, of course, be even more conspicuously the case in nonliterate societies in which failure to learn to read would not be a problem. Even in a literate society the manifest disability may be overcome through great effort and good teaching, so that only the superior talents may be evident. The fact that family members may manifest the high talents without obvious disabilities raises the possibility that serious difficulties may occur in only a fraction of those in whom slowed development in the left hemisphere is of greater degree than in most people. These considerations raise the possibility that the mechanisms which delay left-hemisphere growth have been selected in the course of evolution because they often produce individuals of elevated talent. The advantage of these individuals presumably outweighs the disadvantage of the learning disabilities which probably appear in a small number in whom the slowing on the left is excessive. Furthermore, a disability such as dyslexia would have been of minor importance in nonliterate societies.

## Standard and Anomalous Dominance

As we shall see, individual patterns of brain dominance have important biological associations, e.g., increased susceptibility to certain disorders, and a higher likelihood of possession of certain talents. The classification of individuals according to dominance patterns is, however, difficult, and the simple twofold classification into RH and LH presents many problems which have not received the attention they deserve. This section will discuss some of the differences in dominance patterns. Since the literature is vast, emphasis will be placed on issues relevant to our hypothesis.

### Anomalous Dominance: Definition

Although differences in manual preference were probably recognized in early human societies, it was not until Broca's discovery of cerebral dominance for language that it was appreciated that handedness reflected some aspect of brain organization. Many of the early concepts have, however, turned out either to be incorrect or to be distortions of the true situation.

The discovery that lesions producing aphasia lay predominantly on the left led to the belief in a *single* dominant hemisphere that controlled both handedness and speech. It is now clear that one can no longer speak of a dominant and a nondominant hemisphere since each side of the brain is dominant for certain functions. It is also appropriate to discuss briefly the belief that handedness and language dominance are closely linked.

It may appear at first that this question can be answered by statistical means, i.e., are RH and left-hemisphere speech associated more often than would be expected by chance? The problem is, however, complex since there are degrees of language lateralization and handedness that are continuously distributed. Even if one neglected this and accepted the common view that strong RH is more often associated with left language dominance than strong LH, this would not settle the issue. It would only mean that dominance for handedness and dominance for speech were not *statistically* independent, but would not answer the basic biological question. An example should illustrate this.

Assume that two species of plant are always found in the same geographic locations, i.e., their ranges are strongly associated statistically. The association might be obligatory, i.e., each species might depend on the other for some essential substance. At the other extreme it might be possible to show experimentally that one species could be grown independently of the other. Their common geographic ranges would then simply reflect some common mode of spread or common requirements for certain types of climatic and soil conditions.

In the same manner, the nonrandom association of handedness and language dominance might or might not reflect a deeper physiologic connection. Consider the fact that both the heart and the spleen are almost always located on the left side. The existence of cases in which there is dextrocardia but no reversal of location of the spleen suggests that there is no obligatory link between the sites of the two organs.

Applying these considerations to handedness and speech, one might entertain the possibility that they were intrinsically linked, e.g., they might both be manifestations of the same neural substrate; or the development in the embryo of the substrate for one might inevitably cause the substrate of the other to develop on the same side. On the other hand, they might have independent neural substrates.

The assumption that handedness and speech are intrinsically linked runs into many difficulties. There are occasional strong right-handers who become aphasic after right-hemisphere lesions. Furthermore, while a higher percentage of left-handers than right-handers become aphasic after right-hemisphere lesions, the majority of permanent severe aphasias in sinistrals are the result of left-hemisphere damage.[48] Despite these findings the fact that the great majority of right-handers become aphasic after left-hemisphere lesions has kept alive the idea that speech and handedness are intrinsically linked.

Our thinking has been influenced strongly by the ideas of Annett[33] on random dominance. She postulates the existence of people in whom dominance for handedness and language may be random, i.e., either hemisphere may be dominant for either function. We make the assumption that language and handedness are dependent on separate neuronal substrates that do not necessarily develop at the same periods. It is likely, however, that the basic brain pattern in most humans is one in which the left hemisphere contains the separate brain regions involved in language acquisition and in the learning of certain types of motor skills. The neurologic substrates of these functions probably develop according to different schedules. Certain prenatal retarding influences might be operative to a marked degree during the development of either or both of these functions. If the degree of retardation is sufficiently great, the initial anatomic advantage in the left hemisphere will be diminished and there will be a greater degree of symmetry on the two sides. The more nearly symmetry is achieved in some particular region, the more likely there will be random dominance for the function subserved by that region. In the majority of people both functions will remain left-hemisphere dominant, but there will be a minority in whom either or both will be randomly determined or occasionally clearly shifted to the right. If either can be shifted independently of the other it is likely that there is no strong intrinsic linkage.

It should be clear that our hypothesis as to the cause of random dominance differs in some respects from that of Annett. She believes that in about 18% of the population dominance is random and that in these people accidental factors determine the lateralization of language or handedness. The remainder of the population carry a "right-shift" gene which increases the probability of left-hemisphere dominance for these functions. By contrast, we postulate that in most humans there is an innate bias toward left-hemisphere dominance for both of these functions, and that certain influences during fetal life act to diminish this innate bias and thus to create random dominance. Like Corballis and Morgan,[34] we believe in a "left-shift" factor. This factor is influenced by genetic endowment, but there are large nongenetic components. It should be noted that Annett stressed the importance of nongenetic factors in the determination of dominance patterns.

We do not wish to overemphasize the differences in our interpretation from that of Annett, whose innovative ideas on random dominance have so profoundly influenced our thinking.

The *standard dominance pattern* is found in the majority of the population and, of course, in an even larger majority of right-handers, i.e., strong left-hemisphere dominance for language and handedness and strong right-hemisphere dominance for other functions. Even among these people the degree of dominance of any given function will vary somewhat from person to person.

The term *anomalous dominance* is used in reference to those in whom the pattern differs from the standard form. There is no sharp cutoff point at which one can speak of a shift from standard to anomalous dominance. Our rough estimate is that anomalous dominance will be found in approximately 30% to 35% of individuals, i.e., roughly the percentage in whom the planum temporale is not larger on the left side.

It is important to stress anomalous dominance rather than LH. According to Annett's formulation left-handers comprise about half of those in whom handedness is random. She estimates that random handedness is present in 18%, of whom about half, i.e., 9%, will be left-handed. Our tentative formulation differs from Annett's in one respect. She postulates that the same 18% have random dominance for language. We speculate that in about 30% of the population there will be random dominance (with occasional clear shifts to the right hemisphere) for language or handedness, and sometimes, but not always, for both. We believe that random dominance for language may be more frequent than that for handedness although this remains to be confirmed experimentally. Our basis for this view is again speculative, i.e., that the as yet unknown neural substrate for handedness may develop earlier and over a shorter period than that for language. For this reason the shift from left hemisphere to random (or reversed) dominance for handedness will be present in fewer individuals than a similar shift for language functions. Thus many people in whom language dominance is random will also have random handedness, but the postulated later development of the speech regions will make possible random language dominance despite a standard pattern of dominance for handedness.

There is another much less speculative argument in favor of our belief that individuals need not have random dominance for all functions. As we pointed out in an earlier section, certain aspects of right-hemisphere dominance are very conservative, i.e., they are rarely shifted to the left hemisphere even in cases with anomalous dominance for language and handedness. In our view, expressed earlier, the rarity of anomalous dominance of right-hemisphere functions reflects the earlier and more rapid development of that side of the brain, which is thus less subject to modulating influences.

In the anomalous dominance group there will be various degrees of deviance from the more uniform pattern of the larger group with standard dominance.

Because the anomalous dominance group will consist of people in whom the development of asymmetry has been altered at different periods and to different extents, they will be a more variable population and will have to be considered on a more individual basis.

Annett's concept that in some cases laterality is randomly determined may appear to be daring but, as she herself points out, there is a well-documented example. In hereditary situs inversus in mice[196] only half of the offspring of a mating of parents homozygous for the disorder will have reverse situs. Yet the apparently normal offspring have themselves as high a percentage of affected offspring as do their abnormal littermates. The gene thus appears to determine not reverse situs but rather random situs. Another possibly related example is afforded by Kartagener's syndrome[197] in which one finds repeated bronchial infections associated with situs inversus. There are, however, children with apparently similar disorders of the cilia of the respiratory tracts who lack reversed placement of the viscera. Dahlberg[198] also called attention to genes whose unilateral manifestations may appear on either side.

There have been several attempts to distinguish subpopulations among left-handers. Some studies stress the distinction between *familial left-handers,* i.e., those with LH in close relatives, and *nonfamilial left-handers.* Although we believe that this distinction may be important, we will refer to it only occasionally. Another commonly made distinction is that between *normal* and *pathologic* left-handers. There are, of course, some individuals who have sustained either in utero or in early childhood a considerable degree of damage to the left hemisphere and who therefore necessarily end up having right-hemisphere dominance for language and handedness. Although the term *pathologic LH* is appropriately applied to this group, we agree with Annett that this concept has probably been too widely applied. It should be obvious from the discussions in this article that many left-handers who do have visible abnormalities in the brain, e.g., the childhood dyslexics discussed above, have had their brain organization altered by an extreme case of a mechanism that is producing the majority of normal left-handers. If this hypothesis is correct, then the frequent equation in the literature of "genetic" with "normal" LH and of "pathologic" with "acquired" LH must be erroneous. We do not accept the equation of equating *normal* and *genetic* LH since, as will be made clear later, the intrauterine influences producing LH are only in part genetically determined. Furthermore, those genetic influences that favor the development of LH will also favor, in a small proportion of cases, the development of the anomalies of neural migration that lead to dyslexia. We would not subscribe to the view that our hypothesis is equivalent to that of Bakan,[199,200] i.e., that all sinistrality is pathologic. The essential point is that there is a continuum between the cases of LH with and without accompanying disorders.

We have suggested that a major cause of anomalous dominance is markedly delayed development of a left hemisphere which is initially programmed for strong left-sided dominance for speech and handedness. The effect of the delay is to create primarily individuals who have more symmetric brains, although a few will be reversed. An uncommon cause of anomalous dominance is early extensive damage to the left hemisphere. There is a third possibility to consider. It is conceivable that there exist people who are endowed with a right hemisphere which is, in fact, the mirror image of the left hemisphere of the majority of the population, i.e., people who have true "cerebral situs inversus." We believe that such individuals may exist. This issue will be discussed in the final section of the article.

## The Assessment of Handedness

It is important to comment on the assessment of handedness. Benton et al[201] have stressed that self-described left-handers are a highly variable group. Other investigators, however, argue that it is unnecessary to carry out elaborate measurements of manual preference because there is a high agreement between handedness as measured by test and self-described handedness. It is easy to see why the high correlation between self-described handedness and test scores is of little use. Even if the correlation were high, e.g., 0.8, this would mean, according to accepted standards, that 64% of the variance would be accounted for. This means that a considerable fraction of the variance would be unexplained and that there would be many discrepancies, most of which would be present in exactly those individuals of greatest interest, i.e., those with anomalous dominance.

There is a close parallel between this situation and the relationships between speech and handedness. One can predict the side of an aphasia-producing lesion in a very high percentage of cases if one knows the handedness of an individual. It is precisely the small number of discrepant cases that are the object of interest.

In our own population studies we have used the Oldfield[8] Handedness Battery although in later studies we have modified both the items and the scoring. Although we have postulated that deviations from RH might identify only about one third of the anomalous dominance group, LH is still a very valuable marker, because it is readily measurable. It is probably the case for many reasons, only some of which will be discussed here, that existing tests of handedness have, despite their usefulness, serious shortcomings, and that better tests, incorporating recent conceptual advances, should be developed.

A comment is appropriate on the Wada test,[202] i.e., the intracarotid injection of sodium amytal, frequently used to determine the hemisphere dominant for language. It is often assumed that this is an unequivocal test of unilateral or bilateral speech representation. If this assumption is accepted, one might conclude, for example, from the data of Rasmussen and Milner[203] that LH was more common than anomalous language representation. Of the 214 nondextral epileptics studied by them, 50% had left-hemisphere speech by the Wada test and the remaining 50% had bilateral or right-sided speech. As the authors themselves point out, this population of epileptics cannot be necessarily regarded as typical of the general left-handed population. There is, however, another point to make about the interpretation of the Wada test, i.e., that it underestimates the proportion who have significant degrees of bilateral language representation. Luria[67] reported that aphasia was present in the acute stage in nearly all soldiers with penetrating brain wounds in the primary speech areas in the left hemisphere. At a year, the rate of recovery from these left-sided lesions was much higher in the left-handed and in right-handers with familial sinistrality. One assumes that all of these individuals (had they been tested before their injuries) would have become aphasic after injection of sodium amytal into the left internal carotid, but the test would have given no clue as to which ones would recover from such a lesion, since regression of aphasia in those who improved often took weeks or months. In brief, the Wada test can demonstrate right-hemisphere participation in language but it cannot exclude it, since the right-hemisphere linguistic capacity may become manifest only a considerable time after left-sided damage.

We hope that increasingly more accurate markers of anomalous dominance will be developed. The following individuals are, in our view, more likely to have anomalous language dominance: (a) left-handers, (b) right-handers with first-degree left-handed relatives, (c) right-handers with developmental learning disorders, and (d) right-handers with first-degree relatives with learning disorders. In support of criteria a and b is Luria's[67] finding that individuals in these groups had a higher rate of recovery from aphasia. Gordon[44,45] has found by neuropsychologic testing evidence for anomalous dominance in both dyslexics and their relatives. One implication of this classification is that members of groups c and d should also have higher rates of recovery from aphasia. Preliminary observations suggest that this may be the case, but an extensive study will be necessary.

There are other reasons why measurements of handedness have been problematic. The exclusive reliance on the hand used for writing presents many difficulties. As was pointed out by Gloning et al[50] in a study done about 30 years ago, all of their Austrian left-handers had been compelled to write with the right hand in school, and even today this practice is the rule in many countries. The greater tolerance toward left-handed writing in the English-speaking countries might lead some to assume that in these communities the writing hand could appropriately be used as a measure of laterality. Yet even in these countries many pressures, both explicit and implicit, favor right-handed writing; this is reflected in the fact that this activity is the most right-handed of all.

Another source of difficulty is the common assumption that there are two separate populations, i.e., right-handers and left-handers. Unfortunately, the criteria for separation of the two groups vary from test to test. Even altering some of the items on a test may alter the individual's classification, as was shown by Provins et al.[204]

Furthermore, Annett[205] has stressed that handedness, like height, is a continuous variable. In studying the associations of handedness the appropriate question is therefore not, e.g., "Is left-handedness more common in condition A than in the general population?" but rather, "Is the distribution of handedness scores different in condition A from that in the general population?" A recent example shows the value of this approach. In a study of alcoholics[206] the proportion who were frankly left-handed was the same as in controls (about 7.0% with the test used in this study). The proportion not frankly right-handed was 56% in the 99 alcoholics as against 30% in the 86 controls, a highly significant result.

Another problem stems from the inclusion in some "handedness" batteries of items relating to eye dominance, e.g., "Which eye do you use in looking through a microscope?" This actually may weaken the data since as has often been shown[73] replies on eye dominance questions correlate poorly with items on hand usage. The next section will show that even the use of pure motor dominance items may present difficulties.

A recent study on 1,167 professionals by Schachter et al[207] illuminates several of these points. A modified form of the Oldfield[8] Battery was employed. Instead of setting arbitrary cut offs for left-handedness the numbers of individuals in each range of laterality scores (LS) were counted, adjacent cells being pooled only to meet the requirements of the $\chi^2$ test. It was found that a history of dyslexia was found in 9% to 10% of those with scores in the ranges from –100 (complete LH on this test) through +70 and then dropped sharply to about 3% in the ranges above this level. Thus the data showed that +70 was a cutoff point. Of the dyslexics, 56% scored +70 or less, as against 22% of the nondyslexics. By contrast, 20% of the dyslexics wrote with the left hand, as against 10% of non-dyslexics. Of the dyslexics, 30% were self-described left-handers or ambidexters, as against 15% of the nondyslexics. The data from this study show that the writing hand and self-described handedness are much less sensitive measures than consideration of the entire distribution of LS.

## Some Further Aspects of Motor Dominance

Since the concept of handedness has played so great a role in all considerations of dominance, some potentially important distinctions deserve further discussion.

The very term *handedness* has had an important impact on the directions of research on motor dominance. Manual preference can be assessed relatively easily either by questionnaire or by tests of performance. Adroit use of the hand is a cardinal biologic feature of humans and underlies many skilled activities. Most laterality questionnaires consist primarily of questions about activities carried out with one hand, e.g., writing or using a spoon. Liepmann[208] proposed that handedness was a reflection of the greater capacity of one side of the brain to acquire the programs for particular motor skills. Right-handedness would thus imply that an individual's left hemisphere was more capable of learning how to carry out certain unimanual skilled movements. We accept this formulation and therefore believe that the left-hander is someone whose right hemisphere is superior at acquiring these programs. More generally, the non-right-hander is someone in whom the right hemisphere has some significant capacity for acquiring at least certain motor programs. It should be noted that some investigators would not agree with this formulation, since they believe that even in some left-handers the left hemisphere may be superior at acquiring motor programs.[209]

In contrast to the stress on unimanual skill, there has been much less emphasis on other forms of motor dominance, although one can find data on preferences for using one leg or foot. So-called *eye dominance* is not considered here since it is not clear that it reflects any type of *motor* dominance. There is, we believe, another form of motor learning that may also depend primarily on one hemisphere, although it is not immediately evident to the observer, i.e., the learning of activities that depend to a considerable extent on coordinated movements of the trunk and the limbs.

One might describe an individual as clumsy who could not learn to hold a pencil or a fork properly. Someone who could not readily acquire the coordinations necessary for riding a bicycle, dancing, or polevaulting might also be called clumsy. Since the latter type of skill is not *obviously* lateralized, it has not entered into studies of cerebral dominance. Since muscles of both sides of the trunk, in coordination with limbs on both sides are used in these activities, it may seem odd to postulate dominance for them. Even if they were controlled predominantly from one hemisphere, it would be difficult to determine the leading half of the brain by either questionnaires or tests of performance. That activities dependent on bilateral innervation might be controlled by one side of the brain should not be surprising. The sounds of language, with rare exceptions, are produced by symmetrically innervated muscles and yet are typically programmed unilaterally. Furthermore, in singing the same muscles are innervated bilaterally and yet may be controlled from the side of the brain contralateral to the one controlling speech. In fact, the movements of both speech and singing are far more symmetric than many movements involving the trunk. It is commonly pointed out by coaches that ice skaters commonly find it easier to execute turns in one direction than in the other.

Some people, e.g., those with high athletic or dancing talents, are superior in the acquisition of these truncal skills. Others are particularly adept at learning activities that require high degrees of manual adroitness, e.g., painters of miniatures, or those who carry out delicate dissections. It is a common, although unfortunate, practice to characterize skills involving the trunk as gross and those involving the hand as fine. There is no reason, however, to presume that the skill of the great ballet dancer is less refined than that of the neurophysiologist who places an electrode inside a cell. Everyday observation is consistent with the possibility that the two forms of skill can be independent. Accounts of childhood dyslexics often exemplify this contrast. The first patient studied by Galaburda and Kemper,[16] described as clumsy in gait all through development, became a skilled metalsmith. Another typical case known to us is a female dyslexic described as clumsy and unathletic, i.e., deficient in the handling of the trunk, who is a highly skilled painter of miniatures.

Although there may be several ways to account for these discrepancies, one possible explanation is that there may be more than one form of motor learning. One type might be described as "*pyramidal,*" i.e., the ability to learn programs of complex sequences of separate joint movements especially in the fingers. (For reasons which need not be discussed, the term "contralateral pyramidal" might be more appropriate, but the shorter term will be used here.) Another form of motor learning might be described as "*axial,*" i.e., the ability to acquire programs of movements of the trunk and eyes along with coordinated limb movements. The axial system is also commonly involved in control of proximal movements at the limb girdles. This distinction has been discussed in an analysis of the apraxias.[210] The two types of movements have on the whole quite separate representations in the brain. Complex sequences of finger positions depend primarily on purely contralateral motor systems arising in the precentral gyrus, while axial movements depend on several other cortical areas the outflow from which is distributed bilaterally. The programs for axial learning, like almost all other complex cognitive functions, are probably primarily dependent on one hemisphere. It is therfore reasonable to hypothesize that these two forms of motor dominance are independent and that the degree of intrinsic talent can be different in each system.

We believe that in those with standard dominance the programs for both types of motor dominance lie in the left hemisphere, but under conditions of anomalous dominance, they may lie in separate hemispheres. Evidence to support this view is at present only fragmentary. Gesell and Ames[211] described the tendency of newborn infants placed on the back to turn the head and trunk to one side. Of the children studied by them, 90% were right-handed at age 10 years; all of these had turned to the right at birth. The 5% who at birth had turned to the left were all left-handed at age 10 years. There remained, however, 5% who had turned to the right at birth but were left-handed at age 10 years. One speculative possibility is that in the latter group axial and pyramidal dominance were located in different hemispheres.

There is another set of fragmentary but suggestive observations. We have now found many individuals who write on paper with the left hand but who use the right hand to write at the blackboard or to paint. In ordinary writing, one makes many separate finger movements, but in painting or writing at the blackboard there are few, if any, finger movements and control is predominantly at the shoulder girdle. Some further observations are consistent with this hypothesis. One woman uses the left hand for writing and for sculpture, but the right for painting. The German painter Menzel[212] painted with the right hand but did engraving with the left hand, which he also used for writing. Another person known to us writes on paper with the right hand, but in charcoal drawing produces outlines of figures with the left hand and then fills in details with the right.

These observations are compatible with the possibility that there are independent forms of motor dominance. Lateral discrepancies in the hemispheric localization of the two forms of motor dominance would be most common in the anomalous dominance population. An implication of this hypothesis is that in people in whom different activities are carried out on the left and right there will be a tendency to clustering, i.e., one hand will be used preferentially for pyramidal tasks and the other arm for axial tasks. Studies are underway to test the hypotheses presented here and to apply them to laterality testing. If the data are compatible with this hypothesis, certain conclusions would probably follow. It would be easy to understand why laterality batteries with different items might give different results in some people. Furthermore, it is possible that some individuals who are thought of now as having "mixed" dominance may, in fact, have rather pure pyramidal dominance of one hemisphere and equally pure axial dominance of the other. This is not to imply that there will not be other people in whom there may be truly mixed dominance, e.g., each hemisphere might possess a significant capacity for learning pyramidal or axial movement programs.

Annett proposes that left-handers will tend to come from a group with random dominance for handedness. This raises the possibility that in the random dominance group pyramidal dominance will not on the average be as strongly localized in one hemisphere as in most right-handers. This gains support from Kilshaw and Annett's[213] finding that in actual tests of skill left-handers show, on the average, smaller differences in performance between the two hands than right-handers. This accounts for the fact that many non-right-handers show a high rate of ambidexterity. Furthermore, such a bilateral representation would lead to a higher rate of overall skill in cases when each hand could make a significant contribution, e.g., in bimanual tasks. We suspect that non-right-handers will also show, on the average, a higher rate of bilateral representation of axial control. The less strongly lateralized pattern of motor skill would help to account in part for the elevated rate of non-RH among athletes, in contrast to the common view that this is entirely the result of an advantage in competing against right-handed opponents.

## LH and Congenital Lesions

We have suggested that LH is the result, in many cases, of influences that slow left-hemisphere development. Taylor[214] has presented data that appear to conflict with this interpretation. The cause of temporal lobe epilepsy is in some cases "alien tissue," i.e., various types of cell rest such as the neuronal migration disorders discussed earlier. There is a high frequency of LH in these cases even when the alien tissue is found on the right side.

Left-sided operations for alien tissue were carried out on ten men (four LH), and ten women (three LH); in the right operations there were 27 men (six LH) and nine women (one LH). By contrast, in the mesial temporal sclerosis group there were: (a) left-sided operations, 16 men (two LH), five women (one LH); and (b) right-sided operations, ten men (two LH), ten women (none LH). Mesial temporal sclerosis is now generally regarded as a lesion acquired in early childhood, probably as a sequel of febrile convulsions. (The fact that the majority of operated cases with alien tissue had right-sided foci cannot be used as a measure of the total frequency of such anomalies in all temporal lobe epileptics since the operative selection criteria favored right-sided cases. As will be shown later, large population studies show an excess of left-hemisphere epileptic foci.)

Taylor pointed out that male subjects with alien tissue appear to have an elevated rate of LH regardless of the side of the lesion and, therefore, that one could not accept the simple assumption that only those with left-hemisphere developmental anomalies would manifest an excess of LH. These data are, however, not necessarily incompatible with our hypothesis. They are generally in accord with the proposal that LH is determined by events in utero, since the alien tissue group had a higher rate of sinistrality than the mesial temporal sclerosis group. Since the right hemisphere develops more rapidly than the left, those with right-hemisphere hamartomas are likely to have suffered developmental delays early in pregnancy. The hamartomas found were predominantly in the uncal region that develops much earlier than the superior temporal lobe. It is possible that in many of these individuals the delaying influences were still active at later stages and might thus retard the growth of later developing left-sided cortical regions and thus favor random dominance. Furthermore, the standard operation, especially on the left, was removal of the temporal lobe anterior to the speech regions. Alien tissue in the superior temporal gyrus, as seen in our dyslexic patients, would not have been found by the pathologist. The type of lesion seen in our dyslexics would not in general be visible on the surface of the brain. The uncal lesion might thus have no effect on handedness or language lateralization but might only be a marker of a disturbing influence in development. Future data concerning patients with alien tissue will be required before their high rates of sinistrality can be explained definitively. In particular, to our knowledge there are no data concerning the rates of learning disorders in this population.

## Associations of Anomalous Dominance

Even today an accumulated body of essentially folklore beliefs and prejudices concerning LH continues to exist. In many cultures powerful taboos still persist in relation to use of the left hand for certain activities, e.g., eating. In the United States, with perhaps the highest degree of tolerance of sinistrality, a few people still try to inhibit the use of the left hand by children. Because of this body of inherited myths and prejudices, most scientifically trained persons have an understandable skepticism concerning asserted behavioral or bodily characteristics of left-handers. We will not review the many nonscientific beliefs. On the other hand, it has become increasingly clear that individual differences in cerebral dominance reflect variations in brain organization. Furthermore, anomalous patterns of cerebral dominance have many associations, both favorable, e.g., certain superior talents, and unfavorable, e.g., particular developmental learning disorders and immune diseases. In this section, we will discuss some of these variations that constitute an important body of facts which must be dealt with by any adequate theory.

Before describing some of these associations, we must call attention to some misconceptions that could result from a rapid or superficial reading of our discussion.

Some readers might draw the conclusion that individuals with anomalous dominance, and in particular obvious left-handers, are at a disadvantage for health because of elevated frequencies of certain medical conditions, and at a disadvantage intellectually and psychologically because of higher rates of developmental disorders such as autism, dyslexia, and stuttering.

This conclusion would be erroneous. The fact that one group has a higher rate of certain diseases than another does not mean that it is at an *overall* disadvantage for disability or death. An entire field of medicine and many textbooks are devoted to diseases that occur exclusively or overwhelmingly in women and are important causes of morbidity and mortality. Yet women have lower death rates than men at every age. Despite their elevated rate of many conditions women have lower rates of other disorders, in particular cardiovascular diseases and certain cancers, which more than counterbalance the risk of diseases such as ovarian carcinoma.

A study of patients with celiac disease[215] affords an example of at least a partial balance between risks and advantages. In this condition one finds not only a marked elevation of the frequency of malignant lymphomas and some uncommon gastrointestinal cancers, but also a reduction of the numbers of cancers of lung and breast. In this case there is a net disadvantage since the total prevalence of all malignancies is elevated.

In the past, emphasis was usually placed on disadvantages of LH. This grew out of older prejudices that sinistrals were deviant and out of beliefs that much sinistrality was the result of brain damage. We believe that a full investigation of the disease associations of LH (and, more generally, of anomalous dominance) will demonstrate elevated rates of certain conditions but low rates of others. In particular, we suspect that most infections and many forms of cancer will be less often found in sinistrals than in dextrals, but this remains to be studied. Seltzer and Sherwin[216] have reported that while LH is present in elevated frequency in presenile Alzheimer's disease, it is rare in senile dementia, a far more common disorder. The high frequency of LH in many populations suggests that sinistrals are not at an overall disadvantage. Thus they may have a different pattern of disorders, but there is no reason to believe that they are less healthy.

A similar argument applies to intellectual and other psychologic features in the anomalous dominance population. One cannot conclude that this population is disadvantaged, without surveying the entire array of psychologic attributes. There is increasing evidence that even in the learning disabled certain talents occur in high frequency. Left-handedness is found at elevated rate among architects[46] and among the mathematically gifted.[42] There is no reason to assume that either the RH or LH groups is superior; it is likely that each group has certain talents and disabilities at a higher rate than the other.

It should also be kept in mind that in different societies or in different stages of the history of one society, the relative advantages of the two groups may vary in relation to health or accomplishment. There are several examples in other areas which illustrate this point. When malaria is common a population carrying the sickle-cell gene will have a high degree of protection, but in the absence of malaria it will be at a net disadvantage. Individuals with high serum IgE may be favored when parasitic diseases, to which they are probably more resistant, are common[217] but at a disadvantage, because of their high rate of asthma, when these diseases are rare. Great physical strength was once an advantage in nearly all societies but now is of little importance in technologically advanced communities, while mathematical talent, of minor importance in the past, is in great demand. Dyslexia is of little import in nonliterate societies. It is quite possible that the overall relative advantages of those with anomalous and standard dominance are different in different societies and at different epochs.

A common misconception is reflected in some comments that we have heard frequently, e.g., "I know many exceptions to these findings" or "There are lots of healthy left-handers." It is, of course, clear that most people with anomalous dominance do not suffer from the conditions mentioned and that what is being described are higher relative rates of certain conditions.

## Learning Disabilities and Anomalous Dominance

The term *developmental learning disorders* (LD) is applied rather loosely to a group of conditions, with onset before puberty, characterized by difficulties in acquisition of speech or certain cognitive functions or in anomalies of emotional development. It includes both some disorders recognized by the ancients, e.g., stuttering, and others recognized only in the recent past, e.g., developmental dyslexia. The current list includes developmental dyslexia (which is probably the most common), stuttering, delayed speech, childhood autism, and hyperactivity. Although Tourette's syndrome is usually not listed, it has many of the same features. This list is almost certainly incomplete and there are probably many other conditions with delimited behavioral difficulties. Thus Weintraub and Mesulam[218] have recently described a group in which disorders of social adjustment predominate, but we will not include this in our discussion, since much more information needs to be collected.

These conditions have certain common properties, e.g., a preponderance of males; the greater tendency of female cases in some of these conditions, e.g., stuttering, to improve with age leads to a further increase in the male majority. The available genetic studies reveal a rather similar pattern of inheritance. Affected individuals are more likely to have affected relatives than normal controls. The minority of affected women tend to have more affected relatives and more affected children than the men. These conditions appear to be interrelated, e.g., if one identical twin is autistic, the other twin, when not autistic, is likely to have one of the other learning disabilities.[219] Orton[220] commented on the increased rate of stuttering among dyslexics and Ludlow et al[221] found a similar relationship between Tourette's syndrome and dyslexia.

Another common factor is an elevated frequency of personal and familial non-RH, as noted by Orton in his very first descriptions of dyslexia and as found in many later studies. Porac and Coren[73] point out that while some studies deny an increase in LH in the dyslexic population, no study has ever found the reverse, i.e., a deficiency of LH.

The recent study of Geschwind and Behan[14] lent strong support to the existence of this association. In most earlier investigations patients with some form of LD were assessed for handedness. In our study the reverse was done, i.e., groups chosen for handedness were assessed for personal and family histories of LD. In this initial study we compared only individuals with laterality quotients of −100, i.e., very strongly left-handed persons, and +100, i.e., very strongly right-handed patients. Two separate studies gave very similar results. The pooled figures of the two studies show that 11.8% of the 500 strong LH reported LD, as against only 1.1% of 900 strong RH. In both series there was also a significantly higher frequency of LD in the first- and second-degree relatives of the LH than in those of the RH. A third series has yielded similar results.[15] The rate of dyslexia was 15 times as high in the strong LH as in the strong RH, and stuttering was five times as common in the sinistrals.

A more recent study[207] provides further data in relation to the association of dyslexia and handedness. A group of 1,117 professionals completed a modified form of the Oldfield[8] Handedness Battery. With the scoring method used (slightly modified from the original) a score of greater than +70 was attained by about 75% of the respondents. In order to attain a score above +70 there can be at most one item out of ten in which there is predominant use of the left hand or alternatively at most five items in which the left hand is used occasionally. Dyslexia was reported by 3% of those scoring above +70. In both the ranges from 0 to +70 (about 15% of the population) and 0 to −100 (about 10%) the rate of dyslexia was 9% ($P < .001$). The probability of this distribution was less than .001. In other words, even a minor degree of deviation from full RH was associated with a sharp rise in the frequency of dyslexia. Yet many of the individuals in the 0 to +70 range described themselves as RH and most wrote with the right hand. This illustrates the point discussed earlier that it is important to ascertain whether the distribution of laterality scores in those with a given condition is different from that in the general population. In some cases there may be a marked shift to the sinistral end, but in others, when the shift is of lesser degree, it may be demonstrated only by a significant decrease in the proportion of those at the right hand end and an increase in those in the middle ranges.

It should also be noted that these findings do not imply that NRH is the cause of the LD; we regard NRH only as a marker of an alteration in dominance. Nor do they imply that one should expect the majority of cases of LD to be NRH, although this may turn out to be true in some instances.

We cannot deal here in detail with the reasons for the many disagreements in the literature. Let us recall that our initial investigations in Glasgow, Scotland, used a method different from that used by others, i.e., we studied individuals at the extremes of the handedness scale. Second, the study of Schachter et al[207] was confined to professionals with the majority having completed graduate studies, while most studies in the literature have been carried out primarily in children. Although in our studies the individuals identified themselves as dyslexics, it is difficult to see how such huge differences could have resulted from a concealed selection bias.

The data in the literature on autism and stuttering show less disagreement than those on reading difficulty. Autistic children have a far higher rate of non-RH than normal controls.[222,223] Bishop[224] reports five studies on stammerers or stutterers, all showing a higher rate of NRH than in controls; in three, the differences are very large. Obviously stuttering is diagnosed with less uncertainty than reading disorders.

These data are in conformity with the hypothesis, i.e., that the influences which favor LH will, in extreme cases, lead to an increased frequency of LD. In future research, it will be important to study the brains of patients with conditions other than childhood dyslexia, e.g., autism and stuttering, and especially the brains of frank right-handers and of women who suffered from these conditions.

The onset or worsening of many conditions at or near puberty strongly suggests a major role for sex hormones. Temporal lobe epilepsy resulting from alien tissue commonly starts at this time and neurofibromatosis and scoliosis worsen. Of interest are the behavioral conditions, which appear predominantly after puberty, e.g., anorexia nervosa which is female preponderant. The rarer puberty onset male condition, the Kleine-Levin syndrome,[225] is in many ways the opposite of anorexia nervosa, both in sex distribution and clinical features. Patients with Kleine-Levin syndrome have periodic attacks in which they overeat, sleep excessively, and may be sexually hyperactive; all these in contrast to anorexia nervosa in which the patients eat little, are very active, and are typically hyposexual. A recent postmortem report of a case of Kleine-Levin syndrome reports anomalies of formation of certain thalamic nuclei thought to be of possible viral origin.[226] This raises the possibility that some puberty onset syndromes might also be the result of even earlier defects of neuronal migration or assembly. There are still no handedness data for these conditions.

It is worth noting that by contrast other conditions both neurologic and nonneurologic may improve at puberty, e.g., some cases of the Tourette syndrome. There are other important changes at puberty, e.g., the average superiority of males in certain aspects of spatial function does not become fully manifest until this age.[227] Martha Denckla, MD, (oral communication, April 25, 1981) has commented on the improvement in certain motor functions in many male dyslexics at puberty.

There are other developmental LD that, despite their frequency and theoretical importance, have received little attention, presumably because they rarely come to medical or educational attention, e.g., extreme lack of musical ability. A similar problem is that of lack of artistic ability. Since most people are relatively poor at artistic activities, it might be worthwhile to conduct studies in the reverse manner, i.e., to investigate the handedness and sex distribution of artistically talented children. It would be important from the point of view of any theory to identify conditions that were female predominant before puberty and especially those that were more common among RH than among LH.

It is important to point out that one handedness group might contain an elevated proportion both of those with high talent and of those with distinctly inferior capacities for some particular function. A hypothetical example might be that of mathematical talent. Recent studies have supported the view that superior mathematical talents are more frequent among men,[11,228] who have an elevated rate of LH.[42] It has, therefore, been argued by some that special difficulty in mathematics will be more common in women. This need not necessarily be the case. It is thus conceivable that men and even sinistral men might be found more frequently at both ends of the scale. Only further experimental studies will make it possible to work out the intricacies of some of these relationships.

The genetic pattern of LD is compatible with the thesis presented here. The pattern of inheritance has been generally considered to be compatible with autosomal dominant transmission. It might appear at first that this was in conflict with male predominance. In genetics a distinction is made between *sex-limited* and *sex-linked* inheritance. An example of the former is male-pattern baldness, inherited as an autosomal dominant,[229] which is not expressed in young women because of low levels of dihydrotestosterone. In sex-limited inheritance, a gene is expressed less often in one sex. We have proposed that learning disorders are more common in males because of some male-related factor in development, possibly testosterone. Inheritance will play a role, e.g., genes might affect testosterone levels, sensitivity to testosterone, or a large number of other factors. As noted above, affected women are likely to have more affected relatives and more affected children than affected men. According to the hypothesis a female would be more likely to suffer from a learning disorder if she were subjected to high testosterone effect during development. This would be especially likely if she had inherited high sensitivity to testosterone.

Although fewer females stutter, they have, on the average, more affected relatives and are more likely to have affected children than males who stutter.[230] It is easy to conceive of reasons for this pattern. If, for example, there were large differences in genetically transmitted sensitivity to testosterone, then female subjects who stuttered would frequently have inherited high sensitivity, since in most cases females would not have exposure to very high levels of testosterone. Many of her relatives and, in particular, many of her children, would share this high sensitivity. On the other hand, male subjects with, on the average, higher levels of testosterone would not require as high a level of sensitivity to testosterone to be subjected to an excessive delaying effect. In particular, the female relatives of a man who stuttered but did not have high testosterone sensitivity would be expected to have low rates of the disability. Furthermore, since testosterone levels in male fetuses are sensitive to environmental effects (to be discussed in another section), men could be affected more frequently by environmental causes. There are, of course, other possible explanations for the genetic findings; the above example only serves to illustrate that the greater frequency of LD in men need not imply that affected men will have more affected relatives than affected women.

It should be pointed out that the affected woman may have a higher number of affected children for other reasons. The children might, as already noted, inherit a higher genetic sensitivity to testosterone. In addition, as will be pointed out later, there are animal experiments showing that women exposed to high testosterone in development are likely to have their metabolism permanently altered.[231,232] The child of such a woman is thus possibly more likely to be exposed to high androgen levels and therefore to be affected.

## Immune Disorders

The elevated frequency of *immune disorders* (ID) in LH is also compatible with the theory, since evidence to be given later shows that testosterone affects the development of the immune system.

We use the term ID to mean atopic disorders (i.e., the allergies, typically of childhood onset), autoimmune disorders, and other conditions in which immunity plays a major role in pathogenesis. There are, of course, certain infections in which the manifestations during the acute stage are dependent to a major degree on immune mechanisms. In this section, we discuss only chronic conditions in which immunity plays a major role, but we will return to the question of infection in another section.

Because of the clinical observation made by one of us (N.G.) that certain diseases appeared to be more common in LH subjects, a study was carried out in order to investigate these associations.[14] In our first group of investigations we compared only individuals who on the Oldfield Handedness Battery[8] scored either –100 or +100, i.e., complete LH or RH, respectively. The data concerning the increased frequency of LD in the strongly LH subjects have already been given. In the first series, 27 of the 253 strong LH people reported personal histories of ID vs. ten of the 253 strong RH individuals ($P < .005$). In the second series, the diagnosis of ID was accepted only if it had been made in a teaching hospital. A smaller absolute number of cases were therefore found but the relative frequencies in the LH and RH were comparable with those found in the first study. In each of the studies ID was thus about 2½ times as frequent in the strong LH as in the strong RH. The LH subjects also reported a higher rate of ID in first- and second-degree relatives. A third study[15] has yielded similar results.

Having confirmed the hypothesis that ID was more frequent in the strong LH than in the strong RH, we investigated the reverse association, i.e., the frequency of NRH in different disease groups. Although many different ID were reported by our respondents, we were particularly struck by the apparently high frequency of conditions affecting the gastrointestinal tract (ulcerative colitis, regional ileitis, and celiac disease) and the thyroid gland (e.g., Hashimoto's thyroiditis). We did not at the time of our first study have available to us a large number of cases with these ID, although small numbers of other groups were available. In subsequent studies,[15] we have found that among patients in Scotland with the gut-associated and thyroid ID the rates of personal and familial sinistrality are markedly increased. The same was true for migraine and myasthenia gravis and also for atopic diseases, such as asthma. On the other hand, we again found no difference from the general population in the rates of sinistrality at these laterality quotients in rheumatoid arthritis. It should be noted that in these studies of particular diseases we used an arbitrary cutoff score of zero as the upper limit of LH. In future studies, the procedure to be followed should, however, be a different one. As pointed out in an earlier section the logical procedure is not to assign arbitrary cutoff points but rather to compare the distribution of laterality scores in the patient groups and in the controls. We suspect that when this method is used it will be found that in some of the other IDs there will also be significant shifts of the laterality distributions to the left. The method of using zero as an arbitrary cutoff point would, of course, fail to reveal a marked reduction in extreme right-handed scores with a correspondingly marked rise in the range of scores between 0 and +70.

### Design of Future Studies

On reviewing the studies, it is now clear that many details and interrelationships must be worked out. In studying disease groups, one should employ the strategy just outlined of avoiding arbitrary cutoff points. We expect that the degree of shift to the left will vary with different disorders. The use of a cutoff at zero or below will miss disorders in which the shift is less marked, but still substantial, a point we will discuss again in other connections.

It will also be important to study men and women separately. Marcel Kinsbourne, MD, whose work we will mention in more detail further on, has suggested that important information may be obtained by looking at interrelationships. Thus will the rate of immune disorder be the same in those with, e.g., a laterality quotient of –100 who are dyslexic and those with the same score who are not? Furthermore, will dyslexics with strongly *positive* laterality scores have higher rates of immune disorder than non-dyslexic individuals with the same scores?

It will be particularly interesting to study conditions such as rheumatoid spondylitis (Marie-Strümpell disease), Reiter's syndrome, and enteropathic arthritis, all of them male predominant and all with strong associations with HLA-B 27.

### Implications of the Data

The data presented are compatible with the hypothesis that the factors which influence laterality also affect the development of the immune system and thus lead to a later elevated frequency of ID. An elevated rate of ID was found on strongly LH individuals who would by hypothesis have been subject to a greater male-related effect than the strongly RH group. It would be important to determine whether there is a "dose-effect," i.e., whether the frequency of ID increases with the degree of LH.

Some further light is thrown on these findings by a recent study of Kinsbourne and Bemporad (written communication, July, 1983) who studied a group in a school for LD children. The rate of ID was significantly higher among the families of LH dyslexics than of RH dyslexics without familial LH.

Another confirmation has been afforded by Wood[233] who reported that LH was more common in patients with autoimmune diseases of the thyroid and in their first-degree relatives than in those with nonimmune thyroid disorders (e.g., nodular goiter).

Benbow and Stanley[228] have recently studied a large group of mathematically gifted children. This group, which is strongly male predominant, not only had twice as high a rate of LH as a less gifted group but also five times the rate of allergies.

The inclusion of migraine raises several questions. There is some support for the participation of immune mechanisms in at least some cases, e.g., a reported increase in the rate of migraine in lupus erythematosus. During attacks there is an asymmetric distribution of mast cells.[234] In a recent report[235] of a controlled study of treatment of childhood migraine with exclusion diets, the authors argue for an allergic mechanism. There are, of course, causes of food intolerance other than allergy. Further studies will be needed to confirm the existence of an immune mechanism in migraine.

Our data also show an increased rate of sinistrality among those with atopic disorders such as asthma, eczema, and hay fever. It is of interest that atopic disorders usually begin before puberty and are more common in men,[83] while other common IDs typically begin after puberty and are more frequent in women. This is in accord with the hypothesis that the postpubertal male, despite a possibly greater propensity toward autoimmunity, is protected from it by his own hormones, while this masking effect is weaker before puberty.

The types of ID found most frequently in anomalous dominance populations will be determined more accurately only after more extensive studies. It is worthwhile, however, to speculate briefly on the current findings. According to the hypothesis the increased tendency to ID is the result of suppression of development of the thymus and other immune organs. It is likely that the delaying effects on brain growth will not be uniform throughout pregnancy and that the particular dominance pattern of any individual will be determined by the exact timing and intensity of these effects. One would expect that the pattern of ID would also reflect the timing of the delaying effects in relation to processes of development in the thymus and other organs. One might guess that at any given time the processing within the thymus of lymphocytes which recognize self would be closely coordinated with the organ systems developing at that time, since the characteristic antigens of those systems will not have been present earlier. The high rate of gut and thyroid ID may give important hints as to the usual timing of the disturbing influences in brain development, although other factors, including genetic endowment may determine special susceptibility of certain systems. In any case we do not wish to imply that a general susceptibility to all forms of ID will exist in all those with anomalous dominance. In fact, the possibility exists that particular forms of anomalous dominance will be associated with particular conditions, although the available data at present are, at best, only suggestive. The literature on stuttering repeatedly refers to allergies[72,236]; we have been repeatedly told by pediatric neurologists of the high frequency of migraine in dyslexics; Coleman[237] discusses the high rate of a gut-related disorder in autism.

As a corollary of these findings one might expect that some related conditions would also be elevated in the anomalous dominance population, e.g., lymphoid malignancies which have a close relationship to ID. On the other hand, other more common forms of cancer might well be less frequent in this group.

One must also consider some other hypotheses as to the relationship between ID and LH which may deserve further study. An anomalous endocrine environment in pregnancy might modify the later hormonal characteristics of the individual and these might affect immune competence. Another possibility derives from the known effect of sex hormones on the development of certain hypothalamic nuclei, in view of the fact that several recent studies suggest that the hypothalamus may play a role in immune responses.

A question that has been raised repeatedly is whether those with anomalous dominance might have a different complement of HLA haplotypes from those with standard dominance. The fact that some disorders are so strongly associated with certain haplotypes (e.g., B27 with rheumatoid spondylitis) has led to the frequent presumption that all ID will have such associations. It is, of course, possible that certain haplotypes will be found in elevated frequency in those with anomalous dominance. Even if this were the case this should not be regarded as incompatible with our hypothesis. Since most of those with a particular haplotype do not develop ID, the hormonal atmosphere in utero or early postnatal life may still play a major role. Furthermore, the HLA genes must exert their effects through particular chemical products. As we will discuss later, Ivanyi[34] has shown that certain loci in the major histocompatibility complex (MHC) of gene 17 of the mouse affect several different aspects of testosterone production and action.

It must also be kept in mind that particular haplotype associations have not been demonstrated for several IDs, e.g., the data for lupus erythematosus are not considered as convincing by many investigators. In addition, there are occasional families with an ID in which affected members share the same haplotype, which is, however, not found in high frequency in other individuals or other families. This suggests that a given haplotype may be important only in combination with other factors.

There is still another type of association of HLA haplotypes with ID that does not necessarily entail an elevated frequency of any particular haplotype. Since the fetus receives one chromosome six (which carries the HLA groups) from the mother, it will share at least half its haplotypes with the mother. If the parents share haplotypes, then the proportion of haplotypes shared by mother and fetus will, on the average, be even higher. It has been shown both in experimental animals[238] and in humans[239,240] that the greater the degree of haplotype sharing between parents, the higher the rate of infertility and fetal loss. In addition, Faulk[239] has shown that certain disorders of the offspring are associated with an elevated rate of parental haplotype sharing. Whether shared haplotypes are more frequent in parents of children with anomalous dominance has not yet been determined.

### Learning Disabilities and Immune Disorders

The data concerning the association of ID with LH make it possible to re-evaluate certain findings in the literature on developmental LD. Several articles report an increased frequency of allergies among stutterers[72,236]; a high frequency of celiac disease or some similar bowel disorder among autistic children, and a high frequency of autoimmune thyroid disorders in their parents[237]; and a high frequency of food allergies in hyperactive children.[241] Several pediatric neurologists with extensive experience of dyslexia have told us that migraine is a common problem in the learning disabilities clinic. Our own recent studies[15] confirm a high rate of atopic disorder in hyperactive children.

These data have been interpreted in various ways. It is sometimes assumed that the frequency of these diseases is the result of stress on LD children. This could not, however, explain all the findings, e.g., the increased frequency of thyroid autoimmunity among unaffected parents of autistic children. Nor could it explain the apparent, although not yet adequately documented, tendency of certain disorders to be associated with each other, e.g., allergy with stuttering, and bowel disorder with autism. Another explanation attributes the LD to the ID, e.g., the term *celiac autism* reflects the assumption that autism might in some cases be a manifestation of celiac disease. Similarly, it has been proposed that hyperactivity may be a manifestation of food allergy.

These phenomena can be readily explained. Stuttering, autism, and childhood dyslexia are male-predominant conditions with elevated rates of NRH, in which one would expect high rates of ID both in patients and in relatives. A concordant observation is that autistic children have a high frequency of relatives with Down's syndrome,[237] a condition with an elevated rate of thyroid autoimmunity. Against the common assumption that autoimmunity in patients with Down's syndrome is a secondary result of chromosomal abnormality is the finding that the parents, who have no chromosomal abnormality, also have an elevated rate of thyroid autoimmunity.[242,243] Furthermore, in Down's syndrome one commonly finds that the posterior portion of the superior temporal gyrus is thin,[244] i.e., there is a disturbance of the same region in which disorders of neuronal migration or assembly have been found in childhood dyslexics.[16,17] Fialkow[242,243] presents evidence that the chromosomal abnormality in Down's syndrome is not the cause of the autoimmunity but possibly secondary to it.

### Familial Patterns

This section will offer some tentative general principles concerning familial patterns and possible directions for research. On inspection of family trees we have found that LH, LD, ID, and certain talents may all be present in single individuals, or may be distributed among different family members. Thus one non-RH

LD individual with high artistic talents, suffered from severe ID. Throughout his family one finds different LD, ID, migraine, artistic talents, and NRH, sometimes in the same individual but at other times not clustered in the same person. Another example is a strongly left-handed childhood dyslexic with a right-handed brother and a grandmother each with a different ID. In childhood autism this is a familiar pattern since the patients themselves are often LH, and have a high rate of some type of malabsorption syndrome, while the unaffected parents and siblings have higher rates of autoimmune hypothyroidism,[237] and (although this is controversial) a high rate of superior talents. While genetic mechanisms are obviously at play, there is also a considerable degree of freedom from genetics as will soon become clear. While family members may share common genetic susceptibilities, many other factors, both genetic and nongenetic, modify the expression in any one individual. The family patterns illustrate a point made earlier, i.e., that influences which in one individual lead to high talents may in excess lead to serious disabilities in others. The disabilities tend to persist since the overall Darwinian fitness of the group carrying the appropriate predispositions is high because of the production of individuals of exceptional talent.

This section has dealt with a few of the associations of anomalous dominance. Later sections will discuss other features that we believe to be more common in the anomalous dominance population, including certain patterns of hair color, skeletal and other anomalies, certain alterations in the vestibular system, some psychiatric conditions, and other types of special autoimmune effects. We will discuss the possible role of asymmetric migration from the neural crest in the causation of some of these anomalies.

## References


1. Geschwind N, Levitsky W: Human brain: Left-right asymmetries in temporal speech region. *Science* 1968;161:186–187.
2. LeMay M, Culebras A: Human brain: Morphologic differences in the hemispheres demonstrable by carotid arteriography. *N Engl J Med* 1972;287:168–170.
3. Galaburda AM, LeMay M, Kemper TL, et al: Right-left asymmetries in the brain. *Science* 1978;199:852–856.
4. Galaburda AM, Sanides F, Geschwind N: Human brain: Cytoarchitectonic left-right asymmetries in the temporal speech region. *Arch Neurol* 1978;35:812–817.
5. Wada JA, Clarke R, Hamm A: Cerebral hemispheric asymmetry in humans. *Arch Neurol* 1975;32:239–246.
6. Witelson SF, Pallie W: Left hemisphere specialization for language in the newborn: Neuroanatomical evidence of asymmetry. *Brain* 1973;96:641–646.
7. Chi JG, Dooling EC, Gilles FH: Left-right asymmetries of the temporal speech areas of the human fetus. *Arch Neurol* 1977;34:346–348.
8. Oldfield RC: The assessment and analysis of handedness: The Edinburgh Inventory. *Neuropsychologia* 1971;9:97–113.
9. Maccoby EM, Jacklin CN: *The Psychology of Sex Differences.* Stanford, Calif, Stanford University Press, 1974.

10. Wittig MA, Petersen AC (eds): *Sex-related Differences in Cognitive Function.* New York, Academic Press Inc, 1979.
11. Benbow CP, Stanley JC: Sex differences in mathematical ability: Fact or artifact? *Science* 1980;210:1262–1264.
12. Taylor DC: The influence of sexual differentiation on growth, development, and disease, in Davis JA, Dobbing J (eds): *Scientific Foundations of Paediatrics.* Philadelphia, WB Saunders Co, 1974, pp 29–44.
13. Hecaen H: *Les Gauchers.* Paris, Presses Universitaires de France, 1984.
14. Geschwind N, Behan P: Left-handedness: Association with immune disease, migraine, and developmental learning disorder. *Proc Natl Acad Sci USA* 1982; 79:5097–5100.
15. Geschwind N, Behan PO: Laterality, hormones, and immunity, in Geschwind N, Galaburda AM (eds): *Cerebral Dominance: The Biological Foundations.* Cambridge, Mass, Harvard University Press, 1984, pp 211–224.
16. Galaburda AM, Kemper TL: Cytoarchitectonic abnormalities in developmental dyslexia: A case study. *Ann Neurol* 1979;6:94–100.
17. Galaburda AM: Developmental dyslexia: Current anatomical research. *Ann Dyslexia* 1983;33:41–53.
18. Kemper TL: Asymmetrical lesions in dyslexia, in Geschwind N, Galaburda AM (eds): *Cerebral Dominance: The Biological Foundations.* Cambridge, Mass, Harvard University Press, 1984, pp 75–89.
19. Taylor DC: Differential rates of cerebral maturation between sexes and between hemispheres. *Lancet* 1969;2:140–142.
20. Fontes V: *Morfologia do Cortex Cerebral (Desenvolvimento).* Lisbon, Instituto Antonio Aurelio da Costa Ferreira, 1944.
21. Scheibel AM: A dendritic correlate of human speech, in Geschwind N, Galaburda AM (eds): *Cerebral Dominance: The Biological Foundations.* Cambridge, Mass, Harvard University Press, 1984, pp 43–52.
22. Hamburger V, Oppenheim RW: Naturally occurring neuronal death in vertebrates. *Neurosci Commentaries* 1982;1:39–55.
23. Goldman PS: Neuronal plasticity in primate telencephalon: Anomalous projections induced by prenatal removal of frontal cortex. *Science* 1978;202:768–770.
24. Goldman-Rakic P, Rakic P: Experimental modification of gyral patterns, in Geschwind N, Galaburda AM (eds): *Cerebral Dominance: The Biological Foundations.* Cambridge, Mass, Harvard University Press, 1984, pp 179–192.
25. Dorner G: Sexual differentiation of the brain. *Vitam Horm* 1980;38:325–381.
26. Gorski RA, Harlan RE, Jacobson CD, et al: Evidence for the existence of a sexually dimorphic nucleus in the preoptic area of the rat. *J Comp Neurol* 1980;193:529–539.
27. Pfaff DW: Morphological changes in the brains of adult male rats after neonatal castration. *J Endocrinol* 1966;36:415–416.
28. Raisman G, Field PM: Sexual dimorphism in the neuropil of the preoptic area of the rat and its dependence on neonatal androgen. *Brain Res* 1973;54:1–29.
29. MacLusky NJ, Naftolin F: Sexual differentiation of the central nervous system. *Science* 1981;211:1294–1303.
30. McEwen BS: Neural gonadal steroid actions. *Science* 1981;211:1303–1311.
31. Netley C: Dichotic listening of callosal agenesis and Turner's syndrome patients, in Segalowitz SJ, Gruber FA (eds): *Language Development and Neurological Theory.* New York, Academic Press Inc, 1977.

32. Hier D, Crowley WF Jr: Spatial ability in androgen-deficient men. *N Engl J Med* 1982;306:1202–1205.
33. Annett M: Genetic and non-genetic differences on handedness. *Behav Genet* 1978; 8:227–249.
34. Corballis MC, Morgan MJ: On the biological basis of human laterality. *Behav Brain Sci* 1978;2:261–336.
35. Boklage CE: On the distribution of non-righthandedness among twins and their families. *Acta Genet Med Gemellol* 1981;30:167–187.
36. Nottebohm F, Nottebohm M: Left hypoglossal dominance in the control of canary and white-crowned sparrow song. *J Comp Physiol* 1976;108:171–192.
37. Sherman GF, Garbanati JA, Rosen GD, et al: Brain and behavioral asymmetries for spatial preference in rats. *Brain Res* 1980;192:61–67.
38. Diamond MC, Dowling GA, Johnson RE: Morphological cerebral cortical asymmetry in male and female rats. *Exp Neurol* 1981;71:261–268.
39. Serafetinides EA: The significance of the temporal lobes and of hemispheric dominance in the production of LSD-25 symptomatology in man. *Neuropsychologia* 1965;3:69–79.
40. Glick SD, Meibach RC, Cox RD, et al: Multiple and interrelated functional asymmetries in rat brain. *Life Sci* 1979;25:395–400.
41. Holloway RJ, de Lacoste C: Brain endocast asymmetry in pongids and hominids: The paleontology of cerebral hemisphere dominance. *Am J Phys Anthropol* 1982; 58:101–110.
42. Kolata G: Math genius may have hormonal basis. *Science* 1983;222:1312.
43. Tisserand M: Dominance laterale et becde-lievre. *Arch Fr Pediatr* 1944;2:166–167.
44. Gordon HW: Cognitive asymmetry in dyslexic families. *Neuropsychologia* 1980; 18:645–656.
45. Gordon HW: Learning disabled are cognitively right, in Kinsbourne M (ed): *Topics in Learning Disabilities*. Gaithersburg, Md, Aspen Systems, 1983, vol 3, pp 29–39.
46. Peterson JM, Lansky LM: Left-handedness among architects: Some facts and speculation. *Percept Mot Skills* 1974;38:547–550.
47. Broca P: Remarques sur le siege de la faculte du langage articule, suivies d'une observation d'aphemie. *Bull Soc Anat* 1861;6:398–407.
48. Goodglass H, Quadfasel FA: Language laterality in left-handed aphasics. *Brain* 1954;77:521–548.
49. Zangwill O: *Cerebral Dominance and Its Relation to Psychological Function.* Springfield, Ill, Charles C Thomas, Publisher 1960.
50. Gloning I, Gloning K, Haub G, et al: Comparison of verbal behavior in right-handed and nonright-handed patients with anatomically verified lesion of one hemisphere. *Cortex* 1969;5:43–52.
51. Satz P: Incidence of aphasia in lefthanders: A test of some hypothetical models of cerebral speech organization, in Herron J (ed): *Neuropsychology of Lefthandedness*. New York, Academic Press Inc, 1980, pp 189–198.
52. Milner B: Hemispheric specialization: Scope and limits, in Schmitt FO, Worden FG (eds): *The Neurosciences: Third Study Program.* Boston, MIT Press, 1973, pp 75–89.
53. Benton AL: Visuoperceptive, visuospatial, and visuoconstructive disorders, in Heilman K, Valenstein E (eds): *Clinical Neuropsychology.* New York, Oxford University Press, 1979, pp 186–223.

54. Levy J: Psychobiological implications of bilateral asymmetry, in Dimond SJ, Beaumont JG (eds): *Hemisphere Function in the Human Brain.* London, P Elek, 1974, pp 121–183.
55. Larrabee AP: The optic chiasm of teleosts: A study of inheritance. *Proc Am Acad Arts Sci* 1906;12:217–231.
56. Kappers CVA, Huber GC, Crosby EC: *The Comparative Anatomy of the Nervous System of Vertebrates Including Man.* New York, Macmillan Publishing Co Inc. 1936, vol 2, pp 874–876.
57. LeMay M, Geschwind N: Hemispheric differences in the brains of great apes. *Brain Behav Evol* 1975;11:48–52.
58. Kemali M, Guilielmotti V, Gioffre D: Neuroanatomical identification of the frog habenular connections using peroxidase (HRP). *Exp Brain Res* 1980;38:341–347.
59. Diamond MC: Age, sex, and environmental influences, in Geschwind N, Galaburda AM (eds): *Cerebral Dominance: The Biological Foundations.* Cambridge, Mass, Harvard University Press, 1984, chap 9, pp 134–146.
60. Glick SD, Jerussi TP, Fleisher LN: Turning in circles: The neuropharmacology of rotation. *Life Sci* 1976;18:889–896.
61. Penfield W, Roberts L: *Speech and Brain Mechanisms.* Princeton, NJ, Princeton University Press, 1959.
62. Ojemann GA, Ward AA: Speech representation in ventrolateral thalamus. *Brain* 1971;94:669–680.
63. Ciemins VA: Localized thalamic hemorrhage: A cause of aphasia. *Neurology* 1970; 20:776–782.
64. Naeser M, Alexander MA, Helm-Estabrooks N, et al: Aphasia with predominantly subcortical lesion sites. *Arch Neurol* 1982;39:2–14.
65. Cappa SF, Vignolo LA: 'Transcortical' features of aphasia following left thalamic hemorrhage. *Cortex* 1979;15:121–130.
66. Faden AI, Jacobs TP, Woods M, et al: Zona intermedia pressor sites in the cat spinal cord: Right-left asymmetry. *Exp Neurol* 1978;61:571–582.
67. Luria AR: *Traumatic Aphasia.* The Hague, Monton, 1970.
68. Geschwind N, Galaburda AM (eds): *Cerebral Dominance: The Biological Foundations.* Cambridge, Mass, Harvard University Press, 1984.
69. Glick SD (ed): *Cerebral Lateralization in Nonhuman Species.* New York, Academic Press Inc, in press.
70. Drake WE: Clinical and pathological findings in a child with a developmental learning disability. *J Learn Disabil* 1968;1:9–25.
71. Galaburda AM: Anatomical asymmetries, in Geschwind N, Galaburda AM (eds): *Cerebral Dominance: The Biological Foundations.* Cambridge, Mass, Harvard University Press, 1984, pp 11–25.
72. Diehl CF: *A Compendium of Research and Theory On Stuttering.* Springfield, Ill, Charles C Thomas, 1958.
73. Porac C, Coren S: *Lateral Preferences and Human Behavior.* New York, Springer Publishing Co Inc, 1981.
74. Teszner D, Tzavaras A, Gruner J, et al: L'asymetrie droite gauche du planum temporale; à propos de l'étude anatomique de 100 cerveaux. *Rev Neurol* 1972; 146:444–449.
75. Meyer-Bahlburg HFL, Erhardt AA: Sex hormone administration during pregnancy: Behavioral sequelae in the offspring, in Youngs DD, Erhardt AA (eds): *Psychosomatic Obstetrics and Gynaecology.* New York, Appleton-Century-Crofts, 1980.

76. Stumpf WE, Sar M, Keefer DA, et al: The anatomical substrate of neuroendocrine regulation as defined by autoradiography with $^3$H-estradiol, $^3$H-testosterone, $^3$H-dihydrotestosterone, and $^3$H-progesterone, in: *Neuroendocrine Regulation of Fertility.* Basel, S Karger AG, 1976.
77. MacLusky NJ, Naftolin F, Goldman-Rakic PS: Oestrogen formation and binding in the cerebral cortex and diencephalon of the newborn rhesus monkey. Submitted.
78. Huttenlocher PR: Synaptic density in the human frontal cortex: Developmental changes and effects of aging. *Brain Res* 1979;163:195–205.
79. Warner NL, Szenberg A, Burnet FM: The immunological role of different lymphoid organs in the chicken. *Aust J Exp Biol Med Sci* 1962;40:373–388.
80. Frey-Wettstein M, Craddock CG: Testosterone-induced depletion of thymus and marrow lymphocytes as related to lymphopoiesis and hematopoiesis. *Blood* 1970; 35:257–271.
81. Wasi P, Block M: The histopathological study of the development of the irradiation-induced leukemia in C57BL mice and of its inhibition by testosterone. *Cancer Res* 1961;21:463–473.
82. Talal N: Immunologic and viral factors in autoimmune diseases. *Med Clin North Am* 1977;61:205–215.
83. Crawford WA, Beldham CG: The changing demographic pattern in asthma related to sex and age. *Med J Aust* 1976;1:430–434.
84. Ivanyi P: Some aspects of the H-2 system, the major histocompatibility system in the mouse. *Proc R Soc Lond* 1978;202:117–158.
85. Saxen L, Toivonen S: *Primary Embryonic Induction.* London, Logos, 1962.
86. Jacobson CO: The localization of the presumptive cerebral regions in the neural plate of the axolate larva. *J Embryol Exp Morphol* 1959;7:1–21.
87. Karfunkel P: The mechanisms of neural tube formation. *Int Rev Cytol* 1974; 38:245–271.
88. Weston JA: The migration and differentiation of neural crest cells. *Adv Morphol* 1970;8:41–114.
89. LeDouarin N: *The Neural Crest.* Cambridge, England, Cambridge University Press, 1982.
90. Jacobson M: *Developmental Neurobiology.* New York, Plenum Press Inc, 1978, pp 27–55, 115–217.
91. Marin-Padilla M: Prenatal and early post-natal ontogenesis of the human motor cortex: A Golgi study: I. The sequential development of the cortical layers. *Brain Res* 1970;23:167–183.
92. Cowan WM: Neuronal death as a regulative mechanism in the control of cell numbers in the nervous system, in Rockstein M (ed): *Development and Aging in the Nervous System.* New York, Academic Press Inc, 1973, pp 19–41.
93. Heim LM, Timiras PS: Gonad-brain relationship: Precocious brain maturation after estradiol in rats. *Endocrinology* 1963;72:598–606.
94. Curry J, Heim LM: Brain myelination after neonatal administration of oestradiol. *Nature* 1966;209:915–916.
95. Toran-Allerand CD: Gonadal hormones and brain development: Cellular aspects of sexual differentiation. *Am Zool* 1978;18:553–565.
96. Goldman PS, Galkin TW: Prenatal removal of frontal association cortex in the fetal rhesus monkey: Anatomical and functional consequences in postnatal life. *Brain Res* 1978;152:451–485.

97. Innocenti GM: Growth and reshaping of axons in the establishment of visual callosal connections. *Science* 1981;212:824–827.
98. Schneider GE: Early lesions and abnormal neuronal connections: Developmental rules can lead axons astray, with functional consequences. *TINS* 1981;4:187–192.
99. Goldman PS: Contralateral projections to the dorsal thalamus from frontal association cortex in the rhesus monkey. *Brain Res* 1979;166:166–171.
100. Nottebohm F, Arnold AP: Sexual dimorphism in vocal control areas of the songbird brain. *Science* 1976;194:211–213.
101. Rey P: Du poids des lobes cerebraux (frontaux, occipitaux, et parietotemporaux) d'apres le registre de Broca. *Rev Anthropol* 1885;8:385–396.
102. Pfeifer RA: Pathologie der Horstrahlung und der corticaler Horsphare, in Bumke O. Forster O (eds): *Handbuch der Neurologie.* Berlin, Springer Verlag, 1936, vol 6, pp 534–626.
103. Economo C, Horn L: Über Windungsrelief, Masse, und Rindenarchitektonik der Supratemporaltlache, ihre individuellen und ihre Seitenunterschiede. *Z Neurol Psychiatrie* 1930;130:678–757.
104. Fukui T: Transverse gyri of temporal lobe in the Japanese brain, fifth report. *Hokuetsu Igaku Zasshi* 1934;49:1025–1050.
105. Kakeshita T: Zur Anatomie der operkularen Temporal-Region: Vergleichende Untersuchungen der rechten und linken Seite. *Arb Neurol Inst Wien* 1925;27:292.
106. Von Bonin G: Anatomical asymmetries of the cerebral hemispheres, in Mountcastle VB (ed): *Interhemispheric Relations and Cerebral Dominance.* Baltimore, The Johns Hopkins Press, 1962, pp 1–6.
107. Cunningham DJ: *Contribution to the Surface Anatomy of the Cerebral Hemispheres.* Dublin, Royal Irish Academy, 1892.
108. Eberstaller O: Zur oberflachen Anatomie des Grosshirn Hemispharen. *Wien Med Blatt* 1884;7:479, 642, 644.
109. Hochberg FM, LeMay M: Arteriographic correlates of handedness. *Neurology* 1975;25:218–222.
110. Kopp N, Michel F, Carrier H, et al: Etude de certaines asymetries hemispheriques du cerveau humain. *J Neurol Sci* 1977;34:349–363.
111. Meyer A: *The Collected Papers of Adolph Meyer.* Baltimore, The Johns Hopkins Press, 1950, pp 358–369.
112. Beck E: Typologie des Gehirns am Beispiel des dorsalen menschlichen Schlafenappens nebst weiteren Beitrage zur Frage der Links-Rechtshirnigkeit. *Dtsch Z Nervenheilk* 1955;173:267–308.
113. Campain R, Minckler J: A note on the gross configurations of the human auditory cortex. *Brain Lang* 1976;3:318–323.
114. Broca P: Localisation des fonctions, cerebrales, siège de la faculté de langage articule. *Bull Soc Anteropol Paris* 1863;4:200–204.
115. Falzi G, Perrone P, Vignolo LA: Right-left asymmetry in anterior speech region. *Arch Neurol* 1982;39:239–240.
116. McRae DL, Branch CL, Milner B: The occipital horns and cerebral dominance. *Neurology* 1968;18:95–98.
117. LeMay M: Asymmetries of the skull and handedness. *J Neurol Sci* 1977;32:243–253.
118. Gundara N, Zivanovic B: Asymmetry in East African skulls. *Am J Phys Anthropol* 1968;28:331–338.

119. Satz P, Achenbach K, Fennel E: Correlations between assessed manual laterality and predicted speech laterality in a normal population. *Neuropsychologia* 1967; 5:295–310.
120. Flechsig P: *Die Leitungsbahnen in Gehirn und Ruckenmark des Menschen auf Grundentwicklungs geschlichticher Untersuchungen.* Leipzig, W. Engelmann, 1876.
121. Yakovlev PI, Rakic P: Patterns of decussation of bulbar pyramids and distribution of pyramidal tracts on two sides of the spinal cord. *Trans Am Neurol Assoc* 1966; 91:366–367.
122. Kertesz A, Geschwind N: Patterns of pyramidal decussation and their relationship to handedness. *Arch Neurol* 1971;24:326–332.
123. Smith GE: A preliminary note on an aberrant circumolivary bundle springing from the left pyramidal tract. *Rev Neurol Psychiatry* 1904;2:377–383.
124. Galaburda AM, Sanides F: Cytoarchitectonic organization of the human auditory cortex. *J Comp Neurol* 1980;190:597–610.
125. Galaburda AM: La region de Broca: Observations anatomiques faites un siècle aprés de mort de son decouvreur. *Rev Neurol* 1980;10:609–616.
126. Eidelberg D, Galaburda AM: Inferior parietal lobule: Divergent architectonic asymmetries in the human brain. *Arch Neurol* 1984;41:843–852.
127. Luria AR: On quasi-aphasic speech disturbances in lesions of the deep structures of the brain. *Brain Lang* 1977;4:432–459.
128. Mohr JP, Watters WC, Duncan GW: Thalamic hemorrhage and aphasia. *Brain Lang* 1975;2:3–17.
129. Samarel A, Wright TL, Sergay F, et al: Thalamic hemorrhage with speech disorder. *Trans Am Neurol Assoc* 1976;101:283–285.
130. Graff-Radford NR, Eslinger PJ, Damasio AR, et al: Nonhemorrhagic infarction of the thalamus: Behavioral, anatomic, and physiologic correlates. *Neurology* 1984; 34:14–23.
131. Eidelberg D, Galaburda AM: Symmetry and asymmetry in the human posterior thalamus: I. Cytoarchitectonic analysis in normal persons. *Arch Neurol* 1982; 39:325–332.
132. Glick SD, Jerussi TP, Waters PH, et al: Amphetamine-induced changes in striatal dopamine and acetylcholine levels and relationship to rotation (circling behavior) in rats. *Biochem Pharmacol* 1974;23:3223–3225.
133. Glick SD, Cox RD: Nocturnal rotation in normal rats: Correlation with amphetamine-induced rotation and effects of nigrostriatal lesions. *Brain Res* 1978; 150:149–161.
134. Oke A, Keller R, Mefford I, et al: Lateralization of norepinephrine in human thalamus. *Science* 1978;200:1411–1413.
135. Amaducci L, Sorbi S, Albanese A, et al: Choline acetyltransferase (ChAT) activity differs in right and left human temporal lobes. *Neurology* 1981;31:799–805.
136. Glick SD, Ross DA, Hough LB: Lateral asymmetry of neurotransmitters in human brain. *Brain Res* 1982;234:53–63.
137. Szara S: The comparison of the psychotic effect of tryptamine derivates with the effects of mescaline and LSD-25 in self experiments, in Garattini SA, Ghetti V (eds): *Psychotropic Drugs.* Amsterdam, Elsevier Publishing Co, 1957, p 460.
138. Sai-Halasz A, Brunecker G, Szara ST: Dymethyltryptamin: ein neues Psychoticum. *Psychiatry Neurol* 1958;135:285–301.

139. Gentili C, Tiberi F: Rilievi clinicosperimentali sull'azione neuropsicodislettica della N-N-dietiltriptamina. Atti del 2nd Colloquio Internazionale sull'Espressione Plastica, Bologna, 1963.
140. Mandell AJ, Knapp S: Asymmetry and mood, emergent properties of serotonin regulation. *Arch Gen Psychiatry* 1979;36:909–916.
141. Brumback RA, Staton RD: Learning disability and childhood depression. *Am J Orthopsychiatry* 1983;53:269–281.
142. Freeman RL, Galaburda AM, Diaz-Cabal R, et al: The neurology of depression: Cognitive and behavioral deficits with focal findings in depression and resolution after electroconvulsive therapy. *Arch Neurol* 1985;42:289–291.
143. Waziri R: Lateralization of neuroleptic-induced dyskinesia indicates pharmacological asymmetry in the brain. *Psychopharmacology* 1980;68:51–53.
144. LeMay M: Morphological cerebral asymmetries of modern man, fossil man, and non-human primate. *Ann NY Acad Sci* 1976;280:349–366.
145. Strauss E, Fitz C: Occipital horn asymmetry in children. *Ann Neurol* 1980;8:437–439.
146. Herve G: *La Circonvolution de Broca.* Paris, Delahage et Lecrosnier, 1888.
147. Wada JA, Davies AE: Fundamental nature of human infant's brain asymmetry. *Can J Neurol Sci* 1977;4:203–207.
148. Bracco L, Tiezzi A, Ginanneschi A, et al: Lateralization of choline acetyltransferase (CHAT) activity in fetus and adult human brain. *Neurosci Lett* 1984;50:301–305.
149. DeBassio WA, Kemper TL, Galaburda AM: Asymmetric olfactory migratory stream growth in the rat. *Soc Neurosci Abstr* 1982;8:326.
150. Narang HK: Right-left asymmetry of myelin development in epiretinal portion of the rabbit optic nerve. *Nature* 1977;266:28–29.
151. Manz HJ, Phillips TM, Rowden G, et al: Unilateral megalencephaly, cerebral cortical dysplasia, neuronal hypertrophy, and heterotopia: Cytomorphometric, fluorometric, cytochemical, and biochemical analysis. *Acta Neuropathol* 1979; 45:97–103.
152. Woo TL: On the asymmetry of the human skull. *Biometrika* 1931;22:324–352.
153. Mesulam MM: A cortical network for directed attention and unilateral neglect. *Ann Neurol* 1981;10:309–325.
154. Heilman KM, Schwartz H, Watson RT: Hypoarousal in patients with the neglect syndrome and emotional indifference. *Neurology* 1977;28:229–232.
155. Hecaen H, de Ajuriaguerra J: *Left-Handedness.* New York, Grune & Stratton Inc, 1964.
156. Rogers LJ: Light experience and asymmetry of brain function in chickens. *Nature* 1982;297:223–225.
157. Dewson JH III: Toward an animal model of auditory cognitive function, in Ludlow CL, Doran-Quine ME (eds): *The Neurological Bases of Language Disorders in Children: Methods and Directions for Research.* NINCDS Monograph No 22, Government Printing Office, 1979, pp 19–24.
158. Yeni-Komshian GH, Benson DA: Anatomical study of cerebral asymmetry in the temporal lobe of humans, chimpanzees, and rhesus monkeys. *Science* 1976; 192:387–389.
159. Cain DP, Wada JA: An anatomical asymmetry in the baboon brain. *Brain Behav Evol* 1979;16:222–226.
160. Webster WG, Webster IH: Anatomical asymmetry of the cerebral hemispheres of the cat brain. *Physiol Behav* 1975;4:867–869.

161. Kolb B, Sutherland RJ, Nonneman AJ, et al: Asymmetry in the cerebral hemispheres of the rat, mouse, rabbit, and cat: The right hemisphere is larger. *Exp Neurol* 1982;78:348–359.
162. Diamond MC, Johnson RE, Ingham CA: Morphological changes in the young, adult and aging rat cerebral cortex, hippocampus, and diencephalon. *Behav Biol* 1975;14:163–174.
163. Sherman GF, Galaburda AM: Neocortical asymmetry and open-field behavior in the rat. *Exp Neurol* 1984;86:473–482.
164. Diamond MC, Murphy GM Jr, Akiama K, et al: Morphologic hippocampal asymmetry in male and female rats. *Exp Neurol* 1982;76:553–565.
165. Braitenberg V, Kemali M: Exceptions to bilateral symmetry in the epithalamus of lower vertebrates. *J Comp Neurol* 1970;138:137–146.
166. Engbretson GA, Reiner A, Brecha N: Habenular asymmetry and the central connections of the parietal eye of the lizard. *J Comp Neurol* 1981;198:155–165.
167. Petersen MR, Beecher MD, Zoloth SR, et al: Neural lateralization of species-specific vocalizations by Japanese macaques (*Macaca fuscata*). *Science* 1978;202:324–327.
168. Denenberg VH: Hemispheric laterality in animals and the effects of early experience. *Behav Brain Sci* 1981;4:1–49.
169. Nottebohm F: Brain pathways for vocal learning in birds: A review of the first ten years. *Prog Psychobiol Physiol Psychol* 1980;9:85–124.
170. Rogers LJ: Lateralization in the avian brain. *Bird Behav* 1980;2:1–12.
171. Zimmerberg B, Glick SD, Jerussi TP: Neurochemical correlate of a spatial preference in rats. *Science* 1974;185:623–625.
172. Schneider LH, Murphy RB, Coons EE: Lateralization of striatal dopamine (D2) receptors in normal rats. *Neurosci Lett* 1982;33:281–284.
173. Jerussi TP, Glick SD: Drug-induced rotation in rats without lesions: Behavioral and neurochemical indices of a normal asymmetry in nigro-striatal function. *Psychopharmacology* 1976;47:249–260.
174. Robinson TE, Becker JB, Ramirez VD: Sex differences in amphetamine-elicited rotational behavior and lateralization of striatal dopamine in rats. *Brain Res Bull* 1980;5:539–545.
175. Starr MS, Kilpatrick K: Bilateral asymmetry in brain GABA function? *Neurosci Lett* 1981;25:167–172.
176. Zimmerberg B, Strumpf AJ, Glick SD: Cerebral asymmetry and left-right discrimination. *Brain Res* 1978;140:194–196.
177. Cynader M, Lepore F, Guillemot JP: Interhemispheric competition during postnatal development. *Nature* 1981;290:139–140.
178. Glick SD: Heritable determinants of left-right bias in the rat. *Life Sci* 1983; 32:2215–2221.
179. Mellon DeF: Nerves and the transformation of claw type in snapping shrimps. *TINS* 1981;4:245–248.
180. Govind CK, Kent KS: Transformation of fast fibres to slow prevented by lack of activity in developing lobster muscle. *Nature* 1982;298:755–757.
181. Alderman AL: The determination of the eye in the anuran Hyla regilla. *J Exp Zool* 1935;70:205–232.
182. Kallen B: *Teratology, The Science of Malformations*. Stockholm, Almqvist & Wiksell, 1967, p 239.

183. Galaburda AM, Sherman GF, Rosen GD, et al: Developmental dyslexia: Four consecutive cases with cortical anomalies. *Ann Neurol,* in press.
184. Galaburda AM, Eidelberg D: Symmetry and asymmetry in the human posterior thalamus: II. Thalamic lesions in a case of developmental dyslexia. *Arch Neurol* 1982;39:333–336.
185. Levine DN, Hier DB, Calvanio R: Acquired learning disability for reading after left temporal lobe damage in childhood. *Neurology* 1981;31:257–264.
186. Caron JP, Colin H, Comoy J, et al: Resultats de l'exeoese chirurgicale des aneurysmes arterio-veneux (AAV) des zones rolandique, parietale, occipital, et du pli courbe de l'hemisphere dominant: Å propos de vingt cas. *Neurochirurgie* 1982; 28:295–307.
187. Mori K, Murata T, Hashimoto N, et al: Clinical analysis of arteriovenous malformations in children. *Childs Brain* 1980;6:13–25.
188. Hier DB, LeMay M, Rosenberger PB, et al: Developmental dyslexia: Evidence for a subgroup with reversed cerebral asymmetry. *Arch Neurol* 1978;35:90–92.
189. Hier DB, LeMay M, Rosenberger PB: Developmental dyslexia and unfavorable left-right asymmetries of the brain. *J Autism Dev Disord* 1979;9:153–159.
190. Rosenberger PB, Hier DB: Cerebral asymmetry and verbal intellectual deficits. *Ann Neurol* 1980;8:300–304.
191. Veith G, Schwindt W: Pathologisch-anatomischer Beitrag zum Problem 'Nichtsesshaftigkeit.' *Fortschr Neurol Psychiatr* 1976;44:1–21.
192. Balthasar K: Über das anatomische Substrat der generalisierten Tic-Krankheit (Maladie des Tics, Gilles de la Tourette): Entwicklungs-hemmung des Corpus striatum. *Arch Psychiatrie* 1957;195:531–549.
193. Sano F: James Henry Pullen, The Genius of Earlswood. *J Mental Sci* 1918;64:251–267.
194. Rimland B: *Infantile Autism.* New York, Appleton-Century-Crofts, 1964.
195. Rimland B: The autistic savant. *Psychol Today* 1978;12:69–80.
196. Layton WM Jr: Random determination of a developmental process. *J Hered* 1976; 67:336–338.
197. Afzelius BA, Camner P, Eliasson R, et al: Kartagener's syndrome does exist. *Lancet* 1978;2:950.
198. Dahlberg G: Genotypic asymmetries. *Proc R Soc Edin* 1944–1947;62:20–31.
199. Bakan P: Handedness and birth order. *Nature* 1971;229:195.
200. Bakan P: Left-handedness and birth order revisited. *Neuropsychologia* 1977; 15:837–839.
201. Benton AL, Meyers R, Polder GJ: Some aspects of handedness. *Psychiatr Neurol* 1962;144:321–337.
202. Wada J, Rasmussen T: Intracarotid injection of sodium amytal for the lateralization of cerebral speech dominance. *J Neurosurg* 1960;17:266–282.
203. Rasmussen T, Milner B: The role of early left-brain injury in determining lateralization of cerebral speech functions. *Ann NY Acad Sci* 1977;299:355–369.
204. Provins KA, Milner AD, Kerr P: Asymmetry of mammal preference and performance. *Percept Mot Skills* 1982;54:179–194.
205. Annett M: A classification of hand preference by association analysis. *Br J Psychol* 1970;61:303–321.
206. Nasrallah HA, Keelor K, McCalley-Whitters M: Laterality shift in alcoholic males. *Biol Psychol* 1983;18:1065–1067.

207. Schachter SC, Ransil BJ, Geschwind N: Associations of handedness with hair color and learning disabilities. *Neuropsychologia,* in press.
208. Liepmann H: *Drei Aufsätze aus dem Apraxiegebiet.* Berlin, S Karger AG, 1908.
209. Kimura D, Archibald Y: Motor functions of the left hemisphere. *Brain* 1974; 97:337–350.
210. Geschwind N: The apraxias: Neural mechanisms of disorders of learned movement. *Am Sci* 1975;63:188–195.
211. Gesell A, Ames LB: The development of handedness. *J Genet Psychol* 1947; 70:155–175.
212. Keller R: Two famous left-handers. *Ciba Symposia* 1942;3:1143–1145.
213. Kilshaw D, Annett M: Right- and left-hand skill: I. Effects of age, sex, and hand preference showing superior skill in left-handers. *Br J Psychol* 1983;74:253–268.
214. Taylor DC: Ontogenesis of chronic epileptic psychoses: A reanalysis. *Psychol Med* 1975;1:247–253.
215. Swinson CM, Slavin G, Coles EC, et al: Coeliac disease and malignancy. *Lancet* 1983;1:111–115.
216. Seltzer B, Sherwin I: A comparison of clinical features in early- and late-onset primary degenerative dementia. *Arch Neurol* 1983;40:143–146.
217. Marsh DG, Meyers DA, Bias WB: The epidemiology and genetics of atopic allergy. *N Engl J Med* 1981;305:1551–1559.
218. Weintraub S, Mesulam MM: Developmental learning disabilities of the right hemisphere. *Arch Neurol* 1983;40:463–468.
219. Folstein S, Rutter M: Genetic influences and infantile autism. *Nature* 1977; 265:726–728.
220. Orton ST: 'Word-blindness' in school children. *Arch Neurol Psychiatry* 1925; 14:581–615.
221. Ludlow CL, Polinsky RJ, Caine ED, et al: Language and speech abnormalities in Tourette syndrome, in Friedhoff HJ, Chase TN (eds): *Gilles de la Tourette Syndrome.* New York, Raven Press, 1982, pp 351–361.
222. Boucher J: Hand preference in autistic children and their parents. *J Autism Childhood Schiz* 1977;7:177–187.
223. Colby KM, Parkinson C: Handedness in autistic children. *J Autism Childhood Schiz* 1977;7:3–9.
224. Bishop DVM: How sinister is sinistrality? *J R Coll Physicians Lond* 1983;17:161–172.
225. Oswald I: Sleep and its disorders, in Vinken PJ, Bruyn GW (eds): *Handbook of Clinical Neurology.* New York, Elsevier North Holland Inc, 1969, vol 3, *Disorders of Higher Nervous Activity,* pp 80–111.
226. Carpenter S, Yassa R, Ochs R: A pathologic basis for Kleine-Levin syndrome. *Arch Neurol* 1982;39:25–28.
227. Vandenberg SG, Kuse AR: Spatial ability: A critical review of the sex-linked major gene hypothesis, in Wittig MA and Peterson AC (eds): *Sex-Related Differences in Cognitive Functioning.* New York, Academic Press Inc, 1979, pp 67–94.
228. Benbow CP, Stanley JC: Math talent, in press.
229. Carter CO: Sex-linkage and sex-limitation, in Ounsted C, Taylor DC (eds): *Gender Differences: Their Ontogeny and Significance.* New York, Churchill Livingstone Inc, 1972.
230. Kidd KK, Heimbuch RC, Records MA: Vertical transmission of susceptibility to stuttering with sex-modified expression. *Proc Natl Acad Sci USA* 1981;78:606–610.

231. Edwards DA: Mice: Fighting by neonatally androgenized females. *Science* 1964; 161:1027–1028.
232. Bronson FH, Desjardins C: Aggression in adult mice: Modification by neonatal injections of gonadal hormones. *Science* 1968;161:705–706.
233. Wood LC: Presentation, American Thyroid Association, New Orleans, 1983.
234. Thonnard-Neumann E: Some interrelationships of vasoactive substances and basophilic leukocytes in migraine headache. *Headache* 1969;9:130–140.
235. Egger J, Carter CM, Wilson J, et al: Is migraine food allergy? *Lancet* 1983;2:865–870.
236. Szondi L: Konstitutionsanalyse von 100 Stotterern. *Wien Med Wochenschr* 1932; 82:922–928.
237. Coleman M (ed): *The Autistic Syndromes.* New York, Elsevier North Holland Publishing Co, 1976.
238. Beer AE, Billingham RE: *The Immunobiology of Mammalian Reproduction.* Englewood Cliffs, NJ, Prentice-Hall Inc, 1976.
239. Faulk WP: Human trophoblast antigens: Role in normal and abnormal pregnancies. *Bull Mem Acad Roy Med Belg* 1981;136:379–388.
240. Taylor C, Faulk WP: Prevention of recurrent abortions with leucocyte transfusions. *Lancet* 1981;2:68–69.
241. Tryphonas H, Trites R: Food allergy in children with hyperactivity, learning disabilities, and/or minimal brain dysfunction. *Ann Allergy* 1979;42:22–27.
242. Fialkow PJ: Autoimmunity: A predisposing factor to chromosomal aberrations? *Lancet* 1964;1:474–475.
243. Fialkow PJ: Thyroid autoimmunity and Down's syndrome. *Ann NY Acad Sci* 1970; 171:500–511.
244. Greenfield JG, Blackwood W, McMenemy WH, et al (eds): *Neuropathology.* London, Edward Arnold, 1958, p 353.

This study was supported in part by grants from the National Institutes of Health (NS 14018, NINCDS 06209), the National Science Foundation (BNS 05674), the Orton Research Fund, and the Essel Foundation.

It will be evident in these pages how indebted we are to Peter Behan, MD, of the University of Glasgow (Scotland) and to Dr Thomas Kemper, MD. We would also like to express our gratitude to many other individuals whose work or personal comments have especially influenced our approach to different issues. Much of whatever may be useful is the direct outgrowth of their stimulation, but they are not responsible for any erroneous facts or conclusions. We apologize for any omissions in this list.

We are indebted to the following (in alphabetical order): B. A. Afzelius, MD, Marian Annett, PhD, Charles Boklage, PhD, Patrick Bray, MD, Michael Corballis, PhD, Martha Denckla, MD, Victor Denenberg, PhD, Marian Diamond, PhD, Gunter Dorner, MD, Jack Fishman, MD, Pierre Flor-Henry, MD, Stanley Glick, MD, PhD, Patricia Goldman-Rakic, PhD, Roger Gorski, PhD, J. A. Gustafsson, Paul Ivanyi, Robert Lahita, MD, Nicole LeDouarin, PhD, Jerre Levy, PhD, Christie Ludlow, PhD, Richard Masland, MD, Michael Morgan, Charles Netley, PhD, Fernando Nottebohm, PhD, Christopher Ounsted, MD, Philip Paterson, MD, Geoffrey Raisman, Pasko Rakic, MD, David Rosenfield, MD, Arnold Scheibel, MD, Richard Sidman, MD, John Simpson, MD, David C. Taylor, MD, Juhn Wada, MD, and the late Paul Yakovlev, MD. Special thanks are due to our coworkers Francisco Aboitiz, MS, Heiko Braak, MD, William DeBassio, MD, PhD, David Eidelberg, MD, Olaf Heine, MD, Marjorie LeMay, MD, Deepak Pandya, MD, Glenn Rosen, PhD, Marjorie Ross, the late Friedrich Sanides, MD, Gordon Sherman, PhD, and Steven Schachter, MD, and to our colleagues of the Neurology Department of the Beth Israel Hospital and the Psychology Department of the Massachusetts Institute of Technology. Our indebtedness to those who helped produce the manuscript will be expressed at the end of the third article.

# CHAPTER 16 (II)

# Cerebral Lateralization

## Biological Mechanisms, Associations, and Pathology: II. A Hypothesis and a Program for Research

*Norman Geschwind and Albert M. Galaburda*

### Anomalous Dominance and Special Talents

According to our hypothesis, slowed growth within certain zones of the left hemisphere is likely to result in enlargement of other cortical regions, in particular, the homologous contralateral area, but also adjacent unaffected regions. The influences that favor anomalous dominance may thus favor talents associated with superior development of certain regions, either in the right hemisphere or in adjacent parts of the left hemisphere. Even with excessive retardation of growth and the resultant migration abnormalities and learning disorders (LD), high talents may exist as a result of compensatory enlargement of other cortical regions.

Several types of data are in concordance with these conclusions. Several studies have claimed that the average level of spatial talents is higher in male subjects.[2] Hier and Crowley[3] found that congenitally totally hypogonadal males, who lack testosterone (T), typically had superior verbal scores and low scores on tests of spatial function, unlike normal males. In Turner's syndrome, in which there is a marked lack of all hormones, inferior spatial talents are commonly found while verbal talents are sometimes superior. Taylor[4,5] found that male temporal lobe epileptics with alien tissue (i.e., areas of disturbed neural development) in the *left* hemisphere typically had low verbal scores and high spatial scores, with the reverse pattern in males with alien tissue in the right hemisphere.

---

Reprinted with permission from *Archives of Neurology*. 1985; 42 (6): 521-552. 

This study provides evidence that, in males, prenatal influences may be more important than postnatal, since males with mesial temporal sclerosis (MTS), a postnatally acquired lesion, tended to show patterns similar to those of alien tissue patients, but the effects are less striking. The results in female subjects lend support to the view that postnatal influences may be somewhat more important in them than in males. Female subjects with MTS tended to show greater discrepancies in verbal and performance scores, depending on the side of the lesion, than did those with alien tissue.

Other data support a role of hormonal influences on laterality and associated skills. Women with late menarche tend to have higher spatial scores than those with early menarche.[6]

Several studies have shown an elevated rate of non-right-handedness (NRH) in certain occupations, e.g., among professional athletes,[7] artists,[8] architects,[9] and engineers,[9] although there are some disagreements,[10] i.e., occupations in several of which there is an increased use of spatial talents.[11] A group of particular interest includes mathematicians and the mathematically gifted among whom there is also an increased rate of left-handedness (LH).[12,13] Non-right-handed individuals are superior on several tests of musical ability.[14] Some other articles show an elevated rate of NRH in musicians,[8,15,16] although there is disagreement.[10] One potential objection can be raised against these studies. In order to prove that NRH individuals are found in specially high frequency in occupations requiring high spatial talents, it would be necessary to document a low proportion of them in other occupations. One might otherwise postulate that those with NRH are overrepresented in all populations with high talent, which is a possible interpretation of the existing data. It could be the case that although growth of the left hemisphere is slowed to a greater extent in sinistrals than dextrals, it may attain a greater final size in sinistrals. This could occur when the growth period is prolonged, e.g., when the duration of pregnancy exceeds the average or when puberty is late, which would allow for further development in childhood. This situation would be analogous to that of the greater final average height of males despite their slower rate of bone growth. Left-handers might thus be found in increased numbers in all occupations demanding high talent, including those in which verbal talents were necessary. On the other hand, when full development was not achieved because of excessive retardation of growth or because of early termination of pregnancy or early puberty, one might observe disorders of development such as LD, and in more extreme cases a distinctly inferior overall level of functioning. Those with anomalous dominance could thus be present in excess both at the higher and lower ends of the scale of accomplishment. The very high frequency of LH in cases of mental retardation[17] would be in conformity with this hypothesis. The data necessary for settling these questions are not yet available.

A related issue is that of superior talents in association with childhood LD. There are, of course, many individual examples of such cases. Although some autistic children have widespread impairments, others exhibit dramatically isolated islands of superior behavior, e.g., an autistic girl who at the age of 4 years exhibited remarkable artistic talents. Many idiot savants illustrate this phenomenon." High right-hemisphere talents are common in dyslexic subjects and in their families.[19, 20]

Much research is needed before one can confidently assert the existence of a 'pathology of superiority', i.e., compensatory growth leading to superior development of some portions of the brain as a result of poorer development of others. Goldman-Rakic and Rakic [21] showed that if a cortical area is removed from one hemisphere of a fetal monkey, one observes hypertrophy both of the corresponding area on the opposite side and of areas in the lesioned hemisphere adjacent to the ablated region. It seems likely that at the time of cell death there is competition not only between homologous contralateral regions but also between regions in the same hemisphere.

The situation in which there is delayed development of a cortical region in one hemisphere is not necessarily equivalent in all cases to the ablation of a region. If the delaying influence acts only during the development of a particular cortical area, then one might expect hypertrophy of adjacent regions, i.e., this situation would resemble the one in which a surgical lesion is placed in that area.

On the other hand, if the retarding influence is present over a period, it may affect other areas in the same hemisphere and thus might diminish or prevent the hypertrophy of adjacent areas, although contralateral hypertrophy should still take place and indeed might even be enhanced.

The possibility of hypertrophy of areas adjacent to a zone of retarded growth may help to explain another one of the apparently paradoxical findings in childhood dyslexia. In the adult, the acquired Gerstmann's syndrome (i.e., acalculia, agraphia, right-left difficulty, and disordered finger identification) is almost always the result of a lesion in the left temporoparieto-occipital (TPO) junction region.[22] It may exist in isolation but is usually associated with signs of involvement of adjacent regions, e.g., alexia with agraphia and constructional disorders. Some years ago Hermann[23] reported cases of developmental dyslexia with Gerstmann's signs. Cases of the developmental Gerstmann's syndrome without dyslexia have, however, been reported.[24] Another report[25] dealt with a 14-year-old boy with severe Gerstmann's syndrome who had learned to read precociously and whose current reading abilities were distinctly superior for his age and grade level. Thus the literature contains cases of the developmental Gerstmann's syndrome both with and without dyslexia.

The apparent paradox may have a simple solution. As we have pointed out, the brains of several childhood dyslexics have contained disordered cytoarchitectonic organization at the TPO junction in a region known from studies of adults suffering from alexia with agraphia to be of major importance for reading.[26,27] If the developmental disturbance should extend further into the TPO region, one might expect to find congenital Gerstmann's syndrome. If, on the other hand, there were a clear restriction of the disturbed cortical architecture to the region involved in reading (perhaps because adverse influences were present only over a limited period), then the immediately adjacent region might hypertrophy. Instead of Gerstmann's syndrome one might have superiority of the functions subserved by this region.

This hypothesis immediately suggests certain experiments. Among dyslexic subjects one might find superior "Gerstmann talents" than among controls as well as a higher proportion with poor abilities of this type than among controls. A simple assessment of the mean scores on tests of these abilities might obscure the elevated frequency of dyslexics at both extremes. In particular, this type of study might help in accounting for both the assertion that there is a disproportionately high number of dyslexics with high mathematical ability and for the claim that poor mathematical abilities are found in elevated frequency in dyslexics. Both statements could be correct.

Conversely, if the major impact of delayed migration were on the "Gerstmann's region" with sparing of the area particularly important for reading, one might expect a syndrome like that of the boy described earlier, i.e., a Gerstmann's syndrome with superior reading abilities. A related and perhaps identical problem is that of the child with very poor spelling and writing abilities in the face of high reading scores. It is often assumed that all such individuals were dyslexic at one time, but there are examples in which this appears not to be the case. The type of mechanism discussed here might account for this situation. If this interpretation is correct, then the poor spellers and writers should usually perform poorly on right-left, calculations, and finger identification.

As can be readily seen, the above discussion may be relevant to the difficult problem of subtypes of dyslexia, but this is not within the scope of this article.

Sano[18] described in detail the brain of the "genius of Earlswood" (an English institution for the mentally retarded), who in the face of marked retardation in the development of speech and reading had highly developed artistic abilities, especially in sculpture. In comparison with control cerebra, this brain had very small frontal lobes and small temporal lobes, but the occipital regions were massively developed. The findings are compatible with intrauterine reorganization. It is of interest that the patient's brother had a similar pattern of talents and deficits.

While the idiot savant pattern is found in some autistic children, the majority do not exhibit such spectacular islands of performance. The existence, however, of even a small number of such cases would be unexpected in view of the great obstacles faced by these patients. Cases of this type could easily be overlooked if one simply averaged the scores of many autistic individuals. The mean level of performance has little significance in relation to a population with an excess of members at both the upper and the lower ends of the distribution.

The existence of such distributions may explain some apparently discrepant findings. It has been found that among male architects there is an excess of LH.[9,11] Yet several recent studies of college students found that LH persons scored lower on tests of spatial function than right-handed (RH) males.[28,29] The apparent contradiction in the findings concerning spatial talents of LH might be resolved if they were found in excessive numbers at both high and low levels of spatial function. The preceding discussion deals with one possible mechanism that might account for these findings. There is another type of explanation that deserves brief consideration. Spatial performance may not be related in a simple linear fashion to the magnitude of the male-related effect in development; there may be a U-shaped relationship, with an optimal hormonal level for spatial function. On the average, the effects tend to favor the male population. On the other hand, excessive effects would also occur predominantly in male subjects who would therefore be found in excess number, both among those with high spatial function and those with low spatial function. The effects are less likely to reach an excessive degree in females, so that few would be in a dosage range that would lead to diminution of function. Left-handed females might thus be found in excess in the high spatial talent group but not in the low-scoring group.

It is difficult to carry out experimental studies on the problem in humans, but the existence of high spatial function in male rats which is dependent on the right posterior hemisphere[30] and the existence of anatomic asymmetries in these animals[31–33] that can be modified by early hormonal treatments may provide the possibility of controlled experimentation.

The possible existence of bimodal effects, i.e., the finding of excessive numbers of NRH individuals at both extremes of the spectrum of certain talents is not surprising from the perspective of biological fitness. If two populations share the same *mean* level of performance of some function, the two groups are not necessarily equally competitive. Assume that one population contains a higher percentage than the other of individuals with both very high and very low talents for this function. The population with higher numbers in the extreme ranges may compete more effectively since success often depends primarily on the performance of those individuals in the highest ranges. If in two populations of comparable size talented athletes were present in percentages of 0.2% and 0.1%, respectively, the first group would carry off most of the prizes. It would make no difference whether the mean level of performance of the first population was lower than that of the second, or whether it also contained an excessive number of athletically untalented people. A process affecting brain growth that produced high talents in a large number at the expense of creation of an unusual number of incompetents would be favored in the course of evolution. A mechanism of this type might not readily be detected, because of the small numbers of individuals in the tails of the distributions. An analogous situation exists in the study of the rates of chemical reactions. It was originally believed that the rates were proportional to the mean velocities of the molecules involved. It later became clear that only those molecules with velocities above a certain level (the activation energy) participate in a given reaction. It was, therefore, the tails of the distributions that were important. As long as the theory of reaction rates confined itself to mean velocities, no adequate theory could be constructed.

Another factor, often overlooked in the study of spatial function, may lead to erroneous conclusions. It is often assumed that spatial talent depends only on right-hemisphere function, but in fact each hemisphere contributes. Left-hemisphere lesions affect predominantly the placement of internal details while right-hemisphere lesions tend to affect external configuration. It is possible that some individuals may have high talents in one or the other function, although some are good at both. Tests of spatial function often do not distinguish these capacities, just as handedness tests may fail to distinguish "pyramidal" and "axial" motor dominance, as was discussed in an earlier section. The possibility of dissociation in spatial function is suggested by some data cited earlier, e.g., the dyslexic who was clumsy in trunk movements but who worked as a metalsmith. A metalsmith might need both superior small detail spatial function and high "pyramidal" talents while an athlete might require excellent large spatial relationships and superior axial dominance. A recent study suggests that in early development females may have superior small detail spatial function and males may have superior capacities for large spatial relationships.

Some dyslexics appear to be superior at small detail spatial functions while others are superior in the large ones, e.g., in athletic activity. Unfortunately, these patterns have not yet been studied in adequate detail. If this were true it would suggest that in some cases delayed development of the speech region leads to superior development of the adjacent posterior region in the same hemisphere, while in others the opposite side enlarges. Whether these differences might result from variations in timing or duration of the delaying influences or from other factors is not known.

Animal studies of spatial function probably tap the capacities for spatial orientation, e.g., maze running. If left-sided dominance for small details could be shown in animals, the probability of rapid clarification of these issues would be greatly increased.

## Sex Hormone Influences on Brain Growth

### Fetal Chromosomes and Sex Hormones

One of the major contributions of the Darwinian theory was the elucidation of the importance of sexual reproduction. Although asexual reproduction is found in many species, sexual reproduction is the exclusive form in others, e.g., in all mammals. Since natural selection depends on differences between animals, evolutionary mechanisms that favor diversity have attained central importance. Sexual reproduction, by its mixing of parental genes, is the most important mechanism for achieving diversity although not the only one. It had been known for years that sex hormones play a major role in male-female differentiation, but their effects on neural development have received little attention until recently. The rapid growth of knowledge of these mechanisms has created a revolution in the brain sciences, although they are still frequently neglected.

At fertilization, the male and female zygotes differ on the average in only two chromosomes. Yet these chromosomal differences at conception are the prime movers, the ultimate origin, of all of the striking differences in male and female development. Only the male zygote has a Y chromosome, but it carries only one X chromosome while the female zygote has two.

The Y chromosome is unusual in bearing few genes; it carries, however, a protein, the H-Y antigen,[34] that is essential for development of the testes which will later in fetal life secrete T. This hormone is, in turn, essential for the development of typically male structures in the body and brain. One should not assume that H-Y antigen exerts all its effects only indirectly through the formation of testes and the later production of T; this antigen is expressed on other organs, e.g., the thymus gland, an essential component of the developing immune system.[35] The ovaries appear to play a more limited role in prenatal development.

The significance of the presence of one X in the male and of two in the female zygote is sometimes underestimated because of lyonization, i.e., the random inactivation of one X chromosome in each cell of the female. Inactivation does not, however, take place in germ cells. Thus at conception the female zygote carries twice as many X-linked genes as the male. The X chromosome plays an important role in effects of T since it contains the Tfm locus, one of the genes that controls sensitivity to this hormone.[36] Thus, although the female conceptus is usually exposed later in gestation to a lower level of T than the male, it is probably more sensitive to maternally and placentally produced T especially in the earliest stages of embryogenesis. At the time of lyonization, one might expect loss of this higher sensitivity, but inactivation is not complete, and the female retains a greater dosage of some X-linked products.[37]

The H-Y antigen is essential for the formation of testes. It is intriguing that both the right testis and the right ovum develop before the gonad on the left, and development of the ovary occurs somewhat later than that of the testis.[38] The development of the testes is of cardinal importance for later development. The male fetal gonads produce T in high quantities, i.e., at times the level is comparable with that of adult males. The rate drops late in pregnancy and even more shortly after birth, but then rises again for several months and again declines. As puberty is approached T levels rise again. Testosterone and its metabolites are essential not only for normal development of genitalia and secondary sexual characteristics, but also for the formation of the brain. Sex hormones affect the development of nervous structures involved in the control of reproduction, e.g., the cyclic release of gonadotropins, mating, and lactation. There are, however, also hormonal effects on body and brain systems other than those related directly to reproduction. Males and females differ in almost every aspect of visible body structure, but there are differences that transcend obvious structural features, e.g., gender-related variations in the immune system in responsiveness to drugs and toxins[39] and in metabolism,[40] some of which will be discussed later.

Before the testes begin to produce T most aspects of the hormonal environment are the same for male and female fetuses. The mother and the placenta produce great quantities of estrogens, progesterone, and gonadotropins. The fundamental pattern of the mammal is female, and specific influences must supervene in order to produce male differentiation. As development advances, sex differences increase in number. Thus, although T has a special role as a prime mover, the eventual pattern of possible influences becomes increasingly complex. The female zygote is also exposed to T, little or none of which appears to come from the fetal ovaries or adrenals, but rather from the maternal ovaries, adrenals, and extragonadal structures such as fat. The fetus is protected from much of this maternal T because aromatase in the placenta converts it to estradiol, but the protection is not complete.

The level of ambient T is not the only factor determining T effect. Testosterone-binding globulin (TEBG) lowers the level of active free T. Furthermore, the sensitivity of target tissues may vary. In the syndrome of testicular feminization male fetuses produce T but are insensitive to it. In addition, the rates of reaction in metabolic pathways that can inactivate T probably vary considerably. Thus while male and female zygotes differ on the average in the degree of T effect to which they are subjected, there is no absolute difference between the sexes. There is evidence that T in small amounts may be essential for some aspects of normal female differentiation in the rat.[41]

Another hormone that deserves stress is progesterone which is also present in large amounts during fetal life and which is known to have masculinizing effects in the female, at least at certain periods. Sensitivity is perhaps different in the two sexes. Many of the effects of T may, of course, be mediated indirectly. Biegon and McEwen[42] have found male-female differences in serotonin systems, which might play a special role in laterality. It is worth noting that infants of mothers who have taken LSD (a serotonin derivative) in pregnancy may have missing fingers, especially on the right hand,[43] a finding that also suggests a possible role of serotonin in laterality. As we shall point out later, serotonin derivatives can produce asymmetric pharmacologic effects in adults.

## Hormonal Effects on Brain Structure

Since the 1960s there has been a rapid growth of knowledge concerning the role of early sex hormone exposure in determining later sexual behavior.[37] This remarkable literature has shown the importance of such hormonal effects for the development of normal cycling in the female, for determining the nature of the sex object, and for other aspects of sexual and maternal behavior. It is not possible adequately to review this vast literature, but some of the important principles will be presented. It should be noted that despite many common features, no single set of mechanisms will be universally applicable in all species.[44] Knowledge concerning the details of the process in the human is, of course, limited. Research on sex hormone effects on neural development has dealt primarily with structures in the hypothalamus and limbic system controlling sexual behavior in the rat. Much of it has been on the effects of sex hormones in the immediate postnatal period, when the rat is comparable with a human fetus still within the uterus in late pregnancy, but even in the rat many important developments take place before parturition. Denef[45] showed that the masculinization of the sexually dimorphic ventromedial nucleus of the hypothalamus begins prenatally but continues after birth. Although the human brain at birth is relatively more advanced than that of the rat, recent findings suggest that in the postnatal period, even perhaps up to puberty, important changes, including extensive cell death, are taking place in the human brain.[46]

Many locations in the nervous system contain receptors for the gonadal hormones including estradiol and T.[47] The effects of hormones may be modulated by other influences, e.g., some actions of estradiol in certain locations, e.g., the liver, require the presence of prolactin. Furthermore, not all estrogens or androgens will necessarily share similar actions at a particular site. Dihydrotestosterone, the metabolite that affects many of the secondary male characteristics, does not act in some species in certain locations in the nervous system in which only T may be effective. The actions of T itself vary from location to location within the brain. Certain neurons within the rat preoptic nucleus and amygdala contain aromatase, an enzyme that converts T to estradiol. The action of T within the preoptic nucleus in the rat depends on this conversion. There are other locations in which aromatase is not found even though the target organ contains T receptors, e.g., the pituitary gland.

The sex hormone receptors in the cortex are, of course, of special interest to us. Estradiol receptors are present in the cortex in the postnatal rat, but apparently not in adult life and the same is true for enzymes involved in steroid metabolism, thus suggesting that sex hormone effects are prominent only during a particular period of development.[48] In particular, it should be noted that the rat cortical neurons do not contain aromatase. MacLusky et al[49] have, however, recently found estradiol and T receptors in association cortex of infant monkeys, along with aromatase.

The development of the preoptic nucleus, essential for cyclic release of gonadotropins, is particularly interesting, since it has a distinctly different structure in the adult male and female rat.[50] The male nucleus is larger and contains more neurons than that of the female. If the newborn female is exposed to a single large dose of T before the 15th day of postnatal life, the nucleus assumes the typical male pattern, while in a male castrated at birth it retains the female pattern. The sexual dimorphism of this nucleus is thus dependent on the early hormonal environment. When the female form of the nucleus is present, gonadotropins are released cyclically regardless of whether the animal is a genetic male or female, but when the male pattern is found, cyclic gonadotropin release does not occur.

The literature now routinely distinguishes *masculinization* and *defeminization*. A masculinizing effect is one that leads to male-typical behavior in the female, e.g., mounting other females. A defeminizing effect is one that leads to loss of female-typical traits, e.g., cyclic release of gonadotropins. The two classes of effect can occur independently and depend on hormonal effects at different sites. For convenience we will use the term *masculinization* to mean "masculinization and/or defeminization" except when the distinction is critical to the discussion.

The action of T in altering the structure and function of the preoptic nucleus depends critically on the presence of aromatase, which converts it to estradiol the intracellular action of which is responsible for the change of structure and function to the male form. One might expect the nucleus to be masculinized in both male and female subjects since it is exposed during intrauterine life to massive levels of estradiol. In the case of the rat, the widely accepted explanation is that circulating α-fetoprotein binds estradiol and thus keeps it from crossing the blood-brain barrier and reaching the neurons of the preoptic nucleus. Testosterone, not significantly bound by α-fetoprotein, can reach the nucleus, where it is converted by aromatase to estradiol which then alters the pattern of the cells. The binding to α-fetoprotein also explains another apparently paradoxical phenomenon. The administration of diethylstilbestrol, a powerful estrogenic substance, to the newborn female rat also produces masculinization of the function and structure of this nucleus. Diethylstilbestrol binds only weakly to α-fetoprotein and can therefore reach the neurons of the preoptic nucleus where it acts like estradiol to masculinize structure and function.

Since the binding of estradiol to α-fetoprotein is not complete, some estradiol may enter the nucleus. The administration of very large amounts of estradiol can thus also produce masculinizing effects, presumably because the binding capacity of the ambient α-fetoprotein is exceeded. Pellets of estradiol implanted directly in the nucleus have the same effects.

The multiplicity of mechanisms is illustrated by the finding of Breedlove and Arnold[51] that the male form of a sexually dimorphic nucleus in rat spinal cord is produced by either T or dihydrotestosterone, but not estradiol.

### Sex Hormone Effects on Human Brain

The situation in the human is less clearcut.[52] The sexual dimorphism of the preoptic nucleus that is so evident in the rat is not clear in the human. Second, the human form of α-fetoprotein does not bind estradiol significantly. There is in the human a sex hormone-binding globulin that, however, binds T more powerfully than it does estradiol. Furthermore, the effects of early exposure to androgens in the human are not as dramatic as those seen in the rat. Early exposure to androgens in adequate dosage prevents the appearance of an estrus cycle in the female rat. Human females with congenital adrenal hypertrophy who produce excessive amounts of androgens are virilized in infancy, yet they may have essentially normal sexual function in later life.

It has, therefore, been argued by some that the effects of early androgens in humans are totally different from their effects in the rat. This extreme view is, however, contradicted by others who argue that the effects in the human are in the same direction, although milder. Karsch et al[53] in reviewing the literature point out that in both nonhuman primates and humans, the administration of T in pregnancy fails to alter normal ovarian cyclicity in female offspring, but that in these cases there is pronounced morphologic and behavioral masculinization.

Female mice with early exposure to androgens show permanent alterations in their responses to these substances, e.g., when T is administered to them in adult life they may show increased aggressivity in contrast to the normal adult female.[54,55] Money and Ehrhardt[56] have found that human females with congenital adrenal hypertrophy do show differences from other females later on, e.g., an increased tendency to participation in rough and tumble sports. Although many of these patients marry and bear children, studies are still lacking on large series to determine whether there are changes in menstrual function, fertility, and pregnancy.

Further evidence supports the view that changes in the human are similar to those in the rat, although of lesser degree. For reasons given above, diethylstilbestrol in the female rat resembles T in its central actions; females exposed early have abnormal estrus function in adult life and increased sensitivity to the actions of androgens. Although the majority of human females exposed to diethylstilbestrol resemble other women on the average, there are certain features that are more common in this population, e.g., masculinizing effects of diethylstilbestrol on the structure of the genitalia.[57] Diethylstilbestrol daughters have been reported to have an elevated rate of menstrual difficulties, infertility, and problems during pregnancy including premature and preterm births, prolonged labor, and a higher rate of children with congenital anomalies[58] but agreement on this is not universal. It will be necessary to conduct a study on a large number of diethylstilbestrol daughters in order to ascertain whether they show an increased rate of the changes in the cortex that we have hypothesized would result from high intrauterine T exposure. One might expect diethylstilbestrol daughters to have an elevated frequency of LH, learning disabilities, spatial talents, and the other associations hypothesized to be more frequent with elevated intrauterine male-related effects. Hines[59] has reviewed the effects of diethylstilbestrol. We have carried out a study on a group of 77 adults exposed to diethylstilbestrol in utero, and our preliminary results show a markedly elevated rate of NRH in this population. Nichols and Chen[60] have found that sex hormones administered to pregnant women lead to an elevated rate of hyperactivity in the offspring, especially in the female offspring.

## Sex Hormone Effects on Cortex

There is evidence in support of the possibility that sex hormones might affect cortical structure. Diamond and colleagues[31] have found that in the male rat at birth and in later life the cortex of several areas in the posterior right hemisphere is significantly thicker than in corresponding areas on the left. By contrast, in the female rat there are several thicker areas on the left at the same periods. If the male rat is castrated at birth, many of the differences in favor of the right side are not observed at 90 days of age,[32] while castration of the newborn female rat also alters the typical pattern. In addition, ovarian hormones administered at birth alter the later pattern of cortical asymmetries. These data clearly support a role for sex hormones in postnatal development in the rat, in this case for both ovarian and testicular hormones. No studies of prenatal hormone effects on rat cortical structure are known to us.

Rosen et al[61] have recently reported that prenatal T alters cerebral laterality, as measured by tail posture at birth, in Wistar rats. Female pups show a predominance of tail turning to the left while males show little lateral preference. Prenatal T causes a shift of the tail posture to the right in the female pups but has no significant effect on males. This work, however, needs replication. Brains from these animals will be studied in our laboratory.

Glick[62] has studied the turning tendencies of Sprague-Dawley rats. In litters with an excess of males there is an increase in the number of females rotating to the left, while in litters with an excess of females the reverse is seen. One possible explanation is that higher ambient levels of T in male-predominant litters increase left-turning in females. In these studies the males are unaffected by the male-female proportions in the litter. The possible effects of T on human litter mates will be discussed in the section on twinning.

Data in humans support the existence of hormonal influences on development of the cortex. Taylor[63] studied cases of temporal lobe epilepsy with unilateral MTS, a lesion believed to follow febrile convulsions. Nearly all MTS cases in their series had had a first seizure before the age of 5. Among cases with a first febrile convulsion before the age of 1 there was a predominance of males with left-sided MTS. With increasing age there were fewer new cases that were more equally divided between males and females and the right and left sides. Taylor suggested that (a) seizures tend to invade less active areas in brain, (b) the right hemisphere matured before the left, and (c) maturation was faster in females than in males. Thus the earliest cases of MTS tended to involve the least mature hemispheres, leading to a predominance of males with left-sided lesions. With increasing maturity there were fewer cases and less selectivity between males and females and the right and left sides.

Although data on hormonal effects on cortical development are limited, there is considerable documentation of direct effects of gonadal hormones on the development of neuronal assemblies in such structures as the preoptic nucleus, which has already been discussed above. In most of these experiments T was administered systemically. There are, however, other experiments in which the same effect was produced by direct placement of hormones in the hypothalamus. Of particular interest is the recent study of Nordeen and Yahr[64] who found lateralized effects. Estradiol implanted in females on one side produced masculinization of behavior, i.e., preference for female sex objects and aggressiveness; on the other side it led to defeminization, i.e., loss of the estrus cycle. These data amplify the earlier findings of Gerendai et al[65] who showed that the luteinizing-hormone releasing hormone (LHRH) content of the right hypothalamus in the rat is double that of the left. Toran-Allerand[66] has shown direct effects of estradiol and T on the growth of neurites of preoptic nucleus neurons in tissue culture. Nottebohm[67] has provided a dramatic example of the effects of T on neuronal growth in the hyperstriatum ventrale, pars caudalis (HVc) nucleus, a structure critically involved in the control of bird song. Normally only the male sings since T is required for song production. There is a striking sexual dimorphism, this nucleus being much larger in the male. The nucleus changes in size in the course of the year, growing each spring under the influence of T and regressing in the fall. There is a marked functional asymmetry in this system, with dominance of the left hemisphere. No structural asymmetry has, however, been found in HVc, although a modest asymmetry is found in the nucleus of cranial nerve XII, one of the peripheral components of the song system.

There are thus many neural systems, including lateralized cortical systems in the rat and a lateralized system for singing in the bird, that are sensitive to the effects of T and other sex hormones. Much more experimental evidence will be required in order to confirm the supposition that the left-sided cortical structures underlying language are particularly sensitive to this hormone in utero. The increasing availability of animal models should make it possible to ascertain whether there are significant hormonal effects on the homologues of the postero-superior temporal cortex and the adjacent junctional region of the left parietal lobe.

It is likely that there will be important species differences. The rat data suggest that there are strain differences. It is not unlikely that there will be variations in human populations in the role played by hormones. Sex hormones administered during pregnancy increased the rate of hyperactivity in the offspring, the effects being greatest in black girls and least in white boys.[60]

Agenesis of the corpus callosum, a frequent anomaly in the Bagg-Albino (BALB) mouse strain is another illustration of possible effects of hormones on cortical systems. In his original description, King[68] pointed out the great variability in the expression of this malformation. Wahlsten[69] has clarified this perplexing situation. If BALB female mice become pregnant while still suckling the young of a previous litter, the new litters will, on the average, be smaller in number, but will contain a higher proportion of animals with agenesis. When the female does not become pregnant until the previous litter is weaned, the new litter will, on the average, be larger in number and will have a lower proportion of affected pups. At this time, one can only speculate on the possible causes of this remarkable phenomenon. One of the likely candidates for the effect of lactation on the formation of the corpus callosum is prolactin. It might have a direct effect on migrating axons, or it may alter the effects of either estradiol or T on the process. It is known that in the liver certain effects of estradiol are modulated by the presence of prolactin. Another possibility is that prolactin alters immune mechanisms which in turn affect formation of the corpus callosum. Prolactin receptors are found on lymphocytes and prolactin can disinhibit certain forms of suppression of the immune response.[70] There are, of course, other possibilities to be considered.

While H-Y antigen is expressed on structures other than the testes, e.g., the thymus,[35] it is unlikely that it is the major mediator of sex differences in brain effects. Females do not carry H-Y antigen, but it is clear that many of the effects observed in males are observed in females although less often, presumably because of exposure to androgens at lower levels. In addition, females may have, as we have noted, high sensitivity to T.

**Other Chemical Effects on Brain Development**

Even if it is true that a male-related factor modulates intrauterine growth of certain cortical regions, it is obvious that cortical development will be susceptible to many other influences, some closely related to the hormonal effects, some more remote. Ward and Weisz[71] showed that if a female rat is stressed during the course of pregnancy the male offspring show demasculinization. Following the stress there is a rapid rise of T in male fetuses, followed by a fall to subnormal levels. It is not clear exactly how stress on the mother leads to this sequence of changes. It is interesting to note that the female offspring of such a stressed mother will also tend to have demasculinized male offspring, even though these females are not themselves stressed in pregnancy. Phenobarbital sodium administered during pregnancy has similar effects and the male offspring have permanently low T levels. This is an example of a phenomenon already mentioned, i.e., chemical effects on the fetus may produce permanent alterations in metabolism. When present in the female they can lead to a mechanism of nongenetic transmission to the following generation.

Sherman et al[30] have also demonstrated an environmental effect on lateralization. In studies carried on some years earlier it had been shown that brief periods of handling of newborn rats exerted permanent effects on emotionality and on other traits, e.g., on resistance to infection. In the more recent experiments it was shown that handled male rats showed greater right-hemisphere lateralization in tests of emotionality and spatial performance than animals who had not been handled.

It should be clear that the emphasis on T by those investigators who have studied sexual and reproductive traits in no way implies that it is the only possible mediator of the structural and chemical alterations that follow manipulations of its level. One can be sure that a myriad of chemical reactions are altered by changes in the level of T, and direct manipulation of any one of the steps involved could lead to similar effects. The same must be true of the effects of T on cortical development.

**Seasonal Effects**

A corollary of our hypothesis is that the hormonal effects on the brain of the offspring may vary with the time of conception. The activity of the pineal gland changes seasonally with alterations in day length. As a general rule one may say that during the dark winter months, the pineal gland becomes active and suppresses both ovaries and testes, while in the summer it is inactive and sex hormone levels are higher. For this reason many animals bear young in the spring, an advantageous situation, since temperature and food supplies are more suitable for survival. An example of such seasonal modulation of hormonal effects on the brain is observed in the HVc nucleus of the singing bird.[66]

This description of pineal physiology is, however, somewhat oversimplified. An animal's sensitivity to light may vary through the year. Gonadal hormonal activation may thus occur in the spring, but as a result of loss of sensitivity to light over the summer, hormone levels may diminish as the fall is approached. Despite these facts day length is a powerful influence. Thus, steers increase their weight more rapidly in the winter when artificial light is supplied to lengthen the day. This light-enhanced growth of muscle mass does not take place if the bull is castrated, suggesting that the effect of light is mediated by a rise in production of T.[72]

While seasonal breeding is the rule in many animals, humans tend to bear young in all months of the year. This does not exclude the existence of photoperiodicity in the human, but much more research is needed. If pineal gland effects on sex hormone levels are important, then the months of birth of left-handers and of those with LD might not be uniform throughout the year, since fetuses conceived at different seasons might be subjected to very different hormonal environments. These effects should differ in the northern and southern hemispheres and at the equator, although other factors, such as variations in the ethnic composition of populations would have to be considered. Data are still very sparse. Badian[73] found that in males born in each of the six months beginning in September the rate of NRH was higher than that in any of the other six months, but no clear trend was observed for female births. A possibly related and intriguing observation in the lamprey is the development of an asymmetric pineal gland.[74] We will return later to the seasonal modulation of hormonal effects on brain development.

## Sex Hormones and Immunity

We have hypothesized that the influences which affect brain lateralization also alter development of the immune system. It was pointed out that several genes in the major histocompatibility complex (MHC) of the mouse influence T levels and sensitivity to it. In this section, some of this evidence will be given in greater detail and further theoretical possibilities will be considered.

It is well known that immune disorders (ID) do not in general affect the two sexes equally. The prepubertal allergic disorders such as asthma, eczema, and hay fever are more likely to affect boys,[75] while after puberty the autoimmune disorders are usually, although not invariably, more common in females. Differences in immune responsiveness of male and female subjects have been documented repeatedly. A common, but perhaps too simple, formulation is that females are more immunocompetent than males, as evidenced, for example, by a greater tendency to reject skin grafts. The New Zealand Black mouse and the New Zealand Black/White mouse models of autoimmunity show important sex differences that will be mentioned later.

There is ample evidence that sex hormones have important effects on immunity, both during development and in later life. The greater involution of the thymus in males after puberty is prevented by castration. Wasi and Block[76] studied the leukemia that occurs in rats during regrowth of the thymus gland after involution produced by radiation. The frequency of leukemia was diminished when radiation was followed by administration of T which inhibited thymic regrowth. Several articles document that T diminishes the size of the thymus gland during development.[77,78] Testosterone administration leads to destruction of the bursa of Fabricius in the chick embryo.[79] Orchidectomy in the prepubertal rat delays thymic involution and in the postpubertal state leads to hypertrophy.[80]

The effects of sex hormones on immunity are not confined to estrogen and T. Lymphocytes have prolactin receptors (but not receptors for T or estradiol) and prolactin will reverse the suppression of immune responses by suppressor T cells.[70,81] It is possible that this effect protects the nursing infant. By increasing the immune responsiveness of the mother, prolactin may heighten her resistance to infection, an effect advantageous to the nursling.

The relationship of sex hormones, especially T, to immunity is an intimate one as shown by the studies of Ivanyi[35] on the MHC of the mouse, the group of genes that play so central a role in the control of immune responsiveness. Ivanyi[35] found loci in the MHC that control the weight of the testis, the serum level of T, the level of T-binding globulin, responsiveness to T, and the expression of the H-Y antigen on the thymus gland. The presence of H-Y antigen on the thymus gland suggests that this substance may play a role in male-female differences in immunity, but it cannot be the only determinant since evidence for direct T effects is plentiful. Another locus in the MHC that controls the production of the fourth component of complement also controls the level of sex-linked protein, a substance normally found in the male but not in the female mouse. The thymic epithelium that processes lymphocytes both in development and in later life contains both T and estradiol receptors, which have not been found on lymphocytes, according to Stimson.[81]

There is another locus found in the human on chromosome 15, which controls production of β-2-microglobulin ($\beta_2M$), a protein essential for immune responsiveness. Ohno[82] has suggested that it is also necessary for the expression of the H-Y antigen, which is itself essential for the development of the male gonads. Smith et al[83] have recently reported, on the basis of large family studies, that dyslexia is linked to a locus on chromosome 15. It would, from the point of view of the theory, not be surprising if a locus that is involved in immune response and testicular development is also involved in the predisposition to dyslexia.

There are still other relationships between the sex hormones and immunity. α-Fetoprotein is an estradiol-binding protein in the rat and therefore plays a major role in the processes that lead to sexual dimorphism of the preoptic nucleus and other structures. It also possesses distinct immunosuppressant actions.[84] Unfortunately, it is not clear that one can extrapolate readily from the rat to the human. Although α-fetoprotein is apparently not thought to be a sex hormone-binding globulin in humans, there are some intriguing parallels. α-Fetoprotein is found in elevated quantities in the amniotic fluid of mothers bearing children with neural tube defects and other major anomalies of the central nervous system. In patients with the Louis-Bar syndrome (ataxia-telangiectasia), in which one finds maldevelopment of the nervous system, immune disorders and, in some cases, gonadal dysgenesis,[85] there is also a high level of α-fetoprotein.

Prolactin is another reproductive hormone with immune effects that may perhaps affect neural development. We have pointed out earlier that BALB mice mothers are more likely to produce offspring suffering from agenesis of the corpus callosum if the litters are conceived while the mother is lactating.[69]

The H-Y antigen is expressed on sperm and on the thymus gland.[35] There are common antigens to germ cells and to brain,[86] suggesting a close developmental relationship between the two, which may have important clinical reflections. Schoene et al[87] reported the postmortem findings of a patient who had died after a prolonged neurologic illness that occurred after an orchitis. In addition to typical severe lesions of multiple sclerosis, there was severe hypertrophic peripheral neuropathy. Another patient who had had a vasectomy, developed a similar clinical syndrome. We have recently seen a third patient who had his first attack of multiple sclerosis coincident with a genitourinary infection. Dr Andrew Herzog is now preparing a report on a group of patients seen by him, and by us, who developed a first temporal lobe seizure following an orchitis or an epididymitis or other genital infection. Philip Paterson, MD (oral communication, September 1984) found in experiments with S. M. Harwin that 10% of rats immunized with ground-up testis or ovary develop the histologic changes of experimental allergic encephalomyelitis. The obese (OS) chicken is a strain that develops a rapidly progressive immune thyroiditis after birth, which can be controlled by administration of T.[88] It is, of course, likely that the immune system has a special role in the development of the nervous system. A remarkable feature of the immune system is its tremendous polymorphism so that lymphocytes are produced that can recognize enormous numbers of different antigens. Ohno[82] has suggested that this system is ideally suited to provide markers or "anchoring sites" that enable developing structures to be built up in precisely the correct form. In no organ system can this type of detailed anchorage mechanism be so important as in the developing nervous system in which many millions of nerve fibers traverse great distances and establish connections with particular groups of target cells. Marking by means of histocompatibility antigens might provide exactly such a system. Sperry[89] showed that if a frog's eye was removed and rotated, the nerve fibers grew back to the locations to which they had been connected previously, a finding that suggested the existence of a system of specific markers. Certain viruses appear to attack neurons within connected systems, raising the possibility that the successive axons have similar anchoring sites for the virus. The poliomyelitis virus will attack the Betz cells of the primary motor cortex as well as anterior horn cells, i.e., connected components of the pyramidal system but almost always spares the neurons controlling the extraocular muscles, the movements of which have no representation within the pyramidal system. The herpes simplex virus does not affect the nervous system randomly but tends to concentrate its attack on connected sets of neurons within the limbic system. A recent article[90] documents that certain monoclonal antibodies bind preferentially to the different components of the limbic system.

If the immune system provides anchoring sites for the processes of axons, then sex hormones that affect the immune system could lead to alterations in the formation of the nervous system. If the immune system provides markers for neural development, then immune suppression at a particular period might lead to disordered neural development. These possibilities are susceptible to direct experimental study.

The later occurrence of ID in patients subjected to parallel influences on the thymus and nervous systems might result from diminished production of lymphocytes involved in self recognition of certain organ systems. This suggests that the organ systems most affected would generally be those that were in the process of active development at the time of the disturbing influences on the immune system. The fact that in our studies[91,92] the most common ID found in individuals with strong LH involved the bowel and the thyroid may give important clues as to the timing of the causative events. This possibility might help to explain data suggesting that particular forms of learning disability have strong associations with certain types of immune disorder, e.g., gut involvement with autism[93] and atopic disorders with stuttering.[94]

The hypothesis that suppression of the thymus at a given period will increase the possibility of later immune attack on organs currently undergoing active development may help to explain another curious phenomenon. Certain MHC alleles in the Buffalo (BUF) rat are strongly associated with the development of autoimmune thyroiditis.[88] This raised the possibility that animals with the appropriate haplotype were more likely to produce antithyroglobulin antibodies. Yet when such antibodies were given to rats of another strain bearing the same haplotypes they were much more resistant than BUF animals. This suggested the presence of a tissue factor, i.e., that the thyroid gland of the BUF animal was more susceptible to immune attack; later studies have shown that the thyroid glands of BUF animals differ in several respects from those of nonsusceptible strains. It has also been pointed out that nonimmune thyroid disorders (e.g., nodular goiter) as well as immune disorders are found in elevated frequency in the families of patients with immune thyroid disease. This also suggests the presence of a tissue factor.

These findings are possible examples of the mechanism proposed above. An anomalous hormonal atmosphere at a particular period in gestation will affect both structures being formed and the processing of lymphocytes that would normally recognize those structures. This implies that malformed structures will often be susceptible to later immune attack. The malformed structure may thus be, in classical terms, a *locus minoris resistentiae* (a site of lowered resistance). The same mechanism may affect the simultaneously developing brain structures, a point to which we will return later.

The sex ratios for immune disorders may appear to present a problem since the hypothesis implies that males should be at greater risk for immune disease.

Indeed, before puberty the common immune disorders are the allergies that are male predominant. After puberty the autoimmune disorders are generally, although not universally, female predominant. There is, however, evidence that T in adult life acts to suppress autoimmunity presumably by its effect on the thymus gland. The implication is, therefore, that the male is indeed *more susceptible* to autoimmune disorders, but is protected by his own production of T after puberty. High T effect in utero increases susceptibility to immune disease, but after puberty it diminishes its expression. If this hypothesis is correct, then males subjected to high T effect in utero but who are hypogonadal after puberty should have very high rates of autoimmune disease. The Klinefelter male appears to fit this picture, since they may have high T levels even at birth, but later become hypogonadal. It has been suggested that they have a high rate of autoimmune disorder.

Data on the New Zealand Black mouse are concordant with this hypothesis. The animals develop spontaneous autoimmunity that occurs earlier and with greater severity in the female. Castration of the female at birth has no effect, but castration of the male leads to acceleration of the ID. Conversely, T retards the disease in females. In another recently developed mouse model of autoimmunity, males are more susceptible, but detailed hormonal studies have not yet been carried out.[95]

This hypothesis is in keeping with other findings concerning several autoimmune diseases. Myasthenia gravis is more common in young women and old men, i.e., in those groups in whom androgen effects are the lowest. Lupus erythematosus has a strong female preponderance but with increasing age the percentage of new male cases increases. Furthermore, before puberty the proportion of male cases is higher than it is after puberty. In hereditary angioneurotic edema, an immune, but not an autoimmune disorder, one of the most effective treatments is danazol, a modified T with definite although diminished masculinizing effects.

Many questions remain concerning the relationships between sex hormones and immunity. Not all ID are female predominant, e.g., Marie-Strümpell disease (rheumatoid spondylitis), perhaps ten times as common in male as in female subjects. It has been suggested that the female prevalence is higher than the figure just quoted because many women develop the disorder in mild form, but even if this is the case one must still account for greater severity in male subjects. There are, furthermore, late onset female-predominant ID, such as temporal arteritis. These discrepancies should not be surprising. Immune disorders are not a monolithic category, but rather include many conditions with different mechanisms. It is not unlikely that when more information is available, it will be found that there are certain classes of ID that are most frequent in left-handers, while others are more frequent in right-handers, while in still others there is no difference. Furthermore, sex hormones may play a large role in certain types and not in others.

Differences in the frequency of the allergic and immune diseases may well be paralleled by differences in susceptibility to infection. Females are less likely to die of infection than are males, and this must be in good part attributable to differences in the immune system. This would presumably have made excellent biologic sense in earlier human communities in which the lifestyles of males and females were so different. Females were more likely to be in close contact with children and many members of the community other than males who were more often away from home. Female resistance to infection would protect her, the children, and other members of the community. Resistance to infection may have disadvantages, since the prostrating effects of many illnesses are primarily the result of the immune response. This might have been less of a problem for females surrounded by other family members than for the more isolated males away from home. Lessened male immune response would imply less temporary incapacity, although at the price of increased risk of death from infection itself.

The possibility that decreased risk of infection is the result of a more active immune system is in conformity with recent suggestions that children susceptible to allergic disorders are more resistant to parasitic infection.[96] It has been pointed out[97] that parasitic infection tends to cause immune suppression. It would be interesting to know if this occurs less often in children susceptible to allergic disorders. This raises the possibility that male subjects with anomalous dominance are more resistant to many infections than those with standard dominance patterns.

It is likely that some organisms will have developed special strategies for attacking individuals resistant to most infections. Even under the special conditions of pregnancy, females are resistant to many infections but they may be at elevated risk for some particular disorders. In the great epidemics of poliomyelitis that preceded the introduction of successful vaccination, many observers were struck by the great susceptibility of pregnant women, and the same observation was made during the worldwide spread of epidemic encephalitis in the 1920s. Similarly, the anomalous dominance population may be resistant to most infections but have a heightened susceptibility to others. We have been struck by an apparently high frequency of LH among former victims of poliomyelitis, and are planning to explore this possibility in a formal study.

The interrelationship between laterality and the immune system is highlighted by recent findings that brain lesions in each hemisphere may have different effects on immunity. Renoux et al[98,99] found that left cortical lesions in the rat reduced the number of natural killer (NK) cells while right-sided lesions had no such effect.

## Genetics and Chromosomes

### Genetics of Laterality

Cerebral dominance was described long before general awareness of Mendel's discoveries, but once these had entered the general consciousness of scientists, investigators began to study the possible genetics of handedness. Much of the early success of the mendelian doctrine of segregation of characters and of the later discovery of genes was the result of study of fairly simple systems to which the principles could be readily applied. It has, however, become increasingly clear that there are many phenomena explainable only by complex mechanisms. The simplest forms of dominant or recessive transmission are easily handled, but it is more difficult to deal with polygenic inheritance. Attempts to analyze handedness on the basis of simple classic dominant or recessive inheritance were not successful. Perhaps the most successful theory of the genetics of laterality is that of Annett[100] which attains high agreement with observed distributions. Although, as will become clear, our own views on the detailed genetic mechanisms involved in laterality are different from those of Annett, we must express our debt to her contributions without which we would have been unable to develop our own formulations. Among these important contributions was the concept of random dominance that was discussed in an earlier section. She postulates the existence of a gene that favors left-hemispheric dominance in the absence of which dominance for language or handedness is determined by random effects. Many pieces of evidence are in concordance with this concept. Mice will tend to use one forepaw consistently in a task that must be carried out unimanually, but the distribution of dextral and sinistral mice is approximately equal. Collins[101] mated only mice who used the same paw but after several generations of such selective breeding the offspring still showed an even distribution of dextrality or sinistrality. It is thus evident that in these animals there is random dominance for paw preference.

A similar situation prevails in hereditary situs inversus in mice.[102] Even when homozygous animals are mated, only half the offspring show reversed situs, even though the offspring with normal situs are as likely as the affected offspring to transmit the condition to their own offspring. In this case there is transmission not of reversed situs but rather of random situs.

The major difference between our ideas and those of Annett resides in the fundamental assumptions. She postulates the absence of a gene for right cerebral dominance but the existence of one that favors a "right shift," i.e., it increases the probability of left-cerebral dominance for either language or handedness. The homozygotes will have an even greater probability of left cerebral dominance than the heterozygotes, while individuals who lack the gene will have essentially random dominance. The theory specifically makes allowances for non-genetic effects, so that even among homozygotes there is an increased probability, but not a certainty, of left dominance. The Annett formulation successfully predicts the distribution of handedness under many conditions, although it does not deal explicitly with such phenomena as the greater degree of LH in males and in twins and their first-degree relatives.

Our own formulation is in some respects similar to that of Corballis and Morgan[103] who postulates the existence of a "left shift," i.e., influences that tend to favor right cerebral dominance, but differ in several ways. We begin with the assumption that cerebral dominance is determined primarily by anatomic asymmetry so that language lateralization will depend to a great extent on the size of the planum temporale, which is larger on the left side in about 65% of brains.[104] While the left side can be even ten times larger than the right, one rarely finds the reverse, i.e., it is unusual for the right side to be massive compared with the left. One finds a size distribution that is markedly skewed to the left, and as we have already noted this appears to be the case even in utero,[105] although the right side develops more rapidly.[106] Our presumption is that the basic pattern of most brains includes a larger left side. (We will discuss the possible existence of brains whose fundamental pattern is reversed in part III.) Certain influences in the course of pregnancy tend to slow development on the left side; the greater these influences, the more likely that the brain will be shifted toward symmetry, and in a few cases even to modest asymmetry favoring the right side. Our hypothesis is essentially the mirror image of Annett's, i.e., we presume a strongly left-hemispheric basic dominance pattern, and a set of influences that produce a shift to increasing symmetry, and thus favor random dominance.

We have earlier described several genetic factors that might play a role in this process by controlling the levels of hormones, especially T, as well as sensitivity to it. These include the Y chromosome, several major histocompatibility locus genes, as well as genes on the X chromosome and chromosome 15. There are probably other types of genetic influence, e.g., the baseline level of left-sided asymmetry probably varies in the population.

The hypothesis advanced in this article helps to explain some aspects of the distribution of handedness not dealt with by some other proposals, e.g., the greater frequency of LH in male subjects. We will discuss the elevated rates of LH in twins and their first-degree relatives, another feature that poses a problem for many theories.

There are other features of the familial distributions that present problems for any genetic theory, e.g., a trend for LH mothers to have more LH children than LH fathers. We will argue that the number of nongenetic factors involved in the determination of laterality is so large that no purely genetic theory will be able to deal with them. These factors will not affect all fetuses at random but may preferentially affect a particular group, e.g., males, females, or twins. Further discussion of the existing genetic theories may be found in Porac and Coren[107] and Bryden.[108]

The difficulties inherent in this field are well demonstrated by two sets of breeding experiments. Larrabee[109] described the asymmetry of the completely decussated optic nerves in the trout and cod; the nerve from the right eye crosses dorsal to the one from the left eye in 60% of cases. His attempts to alter this ratio by selective breeding failed. In an ingenious experiment he produced two-headed monsters, the two heads of which have, of course, identical genetic endowments. The distribution of right or left dorsal crossings in the two heads was identical to that found in two individuals chosen at random from the general population.

In flounders both eyes are on one side of the head: in some on the right, in others on the left. The distribution on the two sides varies in the different species that occupy particular geographic niches. Cross-breeding experiments between species have been carried out with findings that did not fit readily into any standard nuclear genetic model.[110] It is possible that the variations in the distribution of asymmetry may be determined to a great extent by differing environmental conditions, e.g., water temperature or food supply. This possibility gains credence from the fact that the sex ratio of the offspring of certain species shifts sharply from female predominant to male predominant depending on the temperature or food supply.[111,112] In several species, the sex ratio can vary considerably depending on the hormonal conditions of pregnancy. James[113,114] has suggested that this may be true even in humans. It is thus also conceivable that there is a genetic bias toward one form of laterality that is modified by environmental conditions that alter hormonal atmosphere or the time of fertilization.

Another problem for any genetic theory of laterality is the existence of genes that may determine the presence of asymmetry but not its direction. Dahlberg[115] pointed out several examples in both animals and humans. Certain unilateral anomalies such as polydactyly or heterochromia iridis (different colors of the two irises) may be found in different members of a kinship sometimes on one side, sometimes on the other. This is in contrast to other unilateral anomalies that may be consistently on one side. Dahlberg suggested the existence of genes determining asymmetry but not direction. Collins[101] has recently suggested that one can breed mice for a strong tendency to use one paw, but not for which paw will be used.

### Cytoplasmic and Maternal Inheritance

One must explain a basic pattern postulated to favor left-hemisphere dominance in the great majority of instances. In our view, the most reasonable hypothesis is that advanced by Corballis and Morgan,[103] i.e., that there is a fundamental asymmetry that is probably in the ovum itself. This fundamental asymmetry may well be determined by maternal cytoplasmic factors, which deserve a brief discussion.

Most accounts of inheritance refer to nuclear genes, i.e., genes located on chromosomes. Another group of genes, overwhelmingly maternally derived, is found in the cytoplasm. The ovum contributes many cytoplasmic genes to the zygote, while the sperm contributes few, if any.[116] These are well known in plant genetics but have received less attention in studies of animal heredity. There has been special emphasis on cytoplasmic genes associated with mitochondria, thus leading to stress on their role in regulation of energy metabolism within the fertilized egg before the conceptus develops its own metabolic systems controlled by its own nuclear genes. Recent studies show that at least in some species maternal cytoplasmic genes are also involved in production of structural proteins, e.g., actin.[117] Furthermore, these genes may be active during development for a much longer period than was previously thought. It is increasingly clear that these genes are important in higher animals.

Cytoplasmic genes are often modulated by nuclear genes. In *Drosophila* the inheritance of the anomaly designated as *tumor head* is jointly controlled by cytoplasmic and nuclear genes.[118] A striking example of another type of cytoplasmic role in heredity is afforded by the snail *Lymnaea peregra,* the spiral patterns of whose shells were studied by Boycott and Diver.[119] In the initial studies the dextral or sinistral spiral patterns of offspring appeared to have little relationship to that of the parents. It eventually became clear that this was an example of *delayed inheritance.* There are nuclear genes for dextral coiling (*d*) that are dominant and for sinistral coiling (*s*) that are recessive. The coiling of the offspring is determined *only by the mother's genotype.* Thus, if the mother carries *ds,* the offspring all coil dextrally regardless of the genes contributed to the zygote by the sperm. If the father were also *ds* in this case, this would thus not affect the coiling of the offspring, some of whom will be *dd,* others *ds,* and still others *ss.* An *ss* female offspring of this union of two *ds* parents would herself coil dextrally, but all her offspring would coil sinistrally. The coiling pattern of the offspring is thus determined by nuclear genes contributed by the ovum that controls the pattern of spiral cleavage. These nuclear genes thus act on the cytoplasm of the zygote, possibly by affecting the expression of cytoplasmic genes. Freeman and Lundelius[120] have shown that the dextral gene carries a product that will cause dextral coiling if injected into the maternal cytoplasm, but the sinistral gene has no effect. Whether such delayed effects on asymmetry are seen in higher animals and in particular, in humans has not, to our knowledge, been studied.

Note that another way to describe these data is that coiling of any individual can be predicted from the genetic endowment of the *maternal grandparents.* The potential application to the human is obvious. It will be important to ascertain whether this type of delayed inheritance plays a role in humans. Another point to stress is that in the situation just discussed the mother's contribution to the offspring's laterality is more important than that of the father. Several studies in humans have shown a closer relationship of the laterality of the offspring to that of the mother than that of the father.[107]

Nance[121] has called attention to a maternal effect in the inheritance of human neural tube defects. Mothers who had conceived an infant with a neural tube defect by one husband were more likely than control mothers to have an affected child by a second husband. By contrast, fathers of a child with a neural tube defect by one wife were no more likely than control fathers to have an affected child in a second marriage. These data suggest a maternal factor affecting neural development.

Although we agree with the basic postulate of Corballis and Morgan[103] concerning a maternal cytoplasmic effect favoring the left hemisphere, we do not agree with their additional assumption that the left hemisphere grows more rapidly. The available evidence that we have reviewed in detail in an earlier section clearly supports the contrary, i.e., that right-hemisphere growth is faster than that of the left.

If cytoplasmic inheritance plays a role in the human, are we to assume that the ovum always carries a bias toward larger speech and handedness regions in the left hemisphere, or is there some minority of ova that carry a bias in the opposite direction? In the studies of Boycott et al[122] most female snails carried a dextral bias while a small number carried the opposite one. Verkoren (personal communication, January 1983) has, for example, argued that right and left biases in cytoplasmic genes may be primary determinants of laterality. If more than one bias is present in the population, are we to assume that all the ova of a particular human female carry the same bias? Although many copies of cytoplasmic genes are found in a cell it is likely, on the basis of recent studies, that different alleles would not be present, or if present, only in very small numbers.[116] The ova of one particular female would presumably, therefore, carry only a single bias. There is no way to deal with these questions at present. The existence of asymmetry in other species should make many of these problems readily accessible to laboratory experimentation. We will discuss the issue of reverse bias in the last section of the article. As we will point out shortly, even if such biases exist in humans, they must be modified to a considerable extent by nongenetic factors.

### Paternal Effects

The father contributes half his nuclear genes to the zygote, but following fertilization has no further influence on its development. Preconception environmental influences can, however, alter the paternal contribution. Some gross effects of this type are easy to understand, e.g., radiation causing damage to paternal germ cells could lead to chromosomal damage and thus to effects on offspring. Some environmental effects may be less crude. A disproportionate number of parents, both fathers and mothers, of autistic children are reported to have had contact with chemicals.[93] It is possible that chemicals might preferentially affect the fertilizing capacity of sperm carrying certain specific genes. Genes on the Y chromosome could be a source of paternal influences on male offspring. It appears likely that the major effects of this chromosome are mediated indirectly via the induction of tests and the production of T. There is evidence, however, that the Y chromosome may have direct genetic effects, as shown, e.g., by the recent work of Maxon[123] on the inheritance of aggressive behavior in rats.

Another possible source of paternal effects is the T/t gene complex located in the MHC in the mouse.[124,125] It has been suggested that a homologue of this gene complex exists in humans, but this is still under discussion.[126] Although the mouse homozygous for the allele *t* does not survive, animals heterozygous for *t* are still found with high frequency. Although only half of the sperm of a *t*-bearing father carry this gene complex, *t* is transmitted to more than half the offspring, presumably because a sperm bearing *t* has a greater chance of fertilizing an ovum than one which does not. Thus the offspring of a father heterozygous for *t* will inherit *t* in a large majority of matings. This group of genes may have a role in neural development since the lethal *tt* homozygote frequently has anomalies thought by some to resemble human neural tube defects. Exposure of the father to chemicals might well alter the expression of *t* in sperm and thus change the proportion of offspring who carried this allele and the genes linked to it. Since *t* not only affects the probability of fertilization by the sperm that carries it but also inhibits recombination in the chromosome on which it is located, it could well play an important role in altering expected standard genetic effects. There is no evidence at present that *t* plays a role in dominance but with the identification of dominance in rodents this possibility could be tested.

Exposure of the father to chemicals might simply modify the genes transmitted to the offspring (e.g., by methylation) and thus alter the environment of the fetus. There is as yet no clear evidence for any of these speculations.

Another speculative possibility is that paternal cytoplasmic genes could be carried into the zygote. There is little information known to us in relation to this possibility, but most authorities on cytoplasmic genes tend to regard it as unlikely. Although some paternal cytoplasmic genes are probably contributed to the conceptus, their number is very small. As has been pointed out, they are likely not to play an important role in mammals.[116]

## The Role of Nongenetic Factors

Annett[100] postulates that possession of the right-shift gene increases the probability of left-hemisphere dominance; the magnitude of the effect, however, varies from individual to individual because of other random influences. One possible source of such effects might be other genes producing small modifications in the effects of some major gene.

Environmental influences can constitute an important source of non-genetic influences on laterality. Since the effect of a gene is to play a role in some form of chemical reaction, it is not surprising that there is no absolute genetic determination. Every chemical reaction is modifiable by alterations in pressure, temperature, pH, light, the presence of other substances, the availability of chemical precursors, and the rate of removal of products. With the growing sophistication of molecular genetics, it has become increasingly clear that non-genetic effects can play a powerful role, e.g., methylation has been shown to suppress expression of many genes. We will now consider some of the random effects that might modify lateralization.

One implication of our hypothesis is that even if one knew precisely the genetic endowment of any particular fetus, one would not be able to predict the exact lateralization pattern of the brain, although one would be able to make predictions concerning the distribution in a population basis. One of the reasons for this relative freedom from genetic determination is that if hormones do play a role in determining laterality, then the effects of T or related substances on the developing brain will be modified by factors not under the control of the fetal genes. Androgens are produced not only by fetal testes and the placenta, but also by the maternal ovaries, adrenals, and nonglandular tissues. The fetus can be influenced by the actions of many of the maternal genes that it does not share. It is reasonable to expect that if a fertilized ovum were transplanted into the uterus of an unrelated female the final pattern of the brain would be quite different because the brain would develop in an environment of hormones and other substances that would certainly differ in many respects.

Therefore, it might be reasonable to study the genetics of many conditions in a different way from that usually followed. One should perhaps not consider the genes carried only by the offspring, but rather the genes of that organism that exists only for the nine months of pregnancy, i.e., the mother and the fetus considered as a unit. This organism contains three groups of different genes, i.e., one paternal set present in the fetus, one maternal set carried only in the mother, while the other maternal set is carried both by the mother and the offspring. The situation is even more complex when there are dizygotic twins since the maternal-fetal organism will contain another group of paternal genes.

The effects of substances produced by the mother will, however, be diminished by the capacity of the placenta to provide a barrier to some maternal hormones. The fetus is protected to a great extent from maternal T that is converted to estradiol by placental aromatase. Dihydrotestosterone, which is not aromatized and therefore crosses the placenta, is, however, usually present in the mother at much lower levels than T. The protection from maternal T is not complete since offspring do show signs of masculinization when mothers are exposed to this hormone. In addition, progesterone administered to the mother may masculinize female fetuses. It is clear that the placental barrier is far from complete. Furthermore, it is likely that there are individual variations in the aromatizing capacity of the placenta.

It is conceivable that some maternal genes not shared by the offspring have greater effects on female fetuses. Thus the T to which female fetuses are exposed comes predominantly from maternal tissues while males produce it in high quantities. In the study of Nichols and Chen[60] sex hormones given to mothers were associated with a higher rate of hyperactivity in female offspring than in male offspring.

Another random factor is stress during pregnancy, which can lead in the rat to demasculinization of male offspring. Exposure of the mother to exogenous chemicals is another source of random effects. Sodium phenobarbital administered in pregnancy also causes demasculinization of male offspring who have permanently low T production.[127] Exogenous sex hormones should, by our hypothesis, lead to modifications in lateralization of offspring. Nichols and Chen[60] found that children of mothers who received sex hormones during pregnancy had an elevated rate of hyperactivity, another condition in which LH is found in elevated frequency.

Denenberg et al[128] have shown a direct effect of postnatal environment on lateralization. Male rats handled in infancy exhibit more conspicuous right-hemisphere lateralization of activity than animals who are not handled. Previous studies on early handling demonstrated a wide variety of later metabolic and hormonal alterations.[129] If metabolic effects alter dominance, then maternal diet may represent yet another nongenetic influence.

The argument of this section might be summarized briefly by a statement made earlier: an individual could have different dominance characteristics if the fertilized ovum were transplanted into another mother's uterus. While this hypothesis cannot be tested easily in the human, it is certainly subject to straightforward study in experimental animals.

### Seasonal Effects

The time of conception is another nongenetic random variable that may well have important influence on laterality. Seasonal effects have often been considered narrowly. The fact that schizophrenics are more likely to be born in January than July, a repeatedly documented finding, has often been interpreted as a result of increased susceptibility to virus infection of newborn infants in the winter. There are many other possibilities, e.g., changes in sex hormones with day length. The pineal gland, activated in the dark months, tends to suppress gonadal hormonal production. When it is suppressed, during periods of long day length, sex hormone levels rise. We have already alluded to Badian's report of a higher rate of NRH in males born from September through February, i.e., conceived from December through May. Day length is at a minimum on Dec 21 and increases for the following six months. A pineal gland role in laterality has no direct experimental support but certainly deserves study. There are ample data showing the importance of seasonal factors. Seasonal variations in congenital anomalies at birth have been repeatedly documented. It is clear that these cannot be attributed to postnatal effects, e.g., susceptibility of the offspring to infection. Births of infants with neural tube defects are most common in the first three months of the year, and twin births show a similar marked seasonal variation. It is known that there is a greater number of dizygotic twin births in mothers given human chorionic gonadotropin. One might expect circumannual variations in sex hormone production would be paralleled by changes in the gonadotropin level, and therefore more twin conceptions in the months in which maternal gonadotropin levels were the highest.

### Transgenerational Effects

There is another possible but surprising source of random variation. If rats are subjected to stress during pregnancy, the offspring show altered emotional behavior. In turn, the offspring of affected female offspring show similar changes in emotional behavior despite the absence of exposure of their mothers to external stress. One does not have to look far for an explanation. The offspring of a mother subjected to stress in pregnancy show permanent alterations in their own behavior and are more susceptible to stress effects than normal animals. Therefore, when the females among them become pregnant even minor stresses will affect them and their offspring will, in turn, be affected. We thus have here an example of what might loosely be termed a "Lamarckian" effect.

There are two mechanisms by which such persistent effects of stress could be mediated. Stress produces either structural alterations in the brain of the offspring and/or permanent metabolic alterations. Thus newborn female rats exposed to T manifest a series of permanent metabolic changes. They are more sensitive in later life to androgens than normal females in later life. They carry sex-linked protein that is normally found only in males,[130] but conversely certain liver enzymes normally found in females disappear.[40] There is thus an increased possibility that the female who was subjected to excessive T effects in utero will herself show an increased tendency to hormonal masculinization that will in turn affect her offspring. In the rat, diethylstilbestrol has masculinizing effects on brain regions involved in reproductive behavior.[131] In the human, diethylstilbestrol also appears to have certain masculinizing effects,[56] and diethylstilbestrol daughters have been reported in some series to have a higher rate of infertility and difficulties in pregnancy, but other series dispute this.[132] We hypothesize that they will have a higher proportion of children with anomalous dominance, i.e., a higher rate of LH and of the other associations of atypical laterality. Preliminary studies now under way appear to be in agreement with this.

There will be certain limitations on such transgenerational masculinizing effects. Even if the mother is masculinized by endogenous or exogenous hormones, the fetus may be shielded from them to a varying degree by the placenta, as has already been noted.

## Age and Parity Effects

Maternal age and parity both influence the outcome of pregnancy, but these two influences are often confused. In order to separate the effects, it is necessary to compare women of the same parity but different ages, and women of equal age but of different parity. Since the two influences might work in opposite directions, failure to separate them may cancel out any positive effects. Twinning in Nigeria increases with both age and parity.[133,134] Twinning is only one example of these effects of age and parity. Certain congenital anomalies, e.g., neural tube defects, also vary with age and parity. Certain other factors thought to influence twinning or neural tube defects may be reducible to these influences.

The exact reasons for these effects are not entirely clear. It has been speculated that parity effects may depend on immune factors. An obvious example is erythroblastosis fetalis occurring in Rh-negative mothers of Rh-positive children, which is more likely to occur in later pregnancies, since the mother is sensitized to fetal red blood cells in the first pregnancy and produces antibodies more rapidly in a second one. Another possibility may be that high parity selects for women who may be particularly fertile as a result of high levels of hormones. The cause of age effects is also not fully clarified, although certain chromosomal changes increase with age.

Do maternal age and parity influence the frequency of anomalous dominance in the offspring? There are many articles both supporting and opposing the hypothesis that maternal age and birth order have an influence on handedness. It is clear that maternal age and parity can have influences on the offspring that are independent to a considerable extent from genetics.

It is interesting that many clinicians believe that dyslexia is more common in adopted children, but we do not know of any definite documentation of this statement. Adopted children include a higher proportion of the offspring of very young mothers. On the other hand, it is conceivable that adopted children are disproportionately often offspring of parents with anomalous dominance, but this is also speculative. This problem deserves more careful documentation and further study.

## Twins and Anomalous Dominance

Even early studies of the genetics of handedness revealed an excess of left-handers among twins, and, even more surprising, among their relatives. The recent work of Boklage[135] has shown that the rate of LH in twins (both monozygotic and dizygotic) and in their mothers, fathers, and siblings is double that of the siblings of the parents. This would appear to support the belief that twinning and sinistrality are associated, since otherwise one would have to argue that the second-degree relatives of twins had lower rates than the general population. The elevated level of LH in both types of twins and their first-degree relatives has no simple genetic explanation and may reflect nongenetic influences.

The distribution of LH among identical twins has typically been one of the major difficulties in the formulation of any genetic theory of handedness. One would expect that in any identical twin pair both would be right-handed or both left-handed. Yet this is conspicuously not the case. A typical distribution might be: both right-handed, 80%; both left-handed, 4%; and one right, one left, 16%. Annett[100] explains this distribution by her genetic theory. A certain number of twin pairs would not carry the right-shift gene and, therefore, in these pairs handedness would be random. In one-quarter of the pairs, both would be left-handed, in another quarter both right-handed, and in half there would be opposite handedness. This is in contrast to other popular theories. One of these is the theory that some twin pairs are mirror images. In general, this notion has not received wide acceptance in recent years in part because it is rare to find situs inversus in one member of a pair of identical twins. It is possible in experimental animals to produce twin pairs, one of whom does show situs inversus, but it is still likely that this is at best a rare event in the human.

The other popular theory, which has been applied to both types of twins, is that of birth trauma. It is well known that twins are more likely to have difficult births, and the argument is therefore advanced that it will not be rare for one twin to suffer some brain damage. As Satz[136] has pointed out, random unilateral brain damage at birth will tend to increase the number of left-handers. Since a majority of the injured children would be right-handed there will be very few cases of shift of handedness in cases with right-hemisphere lesions, but a large number will be shifted as a result of left-hemisphere lesions. Although this mechanism certainly must occur, it is questionable whether it could account for so large a percentage of twins of opposite handedness. It fails, however, to account for the high rate of sinistrality in first-degree relatives of twins. Boklage[135] has pointed out that there is a 15% higher frequency of LH in second-born dizygotic twins than in their cotwins or siblings. This may well reflect birth trauma but, of course, cannot account for the very high rate of sinistrality in twins and their first-degree relatives.

There is a third theory which asserts that the pattern of handedness in twin pairs is no different from that of any pair of individuals chosen at random from the general population, an issue still under dispute.

Before discussing some possible causes of the dominance patterns of twins, let us consider some facts concerning multiple births. Twins may be identical (monozygotic), both arising from the same fertilized egg, or fraternal (dizygotic), usually thought to result from the fertilization of two separate ova. Monozygotic twins share the same chromosomes and, therefore, the same nuclear genes, while dizygotic twins are usually said to resemble each other on the average no more than any two siblings, i.e., they share half their genes. Boklage[135] believes that there may also be polar body twins. Before fertilization the ovum undergoes two divisions. In the first the number of chromosomes goes from the normal diploid number to the haploid number in which each half carries half of the maternal chromosomes. The haploid ovum then undergoes division. One of the ova produced in the first division regresses to form the first polar body, which is then extruded. Similarly, in the second division one ovum regresses to form the second polar body. Boklage[135] has suggested that in some cases the polar body does not regress and may also be fertilized by a different sperm. In this case the twins would be intermediate in genetic resemblance between dizygotic and monozygotic twins, sharing the same maternal chromosomes but, on the average, only half the paternal chromosomes. Polar body twins will thus share on the average three-quarters of their genes.

It is possible, however, that the genetic resemblance of both monozygotic twins and polar body twins may be less than these theoretical figures. Monozygotic twins are the result of cleavage of a fertilized ovum into two zygotes. The maternal genes carried in the cytoplasm of the ovum may be distributed unequally to the two zygotes. If cytoplasmic genes play a role in laterality, the offspring might differ. The same considerations apply, perhaps even more strongly to polar body twins, since the division of the cytoplasm is so unequal.

The rate of monozygotic twinning differs little throughout the world, i.e., about three twin births per thousand. The dizygotic twinning rate, however, varies considerably. Thus some older data showed that among the Japanese there was approximately one dizygotic twin birth out of 165, while in northern Ireland and Scotland the rate was about three times as high. The rates in northern Europe are generally of this order while rates in southern Europe are lower.[133] The highest twinning rates so far observed occur in West Africa, particularly among the Yoruba, especially in the vicinity of Ibadan, where the rate is about one in 18 births. In young Yoruba women of high parity, the rate of twinning may be nearly one in ten births. It is no surprise that twin dolls are a characteristic feature of Yoruba art. In the United States, blacks (mostly of West African descent) have higher twinning rates and Orientals lower ones than whites.[133]

Familial monozygotic twinning is rare and does not share the high rate of congenital anomalies observed among familial dizygotic twins, which are much more common. Some recent data from Italy[137] suggest, however, that monozygotic twinning may occur more often than expected in families in which dizygotic twinning is found. There is also a high rate of neural tube defects in many populations in which dizygotic twinning is common, e.g., northern Ireland and Scotland. In China, with a very low rate of dizygotic twinning, neural tube defects occur about one-tenth as frequently as in northern Ireland.[138] It is very possible that the rate of twin conceptions is higher than is generally appreciated since in some cases one twin may undergo fetal death and be resorbed. The twinning rate has been falling in recent years in Europe as has the rate of neural tube defects, data for which no satisfactory explanation has yet been found.

The possible relationship between twinning and dominance may be revealed in part by consideration of some known influences on twinning. Mothers treated for infertility with either human chorionic gonadotropin (HCG) or clomiphene have markedly increased rates of multiple births.[139] Because of the high gonadotropin levels in both forms of therapy, more follicles mature and release ova, thus increasing the rate of dizygotic twinning. There are other circumstances in which gonadotropin levels can be high. Masculinized females who, by our hypothesis, should have a high rate of personal and familial anomalous dominance, have elevated levels of luteinizing hormone.[140] Since their offspring may have greater exposure to masculinizing effects in utero, they may have an elevated rate of LH. This hypothesis is in conformity with the higher rate of LH in mothers of twins and in the twins themselves.

There are two other reasons for a possible higher rate of LH in twins. Since the mothers will tend to be masculinized, they will, of course, often come from families with a tendency to greater T production or sensitivity and this will be shared by the twins. There is, however, another effect that is essentially nongenetic. Since male twins both produce T, each will conceivably be exposed to higher levels than he would be if he were a singleton. The females of opposite-sex pairs should, by this hypothesis, have a high rate of LH because of exposure to T produced by the male cotwins. This type of effect has been observed in rats. A female rat lying in the uterus with males behind her will show a greater degree of androgen effects than other females, since the vasculature will carry T from the males in an anterior direction.[141] Other articles on the rat also document masculinizing effects by males on females in utero.[142,143] The least T effect should be found in all-female pairs. In all-male pairs one twin should be subjected to a higher level of T than the other. Glick[62] has found that the rate of turning to the left in response to amphetamine is higher in female rats from litters with higher percentages of male siblings.

Another finding in conformity with the hypothesis is the reported higher rates of dyslexia among twins.[144]

Further studies are suggested by these conjectures. Although masculinized women have a low fertility rate, one might expect an elevated rate of twin births. One would expect a higher rate of twin births among pregnant diethylstilbestrol daughters. As we have already noted above, the seasonal variation in twin births is compatible with the hypothesis, since hormone levels may vary seasonally.

Boklage[135] observed an elevated rate of LH among the fathers as well as among mothers of twins. This might occur because some of the sperm of left-handed fathers have special properties, e.g., they might have a higher rate of fertilization of ova that would lead to a rise in dizygotic twinning. The zygotes resulting from fertilization might have a higher rate of cleavage to twin zygotes, and this would favor monozygotic twinning. If the polar bodies of such zygotes regressed less often, polar body twinning would occur more frequently. We have already pointed out that the allele *t* associated with the major histocompatibility complex of the mouse does alter the behavior of sperm and is transmitted to offspring from fathers more frequently than the 50% expectation. If *t*-bearing sperm had an increased potential for fertilization of an ovum then twins might be expected in elevated frequency. If the same effect were found in the human, this could lead to an increased number of twin offspring. Since the T/t locus in the human has not been positively identified it is conceivable that its behavior might be different. As already noted, the allele *t* in the mouse is associated with disorders similar to neural tube defects so that it may place a role in formation of the central nervous system. We have already commented on the association of rates for twinning and neural tube disorders.

A relationship of sperm characteristics to lateralization is strongly suggested by the findings in Kartagener's syndrome in which affected males have situs inversus and abnormalities of the sperm.[145] In patients with celiac disease, who, as already noted, have high rates of sinistrality, abnormalities of sperm are common.[146] The possible relationships of sperm abnormalities and laterality determination will be discussed in the last section.

In any case, the mechanism of the effect of paternal sinistrality on twinning remains unclear. This problem too should be susceptible to study in laboratory animals.

## The Diversity of the Brain

There are critical periods for the development of structures during which they are particularly susceptible to external influences. Radiation will lead to an increased rate of cleft palate only during a particular very short period. This existence of critical periods is a useful strategy for reducing the possibilities of interference with normal development, since a rapidly developing structure will not be susceptible during most of pregnancy, and a deleterious effect manifest at some particular time will damage only a few structures. The development of the cortex, however, does not appear to be an example of this mechanism, since it appears to include much of pregnancy, and also a significant period following birth. The cortex is presumably protected to a considerable extent by the presence of an excess of neurons during intrauterine life (and probably in the early postnatal period) which tends to guard against harmful effects of localized destruction at a particular time. This long period of development may confer benefits that outweigh the disadvantages of exposure to injury over an extended period. If a system is capable of alteration at many different periods by random influences occurring over a long time, then genetic determination of the final form will be much weaker than it is for systems maturing over a very brief span and thus less likely to be modified by outside agents. The genetic determination of lateralization in the cortex will be weaker than that for other structures if even only a few of the nongenetic effects listed earlier are significant. The system is subject to many influences that can alter the process at many times during pregnancy and postnatally. It has recently been pointed out that the appearance of long-fiber tracts in the course of evolution makes the developing nervous system more subject to external influences, since such a process necessarily requires a long period of time.[147]

The pattern of cortical development may well reflect a mechanism that is advantageous to the population, since it leads to a great diversity of patterns of lateralization, and therefore of patterns of talent. Since the cortex deals relatively little with elementary mechanisms immediately related to survival, the organism can tolerate a much greater degree of variation. This fact is probably reflected in different patterns of neuronal maturation. In some cases, e.g., the visual system and skeletal muscle, neurons appear to be directed to very precise targets. By contrast, the development of the cortex appears to allow for a higher rate of remodeling as cell death occurs. This diversity increases the probability that an unexpected problem can be met effectively by the cognitive specialization of some member of the population. A price is paid for this mechanism of diversity, since the possibilities of interference over the long developmental period are great and the way is opened to unpleasant consequences, e.g., childhood autism or dyslexia.

If these speculations are correct, one can be hopeful about possibilities of successful intervention, technically less elaborate possibilities than those required in a situation of more exact genetic determinism. The many routes of access to the system by environmental manipulation make possible relatively simple methods of modification without resort except rarely to more complex possibilities such as genetic engineering. In theory, it should be possible to specify which parents were more likely to have children with serious developmental disorders, and to apply preventive measures. The more precisely the details of the processes are known, the more exactly one could, in theory, prevent deleterious effects without sacrificing the advantages of the diversity of the system. The great diversity of the nongenetic effects on lateralization probably explains most of the difficulties in setting up genetic theories of handedness.

## Age and Ethnic Differences in Lateralization

Recent data suggest that the rate of NRH is higher in the young at least in Europe and the United States.[106,148] It is likely, for reasons we will not discuss, that this does not reflect a tendency of individuals to use the right hand more with increasing age but is rather a reflection of declining pressures against the use of the left hand. It is important to keep these age-related differences in mind in research.

It is often assumed that there has been little variation in LH over history and that there is little ethnic variation. The available data suggest that in historic times LH has been present in some minority, ranging perhaps from 5% to 10%.[106] There is, however, no assurance that the rate of LH is not 30% or 50% higher now in certain populations than it was thousands of years ago. Furthermore, most of the current handedness data have been collected in the United States and in northern European and French-speaking populations. There are very few studies in Asia. A lower rate of LH was found among children in Taiwan than is reported in the West.[149] There is also a report on handedness in Japanese students, but because of the tests used the data are not comparable with Western studies.[150] It is our impression that extreme RH was more common than in the West. It is sometimes asserted that dyslexia is less frequent in Japanese and Chinese because of their ideographic scripts, but fully adequate data are not available. Perhaps the best study would be that of Japanese children studying in English-speaking schools in the United States, since this would remove the questions raised by differences in the written language.

It is likely that on the average, populations will differ in brain development, structure, and metabolism and therefore in lateralization patterns. Some brain diseases show marked ethnic variation, e.g., Tay-Sachs disease and dystonia musculorum deformans occur predominantly in some Jewish populations. In northern Europe there is generally a higher frequency of twinning and of neural tube defects than in southern Europe and the Orient. Since twinning is associated with LH in whites, one might speculate that sinistrality was less common in southern Europe and Japan and that therefore dyslexia and other learning disabilities might be less frequent. There is a high rate of LH[151] and of twinning[152] in the parents of children with neural tube defects. This line of reasoning suggests that West Africa would have a very high rate of LH, learning disabilities, and possibly neural tube defects since this area has by far the highest reported twinning rates. There is evidence compatible with at least parts of this hypothesis. Stuttering is very common among school children in West Africa, the rates often being three times those found in the United States.[153] The hypothesis advanced to explain this was the high prevalence of sickle cell disease. American blacks, mostly of West African origin, have higher stuttering rates than whites. An alternative interpretation is that in West Africa there is a high frequency of anomalous dominance, and therefore learning disabilities, LH, and the other attendant talents and disabilities. We are now cooperating with Femi Fadahunsi, MD, of Lagos, Nigeria on a study of this problem. The very few studies of handedness in Africa have shown very low apparent rates of sinistrality, but it is not clear whether powerful cultural biases might be present.

The discussion of ethnic differences in handedness thus rests at present on mere fragments of information. It should be pointed out, however, that the distinctions so far presented are not between the conventional white, black, and Oriental groups. Thus the blond haired, blue eyed, and fair skinned northern Europeans might resemble West African blacks, whereas the Japanese might bear closer resemblances to southern European whites. There is no information known to us on some of the largest groups, e.g., those found in India or the Arabs, although Indian twinning rates tend to be comparable with those found in Europe.[133] Similarly, East African populations could well be different in the organization of laterality from those in West Africa just as they are in so many other respects. It seems likely that very important information could be obtained by studying isolated populations such as those found in New Guinea or Australia or in other parts of Africa.

There are several reasons for the study of populations carrying different genetic pools. In the first place there is a very high risk of describing as universal human biology the properties of the best studied populations consisting to a very great extent of individuals of northern European descent. Second, differences between populations may cast important light on the mechanisms that produce lateralization and the disturbances that lead to learning disabilities. It is likely that studies of this type will ultimately benefit each group by providing information that will help to prevent or cure some of the brain disorders present in higher frequency in that population.

## Disease Associations With Gender, Laterality, Dominance, and Learning Disabilities

This article has repeatedly stressed certain factors, e.g., selective unilateral developmental effects, hormonal atmosphere in pregnancy, the mechanisms of dominance, and the special association of learning disabilities with unilateral delays in development. Each of these factors may have special disease associations. The hormonal effects imply that many disorders might be related to gender. Certain diseases should show preferential involvement of one side of the brain or the body. The dominance pattern of an individual may be related to many disease susceptibilities, and the LD group has several distinctive disease associations. We have discussed conditions related to these factors in many other locations. The purpose of this section is to call attention specifically to this group of important factors that have often been overlooked in the past, and to awaken the interest of others in them.

The title of this section may suggest that what is to follow is a list of the disadvantages of individuals possessed of particular characteristics. As elsewhere, we would again like to emphasize the frequent occurrence of advantages that often balance or even outweigh unfavorable susceptibilities. The special risk of females for many disorders is far outweighed by their lower rates of coronary disease and lung cancer. It is likely that the same is true for all other groups. Whether a group is at net advantage or disadvantage can be ascertained only by knowing the rates of all cases of morbidity and mortality.

While many of the disease associations of these factors are undoubtedly related to the mechanisms we have discussed, we are, of course, aware that many other factors may be at play.

**Diseases With Unilateral Preponderance**

The possibility of unilateral predominance is often overlooked although data exist for certain conditions. Disorders of any of the unpaired organs, e.g., the heart, spleen, or liver, is necessarily asymmetric but many disorders even in paired organs affect one side preferentially.[154]

Undescended testes are located significantly more often on the right side although the effect is not large. In a Chinese study, the right testis was higher and heavier than the left in most cases.[155] The right testis develops earlier than the left, just as the left ovary precedes the right.[38] In hermaphrodites who have an ovary and a testis, the latter is usually on the right presumably because it develops earlier than the ovary.

Cancers and cysts of the breast are found to a small but significant extent, more frequently on the right than on the left. The same has been reported for supernumerary nipples, breast hypertrophy, and difficulties in lactation.[156]

The curious condition of hemihypertrophy[157,158] deserves comment. In this disorder, one entire side of the body is larger than the other, although in rare cases there is hypertrophy of the upper limbs on one side and the lower on the other. The patients have high rates of mental defect and neoplasms, e.g., Wilms' tumor. Neoplasms occur with higher frequency on the involved side, which may have a higher skin temperature; there may be more rapid growth in tissue culture of fibroblasts from the larger side. Some series suggest a right-sided predominance. Hemiatrophy appears in isolation or as a component of the Russel-Silver syndrome or disorders and is more frequent on the left side.[154] Many other unilateral conditions, e.g., the preferentially left-sided location of papillomas of the choroid plexus and intraventricular meningiomas, will be discussed in other sections.

**Gender-Related Disease Susceptibility**

The statement that disease associations with laterality, gender, dominance, and learning disabilities have been neglected might appear, at least in part, to be incorrect. In any textbook of medicine gender is by far the most commonly mentioned risk factor. Even a brief inspection will show the correctness of this statement. Among the major killers, cardiovascular disease, cancer of the lung, and cancer of the colon are predominant in men while cancer of the breast occurs only rarely in men. Hemochromatosis in strongly predominant in men, photosensitive porphyria is more frequent in men, but the opposite is true for the acute intermittent form. Although examples could readily be multiplied, our point remains valid since the reasons for the male-female differences are rarely discussed, although they must be of great importance. Hormones do not account for all of the differences; other factors especially affecting men include cigarette-smoking, alcoholism, occupational exposure, and dietary habits. Some other differences must relate to adult hormonal factors. Still others, we believe, must be produced by intrauterine or early postnatal hormone effects; in these cases dominance, laterality, and LD associations should also be common.

Gender susceptibility transcends spontaneous disease. There are very large differences between men and women in susceptibility to many drugs and toxins,[39] yet these are generally neglected in pharmacology texts and tend to be overlooked in discussions of drug therapy and its complications. Many of the gender differences in immunity, metabolism, and drug responsiveness are established in intrauterine or early postnatal developmental period, and are often not reversible at later ages by the administration of hormones. Some of these metabolic forms of imprinting will be discussed in a later section.

Administration of the appropriate hormone during some critical period can, in some cases, induce the pattern of responsiveness to drugs or toxins typical of one gender group in individuals of the other group. The rat female exposed early to T will permanently show a pattern of T responsiveness similar to that of males. The pattern of sex hormones in adult life may, however, in some cases mask or alter certain susceptibilities determined in utero. We have proposed that the heightened susceptibility of those with anomalous dominance to certain immune diseases is the result of effects on the developing immune system of a male-related factor. Yet adult onset immune disorders are in general less frequent in males than in females; we have hypothesized that this might be due to a protective effect of the postpubertal rise of T. There must be many other examples of modification by later hormonal environment of the susceptibilities set in utero.

### Relationships of Cerebral Dominance to Disease

The higher rates of immune disorders and migraine in left-handers have already been presented. Parenthetically, one should note that migraine is related to all of the factors discussed, i.e., unilateral predilection, female predominance, and association with LH, and LD. The older literature contains references to associations of handedness with somatic disease, LD, and psychiatric disorders; many of these are discussed in other sections.

### Disease Associations of Developmental Learning Disorders

Several authors have described an elevated frequency of certain disorders in children with LD. One of our hypotheses is that many of the associations of LD are more generally associations of anomalous dominance (AD). It is easy to understand the earlier emphasis on the association with LD rather than with LH or AD. Since LD children are often collected in special clinics or institutions, the other medical conditions present in these patients may more easily come to the attention of physicians.

We believe that the majority, and possibly nearly all LD children are drawn from the AD population. The question must arise whether those with LD are more often subject to these diseases than are those with AD but without LD. Within the LD group, one might expect degrees of AD, perhaps with corresponding variations in disease associations. M. Kinsbourne, MD, and B. Bemporad, MA, (written communication, July 13, 1983) found a higher rate of immune disease in the families of dyslexics who were left-handed or had left-handed relatives than in dyslexics without such histories.

We must also ask whether the elevated susceptibility to certain immune disorders among those with AD is associated with a changed susceptibility to infection, e.g., both a decreased risk of certain infections but increased risk of others. We will return to the question of infection in a later section.

## Vestibular and Eye Movement Disorders

The literature on LD contains many articles that deal with alterations in the vestibular system, and in eye movement.[159] Some have even attempted to link the mechanisms of LD and schizophrenia to these associated anomalies. We suspect, however, that vestibular and oculomotor anomalies in LD and in some psychiatric conditions do not play a role in causing the deviant behavior but are instead parallel effects of the causes of these behavioral disorders. Vestibular anomalies may derive from lateral imbalances produced in normally symmetric neural systems by alterations in hemispheric dominance relationships. It is often stated that there is a high frequency of childhood motion sickness among those with LD, but this has not been documented. A past or current history of motion sickness is common in migraine,[160,161] a condition with an elevated frequency of LH than in the general population. An anomalous vestibular system may well be present in torsion dystonia and spasmodic torticollis[162] since the direction of head turning in any affected individual corresponds to the direction in which induced nystagmus tends to be greatest. This report denied any relationship to the handedness of the subjects but since only five subjects were left-handed, further studies are warranted.

There are several mechanisms that might lead to an elevated rate of vestibular anomalies in subjects with AD, e.g., abnormalities in the formation of the vestibular systems in the brain stem. Another speculative possibility would tie vestibular changes to altered cortical mechanisms. Some authors have suggested that there is a cortical representation of the vestibular system in the temporal lobe in close proximity to the cortical auditory systems.[163] In primates lesions of this cortex can lead to dramatic spontaneous rotation. Temporal lobe epilepsy occasionally produces powerful sensations of rotation that can mimic attacks of acute vestibular dysfunction. This type of sensation would arise from the superior portions of the temporal lobe if the human vestibular cortex were comparable with that of the monkey. Anomalies of development in or near this location should, however, not be rare since the cytoarchitectonic defects in dyslexic subjects appear to have a predilection for this late developing region of the temporal lobe.

Several types of disturbance might result from disturbed formation of the cortex in this region, e.g., seizures with an aura of vertigo, which do occur, although uncommonly. In some cases a spike focus in this location might lead to a distortion of the stimuli reaching the vestibular cortex or to distortion of the response pattern. Even in the absence of abnormal electrical activity anomalous formation of this region might lead to altered responses to vestibular inputs. One might speculate that the normal vestibular system is balanced, i.e., there is little bias in either direction, so that stimuli in one direction will, on the average, be balanced by stimuli in the other direction. Anomalous formation of the vestibular cortex might disturb this balance, thus favoring motion sickness and also a greater bias for eye movements to one side. These considerations are, although speculative, susceptible to experimental study. The existence of a bias of the kind suggested might also play a role in such conditions as spasmodic torticollis.

### Mirror Reading, Writing, and Movements

Orton[164] pointed out that some childhood dyslexics could read better in a mirror, or with a book held upside down (in which case the print is both inverted and reversed). There has been a marked revival of interest in this phenomenon. One hypothesis is that reading is hampered in these patients when eye movements are not in a preferred direction, but there is at least one other possible explanation. In the normal reading of languages such as English, written from left to right, the next words to be read lie to the right of the fixation point, i.e., in the right visual field; they are, therefore, projected to the *left* hemisphere. When words are presented in mirror fashion the next words to be read reach the right hemisphere. If the left hemisphere is less efficient than the right in processing visual language reading might be more adequate if the message could reach the right side of the brain. One might argue that if the left-hemisphere systems were inadequate the callosal projections would simply relay the visual language message to the more competent right side. The anomalous development of the cortex on the left might, however, also lead to disturbance of callosal projections, which, of course, originate in the cortex. We will return to the issue of the anomalous callosal projections in a later section. A possible explanation of superior reading of words presented in mirror fashion is, therefore, that the message is transmitted to the more efficient reading-related areas of the right hemisphere; when words are presented in the standard left-to-right fashion they fail to be transmitted to the right hemisphere because the necessary callosal connections are poorly formed in many dyslexics.

It has been suggested to us by Per Udden, MD, (oral communication, Feb 20, 1985) that those dyslexics who find it easier to read English in mirror fashion might not have been dyslexic in learning to read Hebrew which is written in the reverse direction. This raises the possibility that a different group of individuals would be dyslexic in learning to read Hebrew, which is reading in the left hemisphere. This group would prefer to read Hebrew in mirror fashion, i.e., in the same direction as English. We suspect, however, that those dyslexics who read English better in mirror fashion would still be dyslexic in Hebrew, although probably less so, because even when the right hemisphere has superior capacities for reading it is probably not as competent as a normal left hemisphere. On the other hand, the great bulk of Israelis who have a left hemisphere with superior capacities for reading will not be dyslexic in learning to read Hebrew. Although the written word will typically be projected to the right hemisphere, their normal callosal connections will relay the message to the more efficient left hemisphere. Since our belief is that those dyslexic in learning Hebrew would be drawn from the same population, they too would have an elevated rate of NRH. Udden has suggested to us that the same mechanism might account for the preference of some left-handers to write with a hooked position, or, in the extreme case, in mirror fashion, i.e., in such a manner as to be read more easily by the right hemisphere. The notebooks of Leonardo DaVinci, who was left-handed, were written in inverted and reversed fashion. A finding in conformity with this hypothesis is that in Israel left-handers write much less frequently in the hooked position.[165] The ability to read in mirror fashion and to mirror write are much more common in left-handers. There are even occasional non-RH who can write a sentence with one hand in the forward direction and a *different* sentence with the other in the mirror direction. It was even said of President James Garfield, who was left-handed, that he could do this in two different languages. (There is a hint that Garfield was mathematically inclined since he devised a proof of the Pythagorean theorem.) These findings suggest not only bilateral representation of language and pyramidal motor control but also a lack of interference effects between the two sides as the result of a defect in callosal connectivity.

The hooked writing position is seen in many left-handers, particularly men. We will not, however, go into detail on this fascinating and complex phenomenon to which Levy and Reid[166] drew attention. The studies of Levy and Reid[165] suggest anomalous connectivity in this group. This raises the important possibility that there are multiple forms of NRH varying according to the particular motor systems involved.

Mirror movements represent a disturbance of laterality, of which the mechanism has not yet been worked out. There is a general belief that these are also more common in non-RH and this fits in with our experience. While marked degrees of mirror movement will often attract attention, our experience suggests that minor degrees of it are more common than is generally appreciated. We have also seen individuals with AD in whom mirror movements are found at certain times and absent at others. Two such patients with AD had an intermittent tremor, accompanied by mirror movements that disappeared when the tremor improved. This may suggest participation of subcortical motor mechanisms in mirror movements. It would be of interest to know whether propranolol would diminish some forms of mirror movement.

Congenital mirror movements, which may appear in families, are sometimes so severe as to be disabling. An odd association is the frequent presence of Klippel-Feil syndrome and other bony anomalies of the cervical spine in such patients.[167] This has suggested the likelihood of an associated anomaly in the adjacent region of the junction of the spinal cord and medulla, very possibly in the decussation of the pyramidal tracts. One group has argued for cortical anomalies in these cases.[168] It is possible that there is more than one mechanism of mirror movements and also that affected individuals have several related anomalies. Woods and Eby[169] have found that mentally defective children with mirror movements are more aggressive on the average than those without them.

Acquired mirror movements may throw some light on this problem. We believe, however, that not all acquired mirror movements have the same mechanism. Thus in acquired hemiplegia,[170] mirror movements tend to occur in the *intact* hand on the attempt to move the paretic one. Our guess is that this does not reflect a release of involuntary mirror movements. One possibility is that as a result of damage to the motor systems of one hemisphere the patient attempts to use bilaterally distributed motor systems from the other hemisphere. One occasionally sees mirror movements on the paretic side with movements of the intact one, which presumably have a different mechanism. In unilaterally predominant parkinsonism we have several times seen mirror movements in the *affected* limb on movement of the less involved side.

A progressive syndrome has been described in three patients of Irish-descent, which began with involvement of the left limbs.[171] One may observe pyramidal, basal ganglia, and cerebellar signs. In a case seen by us, there were dramatic mirror movements involving the entire affected left arm when the right arm moved.

No study has yet been made of anomalous dominance in relation to acquired mirror movements, a topic which deserves study.

## Asymmetries in the Neural Crest and Other Systems

In the preceding pages we have developed the hypothesis that variations in asymmetry of neurologic function reflect influences, often of an endocrine or immune nature, acting during the development of the nervous system. We believe that patterns of development of other organs may also be altered along with the structures underlying dominance.

Most of the subsequent sections will be devoted to some of these implications. In some cases, we believe that there is reasonable existing evidence for some of the links suggested while in other cases the discussion will center on topics that can be elucidated only by further study. It is important, in our view, to present these more speculative possibilities which suggest fruitful research areas.

### Asymmetry in the Neural Crest

In this section we discuss the possibility of asymmetry in development of derivatives of the neural crest, which has been suggested to us by both personal clinical observations and findings in the literature.

The neural crest is a particularly interesting structure that develops on the lips of the neural tube.[172] Therefore, it is not surprising that it plays a major role in the formation of the nervous system, giving rise to all the dorsal root ganglia, as well as autonomic ganglia and several of the ganglia of the cranial nerves. It also forms both leptomeninges and dura in the forebrain, but not in hindbrain or spinal cord. Its participation in the formation of nonneural tissues is equally extensive. Nearly every pigmented cell of the body is of crest origin, a point of major importance since so many anomalies of neural crest origin, in whatever tissue they are located, may be accompanied by changes in skin pigmentation, e.g., hyperpigmented or hypopigmented areas, or of other structures within the skin, e.g., vascular nevi.

Derivatives of the neural crest form several other tissues. Of special interest are the connective tissue of the thymus gland (the epithelium that processes lymphocytes being of different origin) and the skin and bones of the face.[172] The importance of this structure actually extends to many other tissues that it does not form directly. In DiGeorge's syndrome, in which there is failure of development of several crest derivatives, there is thymic hypoplasia or aplasia. The absence of the crest-derived thymic connective tissue leads to a lack of the inductive influence necessary for formation of the epithelium. Similarly, tooth development can be impaired. A recent article shows that lesions of the cephalic neural crest lead to aplasia or hypoplasia of the thymus and thyroid glands along with cardiac lesions.[173]

Disorders of crest development may have even more profound effects on the nervous system. The Siamese cat, which is an albino, has an anomalous pattern of decussation of the optic nerves that is probably the result of lack of melanin-bearing cells in the pigment epithelium of the retina. Recent work supports the view that melanin-bearing cells may be necessary to act as guides for migrating optic nerve fibers.[174,175] If the same is true elsewhere failures of neural crest formation or migration may underlie anomalous neural pathway formation in other regions. It would, therefore, not be surprising if one found an elevated rate of disordered neural crest derivatives in the anomalous dominance population. The pigmented cells of the retina are not of neural crest origin.[172] It remains to be shown that pigmented cells elsewhere play a role in migration of axons. There are, however, certain suggestive data, e.g., the higher rate of light hair in harelip patients than in the unaffected.[176] Neural tube defects, e.g., spina bifida, are many times more common in the northern British Isles than in the Orient,[137] and in the United States are more common in white than in black infants.

Indirect evidence exists that sex hormones play a role in crest development although this has, to our knowledge, not yet been studied. Melanomas are known in some instances to carry estradiol receptors, and they have sometimes been treated with the estrogen antagonist, tamoxifen citrate. Intracranial meningiomas may carry estradiol receptors, and we have noted the meninges of the forebrain are crest derivatives. The recently described association of meningiomas with breast cancer raises the possibility of the operation of some common endocrinologic factor in intrauterine life. In any case, one should consider the possibility that hormonal effects on neuronal migration might be accompanied by alterations in crest derivatives. Another possibly relevant fact is that neurofibromatosis, which appears to be predominantly a neural crest disorder, typically worsens at puberty, particularly in females, and in pregnancy. Since adrenal steroids are known to affect certain aspects of neural crest development, it would not be surprising if sex steroids also played a role.

Meningiomas of the lateral ventricle are much more common on the left side, and this raises the possibility of asymmetry in neural crest migrations. Conceivably certain delaying influences produce parallel unilateral effects on both neural tube and neural crest derivatives. Another possibility is that some of the delaying factors act primarily on the left neural crest and thus secondarily lead to failures in neuronal or axonal migration.

### Cardiac Asymmetry and Congenital Anomalies

There are nonneural sites in which the neural crest may well play a role in asymmetry. The connective tissue and muscular walls of the great vessels arising from the aortic arch are of neural crest origin.[172] Interference with the embryonic neural crest leads to anomalies at this site,[173] including transposition of the great vessels, a disorder that, along with congenital heart block, has been described in the children of female patients with lupus erythematosus[177,178]; in preliminary studies we have found a high rate of both of these anomalies in the families of dyslexics (P. Behan, MD, and N.G., unpublished data, April 1984).

### Harelip, Cleft Palate, and Anomalies of the Face and Ears

There are several other examples of asymmetric formation of neural crest derivatives. The skin and bones of the face and part of the skull (but not skin or bone in other regions) are derivatives of the neural crest, and harelip is now regarded as a disturbance of the crest.[172] Two-thirds of cases of harelip lie on the left side. Of 200 patients with harelip, 20% were left-handed vs. 8% of 200 controls.[179] Right-handed patients with harelip had twice as high a number of sinistral relatives as unaffected dextrals. Another relationship to the neural crest may be reflected in the later finding that dark hair was found in only about 6% of cases of harelip but in 28% of controls.

There is, however, one odd feature in the data on harelip. Tisserand[179] found that while two-thirds of all harelips lay on the left, the rate of left-sided involvement was about 50% in the left-handed, and about 70% in the right-handed, a difference that is statistically significant. Put in another form, of those with right-sided harelip, 30% are left-handed, and of those with left-sided harelip, 15% are left-handed. More information is needed concerning details of the times when the anlage of the lip is being formed in relation to when the neural areas that control handedness are being laid down. One must also consider the possibility of a greater fetal loss of those with left-sided harelip and left dominance. It is, however, also possible that these apparently paradoxical data reflect the use of the dichotomous categories of RH and LH. The majority of the harelip patients were either left-handed or had first-degree sinistral relatives. It is quite possible that most of the so-called right-handers among the left-sided harelip patients were actually individuals who, on a handedness battery, would have had scores in the intermediate ranges. If this were true, then there could have been a higher percentage of NRH among the left-sided than among the right-sided harelip group.

In the rat adrenal steroids given at the proper time in pregnancy lead to a high rate of cleft palate in the offspring. We are not familiar with similar studies on the effects of gonadal steroids. There is a high rate of epilepsy among the parents of cleft palate and harelip patients, and anticonvulsant treatment has been suggested as a likely cause of some of the cases. There are other data suggesting that the rate of cleft lip and palate may be elevated even in the absence of such treatment. These findings suggest that disorders of neural migration accompany disturbed migration in the neural crest.

Many syndromes are associated with unusual facial features. Malformed or malpositioned ears, e.g., low-set ears, are commonly seen. The extreme example of low-set ears is otocephaly, which is also a neural crest anomaly.[172] Asymmetry of the external ear canals occurs in normal subjects in less than 30% of cases but is present in over 65% of the mentally retarded and learning disabled.[180] One may well expect such anomalies to be more common in the AD population. There are individuals with markedly asymmetric facial size, which we have seen several times in association with scoliosis, which we will discuss shortly. The extreme case, i.e., facial hypoplasia[181] is more common on the left side. Since this is probably also a neural crest anomaly it provides further evidence for asymmetry of neural crest migrations. In particular, it suggests that these migrations are more likely to be delayed on the left side, just like those in the cortex.

## Scoliosis

Another condition in which neural crest migration may play a role is scoliosis. We cannot review all the theories concerning this disorder but will discuss one particular group of studies. In the young experimental animal, dorsal root destruction is often effective in producing scoliosis.[182–184] One possibility is that spinal curvature is induced by the asymmetric proprioceptive input that is responded to as if the spine were being bent to one side. Another mechanism is suggested by the finding that removal of dorsal root ganglia in the developing frog leads to a reduction in motoneurons in the corresponding segments and possibly to an increased number in adjacent segments.[185] The authors cite another study in which it was found that early neural crest removal in the chick reduced mononeuron populations. Alexander et al[184] found that dorsal rhizotomy lead to scoliosis only when the anterior horn cell changes were produced.

We are indebted to Dr Melvin Glimcher, Professor of Orthopedics at the Harvard Medical School, an outstanding authority on bone, for some comments on this mechanism. He points out that the procedure of cutting posterior roots does not lead to scoliosis as reliably as removal of multiple ribs on one side. The latter procedure may, however, not correspond to the causative mechanism in many cases of clinical scoliosis since absence of ribs is surely a rare accompaniment of this disorder. We will present evidence that, by contrast, scoliosis is often found in clinical situations in which there is clear evidence of alteration of sensory systems, or of anomalies of the neural crest.

If this mechanism is responsible for some and perhaps many cases one can envision that defective unilateral formation of the dorsal root ganglia, which are neural crest derivatives, might lead to scoliosis. This possibility is suggested by the clinical picture of a patient with scoliosis seen by one of us. He had total loss of all modalities of sensation from the nipple to the knee on one side with absent cremasteric and abdominal reflexes on that side. Furthermore, he also suffered from irregular skin pigmentation. This case raises the possibility that there was inadequate formation of dorsal root ganglia and pigmented cells on one side. Another patient was born with a hairy black nevus on one side of the lumbar spine and suffered from scoliosis. In later years he developed marked vitiligo, an immune disorder of melanocytes. Still later he presented with a left frontal convexity meningioma. Both the leptomeninges and dura of the forebrain are neural crest derivatives, but not those of the hindbrain or spinal cord. Two other personal patients with meningiomas had nevi on the face and scalp.

Scoliosis is strongly associated with many hereditary or congenital neurologic disorders affecting sensory systems in the spinal cord, e.g., the spino-cerebellar ataxias, syringomyelia, and spinal gliomas. Scoliosis may accompany familial dysautonomia in which there is deficit of neural crest derivatives, i.e., dorsal root autonomic ganglia. Furthermore, a special type of scoliosis is seen in neurofibromatosis, which, with its affection of pigmented cells and Schwann's cells, both crest derivatives, appears to be a neural crest disorder. In addition there may be lack of bone in the wall of the orbit, also a neural crest derivative. Dr Glimcher informs us that the scoliosis in this condition is distinctive in its pattern of involvement of a delimited number of spinal column segments. In any case, this disorder again illustrates the association of scoliosis with a disorder of sensory systems and clear neural crest disorder. MacEwen[183] found scoliosis in 20% of patients with cerebral palsy, but did not discuss the presence of distinctive clinical features in this group.

A particularly intriguing feature of scoliosis is its relationship to sex and age. The largest group of patients, consisting of female subjects in whom the major (thoracic) curve is typically convex to the left, often worsens at puberty. It is possible that this form of scoliosis is equally common in male subjects but that it progresses much less often after puberty and, therefore, does not come to medical attention. In any case, the typical worsening after puberty, especially in female subjects, strongly suggests a role of sex hormones. By contrast, in infantile scoliosis, a much rarer condition, there is male predominance and the major curve is in the opposite direction, convex to the right.[186,187] In all of these infantile cases there is also underdevelopment of the face on the side of the curve.

The asymmetry of scoliosis is suggestive of unilateral failure of dorsal root formation and, therefore, of unilateral disordered neural crest migrations. Further experimental studies will be required to verify the importance of this process in humans and to work out the details. It will obviously be important to study the handedness distribution in scoliosis of both types. It is our impression that the common later form of scoliosis is associated with an elevated rate of NRH.

Scoliosis is very common among patients with spinal arachnoid cysts.[188] As we shall point out later, cysts of this type may well be caused in many cases by immune attack.

### Pigmented Cells of Skin and Hair

If pigmented cells play an important role as guides to the development of neural (and possibly other) structures, hypopigmented or irregularly pigmented individuals might be more susceptible to influence affecting migration and assembly of nerve cells and fibers. The Siamese cat, in which one finds anomalous visual pathways and strabismus is an example. The same types of effects might perhaps be expected among humans with light hair or eyes. Refraction defects were reported as more common in those with light coloration, but strabismus was not discussed.[189] It has been stated that sinistrality is more common in strabismic patients, but we have not found adequate data. Tisserand[176] found that dark hair was much less common in harelip patients (who also have an excess of LH) than among controls. Studies are now underway to investigate these possibilities. We have found that blonds are significantly more non-RH than brunettes.[190] Thus, of 986 nonblonds, 76% scored more than +70 on a modified Oldfield Battery (i.e., were strongly right-handed), 12% were in the zero to +70 range (i.e., ambidextrous), and 12% were in the zero range (left-handed). The corresponding figures for 131 blonds were 56, 28, and 16, respectively; the differences in the distribution of scores of the two groups was highly significant.

It is our impression, but not yet confirmed, that pigmentary anomalies are more common in the AD population. Several of those we have seen have had facial nevi, either pigmented or vascular. The association of vascular nevi at the same dermatomal level as a spinal vascular malformation was pointed out by Cobb.[191] Cushing[192] had commented on a similar relationship between facial or scalp nevi and intracerebral vascular malformations. As noted earlier, we have now seen several patients with meningiomas with nevi, usually on the face or scalp, but in one instance a black hairy nevus at the base of the spine. We have also seen other patients with epilepsy with a facial nevus on the same side. The most dramatic example of a disorder of this type is the Sturge-Weber syndrome which is predominantly female. It would be important to ascertain whether this affects predominantly one side.

Another important pigmentary anomaly is early gray or white hair. It is commonly stated in the lay literature that early gray or white hair is common in the families of dyslexics. It has been our impression that in fact early gray hair is more common in the AD population and their relatives, which would include those with childhood LD. We are now carrying out a study on a population with early gray or white hair to determine the distribution of handedness, LD, and immune diseases.

Early gray or white hair is of particular interest because of its known association with certain autoimmune diseases, the ones most often noted being pernicious anemia[193] and autoimmune thyroid disorder.[194] It is indeed our impression that it is even more widely associated with immune diseases. Our present study should help to provide further information. The association suggests immune attack on pigment cells in the hair follicles. Wood[194] has recently confirmed the presence of a high rate of non-RH in patients with immune thyroid disease, he also found a high rate of early gray or white hair, but did not, however, report whether this was present more often in the sinistral patients. An elevated rate of dyslexia was not found in the immune thyroid patients, but the series was probably too small.

Certain other features of early gray hair deserve mention. It has important ethnic associations being more common in northern Europeans and, we suspect, blacks of West African descent, but less common in southern Europeans and Far Eastern populations. This deserves further study, since it would be concordant with the possibility that anomalous dominance may be more common in northern Europeans. It should be noted that the Japanese usually have sparse facial hair and early baldness is less common than in northern Europeans. This suggests end-organ insensitivity of the hair follicles to dihydrotestosterone, but it is not clear whether this is related to the low prevalence of early gray or white hair.

There is another striking feature of those with early gray or white hair. It has been our observation that affected men have a low rate of early male-pattern baldness (which is very common in populations of northern European descent) and that affected women tend to show thinning of the hair much less often after menopause. Male-pattern baldness and postmenopausal hair thinning occur only in the presence of androgens. The man with early white or gray hair is not usually hypogonadal or insensitive to androgens. Diminished hair loss therefore suggests low *local* sensitivity of the hair follicles to androgens. As we have noted earlier, T in many instances protects from immune attack. The converse may also be true, i.e., that immune attack on the pigmented cells of the hair follicles may lead to reduced sensitivity to androgenic effects. One single but speculative possibility is that antibodies binding to the hair follicles present a barrier to androgens. We have noted the lower rate of early male-pattern baldness and sparse facial hair of the Japanese, resulting from insensitivity of the hair follicles to dihydrotestosterone. It would be interesting to know whether Europeans or blacks with early gray hair also shave infrequently, i.e., whether the immune protection against androgens also extends to facial hair.

Eye color (i.e., the color of the iris) is another interesting feature. The Siamese cat, which is an albino, has a high rate of strabismus. Some older articles claimed, but without adequate documentation that LH was more frequent in those with strabismus. We are now investigating eye color and motor laterality in strabismus. Korein[195] reported that among patients with dystonia and spasmodic torticollis there was an elevated rate of blue or hazel eyes. This was disputed by Lang et al[196] but as Korein[197] pointed out, their data actually confirmed his conclusions, a view with which we agree. We have been interested in anomalies of iris pigmentation, e.g., a woman (the mother of three left-handed children) with blue eyes, except that her left iris has one spoke of brown pigment. Another woman with AD in her family has one blue and one brown eye. This condition, called *heterochromia iridis*, is usually thought to result either from genetic mosaicism or from damage at birth to the superior cervical ganglion on one side. Since this can occur as a familial anomaly[114] it is likely that it can also result from delayed neural crest migration on one side.

There is another intriguing phenomenon, i.e., asymmetric loss of hair pigment. The most common example is the white forelock seen both in normal subjects and in certain disorders, e.g., Waardenburg's syndrome. There are no data known to us as to lateral predominance or relationship to handedness. Even more common is asymmetric frontal graying, with a sharp division at the midline, most readily observed in those with short curly hair. The possible relationships of this to cerebral laterality or lesions has not yet been investigated. An interesting possible example is that of a male patient in his 60s who suffered a spontaneous intracerebral hemorrhage from a very large aneurysm in the right anterior sylvian fissure. His hair was short and tightly curled and originally black in color. He had a striking pattern of graying of the hair with the right anterior frontal region being visibly much grayer than the left.

The rat treated in early life with cortisone is typically small and dark, even if from an albino strain, showing that steroids can lead to removal of the repression of the melanin-producing enzymes that are present in many forms of albinism. These cortisone-treated animals, as is well known, are immunologically different from others of the same strain. In Addison's disease, with its low rate of adrenal steroid production, the skin also becomes darker. In any case, we believe that skin pigmentation and iris pigmentation reflect immunologic, endocrinologic, and dominance characteristics.

We will comment in a later section (on localized immune effects) on the remarkable phenomenon of new local changes in hair color at sites corresponding to a brain lesion.

## Neurons of the Gut

It is also intriguing that the intrinsic neurons of the gut are of neural crest origin in view of the especially high rate of gut-related immune disorders found in our studies of strong left-handers. In the rat, adrenal steroids increase the amount of catecholamine production in the enteric neurons and may also lead to anomalous placement of cells. It would be interesting to know about the effects of sex steroids.

## Skeletal Anomalies and Neural Tube Defects

We pointed out earlier that AD may be associated with immune disorders. In the preceding section we showed that AD is associated with harelip and blond hair, and may also be linked to anomalies of the facial skeleton, scoliosis, and skin lesions.

We believe that AD is also associated in elevated frequency with disorders in other systems. At the time of the Geschwind and Behan study,[91] a surprising number of left-handers added the notation to the questionnaire that they had situs inversus, but this remains to be studied formally. Alterations in the skeleton may be very common. We have already referred to scoliosis. It should be noted that in most people the right arm is longer than the left, but the left foot is larger than the right, and there are corresponding differences in muscle weight.[198,199] Even in utero the bones of the right arm and left leg are heavier than their opposites.[200] Curiously enough the same pattern is found in the frog and the rabbit.[201] It may seem odd that the left leg is the larger, but it is reasonable teleologically, at least in the human. If someone is rightfooted, e.g., kicks with the right foot, the left leg will be used for bearing weight. In quadrupedal animals this advantage would not appear to be important. On the other hand, it might be related to the typical crossed pattern of locomotion, but it would be difficult to use this to explain the pattern in the frog.

It has been shown that the rate of LH is elevated in Legg-Perthes' disease,[202] which is male-predominant. Dr Melvin Glimcher has reviewed his own cases of this condition and finds a very high rate of LH, particularly in the female cases. It is our impression that anomalies of the vertebral column, e.g., Klippel-Feil syndrome and related disorders, and pilonidal sinus are found in raised frequency in the AD population. Furthermore, we believe that these skeletal anomalies are associated with a high rate of immune disease, but this remains to be documented. Since many of these anomalies of the vertebral column may reflect delayed closure of the neural tube it is possible that the influences which produce them also lead to delayed formation of the left hemisphere and to slowing of immune development. Therefore, one might expect spina bifida and related disorders to have similar associations. Neural tube defects are, in general, more common in populations with high rates of twinning, a condition in which LH, for reasons we have discussed elsewhere, is present in elevated frequency. In fact, there is a high rate of twinning among the parents of children with spina bifida.[151] Fraser[203] has recently found a high rate of LH in families of children with spina bifida. It is of interest that the neural tube defects are female predominant, which suggests a role for hormones. The very low rate of concordance for neural tube defects among identical twins strongly suggests a special role for environmental factors in pregnancy. Nance[121] has brought evidence that neural tube defects are transmitted primarily from mothers. This might suggest cytoplasmic inheritance, but this alone would neither account for female predominance or for low concordance of identical twins. Another possibility is that this condition reflects the action of maternal environmental influences on a genetically susceptible offspring. Some of these influences may be hormonal, possibly reflecting anomalous maternal hormone production. Neural tube defects may also have an immunologic component, since a high rate of histocompatibility antigen concordance has been reported between the mothers and fathers of children with neural tube defects.[204,205] Even in this case hormonal effects may contribute, e.g., in the presence of histocompatibility antigen concordance an anomalous hormonal atmosphere may markedly enhance the probability of neural tube defects. A role for the neural crest is suggested by the markedly higher rate of spina bifida in northern Britain than in the Orient[137] and the higher rate of this disorder in American whites than in blacks.[206] In the case of Klippel-Feil syndrome, pilonidal sinus, and other similar relatively minor disorders, one may be dealing with individuals who have what may be described as larval forms of neural tube defects. This formulation leads to certain implications. Gross failures of fusion of the two sides of the nervous system are obviously disadvantageous either for survival or for normal function. On the other hand, complete fusion does not normally occur, since beyond the midbrain the structures are doubled, with connections via the forebrain commissures. At this upper level excessive fusion can occur, e.g., holoprosencephaly, in which the brain halves are fused with a single ventricle. At the other extreme there may be a gross lack of the normal connectivity of the two sides, e.g., agenesis of the corpus callosum. In most individuals there is a balance between the poles of a highly unitary nervous system and one that has varying degrees of lateral dissociation.

The possibility should be entertained that milder degrees of diminished fusion may be advantageous. One of us (N.G.) has suggested elsewhere that the normal nervous system is far from unitary and that a necessary condition for consciousness may be the occurrence of separated neural events with some degree of independence from each other. Mild degrees of diminished fusion might lead to the formation of superior individuals who may be closer to the goal of optimal cognitive capacity, i.e., the ideal balance between separation and fusion.

It is likely that a diminished degree of unity would be present in one system but not others. The capacity of each half brain to control its motor functions relatively independently may be one of the factors accounting for the high rate of NRH among athletes, and, in particular, very successful athletes, and in fields such as architecture and the other visual arts.

Skeletal anomalies have been said to occur in elevated frequency in children of mothers who were themselves exposed to diethylstilbestrol whose masculinizing effects will be discussed in the next section.[207] If rats are exposed to acetazolamide or other carbonic anhydrase inhibitors, there is a high rate of limb reduction defects (i.e., failure to form the distal portion of the limb) which usually involve the right forelimb in females.[208,209] Galaburda and G. Sherman, PhD (written observations, June 1982) have found that the acetazolamide-exposed animals also frequently have anomalous cortical cytoarchitecture. W. E. Castle, in a signed footnote to an article by Larrabee[109] mentions a strain of guinea pigs in whom the females frequently had right hindlimb polydactyly and Di Paolo[210] found that he could induce the same anomaly with 5-bromodeoxyuridine. In humans limb reduction defects have a predilection for the right arm in male offspring. Among diethylstilbestrol children there is an excess of limb reduction deficits.[207] The condition of right radial aplasia and thrombocytopenia occurs primarily in male children.[211]

Limb reduction defects of other causation may also be lateralized. Thalidomide given to pregnant women usually causes bilateral disorder, but unilateral cases are reported to be located more often on the left.[42] By contrast, LSD produces absence of fingers particularly on the right hand; LSD is, of course, a derivative of serotonin which has been suggested as important in control of sex hormones.

Another condition of interest is mitral valve prolapse (MVP), a female-preponderant condition (with a rate of about 20% in some series) with a remarkable array of associated alterations in other systems.[212–214] A skeletal anomaly, i.e., the straight back syndrome, is often present, as well as abnormal platelets and a high rate of migraine and endocrine disorders. We should note in passing the reported high rate of platelet anomalies in attention deficit disorder.[215] Women with MVP have, on the average, smaller breasts than controls[216] which suggests a masculinizing effect, and therefore raises the possibility that this group will have a high rate of AD. Conceivably, MVP is a common marker of AD females.

Studies of other forms of congenital heart disease also suggest a relationship to AD. In a study of neuropsychological test performances of girls and boys with congenital heart disease[217] the male scores were similar to those of male controls, i.e., performance IQ scores higher on the average than verbal scores. The scores of the girls were, however, unusual, i.e., they were similar to those of males and not to those of most girls, who tend to show the opposite pattern, i.e., higher scores on verbal than on performance IQ tests. The pattern of higher performance IQ scores would be expected more frequently in female patients with AD. The sex differences in the scores of the patients with congenital heart disease suggest hormonal effects. There is an intriguing pharmacologic parallel. Sex hormone receptors have been found in the rat heart and the digitalis glycosides contain a steroid skeleton. One digitalis (tablet) can lead to gynecomastia in men, presumably because the drug or its metabolites have an affinity for estradiol receptors. The possibility that sex hormones play a role in congenital heart disease is suggested by several studies.[218–221]

Certain skeletal features are characteristic of some forms of headache. Cluster headache is, in contrast to migraine, strongly male predominant. Graham et al[222] described the high frequency in cluster patients, of a leonine facies, with orange-peel skin, and a full head of wiry curly hair. Kudrow[223] has found that the height of cluster patients averages three inches greater than that of controls.

The issue of skeletal changes has two important implications. There is a body of literature, much of it from the last century, on the association of skeletal anomalies with disordered behavior, which did not achieve acceptance for several reasons. Cesare Lombroso described an elevated rate of skeletal anomalies, e.g., asymmetric ears, in criminals and mental defectives, and recent authors[180] have revived this notion. One reason for the rejection of these ideas was the observation that the same anomalies might be present in normal subjects or highly superior individuals, which suggested that they might be uniformly distributed in the population. It is possible, however, that there is a bimodal distribution with anomalies found at elevated rate both in the very talented and the very disadvantaged, with a low rate in the general run of the population. This is similar to what has been suggested for the AD population, e.g., LH is very frequent both in mentally defective subjects and in some very talented groups.

There is also a large literature on the association of *somatotypes* (body types) with different behavioral characteristics and diseases. Kretschmer[224] proposed that different body types were associated with different forms of mental illness, a concept that has received greater attention from continental and British than from American psychiatrists. In the United States, Draper et al[225] argued for the association of certain body types with particular diseases, but this did not engender much attention. A typical claim was that patients with rheumatic fever were likely to have irregular teeth, but unfortunately adequate statistical documentation was rarely provided.

There has been a recent dramatic revival of somatotype studies that meet the requirements for reasonable scientific evidence. Women with a tendency to upper-body obesity have a much higher rate of diabetes than those with lower-body obesity, involving especially the buttocks and legs.[226,227] These females, whose pattern of obesity resembles the common male pattern, i.e., broad shoulders and upper body fat tend to have high free T, raising the possibility that this group has an elevated rate of AD. This result gains added interest from the fact that diabetes is generally a male-predominant disorder. Benign intracranial hypertension occurs overwhelmingly in females who are obese with a strong history of menstrual irregularities. This raises the possibility that this condition occurs in the group with upper-body obesity and high free T, which would account for the high rate of menstrual irregularities. If this is the case, then benign intracranial hypertension should occur more often among women with AD. A recent case seen by us falls into this category, but only extensive controlled studies can confirm or refute this speculation. It also raises the possibility that the capacity of upper and lower body fat to produce estradiol differs.

## Bodily Asymmetries and Handedness

We have already commented on the asymmetric pattern of the bones of the limbs. In the next section we will mention the asymmetries of the testis. Studies of fingerprints and other dermatoglyphics have shown less asymmetry on the average in left-handers than right-handers.[228] It should be noted that, in general, left-handers have less anatomic asymmetry in the brain,[229] testes,[154] and skin. Certain other somatic asymmetries are often said to be correlated with handedness, e.g., the hair whorl on the back of the head, but they have not been adequately studied, probably because of the problems in the measurement of handedness that were discussed earlier. The same is probably true for limb asymmetries and possibly for those of the face.

Attention is often called to different patterns of folding the arms, clasping the hands, and crossing the legs; it is argued that these are related to handedness, but no good data exist. Preliminary observations suggest to us that these patterns are the result of differences in lengths of bones on the two sides.

### Sexual and Reproductive Function

We have already pointed out that the high rate of twinning in the left-handed population may well reflect some variation in hormonal endowment. Mothers of twins in Nigeria have high follicle-stimulating hormone levels, but handedness has not been studied in this population. In Scotland, mothers of twins do not have high follicle-stimulating hormone levels.[133] It is, of course, conceivable that there are several different factors that might favor twinning.

A corollary of our hypothesis is that left-handed female subjects are likely to differ endocrinologically, immunologically, or both, from right-handed women. This in turn implies that their gynecologic and obstetric histories may well differ from those of right-handers and we are now carrying out a study of this possibility. Herzog et al[230] recently described a high rate of abnormal responses to LHRH in patients with temporal lobe epilepsy, a condition in which Taylor found an elevated rate of lefthandedness. More recently, Herzog et al[231] have shown that there is a high rate of temporal lobe abnormalities in polycystic ovary (PCO) syndrome. We expect an elevated rate of anomalous dominance in this latter group of masculinized female subjects although we have not yet documented this. It is interesting that those familiar with PCO report a high frequency of migraine in this condition. In the temporal lobe epileptic female subjects, we have also found a high rate of benign endocrine disorders, including ovarian cysts and endometriosis. Diethylstilbestrol was shown years ago to produce masculinizing effects on female offspring.[56] The reasons for this have become clear in recent years with the discovery that T masculinizes the rat brain. Estradiol within certain nuclei in the hypothalamus is actually the final cause of this masculinization, but these nuclei are protected from the circulating estradiol which, in the rat, is bound to α-fetoprotein. Testosterone is not bound by α-fetoprotein and thus reaches these nuclei where it is converted to estradiol by aromatase. Diethylstilbestrol also masculinizes; although it is an estrogen it is not bound by α-fetoprotein, and thus reaches the brain sites within which it acts like estradiol to masculinize. It is not surprising that diethylstilbestrol-exposed daughters have a high rate of gynecologic difficulties, infertility, and an elevated rate of children with congenital anomalies, all of which may reflect this masculinizing effect. We have seen several diethylstilbestrol daughters with features such as facial hirsutism, acne, and unusual sensitivity to the masculinizing effects of phenytoin. One might expect a high rate of anomalous dominance in this group, and our preliminary findings on 77 diethylstilbestrol daughters support this hypothesis. Hines,[59] in psychologic studies of a small sample of diethylstilbestrol children, found some results that she interpreted as consistent with a masculinizing effect on the brain, but other data summarized in her review differ, but the numbers were again small. Further study on larger numbers is obviously warranted.

It is likely, in our view, that sex organ anomalies are more common in male left-handers. The right testis and right ovary develop before the left-sided gonads. In a Chinese study the right testis was found to be usually heavier and higher, but the distribution was altered in left-handers.[154] We have heard but have been unable to verify that undescended testes are common in autistic children. We have seen one young autistic man with a history of an undescended testis, who also had skeletal asymmetry, a pilonidal sinus, an unusual pattern of hair color, and with parents and a sibling with early gray hair. Several left-handers have pointed out to us the occurrence of anomalies of their sperm in association with infertility. In one case the individual (a left-handed childhood dyslexic) had a right-handed brother with celiac disease, a condition with a high rate of sperm anomalies.[145] We shall later mention Kartagener's syndrome which has a high frequency of situs inversus and abnormal sperm. Diethylstilbestrol sons have a diminished rate of marriage.[131] Our preliminary studies also show a high rate of non-RH in nine diethylstilbestrol male subjects, but the sample is too small for confidence.

It is interesting to ask why male infertility might be associated in high rate with LH (although this has not yet been documented). It seems clear that in certain conditions high T levels in utero may be associated with later hypogonadism, e.g., Klinefelter's syndrome. Furthermore, when female rats are stressed in pregnancy the male fetuses have an early T surge but later have permanently low levels of free T. It is possible that in certain circumstances a very high T level in utero at a particular period may lead to damage to the testes in its T producing function or to the process of formation of sperm.

## Diseases With Gonadal, Brain, and Immune Anomalies

There are, as we have noted earlier, several conditions with endocrine and immune anomalies and with abnormal brain development. In dystrophia myotonica in which there is testicular or ovarian atrophy, male-pattern baldness (which suggests, in the face of testicular atrophy, high sensitivity to dihydrotestosterone) disordered neuronal migration may be found.[232] In ataxia-telangiectasia there is neuronal maldevelopment along with gonadal dysgenesis and high $\alpha$-fetoprotein. There are several other conditions of this type.

## Asymmetric Aspects of Sexual Function

In several species, e.g., in most birds, but also in some bats, only one ovary is functional.[132] In some bats ovulation takes place in only the right ovary[233] unless this is removed, in which case it takes place on the opposite side. Humans produce ova from both ovaries, but it is not known whether ovulation is more frequent on one side or whether there are some individuals who ovulate predominantly on one side. Neural control over gonadal function has been amply documented. Gerendai[234] has shown that many lesions of the central nervous system or of peripheral nerves (e.g., the vagus) in the rat lead to alterations in the time of onset of puberty. Furthermore, lesions on one side are often more effective than those on the other. She has also found asymmetric neural control of the ovary. Hypertrophy of the remaining gonad after removal of one ovary is asymmetric, with greater hypertrophy on the right after removal of the left ovary. The left hypothalamus has twice the LHRH content of the left. Whether similar effects occur in humans is not known. Nordeen and Yahr[235] have shown that while implantation of estradiol in the right hypothalamus leads to masculinization of newborn female rats (e.g., preference for other females) implantations on the left lead to defeminization (e.g., loss of the estrus cycle). Cancer of the breast is more common on the left, as is unilateral breast hypertrophy[236]; these facts suggest similar asymmetry of control of the breast as of the ovary.

## Homosexuality

Several homosexuals have written to us suggesting that there is a high rate of LH in this population but no study of this has yet been reported. A high rate of non-RH in this population may seem at first sight to be difficult to explain in the light of some animal experiments. Ward and Weisz[71] and Dorner et al[237] have shown that in rats stress in midpregnancy causes the male offspring to have permanently low free T levels and homosexual behavior. Dorner et al[237] have reported low free T in human homosexuals, but no other group has yet confirmed this. His group has also reported a higher rate of stress in pregnancy in mothers of homosexuals than in those of controls.[238] Low free T has been found in male temporal lobe epileptics in whom altered sexual behavior, including hyposexuality, is frequently seen. The low T-level was independent of drug therapy.[239] If the situation in the human is similar to that in the rat, then one would arrive at the apparently paradoxical conclusion that a group with low free T levels in adult life should have a high rate of AD. The answer is, we believe, given by the experiment of Ward and Weisz[71] showing that when the pregnant rat is stressed T first *rises* to higher than normal levels in male fetuses and then drops to permanently low levels. Infants with Klinefelter's syndrome may also have very high T in cord blood, and only later does the individual become hypogonadal. Handedness would, of course, be determined by the level in fetal life, and not by adult levels. Netley and Rovet[240] have recently reported an elevated rate of sinistrality in Klinefelter's syndrome.

If the above interpretation is correct it opens up another way of looking at acquired immunodeficiency syndrome (AIDS). The rarity of this disorder in female prostitutes renders unlikely explanations based on promiscuity, although those who are more promiscuous obviously have increased exposure. One possible alternative is that AIDS is caused by a virus that has undergone a recent mutation. As a result of the mutation the virus is capable of attacking individuals with a specific immunologic constitution. Some individuals have this immunologic pattern as the result of a particular pattern of intra-uterine hormonal experience. Other vulnerable populations, e.g., Haitian males and Central African females, may have the same immunologic pattern for quite different reasons. Another possibility is that a preexisting virus with these special immunologic properties has only recently been introduced to the susceptible Western homosexual population. In either case it might be useful to study the handedness patterns of homosexuals and, in particular, of those with AIDS. We shall speak in another section about other possibilities of selective susceptibility to certain infections in the anomalous dominance population.

## Pregnancy

*Birth Trauma* A high rate of difficult births has been claimed for many conditions, e.g., LH,[241] autism[91] and other childhood learning disorders, and schizophrenia,[242] although many of these data are in dispute. The usual assumption is that a high rate of birth difficulty implies that trauma to the brain at birth is responsible for many cases of these conditions. The lesions that have, however, been found in several cases of childhood dyslexia are clearly the result of alterations during intrauterine development and cannot be the result of birth trauma. It seems to us that difficult birth is much more likely to be a parallel manifestation, rather than the cause of these disorders, i.e., the same influences that alter brain development also lead to disturbance of the birth process. This view implies that all, or nearly all, the children who later turn out to be autistic would still suffer from this condition even if birth trauma were avoided, e.g., by cesarean section or administration of appropriate drugs. This hypothesis leads to a surprising conclusion. As obstetric care improves with a reduction in frank brain truma at birth, the frequency of gross neurologic damage should drop, but the rate of the childhood learning disorders might well rise. Children whose brian development has been disturbed in such a way as to make them dyslexic are also more likely to undergo difficult deliveries and, therefore, to suffer brain damage at birth. The gross impairments that result may make it impossible to diagnose typical dyslexia or autism at a later date. With better care at birth many of these children will be protected from gross brain damage and will therefore be recognized as typical examples of LD. Improved obstetrical care might thus lead, apparently paradoxically, to a rise in the rate of LD, but to a drop in the coarser forms of brain impairment.

*Anomalous Dominance in Offspring* There are several reasons why parents with AD will have a higher rate of children with AD. In the first place the AD parent will transmit any genetic predispositions to factors that favor AD. These might include increased production of or sensitivity to hormones, immune mechanisms, and undoubtedly many other factors.

There will, however, also be nongenetic effects. Thus when the mother is anomalously dominant she will often be hormonally anomalous in such a way as to favor the production of children with similar dominance patterns. The anomalous hormonal pattern of the mother may reflect her own genetic pattern, but when the responsible genes are not shared with the fetus, then the effects on the fetus will be independent, to a great extent, of its genetic endowment. There will be other cases in which the mother was herself exposed to an anomalous hormonal environment as a result of her own genetic endowment or as a result of nongenetic effects, e.g., hormones controlled by maternal genes that she did not share, or exogenous stimuli that altered the hormonal atmosphere, e.g., sex steroids or other drugs, and even the season of birth, which is discussed elsewhere. Rats exposed to early androgens are permanently altered. Diethylstilbestrol daughters are probably an example of a similar phenomenon in humans, i.e., they have high rates of difficulty in pregnancy. One such diethylstilbestrol daughter who had severe acne and small breasts had unusually marked androgenic responses to phenytoin. The fetus carried by such a mother has a strong chance of being exposed to an anomalous environment.

*Further Implications of Hormonal Atmosphere in Pregnancy* It is important to consider some other implications of the hormonal ambience in pregnancy. Let us consider two examples.

Huntington's disease is transmitted as a mendelian dominant, i.e., on the average half of both male and female children are affected, and the disease is passed on equally often by affected fathers and mothers. Unexpectedly, however, early onset cases of this disorder are overwhelmingly transmitted by the father.[243] One must, therefore, ask why maternally transmitted cases do not have an early onset. One possible explanation is that of higher death rates in utero when the mother is affected, but since there is no overall shortage of maternally transmitted cases this is unlikely.

We will not discuss other explanations that have been advanced, but will offer a possible alternative. Assume that the Huntington's gene produces specific changes in the endocrine or other metabolic characteristics of the mother. The fetus of an affected mother is thus exposed to this anomalous chemical environment which we suggest may act to repress expression of the Huntington's gene, at least for several years.

The implication of this mechanism is that there already exists a measure for preventing the onset of Huntington's disease; learning its exact nature might lead to preventive measures that could be applied to paternally transmitted cases while they are still in utero. Furthermore, it is conceivable that the naturally occurring mechanism could be improved on so as to prevent expression entirely.

The possibility that the mother with Huntington's disease is hormonally anomalous should not be surprising since dopamine has important effects on the hypothalamus, e.g., it inhibits prolactin release. Furthermore, Bird et al[244] found high levels of LHRH in the brains of females with Huntington's disease, although this has not been replicated.

If this speculation is correct then the possibility also arises that maternally and paternally transmitted cases might have different rates of LH.

In *dystrophia myotonica,* also transmitted as a mendelian dominant, the reverse is found, i.e., early onset cases are more likely to be maternally transmitted. Presumably the intrauterine environment provided by an affected mother permits earlier expression of the disease gene. The evidence for hormonal anomaly is clear in this disorder. Ovarian and testicular atrophy are common, and infertility is frequently present.[245] Data on anomalous dominance are not available for maternally and paternally transmitted cases.

*Prematurity* The reasons for a possible elevated rate of prematurity or preterm birth in offspring of parents with AD should be clear from our previous discussions. The male fetus who receives genes from the father that favor anomalous dominance may be a producer of high levels of T, which may lead to premature or preterm delivery. Similarly, AD mothers may have higher rates of prematurity. The elevated rate of later cognitive difficulties in premature births is usually attributed to high rates of difficult birth and postnatal complications. In some cases, however, the later cognitive problems may simply reflect that a higher rate of AD may be present. It should be noted that prematurity is more common in male infants.

There is another reason why brains of premature infants might be atypical. The planum temporale asymmetry is typically seen at about 31 weeks of gestation,[246] i.e., Heschl's gyrus is not seen on the left side until that time, although it appears on the right side seven to ten days earlier. Many premature infants are born before the 31st week, and thus have no visible planum temporale asymmetry at birth. How does this brain develop outside the uterus? It is often said that the premature brain develops normally postnatally and indeed even rapidly so that it "catches up" with the normal brain. If this were correct, then the full normal gestation would not be necessary for the brain. It appears to us unlikely that maturation of the brain is normal, especially in the absence of the normal intrauterine hormonal atmosphere.

The absence of a normal hormonal atmosphere appears indeed generally to be overlooked as a possible cause of the many early postpartum difficulties in the premature infant. In the rat, the final stages of development of the preoptic nucleus take place in the early postnatal period that is analogous to the late stages of *intrauterine* life in the human. Since the proper hormonal atmosphere is essential for the preoptic nucleus, it may well be necessary for other hypothalamic centers. Its absence might play a major role in the poor control of blood pressure and other vital functions in premature infants. If this were correct it might have implications for the treatment of the premature infant.

Prematurity is more common in males and in children of diethylstilbestrol mothers. Hyaline membrane disease, which is more common in premature infants, is strongly male predominant. Adrenal steroids play a role in this disorder since they speed up lung maturation, but we know of no data on gonadal steroids. We have seen a masculinized female with this disorder whose mother took progesterone, which may have masculinizing effects on the fetus,[247] in pregnancy. Sudden infant death syndrome is also male predominant and it has been suggested that its frequency follows the course of the postpartum T level. This is low immediately after birth, rises to a peak in the first year, and then declines again.

The "*speeding up*" of brain development said to occur in premature infants is probably not a true mechanism for catching up but rather a method of protecting the brain, but possibly at the expense of a more refined structure, in an unfavorable atmosphere for development. DeBassio and Kemper[248] have found neuronal migration to be accelerated in the developing olfactory system in fetuses of malnourished rat mothers. Accelerated development was found in brains of infants whose mothers were given adrenal steroids in pregnancy.[249] Heydemann and Huttenlocher[250] found that in cultures of immature cortical neurons cortisone accelerated synaptogenesis.

The lack of a normal hormonal atmosphere may lead to anomalous formation of late developing asymmetric regions. Supplying a normal hormonal atmosphere might, however, be disadvantageous since it may place too great a metabolic load on a fetus who can no longer depend on the mother's heart and lungs to supplement its own immature systems, a problem which could be studied in the animal laboratory.

We know of no studies of brains of premature infants who died several years after birth. Their pattern of asymmetries would be an intriguing subject for study. It is even conceivable that certain patterns of giftedness would be more common.

One must ask similar questions about the preterm infant, in whom one might expect alterations, similar, but less marked to those of the premature infant. Possibly even more intriguing is the *postmature* infant, exposed to hormones over a longer period and thus perhaps possessed of a different family background and a characteristic pattern of psychologic endowment.

## Neoplasia

Asymmetry can be associated in several ways with neoplasia. Certain tumors may be more or less common in those with AD than in those with standard dominance. Some tumors may show a predilection for one side of the body or brain.

In view of the high rate of lymphoid malignancies in autoimmune disorders, one might expect an elevated rate of such malignancies in AD individuals and their families, but this remains to be studied. In view of the relatively low rate of these malignancies it would probably be better not to study their frequency in non-RH, but rather to determine the handedness distribution of a large group of patients with lymphoid malignancies. One might also raise the possibility of a lowered rate of other malignancies in the AD population. In celiac disease (which has a high rate of NRH) there is a higher than expected death rate from all malignancies. This elevated mortality is the result of an increased number of lymphomas and other unusual gut tumors, while the rates of cancer of the lung and breast are diminished.

In Down's syndrome, the superior temporal gyrus is often thinner than normal[251] and there are cytoarchitectonic abnormalities,[252] although whether these are more frequent on one side is not known. There is a high rate of lymphoid malignancies both in the patients and in their relatives. Neoplasia is increased in patients with hemihypertrophy[253] in whom the larger side is typically warmer and shows a higher rate of growth of fibroblasts. Tumors transplanted to rats grow more rapidly on anterior parts of the body,[254] but there are no data on growth rates on the two sides, especially in animals with known laterality patterns. The evidence from hemihypertrophy suggests that such differences might well be found.

Certain brain tumors are asymmetric, e.g., meningiomas of the lateral ventricle and choroid plexus papillomas have a predilection for the left side. Arteriovenous malformations in the left temporal lobe have now been found by us and other observers in four dyslexic patients. Arteriovenous malformations in the primary speech areas on the left side are more common in males than in females.[255] Cavernomas of the temporal lobe are usually found on the left side in females.[256] Since hamartomas, which are embryonic rests may give rise in some cases to gliomas, one might expect a higher frequency of gliomas in patients with neuronal migration defects. We have been struck in several cerebral gliomas by a history of previous lumbar disc disease affecting the leg on the side opposite the tumor. A typical example is a male in early middle life who had a shorter leg on that side which required a special shoe in childhood. We have also seen a higher arch or instep or hammer toes on the shorter side. All these suggest very early, possibly intrauterine abnormality, in at least some gliomas.

Several tumors may carry sex hormone receptors, e.g., cancer of the breast (more common on the left side), melanomas, meningiomas, and astrocytomas, but not oligodendrogliomas.[257] Meningiomas may carry progesterone receptors.[258] It would be interesting to look for lateral predilection or associations with AD in all of these cases. Willis[259] reported that malignant neuroblastomas sometimes mature to benign tumors, and this occurs more often in women.

## Hypertension and Other Vascular Disorders

Quinan[260] described an elevated rate of hypertension in sinistrals, but no one has replicated this study. In a recent set of studies on surgical treatment of several conditions, e.g., trigeminal neuralgia, hemifacial spasm, glossopharyngeal neuralgia, tinnitus, and vertigo, by moving arteries or veins that impinge on the respective cranial nerves near the cerebellopontine angle, a high frequency of hypertension, which was often corrected by the surgical procedure, was found in those with left-sided lesions.[261] The left-sided predilection is attributed to the fact that the left vagus supplies the heart. There are no data on handedness in the patients. If the disorders on the left were somehow related to sinistrality this might be a reason for an elevated rate of hypertension in those with AD; this would, however, lead to a significant difference from dextrals only if this type of lesion were a common cause of hypertension.

There is a possible mechanism that might lead to an elevated rate of angina and myocardial infarction in sinistrals. Individuals with thyroid hormone levels in the normal range with elevated thyroid-stimulating hormone have higher levels of thyroid autoantibodies than controls, and an elevated frequency of coronary disease.[262,263] One might presume that even mild declines of thyroid hormone levels (which, however, still remain in the normal range) could lead to elevations of cholesterol, but one of the studies cited did not find this, at least in females. If this were correct, then sinistrals who have an elevated rate of thyroid immune disease might conceivably suffer from cardiovascular disease on the basis of this mechanism. On the other hand, until one considered the many risk factors for this type of disorder one would not be justified in arguing that this type of disorder was more common in sinistrals than in dextrals.

Another conceivable mechanism of cardiovascular disorder in those with anomalous dominance is insulin-dependent diabetes mellitus, which is often regarded as an immune disorder, but we do not yet have adequate data on its frequency in sinistrals.

We have also noted the high rate of diabetes in women with upper body fat who tend to have high free T levels,[226] a group whom we suspect, for reasons discussed earlier, may have an elevated rate of AD. One might expect elevated rates of cardiovascular disorder in this group.

We have also speculated (but do not yet have the data) that females with mitral prolapse may have a high rate of AD. This group is at risk for strokes, possibly on the basis of a high frequency of platelet anomalies.

Other types of platelet anomalies in AD groups might contribute to a lowered rate of cardiovascular disease by interference with clotting. Patients with attention deficit disorder have been reported to have high rates of platelet anomalies.[215] There is also the curious male-predominant condition of right radial aplasia and thrombocytopenia on which no data as to dominance are yet available.

## References

1. Geschwind N, Galaburda AM: Cerebral lateralization: Biological mechanisms, associations, and pathology: I. A hypothesis and a program for research. *Arch Neurol* 1985;42:428–459.
2. Buffery AWH, Gray JA: Sex differences in the development of spatial and linguistic skills, in Ounsted C, Taylor DC (eds): *Gender Differences: Their Ontogeny and Significance.* New York, Churchill Livingstone, Inc, 1972.
3. Hier D, Crowley WF Jr: Spatial ability in androgen-deficient men. *N Engl J Med* 1982;306:1202–1205.
4. Taylor DC: Developmental stratagems organizing intellectual skills: Evidence from studies of temporal lobectomy for epilepsy, in Knights RM, Bakker D (eds): *The Neuropsychology of Learning Disorders.* Baltimore, University Park Press, 1976.
5. Taylor DC: Brain lesions, surgery, seizures, and mental symptoms, in Reynolds E, Trimble M (eds): *Psychiatry of Epilepsy.* New York, Churchill Livingstone Inc, 1981.
6. Waber DP: Environmental influences on brain and behavior, in Ansara A, Geschwind N, Galaburda A, et al (eds): *Sex Differences in Dyslexia.* Townsen, Md, Orton Dyslexia Society, 1981, pp 73–79.
7. McLean JM, Ciurczak FM: Bimanual dexterity in major league baseball players: A statistical study. *N Engl J Med* 1982;2:1278–1279.

8. Peterson JM: Left-handedness: Differences between student artists and scientists. *Percept Motor Skills* 1979;48:961–962.
9. Peterson JM, Lansky LM: Left-handedness among architects: Some facts and speculation. *Percept Mot Skills* 1974;38:547–550.
10. Oldfield RC: Handedness in musicians. *Br J Psychol* 1969;60:91–99.
11. Peterson JM, Lansky LM: Success in architecture: Handedness and/or visual thinking. *Percept Mot Skills* 1980;50:1139–1143.
12. Annett M, Kilshaw D: Mathematical ability and lateral asymmetry. *Cortex* 1982; 18:547–568.
13. Kolata G: Math genius may have hormonal basis. *Science* 1983;222:1312.
14. Deutsch D: Pitch memory: An advantage for the lefthanded. *Science* 1978; 199:559–560.
15. Byrne B: Handedness and musical ability. *Br J Psychol* 1974;65:279–281.
16. Quinan C: A study of sinistrality and muscle coordination in musicians, iron workers, and others. *Arch Neurol Psychiatry* 1922;7:352–360.
17. Hicks RE, Barton AK: A note on left-handedness and severity of mental retardation. *J Genet Psychol* 1975;127:323–324.
18. Sano F: James Henry Pullen: The genius of Earlswood. *J Ment Sci* 1918;64:251–267.
19. Gordon HW: Cognitive asymmetry in dyslexic families. *Neuropsychologia* 1980; 18:645–656.
20. Gordon HW: Learning disabled are cognitively right, in Kinsbourne M (ed): *Topics in Learning Disabilities*. Rockville, Md, Aspen Systems Corp, 1983, vol 3, pp 29–39.
21. Goldman-Rakic P, Rakic P: Experimental modification of gyral patterns, in Geschwind N, Galaburda AM (eds): *Cerebral Dominance: The Biological Foundations*. Cambridge, Mass, Harvard University Press, 1984, pp 179–192.
22. Strub R, Geschwind N: Gerstmann syndrome without aphasia. *Cortex* 1974; 10:378–387.
23. Hermann K: *Reading Disability*. Springfield, Ill, Charles C Thomas Publisher, 1959.
24. Kinsbourne M, Warrington EK: The developmental Gerstmann syndrome. *Arch Neurol* 1963;8:490–501.
25. Benson DF, Geschwind N: Developmental Gerstmann syndrome. *Neurology* 1970; 20:293–298.
26. Dejerine J: Sur un cas de cecite verbale avec agraphie, suivi d'autopsie. *Mem Soc Biol* 1891;3:197–201.
27. Benson DF, Geschwind N: The alexias, in Vinken PJ, Bruyn GW (eds): *Handbook of Neurology*. New York, Elsevier North Holland Inc, 1969, vol 4, pp 112–140.
28. Berman A: The problem of assessing cerebral dominance and its relationship to intelligence. *Cortex* 1971;7:372–386.
29. Miller E: Handedness and the pattern of human ability. *Br J Psychol* 1971;62:111–112.
30. Sherman GF, Garbanati JA, Rosen GD, et al: Brain and behavioral asymmetries for spatial preference in rats. *Brain Res* 1980;192:61–67.
31. Diamond MC, Dowling GA, Johnson RE: Morphological cerebral cortical asymmetry in male and female rats. *Exp Neurol* 1981;71:261–268.

32. Diamond MC: Age, sex, and environmental influences, in Geschwind N, Galaburda AM (eds): *Cerebral Dominance: The Biological Foundations.* Cambridge, Mass, Harvard University Press, 1984, chap 9, pp 134–146.
33. Sherman GF, Galaburda AM: Cortical volume asymmetry and behavior in the albino rat. *Soc Neurosci Abstr* 1982;8:627.
34. Haseltine FP, Ohno S: Mechanisms of gonadal differentiation. *Science* 1981;211:1272–1278.
35. Ivanyi P: Some aspects of the H-2 system, the major histocompatibility system in the mouse. *Proc R Soc Lond* 1978;202:117–158.
36. Bardin CW, Catterall JF: Testosterone: A major determinant of extragenital sexual dimorphism. *Science* 1981;211:1285–1294.
37. Naftolin F: Sexual dimorphism. *Science* 1981;211:1263–1324.
38. Mittwoch V: Lateral asymmetry and gonadal differentiation. *Lancet* 1975;1:401–402.
39. Selye H: *Hormones and Resistance.* New York, Springer Publishing Co, 1971, vols 1 and 2.
40. Gustaffson JA, Mode A, Skett P, et al: Cerebral control of a cytochrome P-450-dependent steroid hydroxylase in rat liver, in Dorner C, Kawakami M (eds): *Hormones and Brain Development.* New York, Elsevier North Holland Inc, 1978.
41. Dohler KD: Is female sexual differentiation hormone-mediated? *TINS* 1978;1:138–140.
42. Biegon A, McEwen BS: Modulation by estradiol of serotonin receptors in brain. *J Neurosci* 1982;2:199–205.
43. Assemany SR, Neu RL, Gardner LI: Deformities in a child whose mother took LSD. *Lancet* 1970;1:1290.
44. McEwen BS: Neural gonadal steroid actions. *Science* 1981;211:1303–1311.
45. Denef C: Differentiation of steroid metabolism in the rat and mechanisms of neonatal androgen action. *Enzyme* 1976;15:254–271.
46. Huttenlocher PR: Synaptic density in the human frontal cortex: Developmental changes and effects of aging. *Brain Res* 1979;163:195–205.
47. Stumpf WE, Sar M, Keefer DA, et al: The anatomical substrate of neuroendocrine regulation as defined by autoradiology with $^{3}$H-estradiol, $^{3}$H-testosterone, $^{3}$H-dihydrotestosterone, and $^{3}$H-progesterone, in *Neuroendocrine Regulation of Fertility,* New York, S Karger AG, 1976.
48. Kolodny E: A postulated role for neutral hydrolases in developing brain. *Neuroscience* 1984;1:89–91.
49. MacLusky NJ, Naftolin F, Goldman-Rakic PS: Oestrogen formation and binding in the cerebral cortex and diencephalon of the newborn rhesus monkey. Submitted.
50. Raisman G, Field P: Sexual dimorphism in the preoptic area of the rat. *Science* 1971;173:731–733.
51. Breedlove SM, Arnold AP: Hormone accumulation in a sexually dimorphic motor nucleus of the rat spinal cord. *Science* 1980;210:564–568.
52. Baum MJ: Pineal gland: Influence on development of copulation in male rats. *Science* 1968;162:586–587.
53. Karsch FJ, Dierschke DJ, Knobil E: Sexual differentiation of pituitary function: Apparent difference between primates and rodents. *Science* 1973;179:484–486.
54. Edwards DA: Mice: Fighting by neonatally androgenized females. *Science* 1964;161:1027–1028.

55. Bronson FH, Desjardins C: Aggression in adult mice: Modification by neonatal injections of gonadal hormones. *Science* 1968;161:705–706.
56. Money J, Ehrhardt AA: Gender dimorphic behavior and fetal sex hormones, in Astwood EB (ed): *Recent Progress in Hormone Research.* New York, Academic Press Inc, 1972, vol 28.
57. Bongiovanni AM, Di George AM, Grumbach MM: Masculinization of the female infant associated with estrogenic therapy alone during gestation: Four cases. *J Clin Endocrinol* 1959;19:1004–1011.
58. Herbst AL, Hubby MM, Blough RR, et al: A comparison of pregnancy experience in DES-exposed and DES-unexposed daughters. *J Reprod Med* 1980;24:62–69.
59. Hines M: Prenatal gonadal hormones and sex differences in human behavior. *Psychol Bull* 1982;92:56–80.
60. Nichols PL, Chen TC: *Minimal Brain Dysfunction: A Prospective Study.* Hillsdale, NJ, Lawrence Erlbaum, 1981.
61. Rosen GD, Berrebi AS, Yutzey DA, et al: Prenatal testosterone causes shift of asymmetry in neonatal tail posture of the rat. *Dev Brain Res* 1983;9:99–101.
62. Glick SD: Heritable determinants of left-right bias in the rat. *Life Sci* 1983; 32:2215–2221.
63. Taylor DC: Differential rates of cerebral maturation between sexes and between hemispheres. *Lancet* 1969;2:140–142.
64. Nordeen EJ, Yahr P: A regional analysis of estrogen binding to hypothalamic cell nuclei in relation to masculinization and defeminization. *J Neurosci* 1983;3:933–941.
65. Gerendai I, Rosztejn W, Marchetti B, et al: Unilateral ovariectomy-induced luteinizing hormone-releasing hormone content changes in the two halves of the mediobasal hypothalamus. *Neurosci Lett* 1978;9:333–336.
66. Toran-Allerand CD: Gonadal hormones and brain development: Cellular aspects of sexual differentiation. *Am Zool* 1978;18:553–565.
67. Nottebohm F: A brain for all seasons: Cyclical anatomic changes in song control nuclei of the canary brain. *Science* 1981;214:1368–1370.
68. King LS: Hereditary defects of the corpus callosum in the mouse, *Mus musculus. J Comp Neurol* 1936;64:337–363.
69. Wahlsten D: Mice in utero while mother is lactating suffer higher frequency of defective corpus callosum. *Neurosci Abstr* 1981;7:349.
70. Newson-Davis J, Vincent A: Receptors, antibodies, and disease. *Immunol Today* 1982;3:149–152.
71. Ward IL, Weisz J: Maternal stress alters plasma testosterone in fetal males. *Science* 1980;207:328–329.
72. Tucker HA, Ringer RK: Controlled photo-periodic environments for food animals. *Science* 1982;216:1381–1386.
73. Badian NA: Birth order, maternal age, season of birth, and handedness. *Cortex* 1983;19:451–463.
74. Nieuwenhuys R: The brain of the lamprey in a comparative perspective. *Ann NY Acad Sci* 1977;299:97–145.
75. Crawford WA, Beldham CG: The changing demographic pattern in asthma related to sex and age. *Med J Aust* 1976;1:430–434.
76. Wasi P, Block M: The histopathological study of the development of the irradiation-induced leukemia in C57BL mice and of its inhibition by testosterone. *Cancer Res* 1961;21:463–473.

77. Dougherty TF: Effects of hormones on lymphatic tissue. *Physiol Rev* 1952;32:379–401.
78. Frey-Wettstein M, Craddock CG: Testosterone-induced depletion of thymus and marrow lymphocytes as related to lymphopoiesis and hematopoiesis. *Blood* 1970; 35:257–271.
79. Warner NL, Szenberg A, Burnet FM: The immunological role of different lymphoid organs in the chicken. *Aust J Exp Biol Med Sci* 1962;40:373–388.
80. Castro JE: Orchidectomy and the immune response: I. Effect of orchidectomy on lymphoid tissues of mice. *Proc R Soc Lond* 1974;185:425–436.
81. Stimson WH: Steroids and the immune system. *J Neuroimmunol* 1982;1:516.
82. Ohno S: The original function of MHC antigens as the general plasma membrane anchorage site of organogenesis-directing proteins. *Immunol Rev* 1977;33:59–69.
83. Smith SD, Kimberling WJ, Pennington BF, et al: Specific reading disability: Identification of an inherited form through linkage analysis. *Science* 1983;219:1345–1347.
84. Murgita RA, Tomasi TB: Suppression of immune response by alphafetoprotein. *J Exp Med* 1975;141:440–452.
85. Sedgwick RP, Boder E: Ataxia-telangiectasia, in Vinken PJ, Bruyn GW (eds): *Handbook of Clinical Neurology* New York, Elsevier North Holland Inc, 1972, vol 14 *The Phakomatoses,* pp 267–339.
86. Golub ES: Connections between the neurons, haematopoietic, and germ-cell systems. *Nature* 1982;299:483–485.
87. Schoene WC, Carpenter S, Behan PO, et al: "Onion-bulb" formations in the central and periphreal nervous system in association with multiple sclerosis and hypertrophic polyneuropathy. *Brain* 1977;100:755–773.
88. Talal N: *Autoimmunity.* New York, Academic Press Inc, 1977.
89. Sperry RW: Restoration of vision after uncrossing of optic nerves and after contralateral transposition of the eye. *J Neurophysiol* 1945;8:15–28.
90. Levitt P: A monoclonal antibody to limbic system neurons. *Science* 1984;223:299–301.
91. Geschwind N, Behan P: Left-handedness: Association with immune disease, migraine, and developmental learning disorder. *Proc Natl Acad Sci USA* 1982; 79:5097–5100.
92. Geschwind N, Behan PO: Laterality, hormones, and immunity in Geschwind N, Galaburda AM (eds): *Cerebral Dominance: The Biological Foundations.* Cambridge, Mass, Harvard University Press, 1984, pp 211–224.
93. Coleman M: *The Autistic Syndromes.* New York, Elsevier North Holland Inc, 1976.
94. Diehl CF: *A Compendium of Research and Theory On Stuttering.* Springfield, Ill, Charles C Thomas Publisher, 1958.
95. Theofilopoulos AG, Prud'Homme GJ, Fieser TM, et al: B-cell hyperactivity in murine lupus: I. Immunological abnormalities in lupus-prone strains and the activation of normal B-cells. *Immunol Today* 1983;4:287–291.
96. Marsh DG, Meyers DA, Bias WB: The epidemiology and genetics of atopic allergy. *N Engl J Med* 1981;305:1551–1559.
97. Nussenzweig RS: Parasitic disease as a cause of immunosuppression. *N Engl J Med* 1982;306:423–424.
98. Renoux G, Biziere K, Renoux M, et al: The production of T-cell-inducing factors in mice is controlled by brain neocortex. *Scand J Immunol* 1983;17:45–50.

99. Renoux G, Biziere K, Renoux M, et al: A balanced brain asymmetry modulates T cell-mediated events. *J Neuroimmunol* 1983;5:227–238.
100. Annett M: *A Single Gene Explanation of Right and Lefthandedness and Brainedness.* Coventry, England, Lanchester Polytechnic Press, 1978.
101. Collins RL: On the inheritance of handedness. 2: Selection for sinistrality in mice. *J Hered* 1969;60:117–119.
102. Layton WM Jr: Random determination of a developmental process. *J Hered* 1976; 67:336–338.
103. Corballis MC, Morgan MJ: On the biological basis of human laterality. *Behav Brain Sci* 1978;2:261–336.
104. Geschwind N, Levitsky W: Human brain: Left-right asymmetries in temporal speech region. *Science* 1968;161:186–187.
105. Wada JA, Clarke R, Hamm A: Cerebral hemispheric asymmetry in humans. *Arch Neurol* 1975;32:239–246.
106. Fontes V: *Morfologica do Cortex Cerebral (Desenvolvimento).* Lisbon, Instituto Antonio Aurelio da Costa Ferreira, 1944.
107. Porac C, Coren S: *Lateral Preferences and Human Behavior.* New York, Springer Publishing Co Inc, 1981.
108. Bryden MP: *Laterality: Functional Asymmetry in the Intact Brain.* New York, Academic Press Inc, 1982.
109. Larrabee AP: The optic chiasm of teleosts: A study of inheritance. *Proc Am Acad Arts Sci* 1906;12:217–231.
110. Policansky D: Flatfishes and the inheritance of asymmetries. *Behav Brain Sci* 1982; 5:262–266.
111. Clutton-Brock TH: Sons and daughters. *Nature* 1982;298:11–13.
112. Harvey PH, Slatkin M: Some like it hot: Temperature-determined sex. *Nature* 1982;296:807–808.
113. James WH: Gonadotrophin and the human secondary sex ratio. *Br Med J* 1980; 281:711–712.
114. James WH: Race, season, gonadotrophin, and sex ratio. *Lancet* 1980;2:1032.
115. Dahlberg G: Genotypic asymmetries. *Proc R Soc Edin* 1944–1947;62:20–31.
116. Birky CW: Relaxed cellular controls and organelle heredity. *Science* 1983;222:466–475.
117. Davidson EH, Hough-Evans BR, Britten RJ: Molecular biology of the sea urchin embryo. *Science* 1982;217:17–26.
118. Jenkins JB: *Genetics,* ed. Boston, Houghton Mifflin Co, 1979.
119. Boycott AE, Diver C: On the inheritance of sinistrality in *Limnea peregra. Proc R Soc Lond* 1923–1924;195:207–213.
120. Freeman G, Lundelius JW: The developmental genetics of dextrality and sinistrality in the gastropod *Lymnaea peregra. Roux Arch Ent Organ* 1982;191:69–83.
121. Nance WE: Anencephaly and spina bifida: A possible example of cytoplasmic inheritance in man. *Nature* 1969;224:373–375.
122. Boycott AE, Diver C, Garstang SL, et al: The inheritance of sinistrality in *Limnaea peregra (Mollusca pulmonata). Phil Trans R Soc Lond* 1930;219:51–131.
123. Maxon SC, Ginsburg BE, Trattner A: Interaction of Y chromosomal and autosomal gene(s) in the development of intermale aggression in mice. *Behav Genet* 1979; 9:219–226.
124. Andrews PW, Goodfellow PM: Analysing the mouse T/E complex. *Nature* 1982; 299:296–297.

125. Dunn LC: Abnormalities associated with a chromosome region in the mouse. *Science* 1964;144:260–267.
126. Goodfellow PN, Andrews PW: Is there a human T/t locus? *Nature* 1983;302:657–658.
127. Gupta C, Yaffee SJ, Shapiro BH: Prenatal exposure to phenobarbital permanently decreases testosterone and causes reproductive dysfunction. *Science* 1982; 216:640–642.
128. Denenberg VH, Garbanati J, Sherman G, et al: Infantile stimulation induces brain lateralization in rats. *Science* 1978;201:1150–1152.
129. Denenberg VH, Zarrow MX: Effects of handling in infancy upon adult behavior and adrenocortical activity: Suggestions for a neuroendocrine mechanism, in Walcher DN, Peters DL (eds): *The Development of Self-Regulatory Mechanisms.* New York, Academic Press Inc, 1971, pp 39–64.
130. Michaelson J: Genetic polymorphism of B2-microglobulin (B2m) maps to the H-3 region of chromosome 2. *Immunogenetics* 1981;13:167–171.
131. MacLusky NJ, Nafolin F: Sexual differentiation of the central nervous system. *Science* 1981;211:1294–1303.
132. Beral V, Colwell L: Randomised trial of high doses of stilboestrol and ethisterone therapy in pregnancy: Long-term follow-up of the children. *J Epidemiol Community Health* 1981;35:155–160.
133. Bulmer MG: *The Biology of Twinning in Man.* Oxford, England, Clarendon Press, 1970.
134. Nylander PPS: Causes of high twinning frequencies in Nigeria, in Nance WE (ed): *Twin Research: Biology and Epidemiology.* New York, Alan R Liss Inc, 1978, pp 35–43.
135. Boklage CE: Twinning, handedness, and the biology of symmetry, in Geschwind N, Galaburda AM (eds): *Cerebral Dominance: The Biological Foundations.* Cambridge, Mass, Harvard University Press, 1984, pp 195–210.
136. Satz P: Left-handedness and early brain insult: An explanation. *Neuropsychologia* 1973;2:115–117.
137. Parisi P, Gatti M, Prinzi G, et al: Familial incidence of twinning. *Nature* 1983; 304:626–628.
138. Ghosh A, Woo JSK, Poon IML, et al: Neural tube defects in Hong Kong Chinese. *Lancet* 1981;2:468–469.
139. Huppert LC: Induction of ovulation with clomiphene citrate. *Mod Trends* 1979; 31:1–8.
140. Jaffee WL, Vaitukaitis JL: Polycystic ovarian syndrome in Vaitukaitis JL (ed): *Clinical and Reproductive Neuroendocrinology.* New York, Elsevier North Holland Inc, 1982, pp 207–230.
141. Meisel RL, Ward IL: Fetal female rats are masculinized by male littermates located caudally in the uterus. *Science* 1981;213:239–241.
142. Gandelman R, vom Saal FS, Reinisch JM: Contiguity to male foetuses affects morphology and behaviour of female mice. *Nature* 1977;266:722–725.
143. Hauser H, Gandelman R: Contiguity to males in utero affects avoidance responding in adult female mice. *Science* 1983;220:437–438.
144. Bakwin H: Reading disability in twins. *Dev Med Child Neurol* 1973;15:184–187.
145. Afzelius BA, Camner P, Eliasson R, et al: Kartagener's syndrome does exist. *Lancet* 1978;2:950.

146. Farthing MJG, Edwards CRW, Rees LH, et al: Male gonadal function in coeliac disease: I. Sexual dysfunction, infertility, and semen quality. *Gut* 1982;23:608–614.
147. McAllister LB, Scheller RH, Kandel ER, et al: In situ hybridization to study the origin and fate of identified neurons. *Science* 1983;222:800–808.
148. McGee MG, Cozad T: Population genetic analysis of human hand preference: Evidence for generational differences, familial resemblance, and maternal effects. *Behav Genet* 1980;10:263–275.
149. Teng EL, Lee PH, Yang KS: Handedness in a Chinese population. *Science* 1976; 193:1148–1150.
150. Shimizu A, Emdo M: Handedness and familial sinistrality in a Japanese student population. *Cortex* 1983;19:265–272.
151. Fraser FC, Czeizel A, Hanson C: Increased frequency of neural tube defects in sibs of children with other malformations. *Lancet* 1982;2:144–145.
152. LeMarec B, Roussey M, Oger J, et al: Excess twinning in the parents of spina bifida, in Nance WE (ed): *Twin Research: Biology and Epidemiology,* New York, Alan R Liss Inc, 1978, pp 121–123.
153. Goodall HB, Brobby GW: Stuttering, sickling, and cerebral malaria: A possible organic basis for stuttering. *Lancet* 1982;1:1279–1281.
154. Schnall BS, Smith DW: Nonrandom laterality of malformations in paired structures. *J Pediatr* 1974;83:509–511.
155. Chang KSF, Hsu FK, Chan ST, et al: Scrotal asymmetry and handedness. *J Anat* 1960;94:543–548.
156. Howard J, Petrakis NL, Bross ID, et al: Handedness and breast cancer laterality: Testing a hypothesis. *Hum Biol* 1982;54:365–371.
157. Poskanser DC: Hemiatrophies and hemihypertrophies, in Vinken PJ, Bruyn GW, Dejong JMBV, et al (eds): *Handbook of Clinical Neurology.* North Holland Inc, 1975, vol 22 *System Disorders and Atrophies,* pp 545–554.
158. Gesell A: Hemihypertrophy and twinning. *Am J Sci* 1927;173:542–555.
159. Pirozzolo FJ, Hansch EC: The neurobiology of developmental reading disorders, in Malatesna RN, Aaron PC (eds): *Neurolinguistic Aspects of Reading Disorders.* New York, Academic Press Inc, 1982.
160. Barbas G, Matthews WS, Ferrari M: Minor diagnostic criteria in childhood migraine. *Ann Neurol* 1983;14:364.
161. Kuritzky A, Ziegler DK, Hassanein R: Vertigo, motion sickness, and migraine. *Headache* 1981;21:227–231.
162. Stejskal L, Tomanek Z: Postural laterality in torticollis and torsion dystonia. *J Neurol Neurosurg Psychiatry* 1981;44:1029–1034.
163. Crosby CC, Humphrey T, Lauer EW: *Correlative Anatomy of the Nervous System.* New York, Macmillan Publishing Co Inc, 1962, pp 469–470.
164. Orton ST: 'Word-blindness' in school children. *Arch Neurol Psychiatry* 1925; 14:581–615.
165. Moscovitch M, Smith LC: Differences in neuronal organization between individuals with inverted and non-inverted handwriting postures. *Science* 1979;205:710–713.
166. Levy J, Reid M: Variations in working posture and cerebral organization. *Science* 1976;194:337–339.
167. Regli F, Filippa G, Wiensendanger M: Hereditary mirror movements. *Arch Neurol* 1967;16:620–623.

168. Harati Y, Meyer JS, Wheeler AH: Neuroanatomical and neurophysiological explanations for mirror movement in Klippel-Feil syndrome derived from rcBF studies, in International Congress Series. Amsterdam, Excerpta Medica, 1981, Series 548, p 386.
169. Woods BT, Eby MD: Excessive mirror movements and aggression. *Biol Psychiatry* 1982;17:23–32.
170. Woods BT, Teuber HL: Mirror movements after childhood hemiparesis. *Neurology* 1978;28:1152–1157.
171. Rebeiz JJ, Kolodny EH, Richardson EP: Corticodentatonigral degeneration with neuronal achromasia. *Arch Neurol* 1968;18:20–33.
172. LeDouarin N: *The Neural Crest.* Cambridge, England, Cambridge University Press, 1982.
173. Bockman DE, Kirby ML: Dependence of thymus development on derivatives of the neural crest. *Science* 1984;223:498–500.
174. Strongin AC, Guillery RW: The relationship of melanin distribution to cellular degeneration in the developing mammalian eye. *J Neurosci* 1981;1:1193–1204.
175. Witkop CJ Jr, Jay B, Crul D, et al: Optic neurological abnormalities in oculocutaneous and ocular albinism. *Birth Defects* 1982;18:299–316.
176. Tisserand M: Resultats d'etudes statistiques sur les becs-de-lievre. *Sem Hop Paris* 1949;25:2547–2550.
177. Esscher E, Scott JS: Congenital heart block and maternal systemic lupus erythematosus. *Br Med J* 1979;1:1235–1238.
178. Vetter VL, Raskind WJ: Congenital complete heart block and connective tissue disease. *N Engl J Med* 1983;309:236–237.
179. Tisserand M: Dominance laterale et bec-de-lievre. *Arch Franc Pediatr* 1944;2:166–167.
180. Durfee KE: Crooked ears and the bad boy syndrome: Asymmetry as an indicator of minimal brain dysfunction. *Bull Menninger Clin* 1974;38:305–316.
181. Aase JN, Smith DW: Facial asymmetry and abnormalities of palms and ears: A dominantly inherited developmental syndrome. *J Pediatr* 1970;76:928–930.
182. Liszka D: Spinal cord mechanisms leading to scoliosis in animal experiments. *Acta Med Pol* 1961;2:45–67.
183. MacEwen GD: Operative treatment of scoliosis in cerebral palsy. *Reconstr Surg Traumatol* 1972;13:58–67.
184. Alexander MA, Bunch WH, Ebbesson SO: Can experimental dorsal rhizotomy produce scoliosis? *J Bone Joint Surg* 1972;54A:1509–1513.
185. Davis MR, Constantine-Paton M, Schorr D: Dorsal root ganglion removal in *Rana pipieus* produces fewer motoneurones. *Brain Res* 1983;265:283–288.
186. Ponseti IV, Pedrimi V, Wynne-Davies R, et al: Pathogenesis of scoliosis. *Clin Orthop* 1976;120:268–280.
187. Wynne-Davis R: Heritable disorders in orthopedics. *Orthop Clin North Am* 1978; 9:3–9.
188. Cilluffo JM, Gomez MR, Reese DF, et al: Idiopathic ('congenital') spinal arachnoid diverticula. *Mayo Clin Proc* 1981;56:93–101.
189. Mieses-Reif M: Contents of pigment in hair and iris in its relation to refraction. *Folia Ophthalmol Orientalia* 1936;2:258–260.
190. Schachter S, Ransil BJ, Geschwind N: Associations of handedness with hair color and learning disabilities. *Neuropsychologia*, in press.

191. Cobb S: Haemangioma of the spinal cord. *Ann Surg* 1915;62:641–649.
192. Cushing H: Cases of spontaneous intracranial hemorrhage associated with trigeminal nevi. *JAMA* 1906;47:178–183.
193. Minot G: Pernicious anemia, in Cecil RL (ed): *Textbook of Medicine*. Philadelphia, WB Saunders Co, 1948, pp 1091–1098.
194. Wood LC: Presentation, American Thyroid Association, New Orleans, 1983.
195. Korein J: Iris pigmentation (melanin) in idiopathic dystonic syndromes including torticollis. *Ann Neurol* 1981;10:53–55.
196. Lang AE, Ellis C, Kingon H, et al: Iris pigmentation in idiopathic dystonia. *Ann Neurol* 1982;12:585–586.
197. Korein J: Response to Lang et al. *Ann Neurol* 1982;12:586.
198. Chibber SR, Singh I: Asymmetry in muscle weight and one-sided dominance in the human lower limbs. *J Anat* 1970;106:553–556.
199. Chibber SR, Singh I: Asymmetry in the muscle weight in the human upper limbs. *Acta Anat* 1972;81:462–465.
200. Pande BS, Singh I: One-sided dominance in the upper limbs of human fetuses as evidenced by asymmetry in muscle and bone weight. *J Anat* 1971;109:457–459.
201. Singh I: One-sided dominance in the limbs of rabbits and frogs as evidenced by asymmetry of bone weight. *J Anat* 1971;109:271–275.
202. Burwell RG, Dangerfield PH, Hall DJ, et al: Perthes disease. *J Bone Joint Surg* 1978;60B:461–477.
203. Fraser FC: Association of neural tube defects and parental nonrighthandedness. *Am J Hum Genet* 1983;35:89A.
204. Taylor C, Faulk WP: Prevention of recurrent abortions with leucocyte transfusions. *Lancet* 1981;2:68–69.
205. Faulk WP: Human trophoblast antigens: Role in normal and abnormal pregnancies. *Bull Mem Acad Roy Med Belg* 1981;136:379–388.
206. Chung CS, Myrianthopoulos NC: Factors affecting risks of congenital malformations, in *Birth Defects*. New York, Grune & Stratton Inc, 1975, vol 11, No. 10.
207. Janerich DT, Piper JM, Glebatis DM: Oral contraceptives and congenital limb-reduction defects. *N Engl J Med* 1974;291:697–700.
208. Layton WM Jr, Hallesy DW: Deformity of forelimb in rats: Association with high doses of acetazolamide. *Science* 1965;149:306–308.
209. Scott WJ, Butcher RE, Kindt CW, et al: Greater sensitivity of female than male rat embryos to acetazolamide teratogenicity. *Teratology* 1972;6:239–240.
210. DiPaolo GA: Polydactylism in the offspring of mice injected with 5-bromodeoxyuridine. *Science* 1964;145:501–503.
211. Hall JG, Levin J, Kuhn JP, et al: Thrombocytopenia with absent radius (TAR). *Medicine* 1969;48:411–439.
212. Channick BJ, Adlin EV, Marks AD, et al: Hyperthyroidism and mitral valve prolapse. *N Engl J Med* 1981;305:497–500.
213. Devereux RB, Brown WT, Lutas EM, et al: Association of mitral valve prolapse with low body weight and low blood pressure. *Lancet* 1982;2:792–794.
214. Pickering NJ, Brody JI, Barrett MJ: Von Willebrand's syndromes and mitral valve prolapse. *N Engl J Med* 1981;305:131–134.
215. Koike K, Rao AK, Holmsen H, et al: Platelet-secretion defect in patients with the attention deficit disorder. *Blood* 1984;63:427–433.

216. Rosenberg CA, Derman GH, Grabb WC, et al: Hypomastia and mitral valve prolapse. *N Engl J Med* 1983;309:1230–1232.
217. Honzik MP, Collart DS, Robinson SJ, et al: Sex differences in verbal and performance IQs of children undergoing open-heart surgery. *Science* 1969;164:445–447.
218. Heinonen DP, Slone D, Monson RR, et al: Cardiovascular birth defects and antenatal exposure to female sex hormones. *N Engl J Med* 1977;296:67–70.
219. Levy EP, Cohen A, Fraser FC: Hormone treatment during pregnancy and congenital heart defects. *Lancet* 1973;1:611.
220. Lorber CA, Cassidy SB, Engel E: Is there an embryo-fetal exogenous sex steroid exposure syndrome (EFESSES)? *Fertil Steril* 1979;31:21–24.
221. Nora JJ, Nora AH, Perinchief AG, et al: Congenital abnormalities and first trimester exposure to progestagen/oestrogen. *Lancet* 1976;1:313–314.
222. Graham JR, Rogado AZ, Rahman M, et al: Some physical, physiological, and psychological characteristics of patients with cluster headaches, in Cochrane AL (ed): *Background to Migraine: Third Migraine Symposium.* New York, Springer Publishing Co Inc, 1970.
223. Kudrow L: Physical and personality characteristics in cluster headache. *Headache* 1974;13:197–202.
224. Kretschmer E: *Medizinische Psychologie,* ed 5. Stuttgart, West Germany, Georg Thieme Verlag, 1939, p 125.
225. Draper G, Dupertuis CW, Caughey JL Jr: *Human Constitution in Clinical Medicine.* New York, Paul B. Hoeber Inc, 1944.
226. Kissebah AH, Vydeligum N, Murray R, et al: Relation of body fat distribution to metabolic complications of obesity. *J Clin Endocrinol Metabol* 1982;54:253–260.
227. Maugh TH II: A new marker for diabetes. *Science* 1982;215:651.
228. Cummins H, Midlo C: *Finger Prints, Palms, and Soles.* Philadelphia. The Blakiston Co. 1943.
229. Galaburda AM, LeMay M, Kemper TL, et al: Right-left asymmetries in the brain. *Science* 1978;199:852–856.
230. Herzog AG, Russell V, Vaitukaitis JL, et al: Neuroendocrine dysfunction in temporal lobe epilepsy. *Arch Neurol* 1982;39:133–135.
231. Herzog AG, Seibel MM, Schomer D, et al: Temporal lobe epilepsy: An extrahypothalamic pathogenesis for polycystic ovarian syndrome? *Neurology* 1983; 33(suppl 2):189.
232. Rosman NP, Kakulas BA: Mental deficiency associated with muscular dystrophy. *Brain* 1966;89:769–788.
233. Bleier WJ, Ehteshami M: Ovulation following unilateral ovariectomy in the California leaf-nosed bat (*Macrotus californicus*). *J Reprod Fertil* 1981;63:181–183.
234. Gerendai I: Lateralization of neuroendocrine control, in Geschwind N and Galaburda AM (eds): *Cerebral Dominance: The Biological Foundations.* Cambridge, Mass, Harvard University Press, 1982, pp 167–178.
235. Nordeen EJ, Yahr P: Hemispheric asymmetries in the behavioral and hormonal effects of sexually differentiating mammalian brain. *Science* 1982;218:391–393.
236. Haagensen CD: *Diseases of the Breast,* ed 2. Philadelphia, WB Saunders Co, 1971.
237. Dorner G, Gotz F, Docke WD: Prevention of demasculinization and feminization of the brain in prenatally stressed male rats by perinatal androgen treatment. *Exp Clin Endocrinol* 1983;81:88–90.

238. Dorner G, Schenk B, Schmiedel B, et al: Stressful events in prenatal life of bi- and homosexual men. *Exp Clin Endocrinol* 1983;81:83–87.
239. Toone BK, Wheeler M, Nanjee M, et al: Sex hormones, sexual activity, and plasma convulsant levels in male epileptics. *J Neurol Neurosurg Psychiatry* 1983;46:824–826.
240. Netley C, Rovet J: Handedness in 47, XXY males. *Lancet* 1982;2:267.
241. Bakan P: Left-handedness and birth order revisited. *Neuropsychologia* 1977; 15:837–839.
242. McNeil TE, Kaij L: Obstetric factors in the development of schizophrenia: Complications in the births of preschizophrenics and in reproduction by schizophrenic parents, in Wynne LC, Cromwell RL, Matthysse S (eds): *The Nature of Schizophrenia*. New York, John Wiley & Sons Inc, 1978, pp 401-429.
243. Myers RH, Goldman D, Bird ED, et al: Maternal transmission in Huntington's disease. *Lancet* 1983;1:208–210.
244. Bird ED, Chiappa SA, Fink G: Brain immunoreactive gonadotropin-releasing hormone in Huntington's chorea and in non-choreic subjects. *Nature* 1976;260:536–538.
245. Harper PS: *Myotonic Dystrophy.* Philadelphia, WB Saunders Co, 1979.
246. Chi JG, Dooling EC, Gilles FH: Left-right asymmetries of the temporal speech areas of the human fetus. *Arch Neurol* 1977;34:346–348.
247. Ehrhardt AA, Money J: Progestin-induced hermaphroditism: IQ and psychosexual identity in a study of ten girls. *J Sex Res* 1967;3:83–100.
248. DeBassio WA, Kemper TL: Neuronal migration in undernourished rats. *Ann Neurol* 1982;12:222.
249. Barmada MA, Moossy J: Advanced cerebral maturation with intrauterine growth retardation. *Neurology* 1981;31:163.
250. Heydemann PT, Huttenlocher PR: Synaptogenesis, synaptic density, and the effect of cortisol in reaggregated mouse cerebral isocortex: A model for evaluating drug effects on synaptic movement. *Ann Neurol* 1982;12:202.
251. Greenfield JG, Blackwood W, McMenemy WH, et al (eds): *Neuropathology.* London, Edward Arnold, 1958, p 353.
252. Ross MH, Galaburda AM, Kemper TL. Down's syndrome: Is there a decreased population of neurons? *Neurology* 1984;34:909–916.
253. Furukawa T, Shinohara T: Congenital hemihypertrophy: Oncogenic potential of the hypertrophic side. *Ann Neurol* 1981;10:199–201.
254. Auerbach R, Auerbach W: Regional differences in the growth of normal and neoplastic cells. *Science* 1982;215:127–134.
255. Caron JP, Colin H, Comoy J, et al: Resultats de l'exeoese chirurgicale des aneurysmes arterioveneux (AAV) des zones rolandique, parietale, occipital, et du pli courbe de l'hemisphere dominant: A propos de vingt cas. *Neurochirurgie* 1982;28:295–307.
256. Mori K, Handa H, Gi H, et al: Cavernomas in the middle fossa. *Surg Neurol* 1980; 14:21–31.
257. Takei Y, Kurisaka M, Pearl GS, et al: Estrogen receptors in malignant gliomas. *Proceedings of the World Congress of Neurology,* Kyoto, Japan, 1981.
258. Paul KS, Hayward E, Barnes DM, et al: Progesterone receptors in meningiomas. *J Neurol Neurosurg Psychiatry* 1984;47:103–104.

259. Willis RA: *The Pathology of the Tumors of Children.* London, Oliver & Boyd, 1960.
260. Quinan C: Sinistrality in relation to high blood pressure and defects of speech. *Arch Intern Med* 1921;27:255–261.
261. Jannetta PJ, Gendell HM: Clinical observations on etiology of essential hypertension. *Surg Forum* 1979;30:431–432.
262. Masala C, Amendolea MA, Lopes R: Subclinical hypothyroidism. *Lancet* 1981; 1:161.
263. Tieche M, Lupi GA, Gutzwiller F, et al: Borderline low thyroid function and thyroid autoimmunity. *Br Heart J* 1981;46:202–206.

This study was supported in part by grants from the National Institutes of Health (NS 14018, NINCDS 06209), the National Science Foundation (BNS 05674), the Orton Research Fund, and the Essel Foundation.

# CHAPTER 16 (III)

# Cerebral Lateralization

## Biological Mechanisms, Associations, and Pathology: III. A Hypothesis and a Program for Research

*Norman Geschwind and Albert M. Galaburda*

## Other Aspects of Immunity and Infection

In view of the special importance of immune disorders in the anomalous dominance (AD) population, we have devoted a special section to immunity and infection, dealing primarily with some topics not covered earlier.

### Localized and Lateralized Immune Effects

In the AD population, certain immune disorders occur with especially high frequency, e.g., those involving the gastrointestinal tract or the thyroid. There might be several reasons for this, e.g., this population might have a high frequency of genes determining special susceptibilities of certain systems. Another possibility is that the elevated frequency of these disorders may be the result of the timing of suppression of the developing thymus gland by hormonal or other effects. During fetal life, new antigens are produced as development progresses. We have raised the possibility that as each new antigen appears, lymphocytes are processed that recognize it as self and not as alien. Suppression of thymic processing at any given point should therefore lead to susceptibility to later immune attack on the specific systems being formed at that time. Since certain parts of the nervous system will be forming, certain specific brain syndromes might be associated with higher immune susceptibility of certain somatic organs. There are

---

Reprinted with permission from *Archives of Neurology*. 1985; 42 (6): 634-654. Copyright 1985 on, American Medical Association.

suggestive data, but no adequate documentation, of this possibility, e.g., migraine is perhaps especially associated with dyslexia, allergies with stuttering, and some gut disorder resembling celiac disease with autism. This possibility should be studied in a proper controlled study.

Another mechanism for selective immune effects is suggested by the finding that immune attack on a specific system sometimes involves a tissue factor, e.g., it has been proposed that in the spontaneously hypothyroid rat there are not only specific genes favoring antithyroid immunity but also some anomaly in the thyroid itself.[3] One possibility is that the factors that delay thymic development at a particular moment may also alter developing structures in the brain and other tissues. It is also possible that both brain and other tissue anomalies may reflect interference with an immune mechanism. If histocompatibility antigens (HLAs) are necessary for providing anchorage sites for development,[4] altered development of brain or of other tissues might occur when some external factor suppressed the normal cell to cell interactions controlled by immune markers.

The special susceptibility of a particular structure to later immune attack because of any of the above mechanisms is a version of the classic concept of the *locus minoris resistentiae,* the locus of diminished resistance that has a higher susceptibility for later disease. The mechanisms we have discussed raise the possibility of several forms of the locus of diminished resistance. On the one hand, a particular structure may be susceptible to later immune attack. Another mechanism may be operative if a particular structure is actually malformed so that it contains abnormal cells or abnormal patterns of connection that may lead to early death because of marginal metabolic properties. Finally, a structure whose development has simply been retarded may contain a smaller number of cells, and therefore a smaller reserve beyond what is needed for normal function. Although the smaller structure may be no more susceptible to damage than other tissues, the death of cells during normal aging will reduce its complement below the level needed for normal functioning before that of other tissues that have a larger reserve. It is possible that all of these mechanisms could be simultaneously operative in some cases.

Another well-known mechanism may favor later immune attack on a particular site. Antigens not recognized by the immune system as self need not be subject to immune damage if they are located in immunologically privileged regions, i.e., regions without contact with circulating lymphocytes. The central nervous system (CNS) and very likely the testes are examples of such structures. When an injury exposes these antigens to blood-borne immune factors, they may be attacked. Responses of this type are probably not rare, although in many, perhaps most, cases they do not lead to significant disease, e.g., antiheart antibodies are often formed after myocardial damage, but only in a few instances is there a clinically significant immune carditis. There are instances, however, of severe damage by this mechanism, e.g., sympathetic ophthalmia and sympathetic orchitis (i.e., immune damage to the unaffected eye or testis when the corresponding structure on the other side is damaged). Certain individuals are more susceptible to such disorders, including perhaps those in whom the thymus gland was suppressed during the period of formation of the compartmentalized antigens.

Let us now consider certain possible implications of these mechanisms. They imply that later immune attack should be common at sites of congenital malformation. It is conceivable that the growth of gliomas might result from immune attack at a cell rest (it is, of course, also possible that the tumor grows for other reasons and the infiltration of immune cells may be a mechanism for restraining growth). A possible example of this mechanism is afforded by a patient who developed his first temporal lobe seizure on a morning when he had an epididymitis, and who was found to have a right-sided glioblastoma. He had smaller limbs on the side opposite the tumor, which favors the thesis of early development of the anlage of the glioma. Since there are common antigens in germ cells and brain,[5] it is possible that the epididymitis triggered immune attack against the testis that in turn led to attack on common antigens at the glioblastoma site. Alternatively, the tumor growth might have led to an immune response to the tumor and to "sympathetic" attack on the same antigens in the epididymis.

There are other cases that illustrate the possibility of attack on the brain secondary to testicular disorder. We have now seen several cases (which are being prepared for publication by Andrew Herzog, MD) in which epididymitis, orchitis, or genital infection led to the first onset of a temporal lobe seizure. We have also observed two patients who developed multiple sclerosis after an orchitis and a vasectomy, respectively. Changes in the testis are sometimes seen in experimental allergic encephalomyelitis. Conversely, Philip P. Paterson, MD (oral communication, September 1984) informs us that in experiments in collaboration with S. M. Harwin, MD, in the period from 1959 to 1962, it was found that immunization of rats with ground-up testis or corpus luteum produced the typical histologic changes of experimental allergic encephalomyelitis in 10% of cases.

Another feature that we have observed is an apparently high rate of immune disorder in those subjects with congenital skeletal anomalies, e.g., Klippel-Feil syndrome, that still requires documentation. We would suggest that in such individuals there will be disturbances in formation in utero of other organs that are not as readily observed as the clear-cut bony anomaly.

### *Late Onset of Symptomatology in Congenital Lesions*

It is a curious fact that many congenital lesions do not manifest themselves clinically until quite late in adult life. Cavernomas of the temporal lobe, found predominantly on the left side typically became symptomatic only in middle life. For reasons to become clear in the subsequent discussion, we consider it possible that the lesions do not become clinically manifest until immune attack on the abnormal vessels causes them to dilate. The marked enlargement of local vessels as a result of local inflammatory mechanisms is well known. A recent article showed the remarkable response of one of these cavernomas to radiation, an effect greater than that usually seen with radiation of vascular tumors.[6] It is conceivable that the radiation worked by means of destruction of immune cells in the lesion. This unproved possibility deserves consideration because of possible implications for therapy. Another study[7] reported marked reduction in the size of arteriovenous malformations (AVMs) and in the vascularity of meningiomas after local perfusion with estradiol. The authors believed that the estrogens favored clotting directly, but another possibility is that local immune responses were heightened so markedly as to produce a major inflammatory response with subsequent clotting.

Angiomas of the spinal cord are thought to be congenital lesions, yet they manifest themselves clinically in male subjects in middle life. A case whose course is concordant with the type of mechanism suggested was that of a middle-aged man with early gray hair and a history of familial AD. He had been suffering from arthritis coming on after an enteric infection, a condition strongly associated with histocompatibility antigen (HLA-B27). He was admitted because of rapidly progressing spinal signs, and was found to have a large longitudinal spinal angioma. A few days later a subarachnoid hemorrhage suddenly developed in the patient. Two aneurysms were found in very unusual locations distally on the posteroinferior cerebellar artery. We would raise the possibility that a concatenation of coincidences is far less likely than a single pathogenetic process that led to enlargement of the angioma and to formation of the unusual aneurysms. Cerebral aneurysms in unusual locations are well known in subacute bacterial endocarditis, in which they are presumed to be of immune origin.

Another possible example of this mechanism is afforded by the occurrence of arachnoid cysts in cases of the lumbosacral plexus syndromes sometimes seen in rheumatoid spondylitis (Marie-Strümpell disease). Removal of these cysts is not helpful.[8] Since this syndrome is presumably the result of immune attack on the lumbosacral plexus, it is likely that the arachnoid cysts are also immunologically produced. Both the arachnoid cysts and the affected nerve roots are close to the site of early involvement of the skeletal system. In the case of enteropathic arthritis discussed above, the spinal angioma was also in the neighborhood of involved skeletal and neural structures in the spinal column and the cord or roots. In favor of this hypothesis concerning the origin of some (possibly most) arachnoid cysts is their association with many localized congenital anomalies, e.g., scoliosis, pigmented nevi, diastematomyelia, and syringomyelia.[9]

Another case was that of a woman with arachnoid cysts at a level corresponding to her clinical findings and that recurred after surgery (although myelography did not support the possibility that the cysts were compressing the cord). There was a clear-cut relationship of clinical exacerbations to the menstrual cycle. The patient had scoliosis and a pigmented nevus on the left side at the dermatomal level corresponding to the clinical spinal level. We raise the possibility that there was recurrent immune attack at a spinal level affected during intrauterine life and that the arachnoid cysts, like those of rheumatoid spondylitis, were a by-product of the same process.

Another possible example of the same phenomenon is the finding of cerebrospinal fluid (CSF) lymphocytosis in a patient who was later found to be suffering from the Dandy-Walker syndrome. It has usually been assumed that the manifestations of this syndrome are the result of mechanical effects. It is possible, however, that the precipitant of neurologic manifestations is the result of local immune response. This might, in turn, produce local mechanical effects so that surgical amelioration need not be surprising.

A recent patient with a meningioma raises the possibility of a similar mechanism. A man in his 70s with childhood scoliosis and a history of extensive vitiligo for many years, had been born with a black hairy nevus over the base of his spine. He entered with a frontal lobe syndrome of a few months' duration as well as fluently paraphasic spontaneous speech with intact comprehension and repetition. A frontal convexity meningioma was found on the left side that did not impinge extensively on the brain. What was striking, however, was a feature often seen with several other meningiomas, i.e., considerable edema extending well into the adjacent cortex and white matter, which is, in many cases, the primary cause of pathologic effects. In some cases variations in the extent of edema lead to relapses and remissions that may suggest other diagnoses. Several mechanisms might account for the edema, but in our patient, the long history of vitiligo, i.e., autoimmune attack affecting pigmented cells (that are almost exclusively neural crest derivatives) makes it reasonable to consider an immune mechanism, especially since the meninges of the hemispheres are also neural crest derivatives. This raises the possibility of immune attack on two structures of similar origin, i.e., pigmented cells in the skin and the meningioma.

Another patient with several years of personality change, increasing headache, and mild left-sided motor signs was found to have a lipoma of the corpus callosum that was thought at first to be producing local effects by pressure. Computed tomographic scan, however, showed ventricles of normal size with no displacement of structures and on lumbar puncture, CSF pressure was normal. This case also raises the possibility that an immune response was taking place in a region that had been improperly formed in utero. The absence of cells in the spinal fluid need not militate against this possibility since many CNS lesions with significant local lymphocytic infiltration do not produce CSF pleocytosis. Another patient, with a familial history of left-handedness, had suffered for several years from steroid-responsive polymyositis. A myelogram, carried out because of new neurologic signs with extensor plantar responses revealed a large spinal angioma. This may be another example of immune attack on anomalous vessels.

If some of these ideas are correct, then the attribution of many clinical pictures to mechanical causes may be incorrect. In other cases there may well be mechanical effects as a result of growth of the lesion, but the change in size itself may be the result of inflammatory immune response.

Syringomyelia is another syndrome in which such a mechanism may play a role. Although the syrinx itself is generally accepted as a congenital malformation, theories of the pathogenesis have often stressed mechanical forces. Yet in some cases a symptomatic syrinx can be seen without enlargement of the spinal cord, i.e., in the absence of a dilating cyst. Progressive gliosis is thought to occur in the lesions.[10] Lymphocytic infiltration is often observed. Finally, some recent observations suggest that particular HLA are associated with syringomyelia.

We will return later in this section to a further discussion of why immune attack might occur at a site of congenital anomaly.

*Lateralized Immune Responses*

This line of reasoning leads to the expectation of lateralized immune responses both in the brain and elsewhere, as a result of lateral differences in times of development. There are several possible reasons for lateralized immune responses. Some immune responses are facilitated at elevated temperatures.[11] If there were differences in temperature on the two sides, as in patients with obvious hemihypertrophy, one might expect greater immune responses on the warmer side. The worsening of multiple sclerosis at high temperatures is often attributed to altered axonal conduction in demyelinated regions. Myasthenia gravis, however, may also be precipitated or worsened in hot weather, which would not be susceptible to the identical explanation. In both disorders, elevation of temperature might favor immune attack on the susceptible structures, although other direct physiologic effects might also take place.

Lateralized immune response could result from lateral differences in sympathetic innervation. Epinephrine administered locally inhibits many immune responses, and thus greater release of epinephrine on one side might suppress such responses. Furthermore, there are sympathetic noradrenergic fibers in lymph nodes that may well play an important role in local regulation of immune responses.[12] It would be intriguing to know whether Raynaud's phenomenon, when worse unilaterally, had a side predilection depending on the individual's dominance pattern.

Lateralized immune responses could also occur if there were lateral differences in chemical composition as might be expected on the basis of the postulated lateral differences in brain growth in response to hormones. In the last section, we will discuss possible mechanisms of such differences.

Immune disorders may manifest themselves asymmetrically. Rheumatoid arthritis tends to spare a limb previously affected by hemiplegia or poliomyelitis, an effect sometimes attributed to lesser use of the affected limb. The different possibilities are susceptible to experimental study.

Neuralgic amyotrophy is another asymmetric immunologic disorder.[13,14] In its classic form this acute predominantly motor neuropathy followed the administration of horse serum, with a time-course similar to that of serum sickness, which might occur simultaneously. There is a male predominance and a predilection for the motor nerves arising from the upper brachial plexus. Because the phrenic nerve may be affected, with consequent diaphragmatic paralysis, it is fortunate that the condition is typically unilateral. Lumbosacral plexus involvement is rare, and (except for the 11th cranial nerve whose motor neurons lie in the upper cervical cord) there is almost never (any) disturbance of the cranial nerves. Although this neuropathy is presumably the result of circulating immune complexes, 65% of the cases affect predominantly the right side and 12% the left side, with approximate equality in 23%. This lateral predilection is sometimes explained as attack on the arm used most often, but another possible interpretation is a difference in immune susceptibility of the two sides. It would be interesting to know the dominance pattern of patients affected by this disorder, i.e., whether those with AD are attacked especially often, or whether their pattern of side distribution differs from that of the standard dominance group.

There are two other forms of neuralgic amyotrophy in addition to that which follows injections of horse serum. In idiopathic cases, also male predominant, the distribution of lateralization of the neuropathy is essentially the same as in cases following horse serum.[13] In the hereditary form, family members suffer recurrent attacks of neuralgic amyotrophy, usually without an obvious precipitant, although females suffer more attacks in pregnancy.[15,16] While both sexes are affected in these families, male subjects tend to have the same clinical picture as in the two previous forms, again with predilection for the right side. By contrast, the disorder in females is frequently atypical; right-sided predilection is less obvious and the lumbosacral plexus may be involved.

Lateral differences in immunity might be reflected in the pattern of certain CNS infections. Poliomyelitis was also thought to attack the most used arm more frequently, but the considerations raised here suggest other possibilities. It would be interesting to know whether such lateralized conditions as herpes simplex encephalitis have a predilection for one hemisphere and also the relationship of this to individual dominance patterns. Herpes simplex, in the form of the common cold sore, often recurs on the same side in many individuals and the same may be true for herpetic corneal ulcers. Herpes zoster and especially postherpetic neuralgia have a predilection for the left side.[17] Tic douloureux is most common on the right side and it has been suggested, although it is not yet generally accepted, that this may reflect herpes simplex infection of the trigeminal ganglion. Three cases, all of Irish descent, suffered from a curious condition beginning with signs on the left side with involvement of multiple sites.[18] A case of ours had the same ancestry, clinical picture, and lateralization. This may be another example of a condition resulting from lateralized infection, a lateralized immune response, or both.

Aphasia in Alzheimer's disease may be another example of lateralized immune attack at a site of congenital anomaly. Seltzer and Sherwin[19] have found that in the presenile form, aphasia is much more common than in late-onset cases. They have also found in two successive series an elevated rate of left-handedness in the presenile cases, with a low rate in senile-onset cases. If the latter finding is correct, it will be of special importance as the first demonstration of a disorder that attacks those with standard dominance more frequently than those with AD. We suspect that in the early-onset cases with higher rates of aphasia and sinistrality there was delayed development in the speech regions. A patient of ours, a nonrighthander with a history of childhood learning disorder (LD) and Raynaud's phenomenon, was a member of a family in which nonrighthandedness, LDs, and immune disease have occurred over several generations. She manifested a progressive presenile onset disorder with aphasia as its main manifestation, along with striking abnormalities of the antinuclear antibody (ANA) and other immunologic tests.

Pick's disease[20] preferentially attacks the temporal and frontal lobes, often bilaterally. When temporal lobe involvement is unilateral, the left side is more often involved, and unilateral frontal involvement tends to affect the right side. Mesulam[21] has described a group of patients with the unusual clinical picture of progressive aphasia over several years, without other intellectual impairments, but the pathology is not yet known. We have seen other cases in which there is remarkably localized progressive impairment over years.

*Sympathetic Immune Responses*

This discussion raises another possibility. An immune response should occur not only in a susceptible local region but also in other locations that share common antigens with it, as in the examples given earlier. Some viruses have a predilection for well-defined neurologic systems, e.g., poliomyelitis, which attack many interrelated parts of the motor system including Betz' cells and anterior horn cells, but sparing, in most cases, supranuclear nonpyramidal motor systems such as those controlling the eye movements, and almost never affecting the oculomotor nuclei. This suggests that the systems affected share a chemical similarity and therefore common immune susceptibility. Amyotrophic lateral sclerosis might conceivably be the result of immune attack in much the same systems that are attacked by the poliomyelitis virus. Herpes simplex encephalitis has a predilection for connected structures of the limbic system and is much less likely to involve other regions. Rabies virus is another selective pathogen. The existence of similar antigens in chains of neurons raises the possibility that transsynaptic and transneuronal degeneration (which occurs almost invariably in the lateral geniculate nucleus after removal of an eye) may reflect "sympathetic" immune attack on structures containing similar antigens. These degenerations are often attributed to loss of the trophic influence of stimulation, an explanation perhaps difficult to sustain in the case of retrograde transsynaptic degeneration. Thus in the monkey, removal of occipital cortex is followed by a chain of retrograde degenerations eventually extending to the retina.

Trauma to the brain may lead to unusual late effects that have not been explained. One possibility is that in some instances there is immune attack in the damaged region. This may not occur in most cases for the same reasons that cardiac autoantibodies do not produce unfavorable effects in most individuals after myocardial damage. Our experience suggests that this type of localized immune response following trauma may be more common in the right hemisphere in female subjects with AD, but to prove this will require extensive clinical and experimental animal studies.

The occurrence of common antigens in sperm and brain has already been mentioned. The brain and skin may also share common antigens, as is suggested by the close relationship between some developmental anomalies of the CNS and of the skin, e.g., in the Sturge-Weber syndrome. Another example is the association of an angiomatous malformation in the spinal cord and a vascular nevus of the skin at the same dermatomal level,[22] sometimes visible only with ultraviolet light. Although these examples are well known, the possibility of other such associations has generally been neglected. The scalp has rarely been studied, possibly because of the presence of hair. There are two minor abnormalities of the skin that are usually considered to have no pathologic association, i.e., "the stork bite" (a small vascular nevus) at the base of the neck and the mongolian spot (a small collection of melanin) at the base of the spine, although the latter is often found in Down's syndrome. The former may reflect late closing of the upper end of the neural tube, while the latter, a remnant of the neural crest, is at the site of the lower closure of the neural tube. These two locations are classic sites of certain neural-tube defects such as meningoceles and spina bifida and, in lesser degree, the pilonidal sinus.

We have mentioned earlier several examples of the association of various types of congenital skin lesion with CNS disorder. Even more intriguing are *acquired* localized disorders of the skin or hair in association with a CNS lesion. A woman in her 80s with a parasagittal meningioma on the right side had developed, over the previous 15 years, a melanotic keratotic area about 2 cm in diameter that kept recurring after excision. A left-handed woman in her 20s who suffered the slow onset of a left carotid occlusion had several congenital lesions on the same side, i.e., a melanin spot on the conjunctiva, a linear vascular nevus about 3 cm in length in front of the ear, and a more diffuse area of pigmentation of the face. These raised the suspicion that she might have had a congenital anomaly of the carotid artery that led to a dissection. By far the most unusual aspect of this patient was, however, the appearance of a new lesion involving the hair. During the ten days in which the aphasia was developing, the sister, who regularly did the patient's hair, observed a progressive, nearly total loss of hair in a circular region about 4 cm in diameter in the left parietal region. This area of alopecia areata overlay a hypodense region in the computed tomographic scan, presumably a zone of infarction or localized immune attack. Alopecia areata is, of course, well known as a manifestation of certain immune disorders, e.g., lupus erythematosus. We believe that in this patient immune attack in the scalp probably involved a region that shared common antigens with the underlying brain. This patient was left-handed.

Epilepsy developed in another left-handed female patient with an electroencephalograph (EEG) focus in the left posterior temporoparietal region. Within the next few months one patch of hair growing from the parietal region of the scalp on the left side turned silvery gray and by a year later stood out in striking fashion from the surrounding light-brown hair. A similar case was recently observed by one of our colleagues. A third patient was also a left-handed female, a diethylstilbestrol daughter with a history of severe acne in adolescence, thus suggesting either excess production of, or sensitivity to, androgens. At about 20 years of age, she sustained a short left-side temporoparietal skull fracture, resulting in marked local scalp tenderness that disappeared over a few months. Left-sided temporal seizures began about five years later. Following the appearance of these attacks, tenderness returned in the same scalp region along with intermittent boggy swelling and warmth. It is possible that immune attack was simultaneously affecting an area of previous brain injury and a corresponding region within the scalp, possibly with a major effect on blood vessels.

This very small series of cases and other similar ones suggest that the hypothesis presented here is deserving of further investigation.

*Tests of Immune Function*

A possible objection to many of these postulated examples of localized or lateralized immune attack is that in most of these patients the results of such tests as the ANA and the sedimentation rate are normal, although there are exceptions, e.g., the patient cited above with a slowly progressive aphasia. Although her only peripheral immune manifestation was Raynaud's phenomenon, her ANA was 1:1,200 with a speckled pattern. Furthermore, CSF pleocytosis is usually absent in these cases, although again there are exceptions, e.g., the case of Dandy-Walker syndrome mentioned above. There are case reports of migraine with CSF pleocytosis,[23] but the diagnosis of migraine is not always absolutely certain.

These negative findings do not, however, rule out immune disorder. In the first place, in many clearly immune disorders changes in the ANA or sedimentation rate are exceptional, e.g., pernicious anemia, vitiligo, Hashimoto's thyroiditis, myasthenia gravis, and diabetes. It is usually stated that the ANA is positive in the great majority of cases of lupus erythematosus. Two series have, however, found that in lupus erythematosus involving the nervous system the ANA is negative in *most* cases, unless there is active nonneural disease. While chronic meningitis can occur, in most cases with CNS lupus erythematosus the spinal fluid is free of cells. It seems likely, therefore, that when even so clear-cut an immune disorder as lupus erythematosus begins with brain involvement, little help is to be expected from existing immune tests or from the CSF. It is thus not surprising that the origin of many other immune involvements of the nervous system might readily be overlooked, even if such cases occurred in high frequency. Lupus erythematosus is itself of particular interest from the point of view of selective CNS involvement. Thus the vasculitis may well have a predilection for the posterior circulation. We have seen two cases of lupus erythematosus with involvement of the posterior inferior cerebellar artery, and a published article describes aneurysms in the same circulation. Selective vascular involvement occurs in other conditions as well, e.g., in migraine a strong predilection for the basilar circulation, and in particular for the distribution of the posterior cerebral arteries. Temporal arteritis involves predominantly the branches of the external carotid artery. Although we suspect that the results of existing tests of immune function will be normal in most cases with localized or lateralized neurologic immune disorder, we expect that eventually tests will be found that are abnormal in such cases.

After the discussion of infection, we will discuss in more detail reasons for the possible susceptibility to immune attack of sites of congenital anomalies.

*Immune Complications*

The question arises as to whether those with AD have not only a higher frequency of immune disorders but also a higher rate of immune complications or complications of drugs or diseases. There is little information available. We have already discussed neuralgic amyotrophy in response to horse serum and its curious lateralization pattern, but nothing is yet known as to differential susceptibility according to dominance patterns.

A rare complication of phenytoin sodium therapy is lymphadenopathy, and in some instances the affected lymph nodes have the appearance of Hodgkin's disease. In some cases a lupus-like syndrome is seen. We have seen striking masculinization with phenytoin in a left-handed diethylstilbestrol daughter, although this is not an immune complication. We have also seen both lymphadenopathy and a rash in a patient from an AD family. A recent report claimed that phenytoin rashes were more common in patients commencing therapy in the summer than in the winter.[24] This might reflect an effect of temperature, but might also be the result of changes in sex hormone production as a result of alterations in pineal gland function with day length. These isolated instances can at this time only suggest further study.

We have already noted the human CNS disorders after orchitis or epididymitis and the induction of experimental allergic encephalomyelitis by immunization with ovary or testis (Philip Paterson, MD, oral communication, September 1984). Similarly, immune attack on Purkinje's cells may occur with ovarian carcinoma. We have seen a patient with the clinical picture of mild Charcot-Marie-Tooth disease who developed the clinical picture of multiple sclerosis after vasectomy. This case may also illustrate immune attack on an anomalous nervous system. H. R. Tyler, MD, has suggested to us that in his experience high arches and other findings of possible formes frustes of Charcot-Marie-Tooth disease are common in the multiple sclerosis population. The issue of immune reactions after vasectomy still, however, remains in dispute.

As is well known, slow acetylators of procaine amide are more susceptible to the development of lupus erythematosus than rapid acetylators. Studies of spontaneous lupus erythematosus have apparently not revealed an elevated rate of slow acetylation. The proportion of slow acetylators, however, varies greatly among populations, with generally very high rates in Northern Europeans and low rates among the Japanese. We have discussed elsewhere the possibility that AD may be high in northern Europe and low in Japan. It would be fruitful to study acetylation rates among those with AD.

All of these questions remain speculative, but one hopes that they will be investigated formally.

## Infections

Infections might be related to our hypothesis in several ways. Certain infections might themselves set up a chain of immune alterations. On the other hand, patients with altered immune systems might show a complex variety of alterations in response to infection, e.g., resistance to many infections, but increased susceptibility to others. We are planning to follow up the possibility derived from several clinical observations that a history of poliomyelitis is more common among those with AD. A special relationship of poliomyelitis to sex hormones is suggested by the high frequency with which it attacked pregnant women in the last great epidemic. It would be important to study not only the frequency of anomalous dominance in poliomyelitis but also the frequency of predominant involvement of one side in relation to the individual dominance pattern.

The differential development at different periods of structures on the two sides of the body may depend in part on immune mechanisms, especially if Ohno[4] is correct in assuming that the histocompatibility antigens may act as markers for development. Conversely, if development of a structure on one side is delayed by influences that also act on the thymus gland the structures on the two sides may have differential susceptibility to immune attack. If some immune responses are more marked on one side, one might well picture that resistance to some infections might be elevated on the same side.

Patients with AD may well be protected from certain infections while more susceptible to others. Those with high IgE have a susceptibility to allergies but may have an elevated level of protection against parasitic disorders,[25] which raises the possibility that many individuals with AD are resistent to these disorders.

On the other hand, there may be high susceptibility in the AD population to other disorders. We have already speculated on the possibility that acquired immunodeficiency syndrome may attack a particular AD group. B. Quart, MD (written communication, Oct 25, 1983) found an elevated rate of history of dyslexia in a group with Reye's syndrome. This intriguing possibility deserves further study, especially in view of the evidence that this disorder involves disturbance of mitochondrial (cytoplasmic) enzymes. We have already discussed, and will again discuss, the possible role of cytoplasmic inheritance as a determinant of laterality, as suggested by Corballis and Morgan.[26]

Certain infections can, of course, trigger immune disorders, presumably in especially susceptible individuals. It has been suggested that congenital anomalies in offspring of mothers infected with rubella in the first trimester are more common when the mother is especially susceptible immunologically. The high frequency of arthritis in women who develop rubella after deliberate inoculation suggests some special immunologic effects. Some infections produce immune disorders in susceptible individuals, e.g., enteropathic arthritis following intestinal infection with certain bacteria is more common in individuals carrying the HLA-B27.

We will return to the discussion of infections in a later section.

## Mechanism of Immune Attack or Infection at Congenital Anomalies

We have suggested that immune attack at sites of congenital anomalies may account for many cases of localized and lateralized immune disorder even in late life. The modification of susceptibility to certain disorders by intrauterine events is well-documented in certain cases. Medawar found that the carcinogenicity of methylcholanthrene in later life was altered by intrauterine exposure to certain antigens.[27] Tumors may arise as a result of acquired alterations, but may also develop in sites of arrested development, as is likely the case for many glioblastomas. Immune responses to many tumors may be a special case of immune attack on structures formed improperly during development. We have also already suggested that in certain cases, e.g., some meningiomas, the clinical signs may be more dependent on local immune attack than on mass effects.

Some tumors arise from embryonic precursor cells. The immune system may fail to recognize the antigens in these cells as self when they are formed before the development of the immune system. Certain precursor cells probably disappear or are sequestered early in fetal life and do not reappear in later life except when certain tumors develop, a situation in which it is useful to the organism not to recognize these precursors as self. Injection of these embryonic antigens into the fetus after immune development has begun leads to partial protection against later immune attack on tumors containing these antigens.[27]

If embryonic rests are more likely to persist in AD individuals because of delays in development, they may be susceptible to later immune attack in the same manner as tumors containing embryonic antigens. When the delay is predominantly unilateral, unilateral immune attack might be expected.

Because malformed tissues may also be metabolically abnormal, many may die prematurely and release substances normally sequestered from the immune system. Immunologic attack in this case would be similar to that which leads to sympathetic orchitis or ophthalmia after damage to one testis or eye. Furthermore, if one tissue is attacked others sharing common antigens may also undergo immune attack.

There is still another reason, mentioned earlier, for attack on a malformed tissue. We have suggested that testosterone may retard growth of certain brain structures and simultaneously suppress thymic development. Processing lymphocytes to recognize self is a major function of the fetal thymus gland. Since many new antigens are being formed throughout gestation, lymphocytes cannot be processed to recognize them until the antigens are actually present. Suppression of the thymus gland at any given point will prevent the processing of lymphocytes that would recognize the tissues concurrently being formed. Since the influences producing malformed structures are likely to suppress the thymus gland antigens, these structures should be especially susceptible to later immune attack.

Many diseases of late life may thus be the result of immune attack on structures whose development was affected during pregnancy. As we have noted earlier, this may be the case for Alzheimer's disease.

It is a simple step to go from these mechanisms of localized immune attack to lateralized attack. In the first place, structures on one side of the brain or body may be subject to greater delays than those on the other side, e.g., the left temporal cortex and left-sided neural crest derivatives. Since slower development on the left side increases the rate of congenital disorders on that side one might expect an elevated rate of immune attack on the left side.

Other mechanisms may favor unilateral immune attack. In the first place, the peripheral immune system, i.e., the lymph nodes, may develop differently on the two sides. Other systems modulating local immune response may also be asymmetric, e.g., adrenergic innervation. Catecholamines may directly modulate local immune response or may act on the lymph nodes that receive adrenergic innervation.

Another effect may derive from differences of temperature in the limbs on the two sides. In hemihypertrophy tumors are common, especially on the larger side that typically has a higher temperature than the opposite side. It has been shown that fibroblasts from the hypertrophic side grow more rapidly.[28] Similar findings may occur in acquired differences in size, e.g., poliomyelitis or hemiplegia. We have noted that rheumatoid arthritis tends to spare a previously paralyzed limb. We have seen a patient with atrophy of the left side, presumably from childhood poliomyelitis, in whom many basal cell carcinomas and melanomas developed, nearly all located on the larger right side, the skin temperature of which was 1.5°C warmer than that of the other side.

It is, however, not entirely clear why tumor growth should be greater in the limbs with a higher temperature, which may heighten immune responses.[11] One possibility is that this effect is counterbalanced by the tendency to more rapid growth in the warmer limb.

## Brain Disease and Laterality

We have already given many examples of the association of certain disorders with anomalous dominance, or of the unilateral occurrence of many conditions. In this section, we will discuss some other associations of brain disease and laterality.

### Epilepsy

The first dyslexic brain studied by Galaburda and Kemper[29] came from a left-handed male metalsmith with severe developmental dyslexia, who also suffered from seizures. The epilepsy appeared easy to explain, since the brain contained an area of polymicrogyria in the left superior temporal gyrus, and such malformed and misplaced areas of cortex often lead to seizures. The possibility had to be entertained initially that one was dealing with an unusual cause of childhood dyslexia, but this can be dismissed in view of the fact that brains of dyslexic subjects so far examined have demonstrated similar anomalies. In fact, seizures occur in elevated frequency in dyslexia and other language-delayed children,[30,31] stutterers,[32] and childhood autism,[33] and in Tourette's syndrome, abnormal EEGs are common.[34,35] In childhood autism the rate of epilepsy is particularly high. The hypothesis that disturbances of neuronal migration and neuronal assembly are common causes of developmental LD, leads to the expectation of an elevated frequency of epilepsy in these conditions, especially involving the left hemisphere.

The fact that all individuals with LD do not have epilepsy need not be surprising. Neuronal migration disorders may not be the only cause of all cases of these syndromes, and only postmortem examination of large numbers of brains of all these conditions can resolve that question. Second, all potentially epileptogenic lesions do not lead to epilepsy. Veith and Schwindt[36] found a much higher frequency of developmental brain anomalies in a group of derelicts (people with a long history of social isolation, wandering, and homelessness) than in controls, yet epilepsy was not noted in the majority. Tuberous sclerosis, a condition characterized by gross disorders of cellular migration, may never produce seizures. The same is true for other epileptogenic lesions, e.g., arteriovenous malformations and new growths. Some individuals may never seek medical attention for mild attacks or for unnoticed nocturnal seizures, and some may have EEG abnormalities without seizures. Herzog et al[37] found a high rate of polycystic ovary syndrome in female subjects with temporal lobe epilepsy (TLE) and, conversely, about 20% of patients with a polycystic ovary without a history of epilepsy had temporal lobe spikes. Furthermore, as we will indicate later, individuals with childhood LD may develop seizures in adult life, when they would no longer be observed by those who treat LD children.

It is reasonable to speculate on the kind of epilepsy that might be expected in patients with LD. Since many of the lesions will lie near the left sylvian fissure, one might expect an elevated frequency of focal seizures arising from this region. There is one known condition that meets this requirement. In recent years there has been increasing interest in a group of conditions known under different names, i.e., sylvian seizures, centrotemporal seizures, or rolandic seizures. Some epileptologists regard these seizures as identical or related conditions, although others believe they are distinct. This type of epilepsy, beginning in childhood, is probably the most common cause of minor attacks in children, exceeding in frequency, according to some observers, cases of classic petit mal. It is generally regarded as a rather benign form of epilepsy, usually readily controlled, and, a particularly intriguing point, thought to disappear in the great majority of cases at puberty. It may manifest itself by sensations in the opposite side of the face, aphasia, or contralateral convulsive movements; it can also produce major convulsions, especially at night.

The investigations of the genetics of this disorder by Bray and Wiser[38–40] are revealing. Although clinical epilepsy occurred in only a small percentage of the first-degree relatives of affected cases, EEG anomalies were found in half the siblings and also in parents, although less often. These authors argued for mendelian dominant inheritance on the basis of the presence of EEG anomalies in half the siblings. The lower prevalence of EEG abnormalities in the parents than in the siblings could reasonably be explained by the usual improvement after puberty. Among the affected parents, however, about 15% of cases showed anterior temporal spikes that led to the suggestion that classic TLE might arise late in some cases of occult sylvian epilepsy, a finding for which it is not difficult to suggest a mechanism. A seizure focus on the convexity might eventually lead (perhaps as the result of kindling) to an anterior temporal focus, i.e., a secondary or "daughter" focus in a region connected to the original location of abnormal electrical activity.

We suggest that the type of epilepsy that will be most commonly seen in the LD population will be sylvian seizures. Frank Duffy, MD (oral communication, July 20, 1982) has, in fact, frequently found silent sylvian spikes in childhood dyslexics.

This hypothesis has several implications. Sylvian spikes should be more common in childhood dyslexics than in controls. Left-sided foci should be more common than right-sided foci, because of more frequent delays in the formation of the left sylvian cortex, and the condition should be more common in boys than girls, a finding reported in some series.[41] The frequent improvement at puberty suggests that even at this relatively late age, hormones affect the areas of abnormal cortex that are the postulated cause of this form of epilepsy. It would be important to study the mechanisms of such possible hormonal action.

This hypothesis has another potential implication. An earlier section expressed our skepticism about the common tendency to regard minor degrees of malformation or malfunction of the nervous system as normal. A parallel condition exists in the EEG literature in which certain deviant findings are described as normal or benign, a judgment based on the belief that they are often found in "normals." Although the abnormalities in question occur frequently in patients without gross neurologic impairments or manifest epilepsy, there is rarely adequate evidence concerning LD or other such impairments.

Cesare Lombroso, MD (personal communication, July 20, 1982) states that in his experience, sylvian epilepsy is predominant in male subjects, in accord with some series in the literature. At least one series reports a higher frequency of left-sided foci, but the data are not entirely consistent from one series to another, possibly a result of differences in diagnostic criteria. Beaussart[41] stated that a majority of the individuals he studied with sylvian spikes had never had a seizure. In operations on some cases with anterior temporal foci, Falconer found a visible lesion on the temporal convexity, recordings from which showed epileptic activity. These lesions were often not detected preoperatively because of their small spike discharges. The surgeon could detect these lesions on the surface, but small foci of spike activity arising from deeper regions of cytoarchitectonic abnormality would not have been detected. Although careful pathologic study of the excised anterior temporal lobes often revealed congenital anomalies (alien tissue), similar undetected lesions may have been present frequently in the posterior temporal region that lay beyond the borders of the excision. Other data concerning epilepsy and EEG changes are compatible with the hypothesis of the special susceptibility of the left hemisphere to delayed growth. In their study of maturation of the EEG in children, Walter and Dovey[42] found that theta typically disappeared last in the left temporal lobe. A study from Italy of several thousand EEG foci found that in two thirds of the cases the abnormality was exclusively or predominantly on the left side.[43,44]

David Taylor[45] made a major contribution in calling attention to the laterality and gender relations of another form of focal pathology. It is intriguing that febrile convulsions in early life should, despite their generalized character, lead so frequently to a unilateral lesion, i.e., mesial temporal sclerosis (MTS). Taylor and Ounsted[46] noted the predominance of left-sided MTS in male subjects who had had their first febrile convulsion before the age of 1 year. They argued that epilepsy was more likely to invade a less active region and that it was immaturity of the left temporal lobe in male infants that endowed it with special susceptibility. In the baboon, induced seizures in early life also led to unilateral MTS, but we do not know whether there is any sex or side predominance of the lesions. The findings in the baboon led initially to some skepticism about Taylor's interpretations since it was generally believed that cerebral dominance was present only in humans. Asymmetry is, however, present in the baboon brain[47] as is probably the case in all other primates and in many other animals. It would be interesting to ascertain whether the laterality of MTS in the baboon can be correlated with functional behavioral characteristics in the affected animals or their families. Stokes and McIntyre[48] have demonstrated lateralized effects in experimental animal studies of production of epilepsy by kindling, as well as evidence of functional dominance for spatial function.

We have found other data concordant with the hypothesis that delayed development on the left side may lead to the formation of epileptogenic foci. A man in his middle 30s with a history of childhood dyslexia suffered a first seizure that was found to arise from an AVM in the superior temporal gyrus that must, therefore, have contained malformed cortex. We have already noted that AVMs in the primary speech areas occur overwhelmingly in male subjects and are most common in the temporal speech zone.[49] Thus in some cases the malformed cortical regions may give rise to epilepsy in adult life.

The finding of a significant number of cases of anterior temporal EEG foci in the parents of children with sylvian epilepsy raises some important questions.[38–40] The common view concerning the benign character of sylvian seizures may be overstated, since a proportion of people with sylvian spikes in childhood, including some without obvious epilepsy, may develop a secondary lesion in the anterior temporal lobe. Apparently benign sylvian spikes may thus conceivably be forerunners of a large number of cases with temporal spikes in adult life, many with epilepsy. In our own clinical observations of adults with TLE, we have been struck by the frequency of history of childhood LD and evidence of AD; our colleague, Marsel Mesulam, MD, believes that there may be a high frequency of immune disorders in these patients. Studies should be performed to test the validity of these observations. If they are, indeed, correct then AD may well play an important role in the pathogenesis of TLE. We have long been interested in the elevated rate of personality change and frank behavior disorder in patients with TLE.[50,51] Anomalous dominance might, therefore, be associated with a significant number of cases of psychiatric disability on this basis.

### Dementia and Other Progressive Disorders

In Pick's disease, lobar atrophy typically affects the frontal and/or temporal lobes, usually bilaterally. Unilateral temporal atrophy usually involves the left side while a single involved frontal lobe usually lies on the right side.[20] As we have noted earlier, the typical normal pattern of asymmetry consists of a larger left posterior region and a larger right frontal region. It is intriguing that the temporal lobe lesions characteristically show a rather sharp demarcation, typically sparing an area that is often affected in many of the other syndromes that we have discussed, i.e., the posterior and middle portions of the superior temporal gyrus.

The asymmetry in some cases of Pick's disease raises several questions. There are no data to indicate whether the cases with unilateral lesions have any relationship to the dominance pattern of the patient. Our speculation is that in the unilateral cases there is an excess of AD individuals in whom there has been a marked delay in the development of the affected regions. If this were true, it would suggest that intrauterine effects on dominance were not acting to slow development only in the left hemisphere, but were rather acting on selected areas in the two hemispheres, i.e., left posterior regions and right anterior regions. The cases of poor social development described by Weintraub and Mesulam[52] might then reflect impaired right frontal maturation by a mechanism similar to that which causes left posterior slowing in childhood dyslexia.

There is more evidence concerning relationships to laterality in Alzheimer's disease than in Pick's disease. A common definition of dementia is global loss of intellectual function, but this formulation is unacceptable since different types of dementia exhibit distinct patterns of loss and preservation of function. In particular, in presenile Alzheimer's disease, (predominantly female) one often finds early fluent aphasia and constructional and memory difficulties, with relative or complete preservation of emotional behavior. By contrast, aphasia is almost unknown in many dementias, e.g., Huntington's disease, and memory is typically preserved in Pick's disease.[20] Seltzer and Sherwin[19] compared two groups of male patients carrying the clinical diagnosis of Alzheimer's disease. Aphasia was common in 28 cases with presenile onset, but infrequent in 43 patients with onset beyond 70 years of age. Furthermore, six of the 28 cases with presenile onset were left-handed as against two of the 43 senile-onset cases. This suggests that those with AD are more likely to develop the presenile form and to suffer impaired function of the left posterior language regions. This is compatible with the hypothesis that delay in development of the language regions on the left would render them more susceptible to later immune attack. Other data also suggest a predisposition to immune disorder in patients with Alzheimer's disease, e.g., an elevated frequency of relatives with Down's syndrome, who have themselves a high frequency of autoimmunity, as well as maldevelopment of cortex, and, in particular, a thin superior temporal gyrus.

Another recently described group of patients exhibit distinctly focal syndromes over several years; only later do signs of more extensive involvement appear. Mesulam[21] has described patients with slowly progressive and highly selective aphasias. The case of Crystal et al[53] with a focal right-hemisphere syndrome had a biopsy specimen that showed typical Alzheimer's findings, but it is not known whether this type of pathology is typical of all such cases.

We suspect that these patients are probably suffering from focal immune attack on an area whose development was delayed in fetal life. An illustrative example was a middle-aged left-handed artistically talented patient from a family in which left-handedness, artistic talent, LD, autoimmune disease, and migraine were often found. The patient suffered slow development of aphasia, but striking preservation of constructional talents, in contrast to the usual situation in Alzheimer's disease. She was unusual in our experience among the patients with these highly focal syndromes, since the ANA and other immune tests were strongly positive.

Torch and colleagues[54] described a case of dementia that developed slowly over several years after a left hippocampal region infarction. Results of a postmortem examination revealed a series of transsynaptic degenerations that had slowly migrated through the limbic system. This may be an example of focal damage leading to an autoimmune response to previously sequestered antigens with subsequent attack on neuronal systems of similar antigenic composition. Hamlin[55] found that for several years after frontal lobe surgery the results of psychologic testing revealed no differences between patients and controls. Some time later, however, the lobotomized group manifested a decline in performance on certain tests. Paul Yakovlev, MD (oral communication, Feb 16, 1980), believed that this might be the result of transneuronal degeneration. This might represent a progressive immune response in regions connected to the removed prefrontal region and sharing common antigens with it. This hypothesis obviously requires much more study. The possibility should be considered that this type of late phenomenon may occur in individuals with a particular pattern of dominance relationships.

We have already mentioned the progressive syndrome in patients of Irish ancestry, in which pyramidal and basal ganglia signs appear at the beginning on the left side, along with right-sided parietal signs and conspicuous mirror movements.[48]

Parkinsonism may begin unilaterally. It is not clear whether this has any relationship to dominance. It is curious that, as Duvoisin et al[56] have pointed out, there is rarely concordance for this disorder in identical twins, a situation in which the handedness patterns would be of particular interest. Juvenile parkinsonism has a distinct lateralization to one side.[57]

### Laterality in Other Neurologic Disorders

We will list here briefly other neurologic disorder associated with laterality. Many have already been mentioned, e.g., the left-sided predominance of meningiomas of the lateral ventricle and papillomas of the choroid plexus.

Tic douloureux begins more often on the right side than the left side. Jannetta[58] has ascribed this disorder to pressure on the fifth nerve by an arterial loop. The fact that the idiopathic disorder overwhelmingly occurs past the age of 50 years raises some questions. If congenitally anomalous vessels were involved, one might predict a higher proportion of cases with early onset. Normal vessels might become tortuous as the result of atherosclerosis, but this would not account for the lateral predominance. Another possibility is that dilatation takes place predominantly on one side because of lateralized immune attack. Jannetta[58] has called attention to the elevated frequency of hypertension in cases with vascular pressure on nerves in the cerebellopontine angle, especially on the left side. He attributes the lateral predilection to involvement of the left vagus nerve, which provides the predominant innervation to the heart.

In torticollis, the abnormal movements occur more frequently toward the left side than the right side. Stejskal and Tomanek[59] have shown that cases with movements to one side exhibit a predominance of induced nystagmus in the same direction. They deny, however, any relationship to handedness, but the series was too small to permit a reliable judgment.

### Psychiatric Disorders

There is an extensive literature on the relationships of psychiatric disorder laterality. Psychosis in temporal lobe epilepsy is more common with left-sided lesions[60] and, in particular, in left-handed females with hamartomas.[61] There is an extensive literature on the preferential involvement of one or the other side of the brain in schizophrenia and depressive illness.[62] Boklage[63] has reported low concordance for schizophrenia in identical twins if either is left-handed. In addition, when a left-handed twin is affected the illness tends to be relatively mild. Concordance is much higher when both twins are right-handed.

Several authors have studied handedness in various forms of mental illness.[64] In view of the hypothesized relationship of platelet monoamine oxidase (MAO) levels to mental illness, it is intriguing that an excess of left-handers has been found in males with low platelet MAO levels.[65] Males have, in general, lower MAO levels than females.

Mendlewicz[66] has called attention to a pattern of an X-linked *dominant* inheritance in some families with manic-depressive illness. An X-linked disorder whether dominant or recessive cannot be transmitted from fathers to sons since a son cannot receive the paternal X (although Mendlewicz mentions a few exceptional cases of father-son transmission in his series). Dyslexia and stuttering, although strongly male predominant, cannot in general be X-linked because father-son transmission is common although, an X-linked subgroup might exist. If there is relationship to dominance in the group described by Mendlewicz, it would probably be different from that of the other conditions we have described.

Bakan[67] reported an elevated rate of left-handedness in alcoholism and a recent study[68] has found alcoholics to be significantly less right-handed than control subjects. The finding that children at high risk for alcoholism have verbal IQ deficits[69] is concordant with these findings.

## Pharmacology, Metabolism, and Cyclic Phenomena

### Pharmacologic Asymmetry

We have already discussed chemical and pharmacologic asymmetries. The major credit for the establishment of this new field must go to Glick and co-workers, who have produced a series of remarkable articles.[70] Earlier pioneering publications on asymmetric actions of drugs in humans[71–73] were unfortunately generally neglected and the work was not followed up extensively. Some more recent studies are cited by Newlin et al.[74] Important contributions have also appeared recently.[75,76] The presence of these asymmetries implies that certain drug actions will vary in relation to patterns of dominance. In the studies from Glick's group, rats given amphetamines circle to the side opposite the caudate nucleus containing the higher concentration of dopamine. The amphetamines must be acting bilaterally, but the net effect is to reveal only the function of the side with a higher dopamine concentration. If the dominant side is destroyed, the drug will reverse its action, so that amphetamines will produce rotation in the opposite direction.

The situation is complicated by the finding that the dopamine contents of the two sides are not independent. When the dopamine level rises in one caudate nucleus of the rat in response to blockage of dopamine receptors in the ipsilateral substantia nigra, the level of the other caudate nucleus falls. The effect on the opposite caudate nucleus can be prevented by cutting the massa intermedia that connects the two.[77] Glick showed that after sectioning of the cerebral commissures the average difference in dopamine content between the two sides increases. These experiments suggest that the concentrations on the two sides are linked reciprocally.

Mandell and Knapp[78] reported asymmetry of brain serotonin content. Since administration of lithium reduced the average difference between the two sides, they advanced the following hypothesis. The levels on two sides are linked so that as the serotonin level rises on one side it falls on the other. The system is not stable and there is continuous see-saw oscillation. It was proposed that lithium had no effect on total serotonin content but rather, that it acted to diminish the amplitude of the peaks, thus leading to smaller average differences in the content on the two sides. They went on to propose that in the normal subject each hemisphere might, as had been suggested by others, make a different contribution to mood, one tending to produce sadness and the other elation. The spontaneous oscillations would sometimes lead to a high level on one side with resulting elation, while at other periods the opposite side would control mood, thus favoring depression. In cyclic affective illness, lithium might simply reduce the heights of the alternating peaks on the two sides, thus controlling both mania and depression.

Whether or not this particular hypothesis is correct, the postulated mechanism has important implications. Just as in certain cases, e.g., turning to one side or the other, only one movement is mechanically possible. A similar opposition may exist between different types of emotional or cognitive function. *The action of a drug might thus be identical in terms of molecular events in two locations,* and yet the ultimate pharmacologic effect might differ depending on the side predominantly stimulated. A substance might act on one hemisphere to produce elation while the identical chemical action on the opposite side might produce depression. This principle suggests that in many cases the effects of a drug cannot be understood only in terms of its biochemical actions but rather, that connectivity of the regions involved must be taken into account. There are some obvious, but nonetheless important, examples of this principle. The appropriate neurotransmitter placed on the hypoglossal nucleus will produce contraction of one side of the tongue; yet if the proximal hypoglossal nerve were anastomosed to the distal facial nerve, the same transmitter would produce facial movement. This principle also applies to anomalous innervation after nerve injury, but the possibility of its participation in more complex functions has not received wide consideration. It is important, therefore, to look at some further implications.

A drug given systemically is distributed to the corresponding regions on the two sides; its net effect in those cases in which the actions on the two sides are opposed will reflect the action on one side. With spontaneous oscillations of neurotransmitter concentrations or receptors the action of the drug will vary with the phase of the cycle.

Consider the circumstance in which the drug is administered to only one hemisphere, e.g., in the intracarotid amobarbital sodium test of Wada. In most instances injection on the left side produces aphasia, while injection on the right side may affect the ability to sing on key.[79] In this case, of course, the sides are not necessarily in opposition since in singing words there is cooperation between the two sides. The unilateral injection leaves intact only one of the functions. There is also an extensive literature showing a lateral difference in the effects of intracarotid amobarbital sodium on emotion.[80] With injections on the left side, one typically produces a depressive reaction while those on the right typically lead to unconcern.

In the normal state the drug may act predominantly on one hemisphere. Serafetinides[73] administered LSD to patients before and after temporal lobectomy. The typical effects diminished after right but not left temporal lobectomy, which suggests that LSD usually affects certain structures in the right temporal lobe. This result is compatible with clinical findings, since many LSD effects are similar to phenomena occurring during right-sided temporal discharges. In normal subjects Beck[81] found a lower amplitude of the alpha rhythm on the right side and greater suppression of alpha on that side during attentional tasks. Administration of alcohol tended to abolish the lateral differences. These results are compatible with the evidence for a special role of the right hemisphere in attention and with the possibility that the impairment of attention by alcohol may reflect a preferential effect on that hemisphere.

This principle also implies that destruction of the side on which a drug usually acts may lead to a loss or reversal of certain actions. If systemic amphetamine causes turning to the right in a normal rat, it will reverse its action, i.e., produce turning to the left, after destruction of the left caudate nucleus. If the action of the drug is predominantly unilateral, as is perhaps the case of LSD, removal of the target zone on one side may abolish its effects.[73] If a drug produces opposing cognitive or behavioral effects on the two sides, then the net effect will alter when the dominant side is damaged. One might expect that if barbiturates produce depression after left carotid injection and elation after right carotid injection, they will, when given systemically, produce an action reflecting the dominance of one side. Systemic effects may thus vary with individual dominance patterns. If one side is destroyed, then the effect will reflect only the actions on the other side. Pharmacologic dominance might be expected when there is dramatic anatomic asymmetry at the site of action. In one of the brains studied by Galaburda et al,[82] the left area temporoparietal area (TPT) was more than seven times as large as the opposite area. If the two sides were similar in their *concentrations* of receptors and enzymes, then total contents of these substances would differ and one would expect that systemic administration of an active drug would produce predominant effects on the left TPT. The pharmacologic actions on the right side would be revealed only with selective right-sided administration or after destruction of the left side. Recent studies from Bracco and colleagues'[83] group suggest that the situation may be quite complex. While the content of cholineacetyltransferase is higher on the left side, affinity for substrate is lower than on the right side.

Let us consider the possible implications of this principle for particular classes of agents. Because certain drugs are called antidepressants and others are described as antipsychotic, there is a common belief in a chemistry of mood or psychosis. These terms may, however, be misnomers and there may be no special chemistry of mood or psychosis. It is possible instead that the usual actions of these drugs reflect the standard dominance pattern of the majority of the population. Those with different patterns of cerebral dominance might react in a quite opposite fashion.

Anomalous drug actions are well known, i.e., medications sometimes produce unusual effects or even effects opposite to those usually observed. There must be many causes for such effects, e.g., unusual metabolic pathways, or alteration of biochemical actions by the presence of other agents. A drug that acts more strongly on a feedback circuit than on the target neuron may produce a reversed effect. We suspect that in many cases anomalous drug actions are linked to AD, a possibility readily subject to experimental verification. Let us consider some possible examples.

In some cases, the so-called antidepressants, e.g., tricyclics or MAO inhibitors may actually produce or exacerbate depression. A tuberculous patient receiving isonicotinic acid hydrazide therapy, an MAO inhibitor that typically elevates mood, developed a depression that cleared only after the drug was discontinued. The fact that the effective antipsychotic agents are dopamine blockers and the finding that amphetamines typically exacerbate schizophrenia have been advanced as arguments for a dopaminergic theory of schizophrenia. Although most schizophrenics become worse after administration of amphetamines, a significant minority show improvement, sometimes dramatic in degree.

Let us now consider a hypothetical example of a role of AD in the anomalous cases. We will make several assumptions. Activation of a right-hemisphere region produces depression and that of the homologus left region produces elation. The two areas have similar chemical properties. In those with standard dominance, the left-sided area is larger. The net effect of a systemic MAO inhibitor, dictated by the larger left side, will be elation. In a significant number of AD individuals the right-sided area is the larger one. In these people the net effect of the MAO inhibitor will be depression rather than elation. A similar argument could be applied to other paradoxic drug actions, e.g., improvement of schizophrenia by amphetamines, or activating effects of barbiturates. The same mechanism might account for some species differences in drug actions, and for paradoxic drug responses in children. Amaducci et al[84] found that the cholineacetyltransferase level is higher in the left than in the right superior temporal lobe in adult human brains. On the other hand, in fetal life cholineacetyltransferase levels in the right lobe exceeds that of the left and has actually reached its adult level.[85] This means that the left side must reach its adult peak only during postnatal life. Since a similar process is probably going on in many regions, certain drugs should have anomalous actions until the normal adult chemical laterality pattern is attained.

Since the arousal of our interest in anomalous drug reactions, we have carefully observed patients in whom these occur but have not yet carried out a formal controlled study. Our impression is that anomalous drug reactions occur more often in those with personal or familial AD or histories of LD. Those affected appear to have anomalous reactions to a wide variety of medications, and a similar pattern is often seen in relatives. Thus a patient in whom tricyclic therapy increased depression and benzodiazepine therapy produced arousal had a son who developed severe prolonged dystonia in response to a single dose of a dopamine-blocking agent.

What has been discussed is susceptible to experimental test. Schizophrenics who respond anomalously to amphetamine therapy could be compared with those who react in standard fashion in relation to handedness scores, family sinistrality, and personal and family history of LD. It would be of interest to ascertain whether there is a relationship between such patients and the schizophrenic subgroup who are said to have reversed patterns of anatomic asymmetry on computed tomographic scan. Another way to do the experiment would be selection of large numbers of schizophrenics with anomalous responses on a laterality test in order to compare their amphetamine responses with those of patients with standard laterality scores. There is another possible reason for anomalous drug responses in AD individuals. As has been mentioned before, exposure to certain substances during intrauterine or early postnatal life may produce permanent alterations in the metabolic pattern. Those subjected to unusual hormonal influences in pregnancy, who will frequently develop AD, might thus have a different pattern of drug reactions from those individuals not subjected to these influences. This type effect will be discussed further in the next section.

Anomalous drug responses may sometimes reflect individual differences in drug metabolism. Procaine amide-induced lupus erythematosus is seen more frequently in those subjects who acetylate this drug slowly but not in rapid acetylators. By contrast isonicotinic acid hydrazide-induced jaundice occurs predominantly in rapid acetylators. Acetylator status is not, however, distributed equally throughout the world. Among the Japanese and other Asian groups there are few slow acetylators,[86] while in the northern European countries, slow acetylators are extremely common.[87] It would be interesting to know whether acetylator status is related to dominance patterns. The possibility of metabolic differences between those with AD and those with standard dominance derives some support from the finding of a much higher percentage of left-handers among male subjects with low platelet MAO levels.[65]

## Metabolism

It has already been pointed out that influences on the fetus in utero and on the newborn infant may alter chemical reactivity permanently. Exposure during these periods to testosterone (T) may lead to later increased sensitivity to T and to altered metabolism of androgens and other sex hormones. In the rat, one normally finds a different pattern of metabolism of steroid hormones in the liver in adult males and females. The female pattern is shifted to that of the male in females treated with T at birth, while by contrast the female pattern is found in the male castrated at birth.[88,89] Testosterone in adult life alters the metabolic pattern only transiently. Sex-linked protein (SLP), the production of which is controlled by a locus in the major histocompatibility complex of the mouse (which also controls production of a very similar protein, C4, i.e., the fourth component of complement), is normally found in the male but not the female. This pattern is reversed by castration of the male or treatment of the female with T.[90]

These metabolic influences may have very far-reaching consequences. It has already been pointed out that the toxicity of many drugs is sharply different in males and females.[91] It is possible that if the dominance patterns of male and female experimental animals were known, the situation might be further clarified. Many drugs that are more toxic to males might also be more toxic to AD than to standard dominance females. Conversely, males who were hypogonadal during critical earlier periods might well show the female patterns.

Such hormone-induced alterations of metabolism might be more marked in females than in males. The number of hypogonadal males is probably relatively small and many males subjected to excessive T effect in utero may not differ sharply from other males because of ceiling effects. On the other hand, most females subjected to excessive T effects in utero would differ from other females. If this hypothesis were correct, anomalous drug reactions should be more common in the female than in the male, but there are no hard data. Our impression is that females have predominated among the patients we have seen with anomalous drug reactions.

Metabolic effects resulting from intrauterine influences are not confined to the brain, as is clear from the data on the female-related liver enzyme and the male-related SLP. Animals exposed at an appropriate period in fetal life to embryonic tissues on thymus have increased resistance in late life to the carcinogenic actions of methylcholanthrene.[27] Exposure at birth to barbiturates may alter the carcinogenicity of certain agents in later life.[92] Of particular interest is that late prenatal exposure to phenobarbital sodium leads to a decreased concentration of T in plasma and brain that persists into adult life. Reproductive function is altered.[93] We would expect an alteration in dominance properties in these animals. The AD population will, on the average, differ in fetal exposures to many substances from the much larger standard dominance population and may thus have a different distribution of malignancies even in very late life. We have already pointed out that patients with celiac disease have a quite different pattern of cancers from the general population with higher adjusted rates of lymphoid and unusual gut malignancies, and lower adjusted rates of cancers of the breast and lung. There is no conflict between this suggestion and the finding of oncogenes in many cancer groups. The hormonal atmosphere in utero may well permanently alter expression of genes or alter genes themselves, e.g., by methylation.

In the next section we will discuss another set of influences on the fetal environment that may play a role in metabolic alterations.

## Cyclic Phenomena

Allusion has already been made to cyclic variations in sex hormone levels throughout the year. The interest in cyclic phenomena, both short-term and long-term, has recently increased greatly although greater emphasis has been placed on circadian than on long-term rhythms. Animals and plants have two major cycles, the first being that of the day, and the second that of the year, the first corresponding to the rotation of the earth on its axis and the second to the revolution of the earth around the sun. There is also a lunar cycle on which great emphasis has been placed in the folklore of many cultures. While this cycle probably has physiologic importance, but there are only a few convincing data.

*Annual Cycles* The annual cycle is particularly important in reproduction, at least in nonhuman species. Animals in the wild tend to be born in the spring. Even though the cycles have been muted in some domestic animals they are not totally suppressed, as is evident from the familiar association of lambs, calves, and colts with the spring. These yearly cycles may be difficult to alter. As was mentioned earlier, lengthening the day artificially in stables during the winter makes it possible for mares to become pregnant earlier, but there is an increased loss of embryos. Other manipulations may be more consistently successful. When the day is artificially lengthened in the winter, Holstein cows increase their milk production and the steers gain weight faster, but not when castrated, which strongly suggests that the testes play a role. It is likely that a major control is exerted by the pineal gland. During the dark months it is active and suppresses the gonads, but it becomes inactive during the longer days and the production of gonadal hormones therefore rises. This mechanism clearly makes it more likely that an animal will be born in the spring, a useful adaptation since conditions of food and climate are far more favorable for survival. Sensitivity to long days appears to diminish over time so that it is less marked by the end of the summer.[94] Male rats raised in constant darkness show diminished sexual activity, but this is reversed by pinealectomy,[95] presumably because of the removal of pineal inhibition.

The yearly cycle is also attended not merely by changes in the other metabolic alterations. The hyperglycemic response to epinephrine in humans is higher in the winter than in the summer.[96] The mongolian gerbil shows greater thermogenesis in response to a cold stimulus in mid-winter than in mid-summer.[97] While the yearly metabolic cycle can probably not be attributed entirely to activity of the pineal gland, it must play a major role.

It has already been pointed out that cyclic alteration in the production of sex hormones is likely to be of importance in many ways, e.g., it might affect the percentage of children with anomalous dominance born at different seasons. Children conceived in March or April will spend most of their first months in utero at a time when hormones are high. The child conceived six months later, in September or October, will tend to spend their early period in utero under much lower hormonal influences. Obviously, different quarters of the year will give rise to different patterns, but adequate information as to the outcome is still lacking. A recent study found that non-right-handedness was twice as common in boys born in the six months beginning in September (and thus conceived from December through May) than in the following six months. The rate of births of non-right-handers was furthermore higher in each of these months than in every month in the other half year. Similar effects were not found in females.[98] It is intriguing that rabbits raised postnatally in darkness for seven months were found to show an increase, as against controls, of synaptic contact zones in the medial visual cortex and the motor cortex on the left side, but not on the right side, but the authors are cautious in their interpretation of this.[99]

There are other possibly relevant data. It has been confirmed repeatedly that schizophrenics are born predominantly in the first half of the year and particularly in the first quarter. They are thus conceived between approximately the first of April and the first of October, i.e., predominantly during the period in which the days are longer than 12 hours. It is possible that schizophrenia is more common in those people who have spent the first six months of pregnancy under maximal hormonal influences. Mental defectives are also more likely to be born at the beginning of the year. On the other hand, many extensive studies of the months of birth of eminent people have shown that they too tend to be born predominantly early in the year and even more consistently to be born at low rate in the mid-summer months of July and August.[100] In all of these studies the data have been corrected for the normal yearly pattern of births. Other kinds of explanations may, of course, turn out to account for these data. In any case, it appears at first glance that people born early in the year are likely to be more variable, and thus to contain an excess of both eminent and highly disadvantaged individuals. It is of interest that mental defectives contain an excess of left-handers. It is, therefore, speculatively conceivable that one is dealing with an influence on the brain that will, when properly controlled, lead to superiority, but that in excess may lead to deleterious influences. It is obvious that hormonal influences deserve consideration, but they are far from being the only possible candidates.

There are other phenomena that may be related to a cycle of hormonal changes. Suicides tend to be at a maximum in May and June, and generally high from March to October,[101] a pattern that is reversed in Australia. The role of the pineal gland is suggested by recent studies that claim that depressives show anomalous patterns of melatonin release in response to changes in light.[102] Recent data have been published on the effects of drugs given at different times of the day, but there are few data, such as the study of Altschule on variations over the year. Leppik[103] has shown that side effects of phenytoin therapy vary throughout the year. Patients receiving phenytoin therapy in the winter almost never develop rashes that reach their peak in mid-summer. It is known that phenytoin may have both androgenizing and immune effects so that a hormonal component of this cycle deserves consideration. On the other hand, other mechanisms may be at play. Elevated temperatures have been shown to increase immune responsiveness,[104] and this might account for a higher rate of immune reactions to phenytoin therapy in the summer.

*Circadian Cycles* Recent articles have stressed the often dramatic variations in drug responses during the circadian cycle. The levels of enzymes in the pineal gland also have a striking daily cycle.[105] There are many physiologic phenomena, e.g., temperature and hormone levels that change throughout the 24-hour period. In disease, circadian variations are often striking, e.g., the classic patterns of fever in many infectious diseases. Migraine headaches may awaken the sufferer at 5 a.m. but rarely do so at 1 a.m. or 2 a.m., while cluster headaches frequently do so. In many patients, irritable bowel symptoms occur predominantly at night.

It is conceivable that these circadian phenomena may be different in those with AD than in those with standard dominance. There are several suggestions of laterality effects in sleep, e.g., a significantly greater frequency of sleep myoclonus in the nondominant hand. This article also claims that a higher percentage of all sleep myoclonus occurs late in sleep in left-handers as compared with dextrals, but this particular finding does not appear to us to be impressive.[106] Furthermore, in the stages of sleep the maximum amplitudes of EEG waves shift from one side to the other.

*The Menstrual Cycle* The recurrence of menstrual periods is, of course, another example of a cyclic phenomenon. One should, however, keep in mind the possibility that even this cycle may alter in relation to the annual pattern of sunlight. Female rats kept in constant darkness do not become pregnant because the ovaries are suppressed and atrophy, while those continuously in lighted quarters are also infertile because the ovaries are in constant estrus. We do not know of any data on variations in the length of human menstrual cycles throughout the year.

Irregular or absent menses have many causes, e.g., female athletes and those with anorexia often fail to menstruate probably because of loss of body fat that produces estradiol, but in many other cases there is no obvious cause. In view of the frequency of benign reproductive system pathology in women with temporal lobe epilepsy, in whom we believe there is probably a higher rate of AD, menstrual irregularities may be more common in the non-right-handed individual. We are now gathering data on this point.

The recurrence of certain neurologic disorders in relation to the menstrual cycle is intriguing and has therapeutic implications that are often overlooked. Migraine, epilepsy, and symptomatic manifestations of meningiomas may all recur in close relationship to a particular point in the cycle. While this is often attributed to fluid retention other possibilities deserve consideration, in particular, variations in immune responsiveness in response to sex hormone changes. We have now seen this type of menstrually related disorder in several cases with AD, a finding that should not be surprising in view of the demonstrated higher rate of sinistrality in migraine and the probable higher rate in those subjects with epilepsy. It would be well worth studying the handedness of a large cohort of patients with menstrually related disorders.

An important therapeutic implication is that in such patients suppression of periods may lead to improvement. We have now seen a few such cases, treated with progesterone or similar agents, in whom there is striking improvement. This also deserves further study.

## The Fundamental Causes of Asymmetry

This final section presents some speculations concerning the ultimate origins of asymmetry, i.e., mechanisms that permit the development of complex asymmetric biological structures.

In many discussions of cerebral dominance and handedness, it is common to find allusions to other types of asymmetry in nature. Asymmetries in plants are common, e.g., some climbing plants wind to the left while others wind to the right.[107] One finds repeated reference to the optically active compounds first discovered by Pasteur. In more recent writings reference is made to Yang and Lee who won the Nobel Prize for their theory of the nonconservation of parity, in which it was shown there were fundamental asymmetries even at the sub-atomic level. Almost invariably, however, these statements are followed by the disclaimer that these physical and chemical asymmetries are not linked in any way to each other or to the existence of bodily or brain asymmetries. The fact that most natural amino acids are in the l-form is thus regarded as the result of some chance event unrelated to the nonconservation of parity. Similarly, brain asymmetry is usually not linked to the asymmetries of biological molecules, and the asymmetries of growth of plants are usually not linked to asymmetric growth in animals.

Some recent studies have, however, suggested to us that there may in fact be a continuous sequence from asymmetry in the spin of the neutrino all the way to human cerebral dominance. Although the considerations presented here will be highly speculative, they do suggest some simple biological experiments that may supply information directly relevant to the attempt to understand the chemical events that determine the development of an asymmetric organism from the fertilized ovum.

## Mechanisms of Asymmetry

There are undoubtedly many mechanisms that can lead to asymmetry. In this section we will present some possible mechanisms, including some for which strong evidence exists.

*Systems With Initial Symmetry* Functional asymmetry of an area could be the result of larger size, or of greater binding of neurotransmitters, or both. It is even possible that in some cases the larger area may not be dominant, e.g., because of abnormalities of its cells or connections, or because of chemical asymmetry favoring the opposite side. Furthermore, the modifiability of chemical dominance makes possible shifts of dominance from one side to the other. Numbers or affinities of receptors and enzyme activity can often be altered rapidly. Shifts of dominance to the other side may, as we have noted, occur in some cases of cyclic manic-depressive illness. Our guess is that, in general, dominant areas will be larger because a greater number of cells will make possible a higher processing and storage capacity.

In some cases the organism begins as a symmetric structure in which asymmetry is then produced, while in other cases asymmetry is present even at the earliest stages. In other words, the original single cell from which the organism develops may itself be asymmetric, while in other cases it may be symmetric and asymmetry may be induced by the action of external influences at some stage in development. The initial asymmetry of single cells will be discussed in a later section.

*Asymmetry of the Lobster Claw* There are at least two types of mechanism that can induce asymmetry in a symmetric organism. The lobster in early life has two symmetric small claws, called pincers, one of which develops into a larger claw called a crusher, that is found equally often on the left and right sides. Recent experiments have demonstrated the mechanism of this unilateral transformation. If one pincer is permitted to crush oyster shells it then grows into a crusher and the other side remains a pincer permanently.[108] Thus in the wild a chance event, the availability of something to crush, determines whether one pincer or the other is transformed. There is a neural mechanism involved by which the information coming from the pincer that first crushes shells passes centrally and activates a process that suppresses the transformation potential of the opposite side. In the male fiddler crab there is hypertrophy of motor neurons and a larger number of sensory neurons on the side of the larger claw.[109]

This mechanism can easily produce asymmetry in a previously symmetric organism. It should, however, lead to an equal frequency of asymmetry on the two sides, and as such might appear to be irrelevant to the population asymmetries of higher animals. While it cannot thus be the fundamental mechanism of asymmetry in higher forms, it may well play a role as a secondary means of inducing asymmetry. Assume that for some reason a given area of a higher animal is larger on one side at some early stage of development. As this area forms fiber connections to other regions both on the contralateral and ipsilateral sides, it may suppress some regions and facilitate others by a mechanism possibly quite similar to that in the lobster. As a result, a consistent pattern of asymmetries may appear in other regions. This type of mechanism would lead to a pattern of *linked* asymmetries, i.e., the larger size of one area would be associated with larger size of certain other regions on both sides. If two or more regions independent of each other were initially large, one might have more than one pattern of linked asymmetry. We will return later to linked asymmetries. What kinds of suppression or facilitation might occur in this hypothetic case? The outflow from the initially larger region could conceivably even lead to death of cells in another area, or to a suppression of formation of axons from the neurons of that area so that more of them disappeared during the period of cell death. Conversely, the connections from the first area might accelerate the formation of axons in another area thus giving it an advantage in the period of cell death. The asymmetry of the callosal fibers in kittens[110] who have undergone removal of one eye may be an expression of a mechanism of this type, although in this case it is not loss of neurons but loss of axonal collaterals that is at play.

A similar mechanism could be operative even without the presence of larger areas, e.g., the projections from an area with greater binding of neurotransmitters or higher enzyme activity than the opposite one might favor or inhibit chemical or structural changes in regions with which it was connected.

*Physical Forces and Asymmetry* There is another mechanism by which asymmetry could be induced in symmetric organisms. This mechanism, unlike that in the crab, can lead to population asymmetry.

One means of the production of asymmetry is the induction of greater growth on one side by means of unsymmetric external forces. All living things find themselves in an atmosphere of unsymmetric physical forces that are the result of the earth's position in the universe and its geography, Sunlight comes from above. The magnetic field at any point on the earth's surface is asymmetrically disposed, and the force of gravity acts in a downward direction. An organism growing in flowing water will also be subjected to an asymmetric force.

A striking example of the operation of such forces is found in the work of Rogers.[111] When eggs were kept in the dark, the chicks no longer showed the typical pattern of asymmetry. Since sunlight nearly always falls from above on the egg this mechanism produces a population asymmetry.

Could some type of physical effect be relevant to side differences in higher animals? A somewhat similar type of mechanism has been suggested several times as operative in humans. A pattern of asymmetric forces acts on the human brain in its passage through the birth canal. While most infants exit in the left occiput anterior (LOA) position, three other normal birth positions also occur although less frequently. Some authors have argued the position in the birth canal leads to asymmetric forces on the brain that affect later cerebral dominance. Thus two studies[112,113] have shown a strong relationship between birth position and later handedness, with right occiput anterior infants having a much higher later frequency of left-handedness than LOA infants.

Although we believe that the data are convincing, one must raise certain questions concerning the suggested mechanism that would imply that dominance is determined at the time of birth. It could not account for the different patterns of anatomic asymmetries in left-handers, the types of brain anomalies found in the dyslexics, or the association of certain congenital anomalies, e.g., harelip, with sinistrality; all of these must be determined before delivery. Second, it does not address the deeper question as to why LOA is the most common presentation. This fact suggests that the position of the head must depend either on asymmetry in the birth canal or on asymmetry in the skull. As already noted, the fetus has the same pattern of asymmetry as that found in the adult, i.e., left occipital and right frontal regions are wider than their counterparts. When the head rotates into the LOA position, the longest diameter of the head lies in the axis of the birth canal with the narrowest diameter at right angles to this axis, i.e., the head is in the position that offers the least resistance to movement. As the uterus contracts, the head will move into this position of least resistance. The fact that the forces of uterine contraction are powerful and that the head is readily molded need not negate this possibility since even a small deviation from symmetry in the head might still lead to the effect we have postulated.

Our suggestion is, in other words, that the head position at delivery is not the cause of functional asymmetry, but is itself the result of the existing asymmetry of the brain, which will have a distinct association with future handedness. Since left-handed parents will have a greater percentage of left-handed children, one would predict that infants of sinistral parents will present right occiput anterior more often than infants of dextral parents. The data of Churchill et al[112] are in concordance with this prediction. Furthermore, symmetry of the occipital lobes is found more frequently in sinistrals than in dextrals in some, although not all, series.[82] Since symmetric heads should rotate equally to the left or right, one might expect the proportions of left and right occipital presentations to differ less in sinistrals than dextrals.

In any case, it may be stated that at present there is no direct evidence for the role of natural physical forces in the determination of asymmetry in higher animals. The number of hours of sunlight may have an effect, as noted in the section on cyclic phenomena, but this probably acts through alterations in the chemical environment (and especially in hormone levels) rather than by direct influence on local metabolism on one side of the fetal brain. Asymmetries in plants may, at least in some cases, reflect the predominant direction of sunlight.

A third possible mechanism for inducing asymmetry in an initially symmetric structure is called linked asymmetry and will be discussed in a later section.

## Systems With Initial Asymmetry

We will now consider cases in which the organism is not symmetric in its earliest stage, i.e., asymmetry is present even if the single-cell influences the pattern of development. Corballis and Morgan[26] postulated that the development of brain asymmetry depended on asymmetry of the ovum itself. The concept of asymmetry at the single-cell level is one that is likely to appear strange, and even if this were accepted it might still be difficult to understand how this asymmetry was transmitted to the descendants of that cell. It is, therefore, necessary to specify the exact meaning of this concept.

It was found early in the history of biology that the cytoplasm itself contains many internal structures, e.g., the Golgi apparatus. Methods such as electron microscopy show that the internal structure is extremely elaborate, and the picture of the cytoplasm as an amorphous fluid or gel is now completely unacceptable. There has been increasing recent emphasis on the cytoskeleton, the network of protein structures that define the form of the cell. It might be thought that the pattern of the cytoskeleton, although well-defined, might reflect random events in the life of the cell, but this seems not to be the case. Solomon[114] has shown that the same characteristic shape of a cell is preserved in its descendents. An asymmetric configuration of any cell is therefore likely to be preserved in mitosis and passed on to later generations.

The cytoskeletal architecture is determined by the arrangement of the fibrils formed by structural proteins such as actin. The synthesis of these proteins may depend on cytoplasmic genes the expression of which in turn often depends on nuclear genes. It was once commonly believed that the cytoplasmic genes, because of their association with mitochondria, were concerned only with energy metabolism, but it has been found that they may produce structural proteins and thus play a major role in the determination of the initial asymmetry of the cell. The role of cytoplasmic factors in asymmetry is well documented in the case of the left or right spiralling of the shell of the snail *Lymnaea peregra*.[115,116] In higher animals, cytoplasmic genes are derived from the mother via the ovum. The possibility that the sperm contributes cytoplasmic genes to the zygote cannot be excluded, but it is generally believed that if such a contribution exists it is very small.

It might be thought that cytoplasmic factors might therefore play a determinative role in the existence of AD, i.e., dominance might be determined exclusively by these genes.[117] Complete determination of dominance by cytoplasmic factors can be excluded since it implies a dominance pattern determined entirely by the mother, which is in conflict with the fact that the handedness of the father plays an important role in that of offspring. It is also not possible to assert that the dominance pattern is determined entirely by the interaction of maternal cytoplasmic factors and nuclear genes from both parents, since, as we have discussed elsewhere, nongenetic factors appear to play a major role in the laterality pattern.

It does seem likely, however, that the cytoplasmic genes (as well as the nuclear genes) may play a major role in determining susceptibilities to environmental chemical influences, and that those with a certain complement of such genes are more likely to be anomalously dominant. It is even possible that all the anomalous dominance population carry a particular cytoplasmic gene or group of such genes. A particular cytoplasmic gene complement might therefore be a necessary but not a sufficient condition for AD, since many of those with the appropriate endowment of such genes might have standard dominance unless they were exposed to particular intrauterine effects. It would not be possible to account for the nongenetic effects without such a proviso. We have pointed out earlier the finding of Nance that neural-tube defects appear to be transmitted primarily via the mother.

If those with AD carried certain cytoplasmic genes more often than the standard dominant group, then certain infections that attack particular genes of this type might occur more often in one or the other population. We have already commented on the possibility that Reye's syndrome in which mitochondrial disorder is prominent, occurs more often in AD individuals.

We will return later to a further discussion of cellular asymmetry.

*Chemical Asymmetry* Asymmetry present in the single cell, might be structural or chemical, or both. Chemical asymmetry might take several forms. Proteins or nucleic acids might be found on the two sides with identical chemical composition, but with different conformations, e.g., differences in the direction of spiralling fibrils or different proportions of so-called "left-handed DNA" (Z-DNA) on the two sides. There might be differences in chemical composition or in the numbers of receptors on the two sides. We suspect that in all cases of initial asymmetry there is chemical asymmetry with or without structural asymmetry at a more macroscopic level. The lateral differences in conformation or chemical composition are responsible for differential responses to chemicals that facilitate or inhibit growth. Larger numbers of mitochondria on one side could lead to unequal metabolic rates and differential responses to certain chemical influences. In the remaining sections we will present some of our speculations—which are, however, susceptible to experimental test—on the evolution and nature of initial asymmetry.

## The Nonconservation of Parity: Implications for Asymmetric Molecules

*Asymmetries in Physics and Chemistry* The possibility that physical factors play an essential role in the molecular asymmetry of living systems has been raised from time to time. Neville[118] points out that beta particles from the decay of radioactive strontium, phosphorus, or potassium decay are circularly polarized in one direction. He quotes the study of Garay[119] who found that when racemic mixtures of certain amino acids were bombarded by such particles the D-isomers were destroyed more quickly than the L-isomers.

It was held as a fundamental assumption over many years that the laws of physics were symmetric. The existence of any phenomenon that had a particular direction therefore implied the existence of another phenomenon of the opposite direction.

This concept was, however, upset by the epoch-making theory of Yang and Lee and its subsequent theoretical confirmation. In beta decay, an electron is emitted, along with a newly formed particle, the neutrino, that spins at right angles to the direction of movement. Standard assumptions of symmetry led to the expectation that there would be equal numbers of neutrinos with left-sided and right-sided spins. It was found unexpectedly that the neutrinos produced are all "left-handed," i.e., as they move toward the observer, they all spin in the clockwise direction, while the emitted electrons spin in the reverse direction. The asymmetric spins of the particles emitted in beta decay might at first appear to be of little consequence outside of the physics of elementary particles. It has, however, been argued on theoretical grounds that the bombardment of a mixture of equal amounts of L- and D-amino acids by such asymmetric electrons would lead to differential ionization and therefore to greater reactivity of the L forms. Preliminary experimental data appear to support this conclusion.

*Structural Proteins and Z-DNA* Neville[118] called attention to the fact that alpha-helixes formed by L-amino acids have a right-handed twist, superhelixes formed from such proteins have the opposite chirality. He also points out that if all the helical components in what appeared at first to be a symmetric biological structure consisted of sterically similar compounds, then despite apparent macroscopic symmetry one would find asymmetry at the molecular level. Compounds on opposite sides of the structure would have their twists in the same direction and would not necessarily be mirror images. This is easily visualized by considering spiralling molecules on the two sides that are oriented vertically. He goes on to point out that if the taste receptors on the two sides of the tongue were mirror images, then sucrose, a steric compound, could bind to only one side and would thus taste sweet on only one side.

Helicity, or direction of twist, is probably critical since certain structural fibrous compounds grow in the form of a coil. As the coil moves forward, the tip may move in the clockwise or in the counterclockwise direction. Such structural proteins play a role in many structures, e.g., the growing neurite contains actin, and the mitotic spindle appears to contain dynein. The cilia of the sperm that determine its movement also show such a definite direction, while the bronchial cilia beat in the same direction and thus help to clear small particles. Neville points out that in order to avoid entanglement the flagella of a bacterium must have the same twist and the same direction of rotation. It appears likely that cilia must contain structural proteins whose fibrils have a consistent torque. When such a coordinated pattern is not found, as in Kartagener's syndrome, one finds a high rate of respiratory infections, as well as an elevated high rate of infertility as a result of abnormality of the cilia in the sperm. Patients with this syndrome also manifest dextrocardia or situs inversus. This raises the possibility that if the spiralling of structural proteins is abnormal, laterality may also be disturbed. The same situation exists in the growth of the nervous system. A recent study showed that the neurites from goldfish retinal neurons in culture grow consistently in a clockwise direction whether they come from the right or the left eye,[120] suggesting that all the structural proteins have been coded to twist in the same direction.

### Asymmetric Chemical Effects

The structural properties of proteins are ultimately determined by the helix of DNA. A new form, Z-DNA, has been discovered recently, which has a left-handed helix[121] rather than the right-handed helix that had been thought to be the only form for many years. Z-DNA has now been found in many locations and research on its functions is proceeding actively. It should be stressed that although it has a left-handed helix, it is not a mirror image of the standard DNA molecule. It is, therefore, unlikely that it codes for proteins of conformations opposite to those of the standard forms.

We have postulated that certain hormones exert different effects on the two sides of the developing nervous system and the neural crest. This raises the question as to how a compound could affect growth differentially on opposite sides. The simplest mechanism would be that of chemical differences in the corresponding structures. The sex hormones themselves are stereoisomeric compounds. Estradiol-17-beta has much greater estrogenic effect than the alpha isomer that differs in the steric conformation of one hydroxyl group; the 17-beta form of T is similarly more active than the 17-alpha form. It is possible to conceive that T might have much greater chemical affinity with a compound with a torque in one direction than with one with its torque in the opposite direction. This situation might arise if on one side of the brain there were neurites with one orientation and on the other side neurites with the opposite conformation, each with a differential sensitivity to sex hormones. The action of T might be indirect, e.g., on a steric compound that in turn acted on the actin helix. It is known that Z-DNA differs from the corresponding standard form in its chemical reactivity since one can make antibodies specifically against Z-DNA. Differences in chemical structure on the two sides could thus ensure that certain compounds had differential lateral effects on growth. Such a mechanism would be particularly necessary in the brain in which the growth of paired structures must be modified differentially for the development of cerebral dominance. Similar situations may exist elsewhere in other paired organs.

Another possibility is that those forms of certain stereoisomeric compounds that are usually regarded as inactive might in fact have important asymmetric growth effects in development. The 17-alpha form of estradiol is not found in the human, but is found in other species. It is said to have measurable activity in certain test systems for estrogenic action. By contrast, 17-alpha T (epitestosterone) is found in appreciable quantities in humans, but no function has ever been established for it. Is it possible that while it may have little action on peripheral androgen-sensitive systems it is of importance in the mechanisms of asymmetry in development? Conceivably, it might have a greater affinity for compounds in a particular conformation than the more common 17-beta form. Testosterone has important actions on skeletal muscle in which actin is present in high concentration. Furthermore, it has effects on neurites[122] that also contain actin. Is it conceivable that the two forms of T might have differential effects on actin in the neurites of the developing brain on the two sides if the proportions of fibrils spiralling in opposite directions was different on the two sides? This is highly speculative but susceptible of some simple experimental tests. We will return in a later section to the question of the spiralling of structural proteins.

Mechanisms of the type we have discussed might fail in certain ways. Afzelius and Eliasson[123] point out that the pattern of the fibrils in cilia may play a major role in the determination of laterality. They also stress the role of such fibrils in the mitotic spindle. In Kartagener's syndrome there is some mechanism that leads to anomalous formation of fibrils with appropriate helical patterns. As a result, the cilia in the bronchi may have random orientations and a high rate of anomalies of the cilia of the sperm, which accounts for poor sperm motility and therefore the high rate of infertility of these patients. Finally, as a result of a disordered pattern of orientation of fibrils it is possible that they fail to guide development of bodily organs in the correct lateral orientation. If alterations in spiralling of fibrils played a role in the determination of laterality then one might expect that one would find evidence of anomalous formation of the fibrils of proteins involved in structure and motility in elevated frequency in the AD population. We pointed out earlier the high rate of abnormal sperm in celiac disease. A left-handed adult who had been a childhood dyslexic had abnormal sperm—and a right-handed brother with celiac disease. We have also commented on the possibility of a high rate of infertility in the anomalous dominance population.

The previously discussed locus *T* of the MHC complex is a set of genes that might be related to proteins involved in motility. The sperm that carries the allele *t* is much more likely to impregnate the ovum than one that does not. This accounts for the fact that *t* is transmitted to much more than half the offspring of a *t*-bearing father. It has been suggested that this is because the sperm bearing *t* swims more rapidly. If this were the case, it would suggest that *t* might play some important role in the formation of the structural proteins of the cilia.

### Asymmetry in Unicellular Organisms

We support the view of Corballis and Morgan[26] that asymmetry may be coded in the organism at its most elementary stage, i.e., as a single cell. The asymmetry might be coded in the cytoskeleton of the single cell. Cytoplasmic genes might play a role in this process.

Although the concept of asymmetry of *function* in a single cell must appear at first to be difficult to accept, its existence appears to be well documented. In a remarkable article, Schaeffer[124] pointed out the striking asymmetries of unicellular organisms. He quotes Jennings who studied 162 species of ciliates that in swimming rotate in the long axis of the body; in each species of ciliate there is only a single direction of rotation. One hundred species rotated in the right-handed direction while 62 rotated to the left. Schaeffer found over many hours of observation that amoebas swim around a glass rod more frequently in one direction than the other. He gives many other examples of such preferred directions in rotation in unicellular organisms and in multicellular invertebrate species in which all members rotate on the long axis in the same orientation, e.g., the Polo worm. He also discussed asymmetry of rotation in sperm, but gave no details.

These preferential patterns imply that the proteins underlying motility probably have a preferential helix in each of the species involved. There is thus no a priori reason to reject the possibility that similar structures are not present in the ovum, the sperm, and the zygote. We would also suggest that asymmetries in the plant world may have similar fundamental mechanisms, and that therefore studies in plants may give valuable insight into the mechanisms of asymmetry even in humans. Asymmetries of structure and function far from being confined to the human are widespread, and possibly even universal, properties of living things in both the plant and animal kingdoms. They are present in unicellular organisms as well as in the most complex multicellular forms.

### Secondary Mechanisms of Asymmetry

*Shifts of Dominance* When initial asymmetry is present, several mechanisms can play a role in determining the final pattern of asymmetry. Evidence has been presented that asymmetry favoring certain brain regions is present early in fetal life. Since we believe that initial asymmetry implies the presence of chemical asymmetry, it is possible to alter the fundamental pattern. Because chemical difference almost always implies immunologic difference of the immune system, it might lead to slowing of growth on one side. Hormones or other substances might act directly on nerve cells or neurites or might modify immune effects.

Our hypothesis, based on the currently available evidence, is that the brain has intrinsic strong left-hemisphere language and motor dominance and that influences in utero can slow development of the structures underlying these functions on the left side, thus diminishing the magnitude of these lateralizations. Slowing on the left side indirectly leads to diminished cell death on the opposite side and therefore an eventual larger size of areas on that side. With exaggerated slowing the two sides tend to become more symmetric and therefore random dominance will be found. A less common effect is a shift to the point where the right-sided structures actually are larger than those on the left.

There is another possible mechanism for random dominance. In animals with situs inversus,[125] the genetic abnormality appears to lead not to reversed situs, but to random situs so that only half of the bearers of the genetic pattern actually show reverse situs. The same mechanism is probably operative in humans. In Kartagener's syndrome dextrocardia or reverse situs occurs in many cases, but is lacking in many others. This again suggests that situs is random in this situation. Afzelius and Eliasson[123] have argued that the mechanism that leads to ciliary abnormality in the bronchi and sperm also leads to the anomaly of lateralization of the internal organs. We suspect that anomalous dominance will be present in elevated frequency in this population.

Annett[126] was the first to suggest that most left-handedness is the result of a mechanism in which brain laterality is randomly determined. According to her theory some individuals carry a right-shift gene that increases the probability of left-hemisphere dominance for language and speech. In the absence of this gene, laterality for these functions is randomly determined.

Our hypothesis differs from Annett's in one respect. We have accepted what we consider to be the major and seminal contribution of her theory, i.e., that there is a group of individuals with random dominance. We believe, however, that the system in its initial stages possesses asymmetry favoring the language and motor regions of the left hemisphere and that influences that allay development of these regions on the left side can drive the system to symmetry. While she argues for right-shift influences that can drive the system from randomness to left dominance, we argue for left-shift influences (as was proposed by Corballis and Morgan[26]) that drive the system to symmetry. Reverse asymmetry is uncommon. An important reason for our formulation is the fact that fetal brains at very early stages typically show asymmetry favoring the left side.

It is possible, however, that there is a greater variety of initial states than we have assumed. While it seems clear that initial asymmetry favoring the left side is present in most brains one should consider the possibility that in some cases the initial state is one of symmetry or even reverse asymmetry. Obviously, it would be important to determine how often the initial state is one of actual symmetry or reverse asymmetry. The methodology for such a study is straightforward. One would require large numbers of brains of fetuses, at most, let us say, five months' gestational age, in order to determine how many show the typical pattern of asymmetry in the sylvian fissures (with left being lower at its end than the right) and more marked development of cortical markings on the right side. If individuals with reversed cerebral asymmetry existed, they would have a reversal of the usual sylvian asymmetry and more rapid cortical development on the left side. Those without asymmetry would have sylvian fissures of equal height and equally rapid development of cortical markings on the two sides. We would predict that the number of such cases would be small, but the experiment is an important one.

If brains with initial symmetry or reverse asymmetry existed, it would be important to know what effect the delaying influences would have. It is conceivable in the cases of initial reverse asymmetry that environmental influences in utero would lead to slowing on the right side rather than on the left side. A certain percentage of these cases would therefore be shifted to symmetry and some even to left-sided predominance. Conceivably, brains with initial symmetry might lack chemical asymmetry and might therefore remain symmetric. If the pattern of hormonal influences were the same as those in the cases with normal brain asymmetry, then males with initial reverse asymmetry should be more often shifted to symmetry or reversal. If this were true, then we would expect more females among those with strong asymmetries favoring the left hemisphere, as is suggested by the higher average levels of female verbal skills and their higher rate of strong right-handedness, and also more females in the small group with strong asymmetries favoring the right side. Wada et al[127] found that a larger right planum was more common in females than males.

The questions raised in this section are important ones that can be settled only by study of large numbers of early fetal brains. We would like to stress, however, that even if one should find a subgroup of brains with initial symmetry or reverse asymmetry, we would not accept a formulation that stated that the laterality pattern was fully determined by the initial asymmetry. Our basic hypothesis is that there is an initial pattern that is capable of major modifications by environmental influences. This would still be our formulation if there were several different initial patterns. Without involving environmental effects, it would not be possible to explain the larger numbers of males than females with AD, the male predominance in LD, and the elevated rate of AD not only in monozygotic but also in dizygotic twins.

*Linked Asymmetries* A *linked* asymmetry is one that is not present initially nor one that is induced in an initially symmetric structure by physical forces. It specifies an asymmetry that is induced in a given structure as the result of the appearance of or modification of asymmetry in another structure.

We have already discussed two mechanisms of linked asymmetry. When certain structures in the left hemisphere are slowed in their development, the opposite homologous area becomes larger, and we have suggested in our earlier discussions that this is the result of diminished cell death.

As a result of the changes in the nervous system that occur when one pincer of a lobster enlarges, the neural system controlling the other pincer is in some way inhibited, thus preventing it from undergoing a similar transformation. We have already discussed the possibility that similar mechanisms could conceivably be at play in higher animals in producing a pattern of linked asymmetries.

We have suggested that the slowing of growth of one particular region not only leads to enlargement of the opposite homologous area but also leads to enlargement of adjacent uninvolved regions, as shown by the work of Goldman and Galkin.[128] It seems likely that the effects of change in one region may be seen not only in immediately adjacent structures, but also in structures at a distance from the site of slowing or damage, a possibility also suggested by the work of Goldman and Galkin.

The existence of linked asymmetries raises the question as to whether there is only one primary asymmetry in the human brain, all the others being secondary linked asymmetries, or whether there are several primary asymmetries each of which may induce linked asymmetries.

The absence of linkage between two asymmetries is suggested when one asymmetry may be altered independently of the other. Thus although the great majority of humans have a particular configuration of the thoracic and abdominal organs, one finds that dextrocardia can exist in the absence of reversal of the abdominal organs. On the other hand, it is extremely rare to find, let us say an isolated shift of the spleen. This suggests that the asymmetries of the abdominal organs are linked but that cardiac asymmetry is independent.

It is important to be aware, however, that if two functions have their dominance in opposite hemispheres this need not rule out linkage of the underlying anatomic or chemical asymmetry. As we have already noted, when corresponding areas are anatomically symmetric the mechanism suggested by Annett[126] is operative, i.e., dominance for the function subserved is probably random. Hence, when symmetry is present in one pair of areas on opposite sides, the areas linked to this pair will also be symmetric. The functions subserved by the different areas will, however, be randomly controlled by either hemisphere. The final decision as to the existence of linkage may therefore require knowledge of the anatomic or chemical asymmetries in addition to that of functional asymmetry.

The data are therefore not yet sufficient to determine whether any brain asymmetries are linked. Language and motor dominance may be located in opposite hemispheres, but linkage cannot be excluded with certainty for the reasons just given. On the other hand, it is clear, as discussed earlier, that the typical dominance functions of the right hemisphere rarely shift even when language is shifted and this suggests that at least one of the right brain asymmetries is not linked to language.

Some anatomic data concerning linkage are available. In a study of East African skulls, frontal, occipital, and parietal petalias were combined randomly, suggesting an absence of linkage.[129] It would be important to carry on an extensive study with radiologic methods. By contrast, Glick and colleagues[130] found that in the human brain several chemical asymmetries were found to be linked. Furthermore, Eidelberg and Galaburda[131] found that language-related areas had linked asymmetries.

It is likely that partially linked asymmetries are often present. In this case two areas may have their initial asymmetries determined independently. It may be the case, however, that a change in one of these areas may secondarily influence the development of others.

*Postnatal Effects* We have discussed elsewhere possible postnatal influences in the modification of asymmetry. We know much less about these, although many of the same considerations probably apply.

## Conclusion

The speculations in the previous pages are presented not through the conviction that they necessarily represent the true origins of asymmetry, but rather because the realization that cerebral dominance is a biological problem makes it necessary to consider its ultimate cellular origins. The application of the techniques of molecular biology and genetics to this as yet unexplored area will surely lead to dramatic findings and to far more sophisticated theories based on solid experimental data. We hope that our naive speculations will help to stimulate research. The existence of asymmetries even at the single-cell level has been stressed because information of importance may come from even the lowliest forms of animal life and from plants. It has become evident in recent years that biological mechanisms of importance in higher animals often embody processes found in very primitive forms. Dominance was, until very recently, thought to be a feature only of humans, but this is now known to be contrary to the facts. The understanding of the ultimate origins of asymmetry will require study not only of the foundations of biology but, very possibly, also those of physics itself.

## References

1. Geschwind N, Galaburda AM: Cerebral lateralization: Biological mechanisms, associations, and pathology: I. A hypothesis and a program for research. *Arch Neurol* 1985;42:428–459.
2. Geschwind N, Galaburda AM: Cerebral lateralization: Biological mechanisms, associations, and pathology: II. A hypothesis and a program for research. *Arch Neurol* 1985;42:521–552.
3. Talal N: *Autoimmunity.* New York, Academic Press Inc, 1977.
4. Ohno S: The original function of MHC antigens as the general plasma membrane anchorage site of organogenesis-directing proteins. *Immunol Rev* 1977;33:59–69.
5. Golub ES: Connections between the neurons, haematopoietic, and germ-cell systems. *Nature* 1982;299:483–485.

6. Mori K, Handa H, Gi H, et al: Cavernomas in the middle fossa. *Surg Neurol* 1980;14:21–31.
7. Suzuki J, Komatsu S: New embolization method using estrogen for dural arteriovenous malformation and meningioma. *Neurology* 1981;16:438–442.
8. Bartleson JD, Cohen MD, Harrington TM, et al: Cauda equina syndrome secondary to long-standing ankylosing spondylitis. *Ann Neurol* 1982;12:77.
9. Cilluffo JM, Gomez MR, Reese DF, et al: Idiopathic ('congenital') spinal arachnoid diverticula. *Mayo Clin Proc* 1981;56:93–101.
10. Greenfield JG, Blackwood W, McMenemy WH, et al (eds): *Neuropathology.* London, Edward Arnold, 1958, p 353.
11. Rodbard D: The role of regional body temperature in the pathogenesis of disease. *N Engl J Med* 1981;305:808–814.
12. Giron LT Jr, Crutcher KA, Davis JN: Lymph nodes: A possible site for sympathetic neuronal regulation of immune responses. *Ann Neurol* 1980;8:520–525.
13. Gathier JC, Bruyn GW: Neuralgic amyotrophy, in Vinken PJ, Bruyn GW (eds): *Handbook of Clinical Neurology.* American Elsevier, New York, 1970, vol 8, part 2, *Diseases of Nerves,* pp 77–85.
14. Gathier JC, Bruyn GW: The serogenetic peripheral neuropathies, in Vinken PJ, Bruyn GW (eds): *Diseases of Nerves, Part II,* vol 8 of *Handbook of Clinical Neurology.* American Elsevier, New York, 1970, vol 8, part 2, *Diseases of Nerves,* pp 95–111.
15. Taylor RA: Heredofamilial mononeuritis multiplex with brachial predilection. *Brain* 1960;83:113–137.
16. Jacob JC, Andermann F, Robb JP: Heredofamilial neuritis with brachial predilection. *Neurology* 1961;11:1025–1033.
17. Epstein E: Triamcinolone procaine in the treatment of zoster and postzoster neuralgia. *Calif Med* 1971;115:6–10.
18. Rebeiz JJ, Kolodny EH, Richardson EP: Corticodentatonigral degeneration with neuronal achromasia. *Arch Neurol* 1968;18:20–33.
19. Seltzer B, Sherwin I: A comparison of clinical features in early- and late-onset primary degenerative dementia. *Arch Neurol* 1983;40:143–146.
20. Tissot R, Constantinidis J, Richard J: *La Maladie de Pick.* Paris, Masson & Sons, 1975.
21. Mesulam MM: Slowly progressive aphasia without generalized dementia. *Ann Neurol* 1982;11:592–598.
22. Cobb S: Haemangioma of the spinal cord. *Ann Surg* 1915;62:641–649.
23. Bartleson JD, Swanson JW, Whisnant JP: A migrainous syndrome with cerebrospinal fluid pleocytosis. *Neurology* 1981;31:125–162.
24. Leppik IE, Lapora J, Loewenson R: Seasonal incidence of phenytoin allergy unrelated to plasma level. *Arch Neurol* 1985;42:120–122.
25. Marsh DG, Meyers DA, Bias WB: The epidemiology and genetics of atopic allergy. *N Engl J Med* 1981;305:1551–1559.
26. Corballis MC, Morgan MJ: On the biological basis of human laterality. *Behav Brain Sci* 1978;2:261–336.
27. Simpson E: Antigens associated with H-2 embryos and tumours. *Nature* 1983;306:738–739.
28. Furukawa T, Shinohara T: Congenital hemihypertrophy: Oncogenic potential of the hypertrophic side. *Ann Neurol* 1981;10:199–201.

29. Galaburda AM, Kemper TL: Cytoarchitectonic abnormalities in developmental dyslexia: A case study. *Ann Neurol* 1979;6:94–100.
30. Dalby MA: Attentional difficulties and subclinical absences in specific language delayed children, abstracted, in *World Congress of Epilepsy*. Amsterdam, Excerpta Medica, 1981, p 118.
31. Masland RL, Masland MW: Epilepsy and specific learning disability, abstracted, in *World Congress of Epilepsy*. Amsterdam, Excerpta Medica, 1981, p 116.
32. Szondi L: Konstitutionsanalyse von 100 Stotterern. *Wien Med Wochenschr* 1932; 82:922–928.
33. Stefan M, Milea S, Magureanu S, et al: The autistic syndrome and epileptic seizures: Clinical and etiopathogenetic interference. *Rev Med Interna* 1981;26:205–211.
34. Bergen D, Tanner CM, Wilson R: The electroencephalogram in Tourette syndrome. *Ann Neurol* 1982;11:382–385.
35. Shapiro AK, Shapiro E: An update on Tourette syndrome. *Am J Psychotherapy* 1982;36:378–391.
36. Veith G, Schwindt W: Pathologisch-anatomischer Beitrag zur Problem 'Nichtsesshaftigkeit.' *Fortschritte Neurol-Psychiatry* 1976;44:1–21.
37. Herzog AG, Seibel MM, Schomer D, et al: Temporal lobe epilepsy: An extrahypothalamic pathogenesis for polycystic ovarian syndrome? *Neurology* 1984; 34:1389–1393.
38. Bray PF, Wiser WC: Evidence for a genetic etiology of temporal-central abnormalities in focal epilepsy. *N Engl J Med* 1964;271:926–933.
39. Bray PF, Wiser WC: The relation of focal to diffuse epileptiform EEG discharges in genetic epilepsy. *Arch Neurol* 1965;13:223–237.
40. Bray PF, Wiser WC: A unifying concept of idiopathic epilepsy. *Postgrad Med* 1969; 46:82–87.
41. Beaussart M: Benign epilepsy of children with Rolandic (centro-temporal) paroxysmal foci. *Epilepsia* 1972;13:795–811.
42. Walter CW, Dovey VJ: Clinical and EEG studies of temporal lobe function. *Proc R Soc Med* 1947;42:891–904.
43. Paolozzi C, Bravaccio F: Ripartizione tra i due emisferi olelle anormalita elletroencefalografiche focalizzate. *Acta Neurol* 1969;24:13–28.
44. Paolozzi C: Hemisphere dominance and asymmetry related to vulnerability of cerebral hemisphere. *Psychiatry Dig* 1970;31:61.
45. Taylor DC: Differential rates of cerebral maturation between the sexes and between hemispheres. *Lancet* 1969;2:140–142.
46. Taylor DC, Ounsted C: Biological mechanisms influencing the outcome of seizures in response to fever. *Epilepsia* 1971;12:33–45.
47. Cain DP, Wada JA: An anatomical asymmetry in the baboon brain. *Brain Behav Evol* 1979;16:222–226.
48. Stokes KA, McIntyre DC: Lateralized asymmetrical state-dependent learning produced by kindled convulsions from the rat hippocampus. *Physiol Behav* 1981; 26:163–169.
49. Caron JP, Colin H, Comoy J, et al: Resultats de l'excision chirurgicale des aneurysmes arterio-veneux (AAV) des zones rolandique, parietale, occipital, et du pli courbe de l'hemisphere dominant: A propos de vingt cas. *Neurochirurgie* 1982; 28:295–307.

50. Geschwind N: Pathogenesis of behavior changes in temporal lobe epilepsy, in Ward AA Jr, Penry JK, Purpura D (eds): *Epilepsy.* New York, Raven Press, 1983, pp 355–370.
51. Waxman SG, Geschwind N: The interictal behavioral syndrome of temporal lobe epilepsy. *Arch Gen Psychiatry* 1975;32:1580–1586.
52. Weintraub S, Mesulam MM: Developmental learning disabilities of the right hemisphere. *Arch Neurol* 1983;40:463–468.
53. Crystal HA, Haroupian DS, Katzmann R, et al: Biopsy-proved Alzheimer disease presenting as a right parietal lobe syndrome. *Ann Neurol* 1982;12:156–188.
54. Torch WC, Hirano A, Solomon S: Anterograde transneuronal degeneration in the limbic system: Clinical-anatomic correlation. *Neurology* 1977;27:1157–1163.
55. Hamlin RM: Intellectual function 14 years after frontal lobe surgery. *Cortex* 1970; 6:299–307.
56. Duvoisin RC, Eldridge R, Williams A, et al: Twin study of Parkinson's disease. *Neurology* 1981;31:77–80.
57. Hunt JR: Progressive atrophy of the globus pallidus (primary atrophy of pallidal system): A system disease of paralysis agitans type. *Brain* 1917;40:58–148.
58. Jannetta PJ: Vascular decompression in trigeminal neuralgia, in Samii M, Jannetta PJ: *The Cranial Nerves.* New York, Springer Publishing Co Inc, 1981, pp 331–340.
59. Stejskal L, Tomanek Z: Postural laterality in torticollis and torsion dystonia. *J Neurol Neurosurg Psychiatry* 1981;44:1029–1034.
60. Sherwin I, Peron-Magnan P, Bancaud J, et al: Prevalence of psychosis in epilepsy as a function of the laterality of the epileptogenic lesion. *Arch Neurol* 1982;39:621–625.
61. Taylor DC: Factors influencing the occurrence of schizophrenia-like psychosis in patients with temporal lobe epilepsy. *Psychol Med* 1975;5:249–254.
62. Gruzellier J, Flor-Henry P: *Hemispheric Asymmetries of Function in Psychopathology.* New York, Elsevier North Holland, 1979.
63. Boklage CE: Twinning, handedness, and the biology of symmetry, in Geschwind N, Galaburda AM (eds): *Cerebral Dominance: The Biological Foundations.* Cambridge, Mass, Harvard University Press, 1984, pp 195–210.
64. Lishman WA, McMeekan ERL: Hand preference patterns in psychiatric patients. *Br J Psychiatry* 1976;129:158–166.
65. Coursey RD, Buchsbaum MS, Murphy DL: Platelet-MAO activity and evoked potentials in the identification of subjects biologically at risk for psychiatric disorders. *Br J Psychiatry* 1979;134:372–381.
66. Mendlewicz J: Role des facteurs neurobiologiques dans le diagnostic et le traitment des syndromes depressifs. *Bull Mem Acad R Med Belg* 1983;138:169–178.
67. Bakan P: Left-handedness and alcoholism. *Percept Motor Skills* 1973;36:514.
68. Nasrallah HA, Keelor K, McCalley-Whitters M: Laterality shift in alcoholic males. *Biol Psychol* 1983;18:1065–1067.
69. Gabrielli WF, Mednick SA: Intellectual performance in children of alcoholics. *J Nerv Ment Dis* 1983;171:444–447.
70. Glick S, Shapiro R: Functional and neurochemical asymmetries, in Geschwind N, Galaburda AM (eds): *Cerebral Dominance: The Biological Foundations.* Cambridge, Mass, Harvard University Press, 1984, pp 147–166.
71. Sai-Halasz A, Brunecker G, Szara ST: Dymethyltryptamine: Ein neues Psychoticum. *Psychiatry Neurol* 1958;135:285–301.

72. Gentili C, Tiberi F: *Rilievi clinico-sperimentali sull'azione neuropsicodislettica della N-N-dietiltriptamina, ed.2. Bologna, Internazionale sull'Espressione Plastica, 1963.*
73. Serafetinides EA: The significance of the temporal lobes and of hemispheric dominance in the production of LSD-25 symptomatology in man. *Neuropsychologia* 1965;3:69–79.
74. Newlin DB, Carpenter B, Golden CJ: Hemispheric asymmetries in schizophrenia. *Biol Psychiatry* 1981;16:561–582.
75. Gerendai I: Lateralization of neuroendocrine control, in Geschwind N, Galaburda AM (eds): *Cerebral Dominance: The Biological Foundations,* Cambridge, Mass, Harvard University Press, 1984, pp 167–178.
76. Nordeen EJ, Yahr P: Hemispheric asymmetries in the behavioral and hormonal effects of sexually differentiating mammalian brain. *Science* 1982;218:391–393.
77. Chesselett MF, Cheramy N, Reisine TD, et al: Local and distal effects induced by unilateral striatal application of opiates in the absence or presence of naloxone on the release of dopamine in both caudate nuclei and substantiae nigrae of the cat. *Brain Res* 1983;258:229–242.
78. Mandell AJ, Knapp S: Asymmetry and mood, emergent properties of serotonin regulation. *Arch Gen Psychiatry* 1979;36:909–916.
79. Bogen JE, Gordon HW: Musical tests for functional lateralization with intracarotid ambarbital. *Nature* 1971;230:524–525.
80. Gainotti G: Emotional behavior and hemispheric side of the lesion. *Cortex* 1972; 8:41–55.
81. Beck E: Typologie des Gehirns am Beispiel des dorsalen menschlichen Schlafenappens nebst weiteren Beitrage zur Frage der Links-Rechtshirnigkeit. *Dtsch Z Nervenheilk* 1955;173:267–308.
82. Galaburda AM, LeMay M, Kemper TL, et al: Right-left asymmetries in the brain. *Science* 1978;199:852–856.
83. Bracco L, Tiezzi A, Ginanneschi A, et al: Lateralization of choline acetyltransferase (CAT) activity in fetus and adult human brain. *Neurosci Lett* 1984;50:301–305.
84. Amaducci L, Sorbi S, Albanese A, et al: Choline acetyltransferase (ChAT) activity differs in right and left human temporal lobes. *Neurology* 1981;31:799–805.
85. Bracco L, Tiezzi A, Ginanneschi A, et al: Lateralization of choline acetyltransferase (ChAT) activity in fetus and adult human brain. *Neurosci Lett* 1984;50:801–805.
86. Weber WW, Hein DW: Clinical pharmacokinesis of isoniazid. *Clin Pharmacookinet* 1979;4:401–422.
87. Sonnhag C, Karlsson E, Hed J: Procainamide-induced lupus erythematosus-like syndrome in relation to acetylator phenotype and plasma levels of procainamide. *Acta Med Scand* 1979;206:245–251.
88. Denef C, DeMoor P: The 'puberty' of the rat liver: II. Permanent changes in steroid metabolizing enzymes after treatment with a single injection of testosterone proprionate at birth. *Endocrinology* 1968;83:791–798.
89. Gustaffson JA, Mode A, Skett P, et al: Cerebral control of a cytochrome P-450-dependent steroid hydroxylase in rat liver, in Dorner C, Kawakami M (eds): *Hormones and Brain Development.* New York, Elsevier North Holland, 1978.
90. Michaelson J, Ferreira A, Nussenzweig V: *cis*-Interacting genes of the *S* region of the murine major histocompatibility complex. *Nature* 1981;289:306–308.
91. Selye H: *Hormones and Resistance.* New York, Springer Publishing Co Inc, 1971, vols 1 and 2.

92. Faris RA, Campbell TC: Exposure of newborn rats to pharmacologically active compounds may permanently alter carcinogen metabolism. *Science* 1981;211:719–721.
93. Gupta C, Yaffee SJ, Shapiro BH: Prenatal exposure to phenobarbital permanently decreases testosterone and causes reproductive dysfunction. *Science* 1982; 216:640–642.
94. Reiter RJ: The pineal gland and its hormones in the control of reproduction in mammals. *Endocrine Rev* 1980;1:109–131.
95. Baum MJ: Pineal gland: Influence on development of copulation in male rats. *Science* 1968;162:586–587.
96. Altschule MD, Siegel EP: Inadequacy of the glycemic reaction to epinephrine as a measure of hepatic glycogen. *Am J Med Sci* 1951;222:50–53.
97. Pohl H: Temperature regulation and cold acclimation in the golden hamster. *J Appl Physiol* 1965;20:405–410.
98. Badian NA: Birth order, maternal age, season of birth, and handedness. *Cortex* 1983;19:451–463.
99. Vrensen G, deGroot D: The effects of dark rearing and its recovery on synaptic terminals in the visual cortex of rabbits: A quantitative electron microscopic study. *Brain Res* 1974;78:263–278.
100. Peterson JM: Left-handedness: Differences between student artists and scientists. *Percept Motor Skills* 1979;48:961–962.
101. Parker G, Walter S: Seasonal variation in depressive disorders and suicidal death in New South Wales. *Br J Psychiatry* 1981;140:626–632.
102. Claustrat B, Chazot G, Brun J, et al: A chronobiological study of melatonin and cortisol secretion in depressed subjects: Plasma melatonin, a biochemical marker in major depression. *Biol Psychiatry* 1984;14:1215–1228.
103. Leppick I: Seasonal allergy to phenytoin not related to dose. *Ann Neurol* 1985; 42:120–122.
104. Sohnle PG, Gambert SR: Thermoneutrality: An evolutionary advantage against ageing. *Lancet* 1982;1:1099–1101.
105. Black IB, Axelrod J: The regulation of some biochemical circadian rhythms, in Litwack G (ed): *Biochemical Actions of Hormones*. New York, Academic Press Inc, 1983, pp 135–155.
106. Jovanovic VJ: Physiologische Myokloni beim Einschlafen und im Schlaf. *Z EEG-EMG* 1971;2:58–63.
107. Flanders M, Swann D: *The Songs of Michael Flanders and Donald Swann*. New York, St Martin's Press, 1977.
108. Govind CK, Kent KS: Transformation of fast fibers to slow prevented by lack of activity in developing lobster muscle. *Nature* 1982;298:755–757.
109. Govind CK, Young RE: Lateralization of the nervous system to the paired asymmetric chelipedes of male fiddler crabs. *Soc Neurosci Abstracts* 1983;9:383.
110. Cynader M, Lepore F, Guillemot JP: Interhemispheric competition during postnatal development. *Nature* 1981;290:139–140.
111. Rogers LJ: Light experience and asymmetry of brain function in chickens. *Nature* 1982;297:223–225.
112. Churchill JA, Igna E, Seirf R: The association of position at birth and handedness. *Pediatrics* 1962;29:307–309.
113. Grapin P, Perpere C: Symetrie et lateralisation du nourrisson, in *Main Droite et Main Gauche*. Paris, Presses Universitaires de France, 1968, pp 83–100.

114. Solomon F: Detailed neurite morphologies of sister neuroblastoma cells are related. *Cell* 1979;16:165–169.
115. Boycott AE, Diver C, Garstang SL, et al: The inheritance of sinistrality in *Limnaea peregra (Mollusca pulmonata). Phil Trans R Soc Lond* 1930;219:51–131.
116. Freeman G, Lundelius JW: The developmental genetics of dextrality and sinistrality in the gastropod *Lymnaea peregra. Roux Arch Entwickl Organsmen* 1982;191:69–83.
117. Verkoren AC: Oorsprang van links: En rechtshandigheid wordt duidelijker. *Aarde Kosmos* 1983;2:158–160.
118. Neville AC: *Animal Asymmetry.* London, Edward Arnold Ltd, 1976.
119. Garay AS: Origin and role of optical isomery in life. *Nature* 1968;219:338–340.
120. Heacock AM, Agranoff BW: Clockwise growth of neurites from retinal explants. *Science* 1977;198:64–66.
121. Rich A: Right-handed and left-handed DNA: Conformational information in genetic material. *Cold Spring Harbor Symposium on Quantitative Biology* 1982; 47:1–12.
122. Toran-Allerand CD: Gonadal hormones and brain development: Cellular aspects of sexual differentiation. *Am Zool* 1978;18:553–565.
123. Afzelius BA, Eliasson K: Flagellar mutants in man: On the heterogeneity of the immotile-cilia syndrome. *J Ultrastructure Res* 1979;69:43–52.
124. Schaeffer AA: Spiral movement in man. *J Morph* 1928;45:293–398.
125. Layton WM Jr: Random determination of a developmental process. *J Heredity* 1976;67:336–338.
126. Annett M: Genetic and nongenetic differences in handedness. *Behav Genet* 1978; 8:227–249.
127. Wada JA, Clarke R, Hamm A: Cerebral hemispheric asymmetry in humans. *Arch Neurol* 1975;32:239–246.
128. Goldman PS, Galkin TW: Prenatal removal of frontal association: Cortex in the fetal rhesus monkey: Anatomical and functional consequences in postnatal life. *Brain Res* 1978;152:451–485.
129. Gundara N, Zivanovic B: Asymmetry in East African skulls. *Am J Phys Anthropol* 1968;28:331–338.
130. Glick SD, Ross DA, Hough LB: Lateral asymmetry of neurotransmitters in human brain. *Brain Res* 1982;234:53–63.
131. Eidelberg D, Galaburda AM: Inferior parietal lobule: Divergent architectonic asymmetries in the human brain. *Arch Neurol* 1984;41:843–852.


The work reported here was supported by grants from the National Science Foundation, the National Institutes of Health, the Orton Research Fund, and the Essel Foundation.

We express our warm thanks to Loraine Karol for her devotion to the preparation of the many drafts of this article and to Patricia Geschwind for preparing the bibliography.

# PART V

# Epilepsy

*Steven C. Schachter*

Norman Geschwind was fascinated by patients with epilepsy. His best-known contributions to the field of epilepsy derived from his primary interest in behavior. Many of these contributions were credited to his students and colleagues, including David Bear, Stephen Waxman, Donald Schomer, Andrew Herzog, Marc Dichter, Orrin Devinsky, and others. He studied the memory disorders found in patients with epilepsy and emphasized the role of neuropsychologic testing in this patient population. He was intrigued by personality changes and the schizophreniform psychosis which took many years to develop after the onset of epilepsy. He was concerned with language and epilepsy,[1] behavioral changes following temporal lobectomy,[2] and aggression in temporal lobe epilepsy (TLE).[3] Most importantly, he described the interictal behavior syndrome of TLE.[4]

As he did years earlier when he wrote about aphasia, Geschwind drew upon his patients and the foreign medical literature for inspiration. He was impressed by the paper of Slater and Beard in which patients with TLE were described who developed a schizophreniform psychosis with the remarkable feature of well-preserved affect and other features such as religiosity — these behavioral changes developed years after the onset of seizures.[5] This paper was not well-appreciated by psychiatrists in the United States, nor were the behavioral aspects of epilepsy, for that matter. Geschwind felt strongly that psychiatrists should study TLE as reflected by his contention that "the personality changes in TLE may in some sense be the single most important condition in psychiatry."[6] The importance of TLE to psychiatry was not proportional to the frequency of personality changes in patients with TLE. Just as the discovery of corticosteroids arose from the study of the rare disorder Addison's disease, so was there the potential for understanding the mechanism by which personality can change through the study of TLE.[6] For Geschwind, TLE was a neurological model of psychiatric illness.

Stephen Waxman heard Geschwind speak about behavior and TLE in 1972.

"When I first heard his description of voluminous, pathologically detailed writings by patients with TLE, I did not believe him. My entreaty to him for a reference that I could read about the subject was met with a puff on his pipe and a shrug of his shoulders: 'It's not in the literature, Steve, but these patients are a dime a dozen.' It was this simple discussion that led me to take a careful interictal behavioral history from my patients. The results, which provided clear documentation that patients with limbic epilepsy had an unusual, pathologic tendency to produce voluminous writings, were written up and published in two papers[7,8] that are still widely quoted. . . . My role was to listen, to read, to coin the term *hypergraphia*, and to collect and describe the patients that appeared in these papers—the idea was Norman's."[9]

David Bear first heard Geschwind speak of the connection between behavioral changes and TLE when he was a freshman at the Harvard Medical School.[10] Bear recalls that Geschwind emphasized "that the relevant changes in behavior developed gradually, over months or years, after the formation of a TLE focus. The behavioral features became pervasive, *interictal* aspects of the patient's personality, often at a time when the person's seizures were infrequent." Bear describes the controversy over the interictal behavior syndrome theory.

I remember well a clinical conference at MGH (Massachusetts General Hospital) at which Dr. Geschwind's first mention of interictal behavior changes was greeted by a round of obviously rehearsed hisses from a group associated with a visiting epileptologist. This well-known neurologist, who rarely attended Geschwind's case conferences, believed that the proposal of specific behavior changes in TLE could only add to the stigma borne by epileptic patients.[10]

Bear later collaborated with Dr. Paul Fedio, a neuropsychologist at the National Institutes of Health, to develop an instrument[11] that measured and supported "Geschwind's qualitative picture of [the] patient [with TLE]."[10] Bear has written extensively about the possible mechanisms underlying the interictal behavior syndrome, based on Geschwind's "proposal that the temporal lobe is a critical meeting place for sensory percepts and drive representations concerning hunger, fear, sexual desire, or anger" and Bear's hypothesis "that a chronic discharging focus involving the temporal limbic structures might lead to extraneous sensory-emotional connections-hyperconnections."[10,12]

Geschwind was concerned with elucidating the physiology of seizure triggers. For example, in 1967, he and Ira Sherwin published the case of a 47-year-old man with language-induced epilepsy.[1] As noted by Orrin Devinsky, Geschwind carefully studied this single patient, identified unique features of his condition, and as a result, made original contributions to areas that appeared peripheral to his main interests but were nevertheless related to behavioral neurology, while at the same time challenging prevailing wisdom and reinforcing his central theme of the relationship between behavior and anatomy.[13]

As in other disease states, Geschwind was above all responsive to the needs of patients with uncontrolled seizures. He believed that epilepsy therapies could be developed if seizure triggers were better understood. For this reason, he encouraged Andrew Herzog to formally study the relationship between female sex hormones and seizures[14] in order to develop treatment approaches to catamenial epilepsy. He admired the "pioneering work" of the neurosurgeons at the Montreal Neurological Institute (MNI) who performed temporal lobectomies, and he recruited Donald L. Schomer, M.D. from the MNI in 1979 to establish an epilepsy program at the Beth Israel Hospital in Boston.[15]

Geschwind believed that TLE was "a probe for the study of the physiology of emotion"[6] and that there was "no other disorder in which alterations of behavior occur whose neurophysiological mechanisms we understand so well . . . we may not be far from the point where we will be able for the first time to explain one form of human behavior disorder in terms of the functions of the nervous system."[3] As David Bear wrote,[10] before the contributions of Norman Geschwind, emotional behaviors in TLE were typically explained as subcortical "seizure equivalents." His emphasis on interictal behavior change and limbic connections shifted attention to epilepsy as a subtle modulator of the highest levels of integrative cortex. Rather than the "violent automatism," he sought to explain the relentless philosophic and moral ruminations motivating Dostoevsky's prolific writing[16] or the blinding emotional incandescence leaping from the canvasses of Van Gogh.

For Geschwind, epilepsy was a window on the mind. Fortunately for the rest of us, Geschwind gave us a glimpse through that window, too.

## References

1. Geschwind, N, and Sherwin, I. Language-induced epilepsy. Arch Neurol, 1967; 16,25-31.
2. Geschwind, N. Effects of temporal lobe surgery on behavior. N Engl J Med, 1973;289,480-481.
3. Geschwind, N. The clinical setting of aggression in temporal lobe epilepsy. In Fields et al. (eds.), *Neural Bases of Violence and Aggression.* St. Louis: Warren H. Green, Inc., 1975, pp. 273-281.
4. Waxman, SG, and Geschwind, N. The interictal behavior syndrome of temporal lobe epilepsy. Arch Gen Psychiatry, 1975;32,580-586.
5. Slater, E, and Beard, AW. Schizophrenia-like psychoses of epilepsy. Br J Psychiatry, 1963;109,95-150.
6. Geschwind, N. Morning session: Introduction. McLean Hosp J, 1977;June,6-8.
7. Waxman, SG, and Geschwind, N. Hypergraphia in temporal lobe epilepsy. Neurology, 1980;30,314-317.
8. Waxman, SG, and Geschwind, N. The interictal behavior syndrome of temporal lobe epilepsy. Arch Gen Psychiatry, 1975;32,1580-1586.
9. Waxman, SG. Norman Geschwind, temporal lobe epilepsy, and peripheral nerve disease. In SC Schachter and O Devinsky (eds.), *Behavioral Neurology and the Legacy of Norman Geschwind.* Philadelphia: Lippincott-Raven, 1997, pp. 31-34.
10. Bear, DM. Behavior in temporal lobe epilepsy: The seminal contributions of Norman Geschwind. In SC Schachter and O Devinsky (eds.), *Behavioral Neurology and the Legacy of Norman Geschwind.* Philadelphia: Lippincott-Raven, 1997, pp. 195-206.

11. Bear, DM, and Fedio, P. Quantitative analysis of interictal behavior in temporal lobe epilepsy. Arch Neurol, 1977;34,454-467.
12. Bear, DM. Temporal lobe epilepsy: a syndrome of sensory-limbic hyperconnection. Cortex, 1979;15,357-384.
13. Devinsky, O. Other forms of epilepsy. In SC Schachter and O Devinsky (eds.), *Behavioral Neurology and the Legacy of Norman Geschwind.* Philadelphia: Lippincott-Raven, 1997, pp. 207-212.
14. Herzog, AG. Neuroendocrinology of epilepsy. In SC Schachter and O Devinsky (eds.), *Behavioral Neurology and the Legacy of Norman Geschwind.* Philadelphia: Lippincott-Raven, 1997, pp. 223-240.
15. Schomer, DL. Behavioral aspects of temporal lobe epilepsy. In SC Schachter and O Devinsky (eds.), *Behavioral Neurology and the Legacy of Norman Geschwind.* Philadelphia: Lippincott-Raven, 1997, pp. 195-206.
16. Geschwind, N. Dostoevsky's epilepsy. In D Blumer (ed.), *Psychiatric Aspects of Epilepsy.* Washington, DC: American Psychiatric Press, 1984, pp. 325-334.

# CHAPTER 17

# Language-Induced Epilepsy

*Norman Geschwind and Ira Sherwin*

The so-called reflex epilepsies, i.e., those in which the seizures can be precipitated by highly specific stimuli, continue to be of great interest to the neurologist. In discussing this form of epilepsy, we restrict the term "reflex" to those instances in which a highly patterned stimulus regularly leads to a seizure by effects transmitted over nervous pathways. By contrast, in all other forms of epilepsy the seizure-provoking agent is presumed to be a local metabolic change within the focus itself or a change in some blood-borne substance capable of influencing the focus. The ready identification and, to some extent, possible manipulation of the specific stimulus hold forth the possibility of greater insights into the mechanisms of the epileptic process. In those instances where specific language stimuli appear to be the triggering mechanisms, the possibility of further understanding of the neurophysiology subsuming language itself makes a thorough investigation of such epilepsies seem most rewarding. We have recently encountered a unique patient whose seizures could be triggered by three modalities of language, i.e., reading, writing, and speaking. To our knowledge, this is the first case in which language in any of three modalities appeared to be a specific seizure-provoking stimulus and, in particular, the first in which speaking has played a major role in precipitating seizures. It is because of this unique specificity that this case is reported. A preliminary account of our findings appears in an earlier publication.[1]

## REPORT OF A CASE

*History* A 47-year-old man admitted Oct 28, 1964, was referred by his own physician to the Neurology Service of the Boston Veterans Administration Hospital for evaluation of a seizure disorder. He had been a stutterer since early

---

Reprinted with permission from *Archives of Neurology*. 1967; 16 (1): 25–31. 

childhood. The past medical history was otherwise unremarkable. With the exception of the seizure problem, the patient considered himself always to have been in good health. Specifically, he was unaware of any perinatal complications and denied any serious illnesses of childhood, head trauma, or symptoms suggesting infection of the central nervous system. There was no family history of seizures, speech disturbance, or other neurological disorders. He had achieved only a tenth-grade education completed at age 16, which the patient attributed to the speech difficulties previously mentioned. At the time of admission, the patient complained of "blackouts" which he had first noticed approximately 15 years before, when he was in his early 30s. Initially, the spells had occurred once or twice weekly, but there had been some diminution in frequency over the five years preceding admission. For a few months prior to admission, however, they had become more frequent once again. The spells were described as occurring without any warning. The patient would first notice jerking movements of the jaw, followed by some tremulousness of the hands. During this time there was speech arrest. On occasion, this was followed by complete loss of consciousness, but generalized convulsions never occurred. The patient's wife volunteered that some of these spells seemed to occur while the patient was reading, although many had occurred while he was not so engaged. Although the episodes themselves were very disagreeable for the patient, he felt well immediately thereafter without any postictal deficit.

The general physical examination revealed a somewhat asthenic white male with a mild kyphoscoliosis. The rest of the general examination was unremarkable.

*Neurological Examination* With the exception of the obvious stutter, the detailed neurological examination was completely within normal limits. Psychometric examination revealed a Wechsler full scale intelligence quotient of 82, placing the patient in the range of borderline deficiency.

*Laboratory Findings* Routine examinations of the blood and urine were within normal limits. The cerebrospinal fluid was under normal pressure with a protein of 44 mg/100 cc and no cells. Plain x-ray films of the skull revealed no abnormality. A pneumoencephalogram disclosed a normal ventricular system and normal subarachnoid pathways.

*Course* During the periods in which the patient was receiving no anticonvulsant medication, clinical seizures could repeatedly be precipitated by certain language stimuli. These included reading (aloud or to himself), speaking (aloud or whispered), and writing. The clinical seizures were noted to begin with speech arrest, although the patient might produce some guttural sounds. The arrest of speech was accompanied by myoclonic movements of the palate which were followed by jerking of the jaw. The spells were obviously most disagreeable to the patient, and he would resist the urging of the examiner to continue the activity after a seizure had been provoked. During the spell, the patient remained conscious and was able to respond to verbal commands. Other provocative techniques which

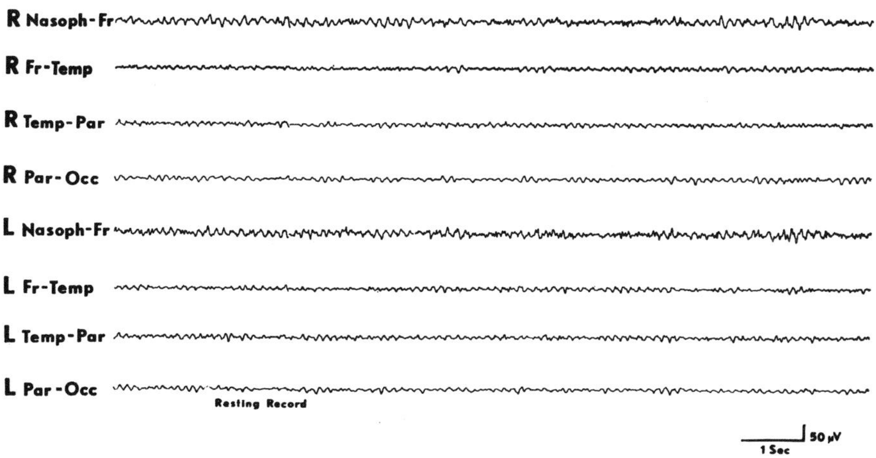


FIGURE 1. Resting record, patient off anticonvulsant medication.

included hyperventilation, as well as intermittent photic and optokinetic stimulation, were all without effect. Although speaking and whispering words were both effective in precipitating seizures, repetitive lip, tongue, and jaw movements and humming of a tune without words were not effective stimuli. Although writing was noted to be an effective stimulus, drawing of geometric forms failed to precipitate seizures. Of the three language modalities reading was the most powerful stimulus. We noted that it was often necessary to provoke one seizure by reading before writing or speaking could be effective in precipitating any further seizures. However, once the patient had been "sensitized" to speaking or writing, he then remained highly susceptible to these forms of stimulation during the remainder of the test period. When sensitization was maximal, a seizure might be provoked by repeating a single word spoken by the examiner. In some instances the seizure activity would begin before the patient had even completed the repetition of the word.

*Electroencephalographic Examination* Several EEGs were recorded both from the convexity and from nasopharyngeal leads. The resting record (Figure 1) revealed a predominance of well-modulated 7 to 9 cycles per second activity bilaterally. Recordings made during sleep revealed no paroxysmal activity. Intermittent photic and opticokinetic stimulation carried out during EEG recordings also failed to produce any paroxysmal activity. During clinical seizures induced by the previously mentioned provocative stimuli, bilaterally symmetrical spike or polyspike and wave complexes, at maximum amplitude in the frontal derivations, appeared in the record (Figure 2). A simultaneously recorded electromyogram from the masseter muscle (not shown) indicated that the cortical discharge did not bear a one-to-one relationship to the muscle potentials. In an

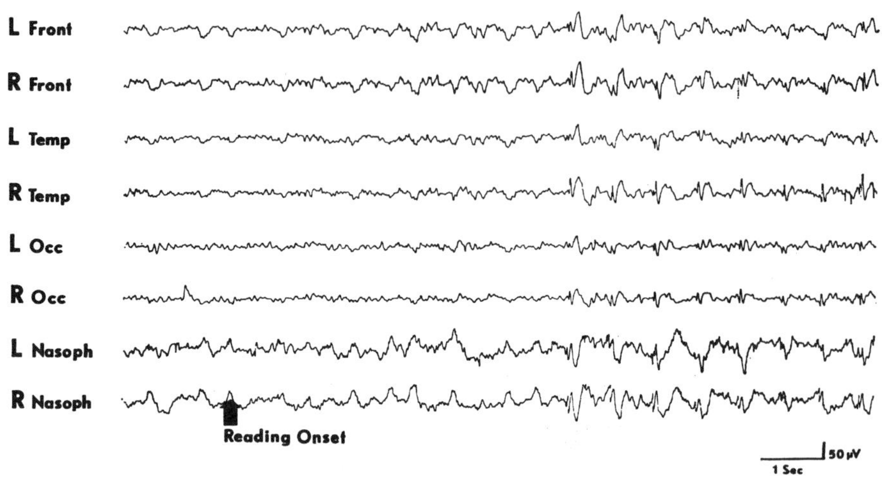


FIGURE 2. Seizure induced by reading; monopolar recording to both ears interconnected. Excess background slowing probably related to several seizures precipitated just prior to this record.

effort to determine, without using one of these "triggering" stimuli, the origin of the initial electrical discharge a pentylenetetrazol- (Metrazol) activated EEG was performed. Following the injection of only 175 mg of pentylenetetrazol, a clinical seizure was provoked. This seizure started with myoclonic jerking of the palate, followed by jerking of the jaw and finally by intermittent contractions of the orbicularis oculi. The patient remained conscious, was able to follow verbal commands, but was unable to speak. The first recorded electrical manifestation of this seizure was rhythmic electromyographical activity picked up from the palate by the nasopharyngeal electrodes (Figure 3A). This was then followed by rhythmic electromyographical activity in the masseter muscles, with only rare spike and polyspike wave complexes appearing over the convexity (Figure 3B). Though distorted by excessively prominent artefacts, this record also showed that a one-to-one relationship between the cortical and electromyographical potentials did not exist. The patient was treated with ethosuximide and phenobarbital with a marked improvement in both EEG and clinical manifestations of the seizure disorder. He has been seen several times in follow-up and continues to do well on this regimen.

## Comment

The patient presents several interesting features. On admission he was thought to be a case of reading epilepsy. Shortly after anticonvulsant medication was withdrawn, one of the house staff reported that the patient was having repeated

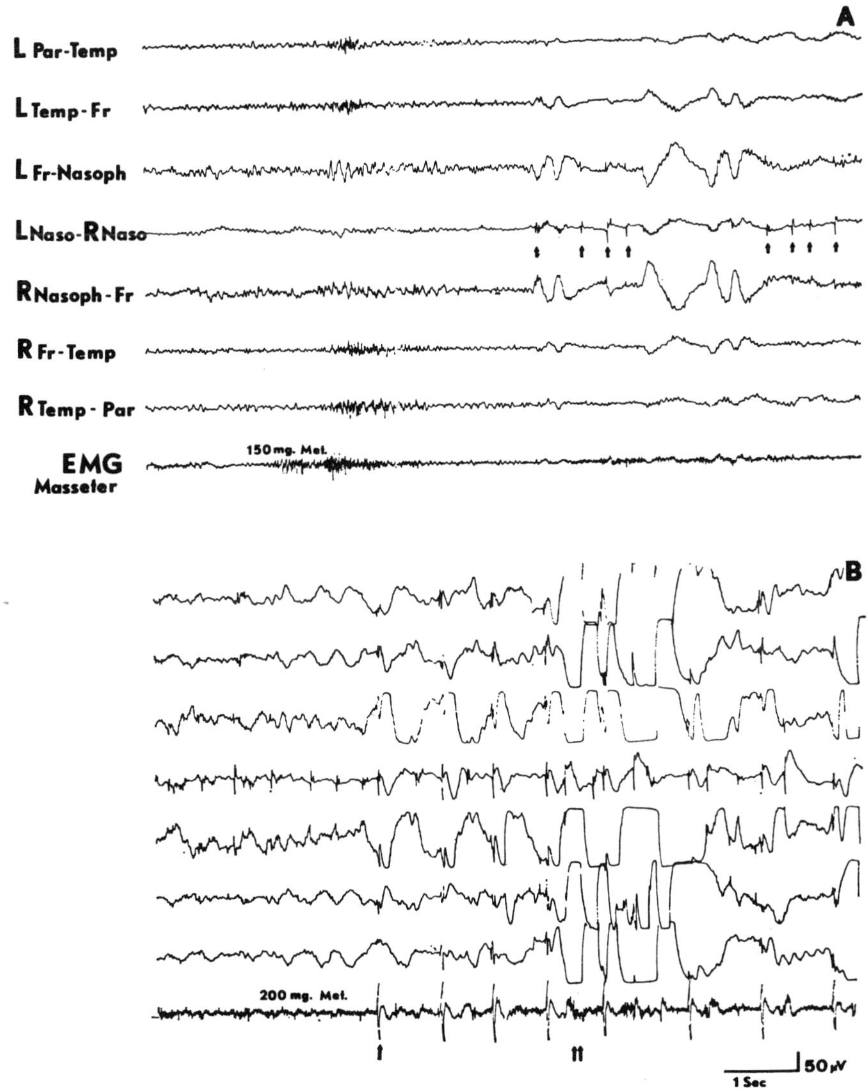


FIGURE 3. Metrazol activated EEG. (A) following intravenous injection of 175 mg, electromyographical potentials recorded from palate (*arrows*); (B) electromyographical potentials from masseter (*single arrow*), onset of jerking of head and eye blinking (*double arrow*).

spontaneous seizures. Careful examination, however, soon revealed that the seizures were not really spontaneous but occurred only when he attempted to speak. As long as he lay quietly, he had only a very occasional mild attack, while attempts at speech, reading, or writing invariably produced a seizure. This observation is in keeping with the increasingly frequent recognition and identification of specific, provocative "triggers" in apparently "spontaneous" seizures.[2]

A second point of great interest was the increased ease of precipitating seizures after at least one seizure had been induced, usually by reading. This feature of sensitization appears to be a most unusual one, for a search of the available clinical literature failed to reveal any discussion of this curious phenomenon. Whether it is present to some extent in all forms of epilepsy or only in certain forms of reflex epilepsy is not known. Since each individual seizure occurs only in response to a specific stimulus, the situation is different from that in status epileticus which it may superficially resemble. In his study of after-burst activity, Burns[3] has suggested that sustained cortical discharge may be due to a chronic differential (surface positive) repolarization of an aggregate of neuronal tissue. Such a state of heightened excitability may in fact be analogous to the dominant focus produced by cortical anodal polarization[4] or by tetanizing stimulation of the cortex.[5] These latter studies indicate that alterations in the regional steady potential may increase the excitability of an area of cortex so that it responds to certain stimulus modalities to which, before sensitization, it was unresponsive.

It would seem possible, then, that a first seizure induced in our patient by reading might alter the steady potential in the focus and thus facilitate the triggering or repetitive after-discharge by related stimuli in a pattern determined by the conditioning process.

To be an effective trigger such a stimulus would have to arrive at the focus during the period that such a regional alteration in the steady potential persists, viz, usually only for a few minutes.[4] It must be acknowledged that such speculations as to the physiologic substrate of this phenomenon of sensitization is purely theoretical and not supported by any direct evidence in this case. However, though the exact mechanism of this phenomenon remains obscure, it seems worthy of further study, since in many cases of reflex epilepsy certain stimuli which might be effective as triggers would be missed should they only be examined for during "interictal" periods, without first subjecting the patient to a sensitization procedure.

The EEG findings were also of some interest. The fast transients, first seen in the nasopharyngeal leads, were soon found to be "muscle artefacts" resulting from palatal movements. The EEG changes found in this case appear to be essentially the same as those reported in primary reading epilepsy.[6–8] This pattern of activity suggests that the electrical focus resides in some portion of the so-called centrencephalon, perhaps at a pontine level.

The most interesting feature of this patient and the one which prompted this report is the ease with which speaking or whispering could induce seizures, although the use of the same musculature in nonverbal tasks had no effect. This case illustrates the great specificity of the stimulus. In evaluating the possible mechanisms involved in this disorder, certain interpretations may readily be rejected. It is extremely difficult to accept the view[9] that these are movement-induced seizures since nonverbal movements of the cranial musculature and limb musculature were both ineffective in inducing seizures, while movement used for the purpose of producing language readily provoked the fits. This is not to dispute the existence of movement-induced epilepsy,[10–12] but only to point out that in the case described movements per se were not the effective stimulus. Proprioceptive feedback[13,14] could similarly not be the provoking stimulus since this would fail to account for the verbal-nonverbal distinction. Furthermore, if proprioception were the essential stimulus, it is difficult to see why in the case of reading epilepsy reported by Stevens[8] different languages showed such marked variation in their ability to trigger seizures. Concentration could hardly be a significant factor since even the most trivial verbal activity was sufficient to produce seizures when the patient was sensitized. Similarly, the view[15] that combinations of such less specific factors might be the responsible triggers is not supported by a critical review[16] of the reported cases of reading and writing epilepsy. Indeed, it is difficult to accept any conclusion other than that the specific seizure-provoking aspect of the stimulus was its verbal character. Further, it is not necessary to be surprised that so specific a stimulus may trigger a seizure, in the light of the fact that one of the most common activities of the nervous system is the linking together of highly specific stimuli. So common is this activity that it is perhaps almost surprising that highly specific reflex epilepsies are not more frequently encountered.

It should be noted that seizures precipitated by speaking may be more common than has been appreciated and that, in particular, many cases of reading epilepsy may also show this disturbance, especially if "sensitization" by reading is first used as a provocative technique. Bickford (written and oral communication to the authors, March 12) has noted occasional provocation by speech in some of his reading epileptics.

We were unable to find a recorded case of epilepsy precipitated by hearing spoken language. It is, of course, difficult to conceive how a patient with such an ictal disturbance would get along since, while it is easy to avoid writing, reading, and speaking to a considerable extent, it is extremely difficult to avoid hearing spoken language. It would therefore seem that such a patient would be bombarded by seizure-provoking stimuli. It is possible, however, that this might eventually result in a "desensitization" to this form of stimulation, so that one might mistakenly assume that the patient was immune to it. A clinical example of such auditory desensitization may be found in Forster's case of musicogenic epilepsy.[17] In any case, one should not exclude the possibility that "heard-word" epilepsy exists without first attempting possible sensitizing procedures. We did not, for example, carefully study our patient to see whether spoken words could provoke seizures in him after a long series of attacks precipitated by reading, writing, or speaking.

One curious aspect of nearly all the cases of primary language epilepsy is that the EEG is nonfocal and that one does not find focal EEG changes in the speech areas of the dominant hemisphere. It differs, therefore, from many cases of reflex epilepsy in which cortical foci are the rule. It appears that there may be two major types of reflex epilepsy. One is the variety in which a simple stereotyped stimulus (e.g., viewing a safety pin in the classic case of Mitchell et al[18]) is seizure provoking. In such cases cortical foci are the rule. The other group comprises those forms of epilepsy in which a highly specific class of stimuli is effective, although the actual individual stimulus may be different in each instance. Thus, in language-induced epilepsy completely different words will be effective on different occasions. In such a case we find no cortical focus. This distinction may well point to some highly significant factors in physiological organization, but it is not possible even to speculate about these at this time.

A final word is appropriate on the patient's "life-long" speech difficulty. Its onset in childhood, the characteristic clonic blocking with grimacing aggravated by any deliberate effort to speak unhaltingly, and its subjectively disagreeable nature, all would seem to identify the disorder as stuttering as opposed to cluttering.[19] That the spontaneous speech difficulty is not identical with the clinical seizure is apparent for the following reasons. The stuttering spontaneous speech was not accompanied by either the clinical manifestation of the seizure, i.e., palatal myoclonus, jaw jerking, or by EEG changes. Secondly, when seizures as manifested EEG changes occurred, the above clinical features were always apparent. The lack of EEG abnormality during the spontaneous stuttering speech further distinguishes the dysphemia from the "cluttering syndrome."[20] Lastly, the differential response of the seizures and the spontaneous stuttering to anticonvulsant medication further served to identify them as distinct phenomena. None of the other patients with reading epilepsy so far reported has been stated to be a stutterer, so that perhaps this association in our case is only coincidental. Our case, however, differs from the others in the ready provocation of seizures by speaking. One could speculate that perhaps the stuttering was instrumental in linking speech production to the patient's epileptic process. Conversely, it is conceivable that the stuttering is, in fact, the result of the seizures. Thus, in our patient at the onset of a seizure induced by speaking, his stutter would worsen. This is highly speculative, of course; and even if true in this case, this mechanism must be a rare cause of stuttering since EEG studies have not in the past revealed such abnormalities in stutterers.

## Summary

This to our knowledge is the first reported case of a so-called reflex epilepsy in which the seizures could be triggered by attempts to use three language modalities, i.e., reading, writing, and speaking, and is also the first case in which speaking has played a major role as a triggering stimulus.

This 47-year-old man who stuttered since childhood gave a history of seizures characterized by speech arrest, jerking movements of the jaw, and, on occasion, loss of consciousness. General physical, neurological, spinal fluid, and pneumoencephalographic examinations revealed no significant abnormalities. With the patient unmedicated seizures consisting of myoclonic movements of the palate followed by jerking of the jaw were repeatedly precipitated by certain language stimuli, i.e., reading (aloud or to himself), writing, speaking, and whispering. Lip and tongue movements, however, and humming (without words) are ineffective. Although writing words was an effective stimulus, drawing of geometric forms was not. Speaking was sometimes not effective in producing a seizure until several seizures had been induced by reading. This phenomenon of "sensitization" has not to our knowledge been described previously. Hyperventilation, intermittent photic and optokinetic stimulation were not provocative. The resting electroencephalogram was normal. During seizures (with retained consciousness) spike or polyspike and wave complexes occurred bilaterally, suggesting a seizure focus in the so-called centrencephalic system possibly at a pontine level. Ethosuximide and phenobarbital therapy produced a marked improvement in the clinical and EEG manifestations of this disorder.

## Generic and Trade Names of Drugs

Pentylenetetrazol—*Metrazol.*
Ethosuximide—*Zarontin.*
Phenobarbital—*Luminal.*

## References

1. Sherwin, I., Geschwind, N., and Abramowicz, A.: Language Induced Epilepsy, *Trans Amer Neurol Assoc* 90:183–188, 1965.
2. Servit, Z. (ed.): *Reflex Mechanisms in the Genesis of Epilepsy,* Amsterdam: Elsevier Publishing Co., 1963.
3. Burns, B.D.: The Mechanism of After Bursts in Cerebral Cortex, *J Physiol* 127:168–188, 1955.
4. Rusinov, V.S.: An Electrophysiological Analysis of the Connecting Function in the Cerebral Cortex in the Presence of a Dominant Region Area, abstracted, Communications of the 19th International Physiological Congress, Montreal, 1953, pp 719–720.
5. Roitbak, A.I.: Primary Responses of the Cerebral Cortex to Sound Clicks and Electrical Stimulation, of the Medial Geniculate Nucleus and Their Changes During Unconditioned Stimulation, Proceedings of the 21st International Physiological Congress, Buenos Aires, 1959, p 234.
6. Bickford, R.G., et al: Reading Epilepsy, *Trans Amer Neurol Assoc* 81:100–102, 1956.

7. Baxter, D.W., and Bailey, A.A.: Primary Reading Epilepsy, *Neurology* 11:445–449, 1961.
8. Stevens, H.: Reading Epilepsy, *New Eng J Med* 257:165–170, 1957.
9. Asbury, A.K., and Prensky, A.L.: Graphogenic Epilepsy, *Trans Amer Neurol Assoc* 88:193–194, 1965.
10. Gowers, W.R.: *Epilepsy,* ed 2, London: J. & A. Churchill, Ltd., 1901.
11. Falconer, M.A., Driver, M.V., and Serafetinides, E.A.: Seizures Induced by Movement: Report of a Case Relieved by Operation, *J Neurol Neurosurg Psychiat* 26:300–307, 1963.
12. Symonds, C.: Excitation and Inhibition in Epilepsy, *Proc Roy Soc Med* 52:395–402, 1959.
13. Bickford, R.G.: Sensory Precipitation of Seizures, *J Mich Med Soc* 53:1018–1020, 1954.
14. Alajouanine, T., Nehlil, J., and Gabersek, V.: A propos d'un cas d'epilepsie déclenché par la lecture, *Rev Neurol* 101:463–467, 1959.
15. Critchley, N., Cobb, W., and Sears, T.A.: On Reading Epilepsy, *Epilepsia* 1:403–417, 1959–1960.
16. Sherwin, I.: Seizures Precipitated by the Use of Language: A Review, *Cortex,* to be published.
17. Forster, F.M., et al: Modification of Musicogenic Epilepsy by Extinction Technique, *Trans Amer Neurol Assoc* 90:179, 1965.
18. Mitchell, W., Falconer, M.A., and Hill, D.: Epilepsy With Fetishism Relieved by Temporal Lobectomy, *Lancet* 2:626–630, 1954.
19. Luchsinger, R., and Arnold, G.E.: *Voice-Speech-Language, Clinical Communicology: Its Physiology and Pathology,* Belmont, Calif: Wadsworth Publishing Company, Inc., 1966.
20. Landolt, H., and Luchsinger, R.: Poltersprache, stottern und chronische organische psychosyndrome, *Deutsch Med Wschr* 79:1012–1015, 1954.

This work was supported in part by grant MH-08472 from the National Institutes of Health to the Boston University Medical School.

# CHAPTER 18

# Hypergraphia in Temporal Lobe Epilepsy

*Stephen G. Waxman and Norman Geschwind*

There is general agreement that specific personality changes are not seen in all forms of epilepsy. Several authors, however, have described certain distinctive personality traits that may be found in patients with temporal lobe epilepsy. Previous reports have dealt with aggressiveness,[1-3] changes in sexual behavior,[4-6] and religiosity[7] associated with temporal lobe disorders. These findings suggest that the behavioral changes in temporal lobe epilepsy do not represent a non-specific "chronic brain syndrome," but rather represent a distinct behavioral syndrome in which affective response is deepened in the presence of relatively preserved intellectual function. We believe that characterization of this syndrome is of importance, not only in terms of understanding the psychiatric implications of epilepsy, but also as an example of a human behavioral disorder associated with damage at specific sites in the central nervous system. The present paper describes still another characteristic of the interictal behavior of patients with temporal lobe disorders, hypergraphia, or the tendency toward extensive and, in some cases, compulsive writing.

In this paper we present seven case histories that illustrate the phenomenon of hypergraphia in temporal lobe epilepsy. In six cases (cases 1 to 6), the patients provided striking documentation of their unusual writing. The seventh patient (case 7) volunteered that he wrote extensively but, as was true of several patients we have seen, was reluctant to exhibit his writings.

## CASE 1

This 24-year-old right-handed woman began to have seizures at age 10 and to exhibit behavioral disturbances at age 15. Her father and paternal aunt were

Reprinted with permission from *Neurology*. 1974;24(7):629-636.

reported to have epilepsy, but her siblings apparently were well. At the age of 10, the patient began to have generalized seizures, often beginning with focal twitching of the left arm and face, on some occasions associated with lip-smacking or chewing movements, and followed by urinary incontinence and tongue biting. Neurologic examination, lumbar puncture, skull films, and brain scan were reportedly normal, but electroencephalogram (EEG) showed a right anterior temporal spike focus. She was treated with various anticonvulsants but continued to have seizures at a frequency of about one per month. At the age of 15, the patient was admitted to a hospital after slashing her wrist. In the following year, her grades in school deteriorated. When she was 17 years old, the patient again was admitted to a hospital because of confused and agitated behavior following two brief left-sided seizures. There was no history of ingestion of drugs, toxins, or hallucinogens. She was noted to be "agitated, crying, incoherent . . . (with) peculiar posturing," and she asked if she were on a spaceship or being controlled by radio.

Neurologic examination at that time revealed slight left facial weakness and slightly greater deep tendon reflexes on the left side. Skull x-rays were normal. A sonar scan was suggestive of some enlargement of the trigone of the left lateral ventricle. EEG showed slow waves and spikes bitemporally, more pronounced on the left. The patient was diagnosed as having an acute schizophrenic psychosis and was treated for several months with trifluoperazine hydrochloride. She was discharged on primidone, diphenylhydantoin, and phenobarbital.

In the ensuing four years, she continued to have seizures several times a month. During this period, the patient became devoutly religious and experienced at least five religious conversions, each of which she felt was of major importance. She also began to experience déjà vu feelings. An EEG at the age of 20 revealed a spike focus in the right anterior temporal lobe.

The patient was admitted to hospitals twice at the age of 21 because of seizures; on both occasions she had failed to take her anticonvulsant medication. She described an aura consisting of a sensation of epigastric distress and a feeling of fear before her seizures. She now admitted to visual hallucinations of blue-green flashing lights moving from left to right in the right visual field. The hallucinations often, but not always, were followed by seizures. The patient professed great interest in mystical issues and in particular in the meaning of her existence and in the fate of the universe. She also complained of having no interest in sexual activities.

Neurologic examination revealed no focal deficits. All language performances were normal; constructions were fairly well done, calculations were performed reasonably well, and memory was normal. Results of hemogram, urinalysis, and routine blood chemistries were normal. Serum thyroxin, cortisol, and $B_{12}$ levels were normal, and serology gave negative results. A chest x-ray and skull x-rays were unremarkable. Results of lumbar puncture were normal. An EEG revealed prominent sharp waves over both hemispheres.

When questioned about writing, the patient stated that she usually spent at least several hours per day writing things down. She dated the onset of this

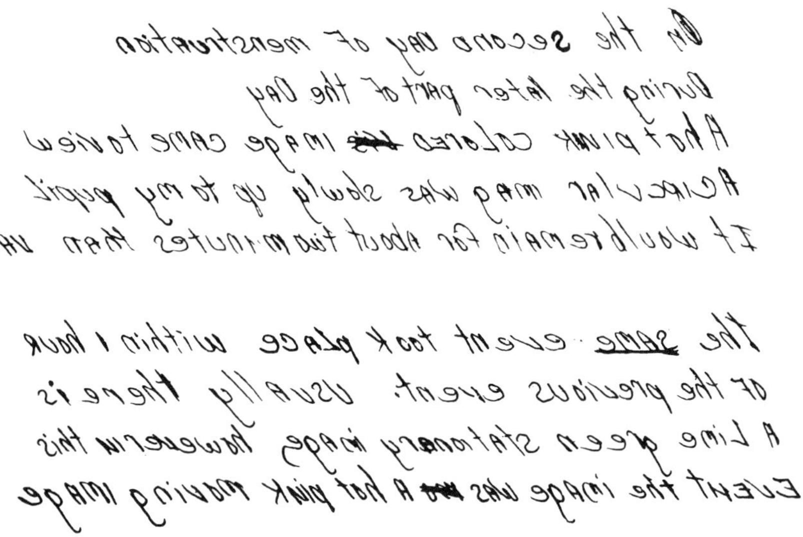

FIGURE 1. Reversed writing of patient 1 describes visual hallucinations. The description may be read by holding the page up to a mirror.

behavior at age 15, and felt that it was nearly coincident with the development of her interest in religion. She stated that she often wrote things down because "I want to be sure of what I do." She carried several tablets of writing paper with her at all times. She often recorded, in her writing pads or scraps of paper, what she had done in the preceding few hours "especially if I believe a seizure is coming on so I couldn't memorize it." She described in detail her seizures, hallucinations, and feelings of déjà vu. She often made lists, and produced catalogs of her records or songs her father could play on the harmonica, of items of furniture in her apartment, of her relatives ("so I will know how many there are"), and of her "likes" and "dislikes." She also often wrote poetry, usually with a moral or philosophical theme. She had the impression that the act of writing might abort her seizures, but did not feel that the content of what she wrote was important in this regard. Usually, she did not interrupt other activites to write, but she did recount having written at least several hundred times the words of a song she had learned at 17, using whatever was available (scraps of paper, napkins) and, in several cases, interrupting other activities to do so. She also reported sometimes feeling compelled to write a word over and over or to copy, once or several times, the printed labels on items she purchased. Some of her writing was reversed (mirror writing) (Figure 1). The patient stated that she had never written in the reversed manner before development of her seizures. She denied other compulsive or ritualistic actions but did describe herself as very meticulous. She claimed to read only rarely.

## CASE 2

This right-handed man began at age five to have "staring spells" lasting about 30 seconds. His father reportedly had had three seizures when he was 20 years old, but his mother and his 12 siblings had no history of neurologic disorder. Petit mal epilepsy was diagnosed initially and was treated with phenobarbital for about two years. The staring spells abated at age six and the patient was well until age 18, when on two occasions he assaulted siblings, claiming afterwards to have no recollection of the assaultive behavior. Between the ages of 18 and 23, he experienced almost daily seizures, consisting of staring spells and stiffening of the body, during which he was aware of his surroundings but was unable to respond; these episodes were preceded by an aura in which the patient experienced a sensation of profound fear and sexual pleasure. He also exhibited occasional psychomotor automatisms, during which he behaved inappropriately with no awareness of his behavior. Surface and depth electrode EEGs revealed bilateral anterior and midtemporal spike activity that in some recordings predominated on the left.

The patient responded poorly to treatment with anticonvulsant medications. At age 23 he underwent a left temporal lobectomy. Pathologic examination revealed a cystic cavity of the temporal white matter with hypertrophy of astrocytes in the neighboring cortex and white matter. After the lobectomy, he was relieved of his staring spells, although he continued to experience episodic sensations of fear and sexual excitement similar to his previous auras. No further psychomotor episodes occurred. Postoperatively, neurologic examination showed a homonymous right upper visual field deficit, and a mild impairment of recent and remote memory (Memory Quotient, Wechsler Memory Scale 103 preoperatively, 86 postoperatively; Wechsler Adult Intelligence Scale (WAIS) Full Scale IQ 90 preoperatively, 99 postoperatively) that did not interfere with his performance as a truck loader. The patient was married, but has experienced difficulty in deriving pleasure from sexual intercourse with his wife.

The patient has kept copious notes on his disorder. At age 23, several months before his lobectomy, the patient's notes contain entries primarily on the days of seizures, and the descriptions are of the form: "_____ said I had another seizure in my sleep. Matches on night table gone in morning. I found empty match pack by bed. I had to have touched them in my sleep," or "I had a seizure while sitting on the toilet." There are also some lists with dates, followed either by the word "seizure" and the time of day it occurred, or by the word "OK" if there was no seizure. One year after surgery (age 24) the lists appear more ritualized and have clear religious overtones. Thus, each day of the month is listed on a separate line, followed either by the time of the seizures (which occurred less than 10 times per month) or by the carefully and stereotypically written phrase "Thank "GOD"—none." The words on each line are in nearly perfect register with the words of the lines above and below. Each page is signed by the patient. Each month's list is followed by a total "_____ seizures" and by a summary, e.g., "For this month of _____ I have had only one (1) sexual fear seizure which only lasted five (5)

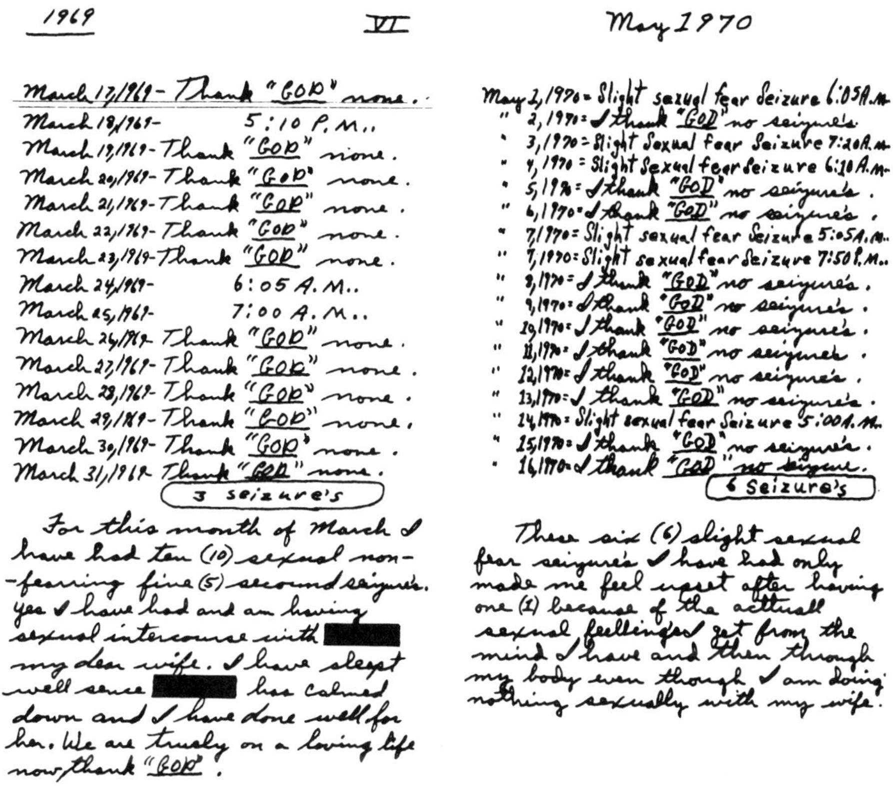

1969 VI May 1970

March 17/1969 - Thank "GOD" none.
March 18/1969 - 5:10 P.M.
March 19/1969 - Thank "GOD" none.
March 20/1969 - Thank "GOD" none.
March 21/1969 - Thank "GOD" none.
March 22/1969 - Thank "GOD" none.
March 23/1969 - Thank "GOD" none.
March 24/1969 - 6:05 A.M.
March 25/1969 - 7:00 A.M.
March 26/1969 - Thank "GOD" none.
March 27/1969 - Thank "GOD" none.
March 28/1969 - Thank "GOD" none.
March 29/1969 - Thank "GOD" none.
March 30/1969 - Thank "GOD" none.
March 31/1969 - Thank "GOD" none.
3 seizure's

For this month of March I have had ten (10) sexual non-fearing fine (5) secound seizure's. yes I have had and am having sexual intercourse with [redacted] my dear wife. I have slept well sence [redacted] has calmed down and I have done well for her. We are truly on a loving life now, thank "GOD".

May 1,1970 = Slight sexual fear Seizure 6:05 A.M.
" 2,1970 = I thank "GOD" no seizure's.
" 3,1970 = Slight Sexual fear Seizure 7:20 A.M.
" 4,1970 = Slight Sexual fear Seizure 6:10 A.M.
" 5,1970 = I thank "GOD" no seizure's.
" 6,1970 = I thank "GOD" no seizure's.
" 7,1970 = Slight sexual fear Seizure 5:05 A.M.
" 7,1970 = Slight sexual fear Seizure 7:50 P.M.
" 8,1970 = I thank "GOD" no seizure's.
" 9,1970 = I thank "GOD" no seizure's.
" 10,1970 = I thank "GOD" no seizure's.
" 11,1970 = I thank "GOD" no seizure's.
" 12,1970 = I thank "GOD" no seizure's.
" 13,1970 = I thank "GOD" no seizure's.
" 14,1970 = Slight sexual fear Seizure 5:00 A.M.
" 15,1970 = I thank "GOD" no seizure's.
" 16,1970 = I thank "GOD" no seizure.
6 Seizure's

These six (6) slight sexual fear seizure's I have had only made me feel upset after having one (1) because of the actuall sexual feelings get from the mind I have and then through my body even though I am doing nothing sexually with my wife.

FIGURE 2. Two pages from the extensive notes kept by patient 2. The page on the left was written at age 24, one year after temporal lobectomy. The page on the right was written one year later. Note the more elaborate entries in the latter record.

seconds. . . ." [parentheses and misspellings as in the patient's original notes]. One year later (Figure 2) the references to days without seizures are still ritualized but more elaborate: "I thank "GOD" no seizures." There are now elaborate addenda to each month's record, with frequent use of underlined words, and words written entirely in capital letters or in red so as to stand out from the remainder of the text. Five years after the operation, the diary is much the same, although the daily entries ("I do thank dear "GOD" above, no seizures") are slightly more elaborate.

## CASE 3

This right-handed man suffered from grand mal and psychomotor seizures beginning at age 13. A cousin had a history of epilepsy. EEGs revealed a spike focus in the right temporal tip with lesser spike activity in the right posterior temporal area. Seizures were not adequately controlled with anticonvulsant medication, and a right temporal lobectomy was performed at the age of 40. Postoperatively, the EEGs showed spike activity over the right low central area. Grand mal seizures no longer occur, but psychomotor seizures occur nocturnally once every 7 to 10 days. The patient has been followed psychiatrically by Dr. D. Blumer for a period of eight years beginning seven years after the operation. The patient volunteered a log of his daily events, and was noted to be "verbose but at the same time highly circumspect and meticulous in his statements. Thus, when he was asked what he would do if he saw a fire in a theater . . . he answered with good judgment but made sure he had pinned down all the possibilities, such as . . . whether the fire was large or small, had just begun or had been going on for some time."[11]

Examination of this patient's daily notes showed them to be highly meticulous, with great attention to detail. Each sheet records in carefully typed text, a day-by-day account of the patient's experiences. For example: "It was cool last night so I opened the windows and left the air conditioner off. I had a very bad night. I was awake about every two hours. I hung three pictures today on three 3/4 screws I put in the wall. It made me so weak I had to lay down. I slept for two hours." Some phrases are underlined or typed in red for emphasis. As in case number 2, there is frequent use of parenthetical expressions to qualify or clarify the meaning of words; thus, "On weekends (Sat. and Sun.) I don't go walking." The single-spaced, typed record of daily events is 1,000 to 2,000 words in length for most months and often has pencilled notes following it. In addition, typed addenda to each month's record, in many cases 450-500 words long, describe in greater detail the patient's dreams. There are also lengthy, detailed accounts of experiences or "incidents" that the patient felt were of specific importance. At the end of each month's day-by-day account, a summary includes detailed "generalizations" (Figure 3).

## CASE 4

This right-handed man began to have seizures at age 18, several months after being struck on the head with a heavy metal object. One brother died shortly after birth; there were no other siblings, and neither of the parents had epilepsy.

The patient had a history of numerous assaultive episodes for which he had spent several years in prison. The patient's seizures, which were generalized and included tongue-biting and incontinence, were preceded by either a "rising" or "fluttering" epigastric sensation or by a tingling sensation over the lips and face, sometimes associated with a feeling of derealization or falling or rising off the ground. Lip-smacking was observed during some seizures. The patient often experienced feelings of déjà vu but denied olfactory or gustatory hallucinations. There had been one episode of auditory hallucinations, thought to be due to acute alcohol withdrawal. The patient was treated with diphenylhydantoin and chlordiazepoxide. His seizures occurred up to two times per month.

June 5 - I have taken Valeum as perscribed. one morning and one evening. I slowly became less irratible and less nervious. [redacted] noticed the change also. The pain in my right chest almost gone. Only slightly sore when pressed on. My legs still quiver when I lay down.

June 9 - I took a walk this morning (8:30 to 9:30) when the sun was week. This afternoon I had to take a nap for an hour ( 1:00 to 2:00) I was too sleepy to stay awake I will be glad when I can stop taking this valeum. It makes me awful sleepy and tired. I will be glad when I can stop taking it.

June 11 - This is the last night I am to take Valeum. Only one at 8:00 A.M. untill my next visit. I am glad . They make me feel sleepy and slow. The slowness I can fight off. The pain in my chest is gone and I feel much better,more quiet and a lot less irratible.

June 12 - This morning I woke with a slight pain in my right chest (center and botten) and a slight warning pain in my heart. As I became fully awake and had breakfast the pains left.(Valeum at 8:00). I also rember Post nasel drip in my sleep.

June 13 - No pain in my chest this morning. Doing fine on one pill at 8:00 A.M.

June 14 - The sun is rising earler each day giving me less time to go out in the morning Today I was out too long (8:30 to 11:00). When I came in I ate lunch and went to bed. I slept for two hours. I felt better wher I woke. At bedtime my face and head felt hot (like sunburn)

June 15 - Today was a cloudy and cool day. A beautiful day for a walk. This afternoon the sun came out. By the time I got home , then met [redacted] (in the shade of a big tree). I was tired when I got home and went to bed for 1½ hours.My chest cavity and lungs quivered. I had supperand rested in bed . By bed time (9:30) most of the quivering was gone and I was tired.

June 21 - This morning it was 9/10 cloudy and looked like rain. I dresses and caught the 9:20 bus and went to the Post Office.The sun came out as I was waiting for the buss to come home. I stood in a doorway out of the sun and cought the buss. I got home at 11:20., had lunch at 12:00 and worked on stamps in my bedroom all afternoon . I met [redacted] at 5:15 and we came home. I felt fair.

June 22 - I woke at 3:00 A.M. I felt slept out. Just a very slight quiver in my legs. I fell back to sleep for a few naps and got up at 6:15. I stayed in today (sunny). The air conditioner did so much good yesterday I have it on this afternoon again. I took a nap after supper and slept untill 11:00 when [redacted] woke me for pills (which I forgot). I turned the conditioner off then went back to sleep untill 3:00 A,M. then cat naped untill 6:10.

June 23 - Another cloudy day which I took advantage of. Walked from 9:30 untill noon. then had lunch andafter a little rest walking again untill 2:00 when the sun came out. I came in and had a short nap (1 hour) with the air conditioner cooling things off.At bedtime the quivering in my legs was almost gone leaving them feeling thick and week.

Genelarisation

The sunshine makes me week in general and the nerve in my limbs, mostly legs, quiver. The severity depending upon exposer to sun (length of time and strength of the suns rays) .A nap in a rather cool air conditioned room will bring back my strength. The quivering of the nerve takes longer to stop. Very greduall becoming weker. This takes two or three days depending upon severity.My skin also feels like sunburn even where not exposed (mid section of body) When the quivering lets uo I t leave my limbs feeling week espicially my hands if exposed The days are getting longer and the sun stronger. This gives me less time for walking or going outside at all.

The pains in my chest are gone and I am not as irratible. Only a very slight warning pain in my heart when I wake after recovery from a sun exposure. Please look at eyeye.

FIGURE 3. One of the monthly records produced by patient 3. The patient kept several copies of each page. Note the frequent use of parenthetical expressions. Following the day-by-day account is a set of "generalizations."

At the age of 31, normal results on cranial nerve, motor, and sensory examinations were recorded. There was mild dysmetria on finger-nose testing bilaterally. Lumbar puncture and skull x-rays were normal. An EEG showed bilateral slow waves, with sharp waves over the right anterior temporal region.

A brain scan four years later was normal. Neurologic examination showed intact cranial nerves and motor and sensory function. The patient's speech and memory were normal. Calculations were performed fairly well and constructions were done well. Moderate concreteness was noted in the interpretation of proverbs and in the judgment of similarities. The patient had attended art school for several years. At age 19, he was married and later had two children, but he was divorced five years later. He became deeply interested in "black magic," but limited his participation in this because he believed occult practices might cause "funny things to happen." The patient stated that he began writing extensively at the age of 17 or 18, keeping a diary and writing songs and poems. One of the songs, he stated, had been "taken" from him and published by a friend. Subsequently, he concealed most of his writings in various locations in his home. He often wrote aphorisms, on some occasions writing for several hours at a time and filling one of more sheets of paper (Figure 4); he stated "once I start, I can't stop." He usually kept a pencil and paper with him, and reported having written the sentences "Why Can't A Man Live Before He Dies?" and "God Bless The Child That Has Its Own" many hundreds of times, on several occasions on newspapers or on the pages of books when blank paper was not available. He was unable to explain why he wrote these sentences, but stated that he felt they concerned "basic questions of life" that had interested him for many years. He denied ever having written anything during his seizures, but did report finding, in various hiding places in his home, notes that he did not recall having written.

## CASE 5

This ambidextrous man was well until he was 34 years old, when he developed headache, nausea, vomiting, and a right hemiparesis; he underwent multiple craniotomies for excision of a left temporoparietal brain abscess. Postoperatively he exhibited a right hemiparesis and sensory loss, right homonymous hemianopia, and a global aphasia. EEGs revealed left-sided theta activity; over the left anterior temporal leads, there was a marked delta-theta focus. He was treated initially with diphenylhydantoin and later phenobarbital. Three years after surgery, he was noted to have a mild right hemiparesis and sensory loss, with persistence of the right homonymous hemianopia. He exhibited an anomic aphasia, with difficulties with simple calculations and recognition of fingers, mild confusion between left and right, and dysgraphic writing. At this time, his hospital records noted that "he now expresses interest in religion and possibly in becoming a minister, and hopes to increase his 'use of good words' toward that end." He initially had occasional grand mal seizures, but beginning seven years postoperatively had episodes in which he was "dazed" and unaware of his surround-

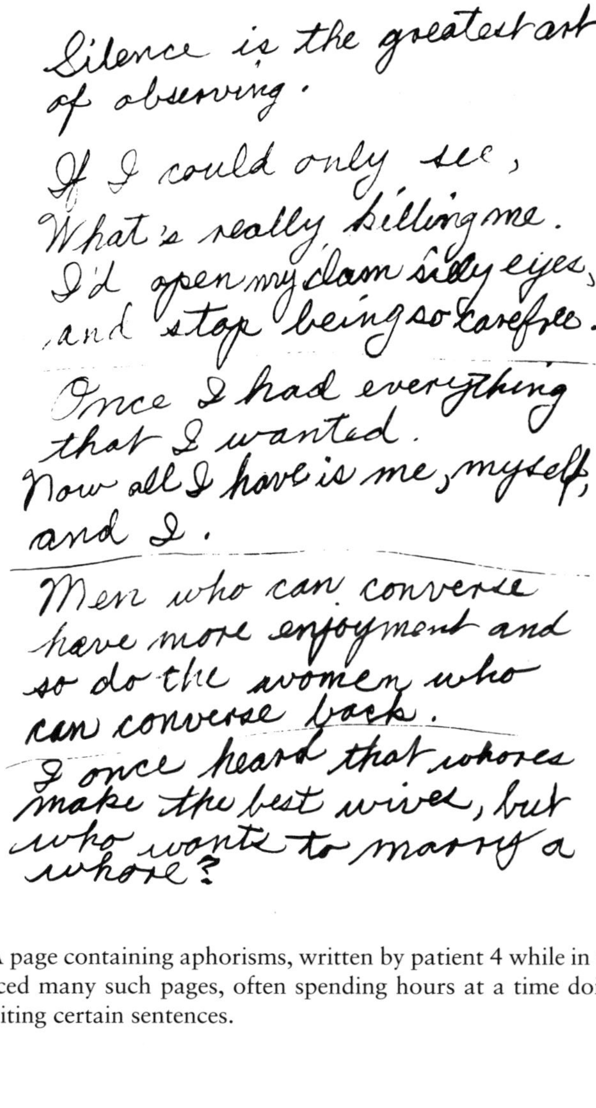

Silence is the greatest art
of observing.

If I could only see,
What's really killing me.
I'd open my dam silly eyes,
and stop being so carefree.

Once I had everything
that I wanted.
Now all I have is me, myself,
and I.

Men who can converse
have more enjoyment and
so do the women who
can converse back.

I once heard that whores
make the best wives, but
who wants to marry a
whore?

FIGURE 4. A page containing aphorisms, written by patient 4 while in the hospital. This patient produced many such pages, often spending hours at a time doing so, as well as recurrently writing certain sentences.

ings, with tremors of the right face, arm, and, to a lesser degree, leg, without loss of consciousness. At this time he also reported seeing "multicolors," especially green and purple flashes, over the entire visual field. He denied visceral, gustatory, or olfactory hallucinations. The patient complained to his physicians of loss of interest in sexual activities. One year later the patient was still unemployed but was spending many hours per day in volunteer work for religious organizations, where he was involved primarily in making charts and graphs. He subsequently at his own suggestion delivered several sermons at his church. He spontaneously volunteered typed copies of the texts of these sermons to his physician. The sermons concerned highly moral issues, which were dealt with in highly circumstantial and meticulous detail.

Specific reference is made in his writings to an "inner meaning" for certain events. Some words are underlined for emphasis, and others are written entirely in capitals. The meaning of words is emphasized and detailed, with frequent use of qualifying expressions in parentheses and with frequent digressions along secondary themes, which are often concerned with precise definitions or qualifications.

## CASE 6

This right-handed man with unilateral temporal lobe atrophy had episodic behavior disturbances. No family history of neurologic or psychiatric disease was elicited. The patient performed well in school until the age of 11, when his grades deteriorated. One year later, there was an episode of fuguelike state in which the patient walked 150 yards across a field, then pedaled his bicycle for a distance of four blocks with no awareness of his surroundings.

From the age of 11, he did poorly in school until age 17, at which time he enlisted in the armed services. He did well during his first three years, but at age 20 became involved in several altercations and subsequently was discharged. After his discharge, he began to experience episodes in which he was unaware of his behavior. During one of these episodes, without apparent aggravation, the patient continuously struck his head and fists against a brick wall for between three and five minutes. Shortly thereafter, he began to exhibit easily provoked rage. He was arrested on several occasions, charged with assaulting an officer and with causing considerable property damage. He was subsequently admitted to several psychiatric institutions, where he was treated with thioridazine and perphenazine. At age 24, he was evaluated neurologically. Cranial nerves and deep tendon reflexes were normal. Motor and sensory examination were unremarkable. Cerebellar function was thought to be normal, but the patient deviated slightly to the left in tandem gait. The full scale WAIS IQ estimate was 109. A brain scan and skull x-rays were normal. A pneumoencephalogram with satisfactory ventricular filling showed enlargement of the lateral recess of the left temporal horn (10 mm in width anteriorly and posteriorly), while the remaining portions of the lateral ventricles, the third and fourth ventricles, and the cerebral gyri appeared normal. EEG recordings from sphenoidal electrodes revealed moderate to high amplitude sharp and spike discharges persistently from right and left temporal regions. The patient was treated with diphenylhydantoin and primidone, 750 mg per day, with only slight improvement, but following treatment with primidone 1,500 mg per day he has experienced a markedly decreased frequency in his seizures. He has had no further episodes of rage, but remains very sensitive to environmental stress.

At age 27 the patient recorded his subjective impressions of his illness. This was done by dictating to a public stenographer, "because I couldn't write fast enough." He dictated for a period of 17 hours beginning at 5 P.M. without stopping to eat and with only several brief intermissions of several minutes duration. The result was a 56 page typed account, in meticulous and deeply emotional detail, of the patient's military service and subsequent hospitalizations. The patient reports having been fully aware of his behavior while dictating and denies any relation to a seizure. He reports having specifically omitted profanity from his account because the stenographer was a female. There have been no other episodes similar to the foregoing, but the patient claims to keep detailed lists of things he must do, and often makes written records of telephone calls.

## CASE 7

This right-handed man was well until age six, when he reportedly had a meningitis secondary to sinusitis, during which he had at least one convulsion. There was some question as to whether he may have had some minor spells of speech arrest for several months after this illness. The patient then remained in good health until age 14, when he contracted poliomyelitis with paralysis of his legs lasting two months, which resolved without neurologic sequelae. He received formal education in law and accountancy and as a clergyman.

At age 21 he was beaten around the head and rendered unconscious. Five years later, the patient began to have minor motor seizures, characterized by an absence spell preceded by an aura of a "vision of light." These spells occurred several times per week. Sometimes they were associated with a feeling of fear or sadness. A year later he began to have grand mal seizures, which occurred about once a month. Findings on general physical and neurologic examinations were normal. Skull x-rays suggested atrophy or hypoplasia of the left frontotemporal region. Electroencephalography initially showed bilateral temporal discharges, predominant on the right. A subsequent EEG with nasopharyngeal and sphenoidal leads revealed an active right anterior spike focus, and intravenous pentylenetetrazol (200 mg) resulted in a verbal report of the patient's visual aura, followed by an absence seizure during which the patient raised his trunk, rubbed the examiner's arm, and made chewing motions, with EEG activation in right sphenoidal electrodes. The patient's seizures were poorly controlled with medication, and at age 37 a right anterior temporal lobectomy was performed. Postoperatively, the patient no longer had major motor seizures, but did have occasional minor spells generally without aura, consisting usually of a brief absence seizure or, in some cases, of automatisms (on one occasion the patient disrobed in public). After the lobectomy, the patient showed markedly decreased interest in his law practice, and spent much of his time at home reading magazines and prayer books and listening to records. The patient was hospitalized one year later because of "paranoid outbursts" and "bizarre behavior." In the following four years, he was investigated at several hospitals because of a "generalized slowing down" and "less initiative." EEG revealed residual epileptic activity over the right midtemporal region. Five years after the operation, psychometric testing revealed a WAIS full-scale IQ of 109 (verbal 112; performance 104; memory quotient 114), normal performance on the Bender-Gestalt test, and a T-score of 79 on the Hunt-Minnesota Test for organic brain damage. Neurologic examination showed a slightly widened left palpebral fissure, mild left-sided hyperreflexia, and slight downward drift of the extended left arm. When asked to write a sentence about the weather, the patient wrote "Today's weather seems to be the epitome of 'April showers bring May's flowers,' with rain and nasty weather all day." When asked about writing, the patient showed his physician a copy of an outline for a novel. He refused, however, to discuss this further or to show a copy of the manuscript to his physician, stating that a previous novel he had written had been plagiarized by the faculty of a foreign university.

## Discussion

The case histories summarized above are striking in that in each case there was an unusual tendency for the patient to write extensively, typically in a meticulous manner. Each of the authors has observed many other patients besides these seven in whom there was evidence for a temporal lobe disorder and who also wrote to an unusual degree. The literature contains numerous references to the circumstantial and pedantic character of the speech of temporal lobe epileptics. In describing a patient with psychomotor seizures, Kraepelin,[8] in 1906, noted that the patient "gives a connected, though very long-winded account of his condition." Similarly, Beard,[9] in his description of the schizophrenia-like psychoses in epilepsy, noted the speech of his patients to be "ponderous, circumstantial, pedantic, long-winded." Glaser,[10] in describing the performance of 37 patients with psychomotor temporal lobe epilepsy on a battery of psychologic tests, noted a pattern of striking similarities in the manner in which the patients responded to and performed the various tests, rather than a characteristic pattern of scores. Thus, Glaser notes that "many of the patients were concerned with clarity of their thinking, and made significant efforts to control, restrict, or contain emotions and actions in order to become clear, accurate, and realistic." However, with the exception of a report by Blumer,[11] which includes examples of the written material produced by the patient described in case 3 above, we are aware of no studies that document the extensive writing of patients with temporal lobe disorders.

There is now a strong body of evidence indicating the existence of a striking syndrome of interictal personality changes characteristically occurring in temporal lobe epilepsy. Gibbs[12] reported an incidence of 49 percent of psychiatric disorders (32 percent "severe personality disorders," 17 percent "psychosis") among 163 patients with anterior temporal epileptic foci; psychiatric symptoms were three times more common than in patients with foci in other areas. Beard,[9] in a study of epileptics in whom schizophrenia-like psychoses had developed, noted a disproportionately high number of patients with temporal lobe disorders

(48 of 69 patients exhibited electrographic evidence of temporal lobe foci). Other authors have questioned the presence of distinct personality changes in temporal lobe epileptics as compared with "non-psychomotor"[13] or "grand mal-petit mal" epileptics.[14] However, even in the study of Guerrant and associates,[15] which questions the presence of personality alterations in patients with temporal lobe epilepsy as compared with a nonepileptic hospital population, results show a striking difference between the psychologic "profiles" of temporal lobe epileptics and controls (Minnesota Multiphasic Personality Inventory profiles were judged as psychotic in 23 percent of the temporal lobe patients, as opposed to 4 percent of the controls).

The interictal personality changes often become manifest some years after the onset of seizures. Slater and Beard[16] reported a latency of 12.8 to 15.6 years (14.1 years average) between the onset of epilepsy and the onset of overt psychiatric symptoms. Glaser[10] reported a latency of six years. The behavioral alterations appear to reflect changes in affective or experiential function and specifically changes in the depth of emotional experience. Thus, a number of studies have reported changes in sexual function,[4-6,17] the frequent presence of religiosity,[7,18] and often a deepened interest in moral and ethical issues.[3] In addition, evidence for an unusual degree of aggressiveness exists in the interictal behavior of some patients with temporal lobe foci.[1,2,19] In this regard, it is interesting that the behavior of these patients is often remarkably well tolerated by their families, a fact that may reflect the capacity of these patients for striking emotional warmth as another aspect of their deepened emotional responses.

The extensive writing we have observed in temporal lobe patients may be explained, in part, on the basis of the above. The writings of four of the patients described have clear moral or religious overtones. The striking preoccupation with detail appears to reflect the importance accorded by the writer to his material. Little room is left for error. Thus, three of the patients (cases 2, 3, and 5) commonly use parenthetical expressions ("On weekends [Sat and Sun] . . . ," or "five [5] seconds") to make the meaning of words absolutely clear. Words are defined, and sometimes redefined, several times. Underlining or writing in all capitals or red for emphasis is common in the material produced by three of the patients. Even minute details (for instance, the number and size of screws used to hang a picture) are accorded importance.

There is a compulsive quality to much of the written material we have examined. Patient 1 wrote down the words to a single song at least several hundred times. Similarly, patient 4 wrote two sentences repetitively. Patient 2 recorded, in a highly ritualized and compulsive fashion, the dates of his seizures. In the context of highly moralistic and/or religious beliefs in these patients, such compulsive acts are not unexpected. In this regard, it is interesting that one patient (case 4) concealed many of his writings, and another (case 7) was reluctant to show his writings to his physicians.

A number of studies indicate the presence of memory deficits in patients with temporal lobe damage. This has been noted not only when bilateral lesions are present[20-22] but also has been seen after unilateral temporal lobectomies[23-25] and proven unilateral temporal infarction.[26] It might be argued that the extensive writings of our patients represent a compensatory mechanism for deficits in memory. This theory, however, does not explain the *content* (for instance, recurrently written words to songs) or the *form* ("I do thank dear "GOD" above, no seizures") of the writing. In addition, we have not observed extensive or compulsive writing in patients with other types of memory disorder.

We believe that the extensive and in some cases compulsive writing we have observed in temporal lobe epileptic patients reflects the previously documented deepening of emotional response in the presence of relatively preserved intellectual function. In this context, it is not surprising that, in speech, some temporal lobe epileptics are described as circumstantial or pedantic or as exhibiting "stickiness" or "viscosity."

The constellation of interictal behavioral changes in temporal lobe epilepsy is of interest for several reasons. Documentation of interictal changes may be as relevant to an understanding of epilepsy as a description of the seizures themselves. The occurrence of a well-defined syndrome of interictal personality changes in many cases of temporal lobe epilepsy suggests that the assessment of behavior itself may be of great value in diagnosis. In addition, the behavioral changes are of considerable theoretical interest, because they occur in association with disorders at *specific anatomic loci.* Similar changes commonly occur in patients with functional psychiatric disorders, particularly in schizophrenia. Indeed, a number of patients subsequently found to have temporal lobe disorders have been initially diagnosed as exhibiting "functional psychoses[27] (see also cases 1 and 6 above). Our understanding of the pathogenesis of the functional psychoses, and of schizophrenia in particular, is very incomplete at the present time. We believe that it is not unreasonable to expect that further clinical studies on temporal lobe epilepsy may yield information relevant to a fuller understanding of the mechanisms involved in some of the functional psychoses.

## Abstract

The phenomenon of hypergraphia, or the tendency toward extensive and, in some cases, compulsive writing in temporal lobe epilepsy is described in seven patients, in each of whom there was electroencephalographic demonstration of a temporal lobe focus. Unusually detailed and strikingly copious writing was evidenced in each patient. Six patients provided documentation of their extensive writing, which often was concerned with religious or moral issues. A seventh patient claimed to have written extensively, but refused to exhibit his writings. Aggressiveness, religiosity, and changes in sexual behavior in temporal lobe disorders have been described previously. The hypergraphia of temporal lobe epilepsy appears to be part of a specific behavioral syndrome of special interest because of its association with dysfunction at specific anatomic loci.

## References

1. Davidson GA: Psychomotor epilepsy. Can Med Assoc J 53:410-414, 1947
2. Serafetinides EA: Aggressiveness in temporal lobe epileptics and its relation to cerebral dysfunction and environmental factors. Epilepsia 6:33-42, 1963
3. Geschwind N: The clinical setting of aggression in temporal lobe epilepsy. In Fields WS, Sweet WH (Editors): The Neurobiology of Violence. St. Louis, Warren H. Green, 1974
4. Mitchell W. Falconer MA, Hill D: Epilepsy with fetishism relieved by temporal lobectomy. Lancet 2:626-629, 1954
5. Davies BM, Morgenstern FS: A case of cysticercosis, temporal lobe epilepsy, and transvestism. J Neurol Neurosurg Psychiatry 23:247-249, 1960
6. Blumer D: Hypersexual episodes in temporal lobe epilepsy. Am J Psychiatry 126:1099-1106, 1970
7. Dewhurst K, Beard AW: Sudden religious conversions in temporal lobe epilepsy. Br J Psychiatry 117:497-507, 1970
8. Kraepelin E: In Johnstone T (Editor): Lectures in Clinical Psychiatry. New York, William Wood and Co., 1906
9. Beard AW: The schizophrenia-like psychoses of epilepsy. II. Physical aspects. Br J Psychiatry 109:113-130, 1963
10. Glaser GH: The problem of psychosis in psychomotor temporal lobe epileptics. Epilepsia 5:271-278, 1964
11. Blumer D: Organic personality disorder. In Lion J (Editor): Severe Personality Disorders. Baltimore, The Williams & Wilkins Company, 1974
12. Gibbs FA: Ictal and non-ictal psychiatric disorders in temporal lobe epilepsy. J Nerv Ment Dis 113:522-528, 1951
13. Mignone RJ, Donnelly EF, Sadorosky D: Psychological and neurological comparisons of psychomotor and non-psychomotor epileptic patients. Epilepsia 11:345-359, 1970
14. Stevens JR: Psychiatric implications of psychomotor epilepsy. Arch Gen Psychiatry 14:461-471, 1966
15. Guerrant J, Anderson WW, Fischer A, et al: Personality in Epilepsy. Springfield, IL, Charles C Thomas, 1962
16. Slater E, Beard AW: The schizophrenia-like psychoses of epilepsy. I. Psychiatric aspects. Br J Psychiatry 109:95-112, 1963
17. Hierons R, Saunders M: Impotence in patients with temporal lobe epilepsy. Lancet 2:761-764, 1966
18. Geschwind N: Effects of temporal lobe surgery on behavior. N Engl J Med 289:480-481, 1973
19. Taylor DC: Agression and epilepsy. J Psychosom Res 13:229-236, 1969
20. Scoville WB, Milner B: Loss of recent memory after bilateral hippocampal lesions. J Neurol Neurosurg Psychiatry 20:11-21, 1957
21. Victor M, Angevine JB, Mancall EL, et al: Memory loss with lesions in hippocampal formation. Arch Neurol 5:244-263, 1961
22. DeJong RN, Itabashi HH, Olson JR: Memory loss due to hippocampal lesions. Arch Neurol 20:339-348, 1969
23. Walker EA: Recent memory impairment in unilateral temporal lobectomies. Arch Neurol Psychiatry 78:543-552, 1957

24. Serafetinides EA, Falconer MA: Some observations on memory impairment after temporal lobectomy for epilepsy. J Neurol Neurosurg Psychiatry 25:251-255, 1962
25. Dinsdale H, Logue V, Piercy M: A case of persisting impairment of recent memory following temporal lobectomy. Neuropsychologia 1:287-298, 1964
26. Geschwind N, Fusillo M: Color-naming defects in association with alexia. Arch Neurol 15:137-146, 1966
27. Malamud N: Psychiatric disorder with intracranial disorders of limbic system. Arch Neurol 17:113-123, 1967

We wish to thank Drs. D. Blumer and V. Mark for making available case records on their patients.

Supported in part by NINDS grants NS 06209 and NS 5074.

## CHAPTER 19

# Effects of Temporal-Lobe Surgery on Behavior

*Norman Geschwind*

When Mr. Murray Falconer moved from New Zealand to London, his neurosurgical unit based jointly in two major London teaching hospitals and at the Maudsley Hospital, one of the leading psychiatric centers of the world, began a methodical study of surgery in the control of temporal-lobe epilepsy. Although the primary indication for surgery was uncontrolled seizures, the presence of behavioral changes in a large fraction of the 250 patients operated on has permitted the accumulation of considerable data on the clinical pictures of these personality changes and the effects of surgery. This study has had the advantage of independent assessment by psychiatrists with a special interest in this area, as well as strong electroencephalographic and neuropathological support.

The total results of these investigations constitute an important landmark in the field of behavioral neurology. Our admiration for this important body of knowledge should in no way, however, temper our realization that these results have probably been more fruitful in raising questions than in resolving problems.

Thus, the data suggest that psychosis is not often associated with mesial temporal sclerosis, but is more frequently seen with hamartomas or tumors. It is not clear that this difference in type of personality disorder, however, is in fact related to type of pathology rather than to age at onset of epilepsy, which is typically early for mesial sclerosis and late for the other forms of histologic abnormality.

Another problem that the series raises is that of the description of the behavioral changes. Falconer's psychiatric colleagues appear on the whole to have used standard classifications. The risk of such an approach, which has also been used by other authors, is that it may fail to reveal, or might even obscure, the presence

Reprinted with permission from *The New England Journal of Medicine*. 1973;289:480-481.

of distinctive psychiatric syndromes in temporal-lobe epilepsy. Furthermore, even the stress on behavior disorder might lead to the failure to overlook patterns of personality alteration that were characteristic, even if not pathologic in the sense that they did not lead to gross difficulties in personal life. Clearly, in other fields of medicine one characteristically is on the alert to find distinguishing features in disorders of different mechanism. Hematology would have been retarded in its development if all anemias had been classified as resembling iron deficiency or pernicious anemia, or all bleeding disorders as resembling hemophilia or thrombocytopenia. Thus, many students of temporal-lobe epilepsy would regard many of the personality disorders as having a pattern qualitatively distinctive from schizophrenia. One need only mention the combination of marked religiosity,[1] striking changes in sexual behavior,[2–4] cosmic and moral concerns, and a remarkable tendency for the patient to turn to writing, all against a background of well preserved and deepened affect.[5] It will be important to document or refute the existence of such distinctive alterations.

The question of the cause of the behavioral changes remains open. Falconer cautiously mentions only two theories, of which one appears to attribute one group of behavioral alterations primarily to social and environmental pressures, and the other raises the possibility that the disorders associated with hamartomas are related to chromosomal abnormalities. It is surprising that nowhere in the paper is the possibility raised that the behavioral changes may be related to abnormal activity in the limbic system, despite its close anatomic relation to the medial temporal lobe, and despite its major importance in emotional behavior.[6]

This study suggests that certain types of abnormal behavior in temporal-lobe epilepsy may improve with surgery. Furthermore, other reports, particularly those of Blumer and Walker,[2,6] show dramatic improvements in sexual disorders after surgery for temporal-lobe epilepsy, a finding also recorded in a patient[3] operated on by Falconer himself. These favorable results will undoubtedly raise another question in the minds of many who have been aware of recent controversies in the press. If surgery on the brain can lead to improvement in behavior in temporal-lobe epilepsy, might not similar surgical procedures be beneficial in other cases with temporal-lobe foci in which control of overt seizures is not a problem, or indeed even in patients without obvious signs of temporal-lobe disease? Although this careful but uncontrolled series would hardly lend support to an indiscriminate use of brain surgery for management of disordered behavior, it lends equally little support to those who would forbid any surgery of this type under all circumstances. It seems to me that the avenues for resolution of this problem are obvious. On the one hand all patients for whom behavior-changing surgery is contemplated should be reviewed by independent committees consisting of both professionals and laymen, including women and minority members. On the other hand, the time is clearly appropriate for a careful, scientifically controlled study of behavior-modifying surgery.

## References

1. Dewhurst K, Beard AW: Sudden religious conversions in temporal lobe epilepsy. Br J Psychiatry, 117:497–507, 1970
2. Blumer D: Hypersexual episodes in temporal lobe epilepsy. Am J Psychiatry 126:1099–1106, 1970
3. Mitchell W, Falconer MA, Hill D: Epilepsy with fetishism relieved by temporal lobectomy. Lancet 2:626–630, 1954
4. Davies BM, Morgenstern FS: A case of cysticercosis, temporal lobe epilepsy, and transvestism. J Neurol Neurosurg Psychiatry 23:247–249, 1960
5. Geschwind N: The clinical setting of aggression in temporal lobe epilepsy. The Neurobiology of Violence. Edited by W Fields, W Sweet. Springfield, Illinois, Charles C. Thomas (in press)
6. Walker AE: Man and his temporal lobes. Surg Neurol 1:69–79, 1973

## CHAPTER 20

# The Interictal Behavior Syndrome of Temporal Lobe Epilepsy

*Stephen G. Waxman and Norman Geschwind*

This article deals with the syndrome of behavioral changes that occur in many patients with temporal lobe epilepsy. The changes are interictal in that they are manifest between those events that are clinically designated as seizures. Ictal events, which occur during manifest seizures, apparently represent only one clinical manifestation of the abnormal physiologic process in temporal lobe epilepsy. Although the available evidence suggests that specific personality changes are not observed in all forms of epilepsy, previous reports have verified a constellation of characteristic changes in temporal lobe epilepsy. These include changes in sexual behavior,[1–3] religiosity,[4] and a tendency toward extensive, and in some cases compulsive, writing.[5] The specificity of the changes suggests that there is a characteristic syndrome of interictal personality changes in some patients with temporal lobe epilepsy. These changes are of considerable theoretical interest because they provide an example of a human behavioral syndrome associated with dysfunction at specific anatomic loci. They may also be of diagnostic value; we have seen several patients in whom the diagnosis of temporal lobe epilepsy was first suggested by interictal behavior changes, and in whom electroencephalograms subsequently revealed temporal lobe abnormalities. This article presents three typical reports of cases and describes a previously unreported feature of this syndrome—the tendency toward compulsive drawing and writing that appears in some patients. We also discuss possible mechanisms underlying the cause of this unique syndrome of behavioral changes.

---

Reprinted with permission from *Archives of General Psychiatry*. 1975;32(12):1580-1586. 

## Report of Cases

### CASE 1

A 25-year-old right-handed woman had seizures that had begun at the age of 10. The seizures were usually generalized, often beginning with focal twitching of the left arm and face, and on some occasions, were associated with lip-smacking or chewing movements that were followed by urinary incontinence and tongue-biting. Her father and a paternal aunt reportedly had epilepsy, but siblings were apparently well. Results of neurologic examination, lumbar puncture, skull roentgenograms, and brain scan were normal, but a right anterior temporal spike focus was present on EEG. The patient was treated with anticonvulsants but continued to have seizures approximately once per month. When she was 15 years old, the patient was admitted to a psychiatric hospital after slashing her wrist with a razor blade after a fight with her sister. While in the hospital, the patient had difficulty with female attendants and accused several nurses and attendants of trying to persecute her. In the following year, the patient's school grades deteriorated. The patient was again admitted to a hospital at the age of 17 after two brief seizures on the left side. At the time of admission, she was confused and agitated. There was no history of the ingestion of drugs, toxins, or hallucinogens. Hospital records described the patient as "agitated, crying, incoherent . . . [with] peculiar posturing," and noted that she asked if she were on a spaceship or being controlled by radio. The patient recalls feeling as if events around her were "not really happening."

Results of a neurologic examination were normal except for slight facial weakness on the left side and deep tendon reflexes that were slightly more active on the left side. Visual fields were normal. Electroencephalogram revealed slow waves and spikes bitemporally that were more pronounced on the left side. Skull roentgenograms were normal. Sonar scan suggested some enlargement of the trigone of the left lateral ventricle. The patient was diagnosed as having an acute schizophrenic psychosis and was treated for several months with trifluoperazine hydrochloride. She was also treated with primidone, phenytoin sodium (diphenylhydantoin sodium), and phenobarbital. In the next four years, the patient became devoutly religious and experienced at least five religious conversions at a time when her family did not increase its participation in religious activities. On one occasion, she described her conversion as "like seeing God . . ." She denied any relation of these events to major seizures. She also began to experience frequent sensations of déjà vu. She noted a decrease in her interest in sexual activities and engaged in sexual intercourse only several times a year, much less than previously.

An EEG at the age of 20 revealed a spike focus in the right anterior temporal lobe. The patient was admitted to hospitals twice at the age of 21 because of seizures. She described an aura consisting of sensations of epigastric distress and a feeling of fear before her seizures. At this time, the patient described visual hallucinations of colored flashing lights that moved from left to right in the right

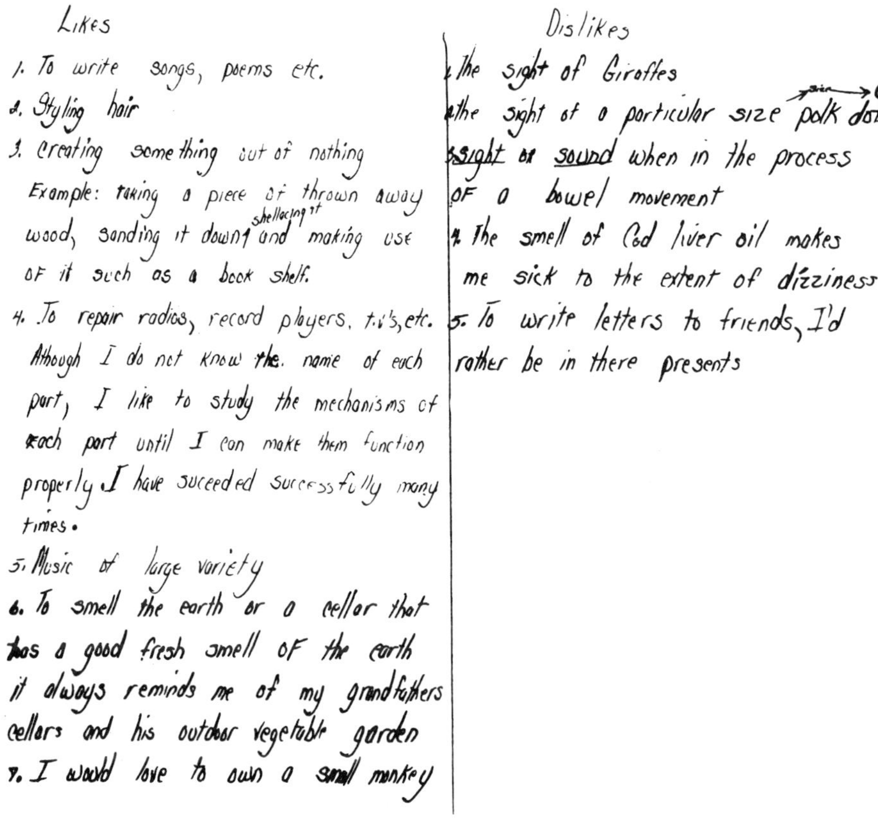

Likes

1. To write songs, poems etc.
2. Styling hair
3. Creating something out of nothing Example: taking a piece of thrown away wood, sanding it down, shellacing it and making use of it such as a book shelf.
4. To repair radios, record players, t.v's, etc. Although I do not know the name of each part, I like to study the mechanisms of each part until I can make them function properly. I have suceeded successfully many times.
5. Music of large variety
6. To smell the earth or a cellar that has a good fresh smell of the earth it always reminds me of my grandfathers cellars and his outdoor vegetable garden
7. I would love to own a small monkey

Dislikes

1. The sight of Giraffes
2. the sight of a particular size polk dot.
3. sight or sound when in the process of a bowel movement
4. The smell of Cod liver oil makes me sick to the extent of dizziness
5. To write letters to friends, I'd rather be in there presents

FIGURE 1. One of many lists produced by patient 1.

visual field. These hallucinations were on some occasions followed by seizures. Results of a neurologic examination revealed no focal deficits. There was no aphasia, constructions were fairly well done, and calculations were performed reasonably well. Roentgenograms of the chest and skull were normal, as were results of lumbar puncture. An EEG revealed prominent sharp waves over both hemispheres. Results of hemogram, routine blood chemistry studies, and urinalysis were normal. Levels of serum thyroxin, cortisol, and vitamin $B_{12}$ were within normal limits; results of serological study were normal. During this hospital admission, the patient also stated that she had begun to write extensively when she was 15-years-old, often spending several hours per day writing, and that she kept a pencil and paper with her at all times. While in the hospital and on subsequent clinic visits, she produced examples of lists she had made of items of food and furniture in her house, of her records and books, of her friends, of her relatives ("so I will know how many there are"), of places she had been, of her "likes" and "dislikes" (Figure 1), and of songs her father could play on the harmonica. She

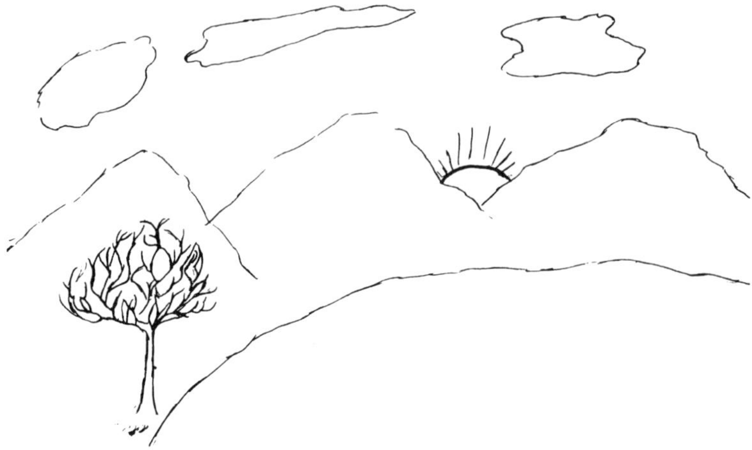

FIGURE 2. Sketch of one of the recurrent pictures of religious conversion sites of patient 1.

also produced detailed descriptions of her seizures, hallucinations, and sensations of déjà vu. She stated that she wrote things down "to be sure of what I do," and noted that she often felt compelled to write down on whatever material was available (napkins, scraps of paper) those events that had occurred in the preceding several hours, "especially if . . . a seizure is coming on so I couldn't memorize it." Much of her writing was concerned with global or mystical issues, such as the meaning of her existence. She stated that she did not usually interrupt other activities to write, but that on some occasions she felt compelled to write a word over and over, or to copy once or several times the labels on items she owned. She recounted having recurrently written "at least hundreds of times" the words to a song she had learned when she was 17. She also recurrently drew sketches of the site of one of her religious conversions. Figure 2 shows one of these sketches; the patient produced a number of others that were almost identical while she was waiting for her clinic appointments. Some of the patient's writing was reversed and could be read only when held up to a mirror (Figure 3). The patient denied having written anything during a seizure, and in fact had the impression that writing or drawing might abort her seizures. She denied other ritualistic or compulsive actions, but did describe herself as highly meticulous. She claimed to read only rarely.

## CASE 2

A right-handed man was admitted to the hospital at age 20 because of "blackout" spells. He had reportedly contracted poliomyelitis at the age of 3, with residual paresis of the right lower extremity. There was no history of head

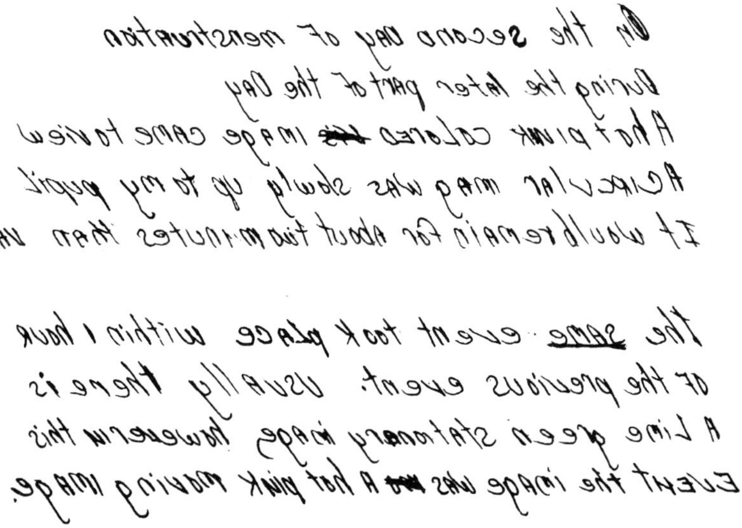

FIGURE 3. Reversed writing of patient 1 describes visual hallucinations. Description may be read by holding the page up to a mirror.

trauma. Neither the patient's parents nor his nine siblings had a history of seizures. The patient earned a high school degree after being dismissed from several schools because of alleged disciplinary problems. He worked as a file clerk. In the year prior to admission, the patient had at least three episodes of loss of consciousness that were preceded by nausea and a sensation of having to vomit. A witness reported that the patient became limp and fell to the floor "as if he were sleeping" but was not arousable. There were no convulsive movements and no incontinence was observed. Similar blackouts had occurred at intervals of several months for at least three or four years prior to hospitalization. The patient reported frequent sensations of déjà vu, and often believed that he had dreamt of events before they occurred. The patient, who frequently wrote poetry or short stories (Figure 4), reported that on several occasions, he "could not stop" writing and filled 30- to 40-page notebooks at a single sitting. He stated that none of his siblings, parents, or friends wrote stories or poetry or kept a diary, but that he had begun to write extensively several years prior to admission. Examination of one of his notebooks revealed that the themes of "love," "life," "God," and "why?" were recurrent. Although the patient denied being religious, his writings contained numerous religious references, and some pages were adorned with religious symbols. Astrological signs were affixed to other pages.

While in the hospital, the patient requested paper and continued to write; he also made crude drawings of each of the other patients in his room. He stated that he often drew pictures of people he met, so as to "portray their inner self." General physical examination was unremarkable, except for atrophy of the right

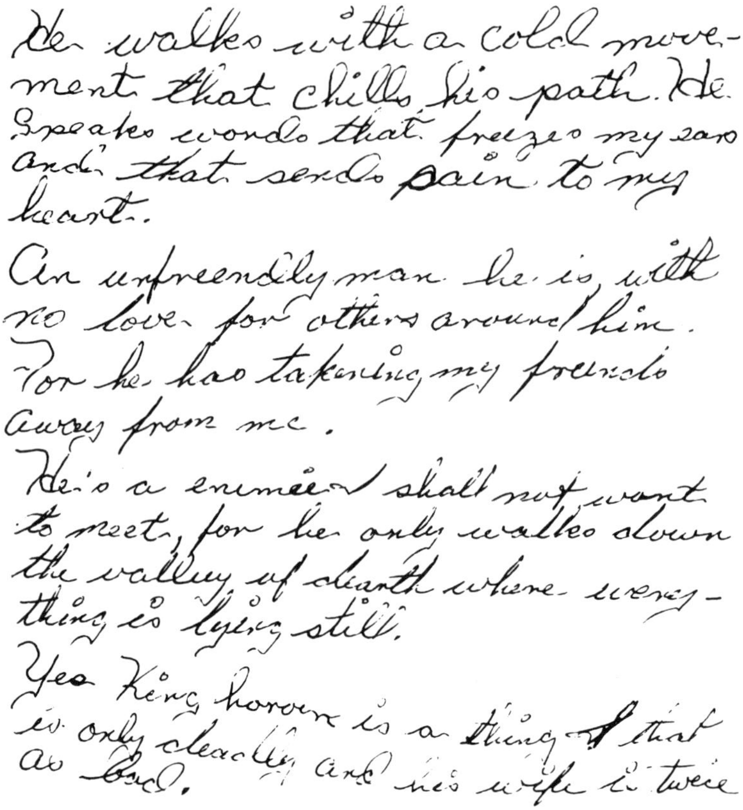
He walks with a cold move-
ment that chills his path. He
speaks words that freezes my ears
and that sends pain to my
heart.
An unfreendily man he is, with
no love for others around him.
For he has takening my freinds
away from me.
He's a enimee I shall not want
to meet, for he only walks down
the valley of death where every-
thing is lying still.
Yes King horor
is only deadly is a thing that
as bad. and his wife is twice

FIGURE 4. Part of a story produced spontaneously by patient 2 while in the hospital. Note reference to the "Valley of Death."

lower extremity. Cranial nerves were intact. Motor examination revealed normal bulk, tone, and strength except for weakness of the anterior tibial muscles on the right, absent right ankle jerk, and decreased knee jerk. Finger-to-nose and heel-to-shin movements were normal. The patient was alert and oriented, and the aphasia examination results were normal. He was able to repeat six to seven numbers forward and three numbers backward. Calculations were performed well. When asked how an apple and an orange were alike, the patient stated that they were "both fruit." However, when asked how a man and a plant were alike, he stated that "some men are actually vegetable." Laboratory findings revealed normal results from hemogram, urinalysis, and nonreactive serological studies; serum electrolytes and calcium levels were within normal limits. The blood sugar and liver function test results were normal. Chest and skull roentgenograms were unremarkable and lumbar puncture was normal. The brain scan was normal, but

EEG revealed theta-slowing in right temporal and parietal regions, more marked in the temporal derivations.

While in the hospital, the patient demonstrated a low threshold for rage. On several occasions he threatened to assault ward personnel. Concomitantly, he exhibited an unusual degree of interest in his fellow patients, volunteering to help with their daily care. He was treated with 300 mg of phenytoin sodium per day, and has reported no further seizures. He continues to visit the hospital periodically, spending time with other patients on the neurology service, and has also continued to volunteer poems, short stories, and drawings to his physicians.

It is not uncommon for the surface EEG to fail to record epileptic activity in deep structures, in particular in deep temporal structures. In the following patient, the EEG results were normal. However, we believe that his interictal behavior and his seizures are consistent with the diagnosis of temporal lobe epilepsy.

## CASE 3

A 28-year-old man was admitted to the hospital because of blackouts that began at the age of 26. These episodes were preceded by tingling paresthesias initially in the chest, radiating to the neck and face, followed by the sensation of an odor "like burning rubber," and in some instances by a sensation of "flashing lights" before his eyes. Observers described the blackouts as generalized convulsions. The patient furthermore stated that for several months previously, he had experienced feelings of déjà vu "99%" of the time. He also reported that reading or writing for more than an hour or emotional stress on some occasions were followed by a feeling of tilting or rising; on two occasions, this was followed in turn by paresthesias in the chest, face, and neck, the olfactory sensation of burning rubber, and a loss of consciousness. The patient volunteered that he had become increasingly irritable during the year prior to admission. He also stated that he recently preferred to be alone much of the time so that he could write or think about issues such as the ultimate goal of mankind. He volunteered that he had noted a decreased interest in sexual activities during the preceding several months. He had left college after two years, and was dismissed from a job after an argument with his supervisor. The patient had struck his head and lost consciousness briefly two years before admission, but there was no other history of head trauma. He reported being quite ill as an infant, but no details of this illness were available. Neither the patient's parents nor his ten siblings had a history of seizures.

When the patient was initially seen in the outpatient clinic, it was suggested that he be admitted to the hospital for evaluation. The patient requested that admission be deferred for several days so that he could put his papers, which he stated occupied much of his apartment, in order. He stated that he had written extensively, mostly poems, essays, and prayers, for three years, but that the volume of his writing had increased greatly approximately six months prior to admission. He also stated that although he had consumed large amounts of alcohol in the past, he had stopped drinking several months before admission, because "it interfered with my writing."

Results of physical examination were normal except for the sequels of an injury to the right axilla and multiple infected teeth. Results of cranial nerve examination were normal and no field cut was detected. Deep tendon reflexes were intact and symmetric; plantar response was flexor bilaterally. Motor examination results were normal, and heel-to-shin and finger-to-nose tests were performed well. There was a mild tendency to fall to the right on tandem gait. Sensory examination results were normal. The patient was awake and fully oriented, with normal speech and memory. Constructions were well performed and calculations well done. Results of hemogram, urinalysis, blood sugar studies, and chemistry studies were normal. Skull and chest roentgenograms were normal. Lumbar puncture was normal, with a cerebral spinal fluid protein value of 44 mg/100 ml. Results of brain scan and several EEGs were normal. Perimetric study revealed a constriction of the visual fields that did not change with distance, which was believed to conform to no anatomic pattern.

While in the hospital, the patient continued to write and kept a pencil and writing pad in a briefcase at his bedside at all times. He carried the briefcase with him much of the time and it was not until his confidence had been won that he showed any of his written material to his physicians. He had produced a series of devotional poems and wrote several poems exalting the devotion of his physicians. He had also produced several "personal prayers." He was reluctant to take anticonvulsant medication because he regarded his spells as "important to him," but agreed to periodic follow-up in the outpatient clinic.

## Comment

Despite the detection of subtle morphologic abnormalities in patients with schizophrenia,[6,7] there is little information concerning the localization of dysfunction in the major psychoses. Thus, the number of human behavioral syndromes for which there are clear neuroanatomic substrates is quite small. One example is provided by the "frontal lobe syndromes" of either apathetic indifference or euphoria and relative release from social inhibitions.[8–10] These syndromes present clinical pictures that are generally quite dissimilar to those observed in the major psychoses. A second example is provided by the small number of patients with herpes simplex encephalitis who develop a clinical picture similar to that described in the Kluver-Bucy syndrome resulting from bilateral temporal lobe damage, with hyperphagia and marked distractability in addition to disorder of memory.[11] A third example is provided by the patient of Reeves and Plum,[12] a 20-year-old woman with hyperphagia, rage, and dementia accompanying a ventromedial hypothalamic neoplasm. In this article, we wish to describe another example of a human behavioral syndrome associated with dysfunction at specific anatomic loci, the constellation of *interictal personality changes* associated with temporal lobe epilepsy. We emphasize this interictal behavior syndrome for two reasons. First, the existence of such a syndrome has clear implications in terms of diagnosis; we have seen several patients in whom the primary diagnosis of "functional" psychosis had been made, and several others in whom the question of temporal lobe seizure disorder was initially raised primarily on the basis of a description of interictal personality changes, and in whom subsequent EEG studies revealed temporal lobe foci. Second, we believe that the syndrome may be of considerable theoretical interest and may provide a useful model for the major psychoses because of its association with dysfunction at specific loci in the central nervous system.

The religiosity associated with the interictal syndrome of temporal lobe epilepsy has been commented on in several studies[13–15] and may take a number of forms. Dewhurst and Beard[4] described sudden religious conversions in temporal lobe epilepsy. In some cases, the patient will have undergone multiple religious conversions; case 1 in our study described a patient who experienced at least five religious conversions during an 11-year period. The preoccupations of the patients often have a cosmic or global flavor, and may transcend the limits of established religions; we have seen a patient who, when asked if he were religious, replied that he was "beyond religion" and that he was a "cosmic minister to the world."

Denial of religion in some patients may in fact belie deeply held convictions. For example, one patient, who initially stated that he was not religious, on further questioning stated that he had rejected religion because he felt that the clergymen he encountered were not devout enough. Another patient, when asked if he was religious, replied, "Absolutely not." When asked why, he stated, "I am sure that God would strike me dead if I were to set foot in church!" A third patient interrupted a religious service by ascending the pulpit to debate certain liturgical points with his clergyman. Deeply held ethical convictions and a profound sense of right and wrong are observed in these patients. It is not unusual for them to exhibit interest in global issues such as national or international politics. They also become involved in issues that are not so global. Several patients exhibited an unusual degree of concern for the welfare of other patients, voluntarily helping with their nursing care while in the hospital and offering to visit them after discharge.

"Stickiness" or "viscosity" have in the past been considered an important part of the "epileptic personality." Although it is now generally agreed that these traits are not seen in all forms of epilepsy, they are characteristic of the interictal behavior of patients with temporal lobe epilepsy. There is often a striking preoccupation with detail, especially as concerns moral or ethical issues or both. There are no trifles for these patients, and humor, if present at all, tends to be heavy-handed.[16] In a study on the performance of patients with temporal lobe epilepsy on a battery of psychological tests, Glaser[14] commented on a pattern of similarity, not in terms of actual scoring of test results, but rather in the way in which patients responded to and performed the various tests; thus, "many of the patients were concerned with the clarity of their thinking, and made significant efforts to control, restrict, or contain emotions and actions in order to become clear, accurate, and realistic." Preoccupation with detail and clarity and a profound sense of righteousness are evident in the speech of many of our patients. One patient, when informed that smoking was not permitted on the medical wards, inquired at length as to whether his physician had personally ascertained that no other patients in the hospital were allowed to smoke. Speech often appears circumstantial because of the tendency of these patients to digress along secondary or even tertiary themes. The meticulousness and attention to detail implicit in this viscosity also appear in the writings that are characteristically produced by patients with temporal lobe epilepsy.

The hypergraphia of temporal lobe epilepsy[5] may take a number of forms, but is usually characterized by strikingly voluminous writings, often of an unusually meticulous or compulsive nature. The degree to which the patient writes is often out of proportion to his educational background. One patient who had been confined to state institutions for most of her life had been taught to add but could not perform simple subtractions or multiplications. This patient volunteered copious handwritten notes on religious topics. Some pages were written in alternate lines of red and blue, other pages were written in a highly stylized script, and some passages were written in code.

The writings of patients with temporal lobe epilepsy are characteristically highly meticulous and unusually detailed. One patient volunteered to his doctor carbon copies of a typewritten day-by-day account of the events between each office visit. The record is 1,000 to 2,000 words in length for most months. Pencilled notes and detailed typed addenda that describe dreams and special "incidents" follow the daily entries. Each month's record concludes with a detailed summary that includes "Generalizations" and often an analysis of causal relationships (see box).

Parenthetical expressions [e.g., "Six (6) seizures" or "On weekends (Sat and Sun) . . ."] appear commonly in the writings of our patients with hypergraphia. Words are often underlined, written entirely in capital letters, or written in red ink for emphasis. Two of our patients have recurrently written the same lines many hundreds of times.

The writings are often concerned with moral, ethical, or religious issues. One patient wrote a "personal prayer" and a series of devotional poems. A second brought to his physician typed copies of two sermons that he had delivered in his church at his own request. Several patients adorned their writings with religious or mystical symbols. In their preoccupation with moral and philosophical issues, the writings of patients with temporal lobe epilepsy appear to reflect a deepening of emotional response in the presence of relatively preserved intellectual function.

The degree of hypergraphia may be somewhat greater than would be anticipated on the basis of the writings that the patients exhibit. One patient showed his physician an outline for a novel, but refused to exhibit or discuss the manuscript, stating that a previous novel had been plagiarized by the faculty of a

*GENERALIZATION: CAUSE*

Exertion, excitement (especially if I am responsible or have a part of it). Weather changing for the worse. Below freezing or too high temperature, especially if humid, strong wind.

*RESULT:*

I begin to tremble and get nervous, a pain starts in my heart. At this point, I have to stop and rest or the pain gets worse. I have been given nitroglyerin tablets which I always have with me in case of emergency. Rest is imperative at this point.

As the pain in my chest clears up, the front of my neck gets sore and draws especially in the hollow at the base of the throat. The pain works in back of my shoulder and down my left arm, also up to my head resulting in a headache. My arm has lost most of its strength and agility. The headache clears up much faster than my arm, usually 6 hours at the most.

All this leaves me in a weakened condition and very hungry. I eat my meals and try to exercise to get my strength back and into condition which to me takes a long time. At this stage, I am very susceptible to seizures — frequent light ones and mild ones. It usually takes 1 to 14 days before I am back to myself.

The severity of the pain and length of time to get back in shape is dependent on the harshness and length of time the cause persisted. I have a tranquilizer which I take when I know I must do something that will overtax me, make me nervous or excited. These I try to avoid.

foreign university. Another patient admitted to concealing many of his writings in various hiding places in his home.

In some patients, the urge to record may take forms other than writing. One patient hired a public stenographer and dictated for a period 17 hours with only several brief intermissions. Another requested a tape recorder while in the hospital. Still other patients record their feelings by drawing or painting. One patient recurrently draws the site of one of her religious conversions. Another patient draws "cosmic paintings," stating that words cannot convey the depth of his feelings.

Although there is evidence for memory deficit after unilateral temporal lobectomies,[17–19] unilateral temporal infarction,[20] and bilateral temporal lesions,[21–23] the hypergraphia of temporal lobe epilepsy cannot be accounted for as a simple compensatory mechanism for memory deficits, since this would not explain the content (Figures 1, 3, and 4) or often unusual form of the writing, and since we have not observed hypergraphia in patients with other types of memory disorder.

We stress that we have described this syndrome as that of behavioral change in temporal lobe epilepsy rather than as a syndrome of behavior disorder. Many patients may show the kinds of changes we have described and yet remain functional and productive. The changes are therefore not necessarily maladaptive. We would also stress that while behavioral changes are often present, they are not necessary concomitants of epilepsy arising in the temporal lobe.

The temporal relationship between behavioral changes and onset of seizures varies in different studies. For example, Slater and Beard[13] reported a latency of 14.1 years from onset of seizures to onset of psychosis; however, all of their patients had been regarded as schizophrenic. In our experience, behavioral changes may occur with much shorter latency after onset of seizures, and in a few patients, these changes have antedated the onset of seizures. However, the patients we have described, who characteristically exhibit a preserved or even deepened affect, do not fall into any established nosologic category and often do not appear schizophrenic.

Some studies have questioned the occurrence of distinct personality changes in patients with temporal lobe epilepsy as compared with patients with other types of epilepsy.[24,25] However, even in these studies the data in fact suggest substantial differences in patients with temporal lobe epilepsy. For example, in the study of Guerrant et al,[24] 94% of the patients with temporal lobe epilepsy demonstrated behavior disorder, while 92% of patients with grand mal epilepsy and 88% of hospital control patients without epilepsy were diagnosed as showing behavior disorder. The figure of 88% for the hospital control patients is so high that no conclusions can be drawn from these data except that possibly too weak a criterion for behavior disorder was used. Furthermore, while the overall incidence of abnormal Minnesota Multiphasic Personality Inventory Profiles was similar for patients with temporal lobe epilepsy and the medical illness group, the incidence of psychotic profiles in the temporal lobe group was 23% as opposed to 4% in the medical illness group, whereas the incidence of neurotic profiles in the temporal lobe group was 33%, compared with 70% for the medical illness group. Thus, even these authors are led to conclude that "the hypothesis that the Psychomotor Group will display different *kinds of disturbances* than the other two groups is supported" [italics added].[24]

It should be stressed at this point that the behavioral syndrome of temporal lobe epilepsy is manifest as an *interictal* phenomenon in that the changes occur between those episodes that we have come to designate as seizures on the basis of clinical observation. More explicitly, it should be noted that we have defined as interictal those events that occur between clinically observed seizures. Might the behavior change in temporal lobe epilepsy represent ongoing seizure activity? Although there are cases with purely paroxysmal behavior changes, the behavioral alteration in most patients is chronic and not paroxysmal. It seems highly unlikely that the change in behavior is a direct result of constant ongoing seizure activity, since this would imply status epilepticus that endured for periods of years, during which some patients perform at an extremely high level.

Several alternative hypotheses concerning causation appear tenable. The observation of interictal spike discharges in patients with epilepsy is common. In many patients with temporal lobe epilepsy, spike activity can be recorded from temporal derivations much more frequently than seizures are observed.[26] Spike discharges in deep structures, such as amygdala and hippocampus, are often not reflected in surface abnormalities.[27] At the intracellular level, interictal spikes associated with paroxysmal depolarization shifts followed by hyperpolarization have been demonstrated in several laboratories.[28,29] While clinically observable seizures represent the most dramatic event related to abnormal discharges, they are not necessary concomitants of or markers for all abnormal electrical activity. While clinical observations have compelled the classical characterization of ictal and interictal states in the patient with epilepsy, the dichotomy is less clear at the level of electrophysiologic process, where frank seizure activity may be superimposed on a background of frequently occurring, paroxysmally abnormal discharges.

The available evidence suggests that spike discharges in the temporal lobe and related structures may have profound effects on behavior. For example, there is evidence that amygdaloid activity may modulate the secretion of gonadotrophin and adrenocorticotrophin[30,31] and that gonadal hormones in turn alter neural thresholds involving the amygdala and rhinencephalic pathways.[32] Experimental evidence also suggests differential facilitating and inhibitory effects of stimulation of various regions within the amygdala on hypothalamically elicited attack behavior in cats.[33] On the basis of these and similar findings, we might in theory expect temporal lobe stimulation to alter limbic function in a relatively immediate fashion. Ongoing interictal activity in the temporal lobe would then become manifest as a chronic behavior syndrome reflecting these immediate changes. Might more delayed and cumulative changes also constitute a theoretical basis for the behavioral alterations? The available experimental evidence suggests that long-term changes in physiologic properties may occur as a result of repeated stimulation. For example Goddard and co-workers[34] showed progressive changes in response to electrical stimulation as a result of repeated subthreshold amygdaloid stimulation. The progressive dissemination of epileptoid abnormalities in the form of "mirror" and "projection" foci has also been found after the production of primary neocortical epileptogenic lesions.[35,36] At the behavioral level, Belluzi and Grossman[37] demonstrated that bilateral injection of carbachol into rat amygdaloid complex is followed by alterations in avoidance learning that persist for several weeks after seizures have subsided. Thus, a second hypothesis is that of "cumulative" effects of interictal spike activity in temporal structures, or of long-lasting effects of clear-cut seizure discharges. We do not know the degree to which such changes depend on or are determined by external events. Such information is clearly crucial to a theory of behavior in temporal lobe epilepsy. However, it seems to us not unreasonable to expect that the pairing of periodic changes in limbic activity, with temporally coincident events in the external world might lead to altered modes of "learning" about external events, in which the unconditioned stimulus is endogenous, in the form of paroxysmal, abnormal limbic activity.

Another possibility that appears less likely to us is that the syndrome is the direct effect of temporal lobe damage. We tend to support the hypothesis that the behavioral changes are the effect of abnormal excitation or responsiveness. We would stress, however, that this issue is not settled. In some series, patients subjected to surgical treatment for temporal lobe epilepsy reportedly show diminution in the behavioral changes[38,39] despite the fact that there has been increased destruction of temporal tissue; however, there are some conflicting reports.[40]

We believe that the interictal syndrome of temporal lobe epilepsy may prove to be a useful model in the investigation of other behavioral syndromes. There are few functional disorders for which distinct anatomic substrates have been demonstrated. The interictal behavior syndrome of temporal lobe epilepsy at least partially fulfills this criterion. Further studies on this syndrome, with particular reference to the behavioral effects of interictal spike activity in limbic structures, and to the continuum of physiologic states between ictus and normalcy, may well prove to be of major value in clarifying our understanding of the neural basis of behavior.

## Abstract

A distinct syndrome of interictal behavior changes occurs in many patients with temporal lobe epilepsy. These changes include alterations in sexual behavior, religiosity, and a tendency toward extensive, and in some cases compulsive, writing and drawing. The concomitants of abnormal limbic activity therefore include behavior alterations as well as manifest seizures. The demonstration of interictal spike activity in temporal structures provides a pathophysiologic basis for this syndrome. The constellation of behavioral changes may be of great diagnostic value. In addition, it provides an example of a human behavioral syndrome associated with dysfunction at specific anatomic loci. The behavior syndrome of temporal lobe epilepsy may prove to be a useful model in studies on the neural substrates for behavior.

## References

1. Mitchell W, Falconer MA, Hill D: Epilepsy with fetishism relieved by temporal lobectomy. *Lancet* 2:626-629, 1954.
2. Davies BM, Morgenstern FS: A case of cysticercosis, temproal lobe epilepsy, and transvestism. *J Neurol Neurosurg Psychiatry* 23:247-249, 1960.
3. Blumer D: Hypersexual episodes in temporal lobe epilepsy. *Am J Psychiatry* 126:1099-1106, 1970.
4. Dewhurst K, Beard AW: Sudden religious conversions in temporal lobe epilepsy. *Br J Psychiatry* 117:497-507, 1970.

5. Waxman SG, Geschwind N: Hypergraphia in temporal lobe epilepsy. *Neurology* 24:629-637, 1974.
6. Meltzer H, Moline R: Muscle abnormalities in acute psychoses. *Arch Gen Psychiatry* 23:481-491, 1970.
7. Meltzer HY, Crayton JW: Subterminal motor nerve abnormalities in psychotic patients. *Nature* 249:373-375, 1974.
8. Kleist K: *Gehirnpathologie*. Leipzig, Germany, Barth Verlag, 1934.
9. Goldstein K: *After-effects of Brain Injuries in War*. New York, Grune and Stratton Inc, 1948.
10. Blumer D: Organic personality disorder, in Lion J (ed): *Severe Personality Disorders*. Baltimore, Williams and Wilkins Co, 1974.
11. Gascon GG, Gilles F: Limbic dementia. *J Neurol Neurosurg Psychiatry* 36:420-430, 1973.
12. Reeves AG, Plum F: Hyperphagia, rage, and dementia accompanying a ventromedial hypothalamic neoplasm. *Arch Neurol* 20:616-624, 1969.
13. Slater E, Beard AW: The schizophrenia-like psychoses of epilepsy: I. Psychiatric aspects. *Br J Psychiatry* 109:95-112, 1963.
14. Glaser GH: The problems of psychosis in psychomotor temporal lobe epileptics. *Epilepsia* 5:271-278, 1964.
15. Geschwind N: Effects of temporal lobe surgery on behavior. *N Engl J Med* 289:480-481, 1973.
16. Geschwind N: The clinical setting of aggression in temporal lobe epilepsy, in Fields WS, Sweet WH (eds): *The Neurobiology of Violence*. St. Louis, Warren H Green Inc. 1974.
17. Walker EA: Recent memory impairment in unilateral temporal lesions. *AMA Arch Neurol Psychiatry* 78:543-552, 1957.
18. Serafetinides EA, Falconer MA: Some observations on memory impairment after temporal lobectomy for epilepsy. *J Neurol Neurosurg Psychiatry* 25:251-255, 1962.
19. Dinsdale H, Logue V, Piercy M: A case of persisting impairment of recent memory following right temporal lobectomy. *Neuropsychologia* 1:287-298, 1964.
20. Geschwind N, Fusillo M: Color-naming defects in association with alexia. *Arch Neurol* 15:137-146, 1966.
21. Scovill WB, Milner BN: Loss of recent memory after bilateral hippocampal lesions *J Neurol Neurosurg Psychiatry* 20:11-21, 1957.
22. Victor M, Angevine JB, Mancall EL, et al: Memory loss with lesions of hippocampal formation. *Arch Neurol* 5:244-263, 1961.
23. DeJong RN, Itabashi HH, Olson JR: Memory loss due to hippocampal lesions: Report of a Case. *Arch Neurol* 20:339-348, 1969.
24. Guerrant J, Anderson WW, Fischer A, et al: *Personality in Epilepsy*. Springfield Ill, Charles C Thomas Publisher, 1962.
25. Stevens JR: Psychiatric implications of psychomotor epilepsy. *Arch Gen Psychiatry* 14:461-471, 1966.
26. Jasper H, Pertuisset B, Flanigin H: EEG and cortical electrograms in patients with temporal lobe seizures. *AMA Arch Neurol Psychiatry* 65:272-289, 1951.
27. Crandall PH, Walter RD, Rand RW: Clinical applications of studies on stereotactically implanted electrodes in temporal lobe epilepsy. *J Neurosurg* 20:827-840, 1963.

28. Ayala GF, Dichter M, Gumnit RJ, et al: Genesis of epileptic interictal spikes: New knowledge of cortical feedback systems suggests a neurophysiological explanation of brief paroxysms. *Brain Res* 52:1-17, 1973.
29. Matsumoto H, Marsan CA: Cortical cellular phenomena in experimental epilepsy: Interictal manifestations. *Exp Neurol* 9:286-304, 1964.
30. Eleftheriou BE, Zolovick AJ, Norman RL: Effects of amygdaloid lesions on plasma and pituitary levels of luteinizing hormone in the male deermouse. *J Endocrinol* 38:469-474, 1967.
31. Solovick AJ: Effects of lesions and electrical stimulation of the amygdala on hypothalamic-hypophyseal regulation, in Eleftheriou BE (ed): *Neurobiology of the amygdala*. New York, Plenum Press Inc, 1972.
32. Kawakami M, Sawyer CH: Neuroendocrine correlates of changes in brain activity thresholds by sex steroids and pituitary hormones. *Endocrinology* 65:652-668, 1959.
33. Egger MD, Flynn JP: Effects of electrical stimulation of the amygdala on hypothalamically elicited attack behavior in cats. *J Neurophysiol* 26:705-720, 1963.
34. Goddard GV, McIntyre DC, Leech CK: A permanent change in brain function resulting from daily electrical stimulation. *Exp Neurol* 25:295-330, 1969.
35. Wilder BJ, King RL, Schmidt RP: Comparative study of secondary epileptogenesis. *Epilepsia* 9:275-289, 1968.
36. Wilder BJ: Projection phenomena and secondary epileptogenesis: Mirror foci, in Purpura DP, Penry JK, Tower D, et al (eds): *Experimental Models of Epilepsy*. New York, Raven Press, 1972.
37. Belluzi JD, Grossman SP: Avoidance learning: Long-lasting deficits after temporal lobe seizures. *Science* 166:1435-1437, 1969.
38. Falconer MA: Reversibility by temporal-lobe resection of the behavioral abnormalities of temporal-lobe epilepsy. *N Engl J Med* 289:451-455, 1973.
39. Blumer D, Walker AE: Sexual behavior in temporal lobe epilepsy: A study of the effects of temporal lobectomy on sexual behavior. *Arch Neurol* 16:37-43, 1967.
40. Glithero E, Slater E: The schizophrenia-like psychoses of epilepsy: IV. Follow-up record and outcome. *Br J Psychiatry* 109:95-150, 1963.

This study was supported in part by National Institute of Neurological Diseases and Stroke grants NS 06209 and NS 05074.

Figure 3 is reproduced with permission from Neurology (24:629-636, 1974), Copyright The New York Times Media Company, Inc.

# CHAPTER 21

# Introduction to McLean Hospital Journal Supplement

*Norman Geschwind*

## Psychiatric Complications in the Epilepsies: Current Research and Treatment

**A Conference Organized by the McLean Hospital Treatment Center for Psychiatric Disorders in Epilepsy. November 15, 1976**

Dr. Blumer has asked me to make some opening remarks for this session. Let me begin with the following statement which some of you may have heard before. I would like to suggest that the personality changes in temporal lobe epilepsy may in some sense be the single most important condition in psychiatry. Let me try to explain this assertion which, if correct, should justify strongly the attendance at this meeting. "Important" diseases have not necessarily been the most common ones. That there are many illnesses which are extremely frequent but which have not been critical in the advancement of clinical science, I think we would all concede. On the other hand, there have been some rare diseases which have been of major importance because they have opened the way to the study of physiological mechanisms, the understanding of which has had an impact on all the rest of medicine. Let me cite an example of such a disorder which despite its rarity has been of such major importance. Those of us who are in our fifties may recall that when we were in medical school there was an enormous amount of work on Addison's Disease in many centers in the world. Since most physicians will in their medical careers never see a case of Addison's Disease, it certainly might have seemed in the period before 1950 that this great interest in such a rare disorder was inordinate. Yet the great concentration on the elucidation of the

Reprinted with permission from *McLean Hospital Journal, Special Issue*. June, 1977; 6-8.

mechanisms of this clinical curiosity led eventually to the isolation of the adrenal hormones and of ACTH, and to the subsequent clinical application of these substances. It would of course be difficult to state adequately the impact on medicine of ACTH and the steroids. Addison's Disease, although rare, was a model disorder. Although allergic diseases are immeasurably more frequent and cause much more death and disability, it is unlikely that, had the same effort been devoted to the study of asthma, it would have paid off as handsomely as the study of Addison's Disease has.

Temporal lobe epilepsy is not a rare disease. It is a common disorder, and I believe that personality changes with it are not rare, although their exact frequency is still unknown. On the other hand, its major importance does not derive from its frequency, either great or limited. It is the best example that we have at this moment of a disorder which regularly causes changes in personality and in which we have the possibility of working out a mechanism for that change. I would suggest to you that there may be no other condition for which this statement is true at the present moment. We know that an overdose of atropine may lead to paranoia but we do not understand the brain mechanisms which are disturbed. We may say that nearly all antipsychotic drugs are dopamine antagonists and we may even speculate that they are acting at a specific site. These are facts of major importance, but we cannot yet integrate them into our understanding of how the nervous system controls behavior.

Temporal lobe epilepsy is a probe for the study of the physiology of emotion, and opens to us many possibilities for research. We can, in temporal lobe epilepsy, specify the sites of disorder in the nervous system, and we know a great deal about the anatomical connections of these sites, something which we cannot yet do for depression, mania, or schizophrenia. Yet despite this important basic information, I do not believe that careful, controlled pharmacological studies of the effects of phenothiazines, antidepressants, lithium, or of other psychotropic drugs, have ever been carried out in this condition. The fact that ACTH and adrenal steroids, agents whose positive and negative psychotropic effects have been somewhat neglected in recent years, have electrophysiological effects on medial temporal structures, opens further possibilities for study. Furthermore, temporal lobe epilepsy opens the way to study the different emotional specializations of the two halves of the brain, and even the possible specificity of pharmacological agents for one side or the other. I will not list the many other possibilities for investigation provided by this disorder.

Personality change in temporal lobe epilepsy is important, whatever its frequency, as a model disorder. But it may in fact be a very common disorder. Falconer has pointed out that many cases of temporal lobe epilepsy are the result of mesial temporal sclerosis, a lesion which may result from severe and prolonged febrile convulsions in childhood. But since febrile convulsions occur in about 5% of children, the presence of mesial temporal sclerosis even in a small percentage of these cases might mean that there is a large group at risk for temporal lobe epilepsy. Furthermore, I believe that Rosman's recent evidence that childhood autism is often accompanied by medial temporal lesions raises the possibility that the same lesion (perhaps bilateral) underlies many cases of this disorder. It also raises the possibility that study of temporal lobe epilepsy may illuminate our understanding of autism.

Let me make two final points. Research on the effects of temporal lobe epilepsy on behavior has been held up by the wrong questions. We have kept asking the question, "What are the behavior *disorders* associated with temporal lobe epilepsy?" Let me suggest that the proper question is, "What are the behavioral *changes* produced by temporal lobe epilepsy?" It is not always easy to decide whether a change in behavior is beneficial, neutral, or deleterious. When many of the psychiatrists in this room practice "reversible psychosurgery" by using major tranquillizers to block transmission at specific sites in the nervous system, they are producing an organic change in behavior which by social standards might often be judged as good, while other substances might produce effects that are socially disapproved. The fundamental question scientifically is the mechanism of change. A very large number of people with temporal lobe epilepsy may undergo changes in behavior that will not lead them to the psychiatrist or to the lawyer. Yet the mechanisms of these behavioral changes are of major significance.

I would also like to suggest to you that we should be wary of describing these behavioral changes by means of the standard names of other psychiatric conditions. We should treat behavior change in TLE as a phenomenon in its own right. It is probably not reasonable to compare the mechanism of a disease of known pathophysiology to others of different or unknown pathophysiology. I think it is a real possibility that one day we will ask, not "Do the behavioral changes of TLE resemble schizophrenia?" but rather "Are there some aspects of some disorders now called schizophrenia which resemble the changes seen in temporal lobe epilepsy?"

# PART VI

# Other Neurobehavioral Disorders

## *Steven C. Schachter*

Frank Benson had a long and fruitful friendship with Norman Geschwind. Benson maintained that one of Geschwind's most significant strengths was "a distinctly superior grasp of neuroanatomy. He not only used the basic neurologist's knowledge of neuroanatomy but maintained an active interest in anatomic research and carefully studied the areas of structural damage in the relatively few individual patients with language disorders whom he was able to follow to postmortem study."[1] Indeed, Geschwind utilized his knowledge of neuroanatomy in conjunction with careful neurologic examinations in pursuit of his conviction that "every behavior has an anatomy."[2]

This dictum figures prominently in each of the selections in this section. The implications of this viewpoint for psychiatrists,[2,3] pediatric neurologists[4,5] and cognitive scientists[6] are developed by Geschwind in this group of papers. An additional strength of Geschwind that is found in this section is his use of the case report.[5] As Tom Sabin commented, Geschwind "believed that thoroughly studying a single case was more valuable than statistically analyzing a large number of poorly studied cases, and he was fond of citing many instances in which a single case report had resulted in an incremental step forward in neurology. Some of his own case descriptions can be counted among them."[7]

These papers reflect many of Geschwind's attributes that were treasured by his colleagues and students. Some of his former residents and fellows may be initially surprised at his knowledge of aphasia[4] and developmental disorders[5] in children. These papers explore Geschwind's prowess in teaching about aphasia,[4] his grasp of the wide-ranging disciplines intrinsic to cognitive science,[6] his chastisement of an overly simplistic approach to patients with psychiatric illness,[2] and his remarkable overview of a field which we know today as behavioral neurology.[3]

These selections encapsulate many of the concepts that Geschwind conveyed in lecture halls and to scores of trainees. Readers will sample the essence of Geschwind's entertaining, engaging, and educational professorial style, which always emphasized the neurologic exam, underlying neuroanatomy, and above all, respectful consideration for the patient.

## References

1. Benson, DF. Norman Geschwind's influence on the study of aphasia. In SC Schachter and O Devinsky (eds.), *Behavioral Neurology and the Legacy of Norman Geschwind*. Philadelphia: Lippincott-Raven, 1997, pp. 71-78.
2. Geschwind, N. The borderland of neurology and psychiatry: some common misconceptions. In DF Benson and D Blumer (eds.), *Psychiatric Aspects of Neurologic Disease*. New York: Grune & Stratton, 1975, pp. 1-9.
3. Benson, DF, and Geschwind, N. Psychiatric conditions associated with focal lesions of the central nervous system. In MF Reiser (ed.), *Organic Disorders and Psychosomatic Medicine*. New York: Basic Books, 1975, pp. 208-243.
4. Geschwind, N. Disorders of higher cortical function in children. Clin Proc Children's Hosp Natl Med Center, 1972;28,261-272.
5. Benson, DF, and Geschwind, N. Developmental Gerstmann syndrome. Neurology, 1970;20,293-298.
6. Geschwind, N. Neurological knowledge and complex behaviors. Cog Sci, 1980; 4,185-193.
7. Sabin, TD. Colleague. In SC Schachter and O Devinsky (eds.), *Behavioral Neurology and the Legacy of Norman Geschwind*. Philadelphia: Lippincott-Raven, 1997, pp. 21-26.

# CHAPTER 22

# Developmental Gerstmann Syndrome

*D. Frank Benson and Norman Geschwind*

During the past decade increasing interest has been given to the existence of specific learning disorders in children. Childhood dyslexia has been the most studied and discussed of these syndromes, but other varieties of learning disorder have been suggested. This paper will present a well-defined developmental syndrome which can be differentiated from other learning disorders of early life. We will stress, in particular, the absence of dyslexia in this syndrome.

## CASE 1

A 12-year-old boy was referred to the Aphasia Research Center of the Boston University School of Medicine because of threatened school failure. In particular, significant spelling disability jeopardized continued school promotion. He was the oldest child in a family of 4, the 3 younger siblings having no recognized learning difficulty. Both parents were well educated, and the father was a highly successful professional man. Birth and developmental history were entirely without abnormality. He was fully right-handed although the father was left-handed. The patient had attended and performed adequately in both private and public schools; his achievements, however, were considered poor when compared with those of his brother, who was one year younger and rated "near genius" by psychological testing. Spelling difficulty was first recognized in third grade and has persisted despite family and school efforts toward improvement. In striking contrast to the disturbance in spelling, reading ability has always been superior. In a test given in an excellent public school system, he was found to read 360

Reprinted with permission from *Neurology*. 1970; 20 (3): 293-298.

words per minute with 82% comprehension and thus ranked as the best reader in the school system for his age group. At the time of evaluation his reading activities were precocious. He had just finished reading *The Rise and Fall of The Third Reich* and was reading *Silas Marner.* He had read nearly all of the works of Poe, his favorite author. His hobby was stamp collecting but he enjoyed many participation sports including tennis, basketball, swimming, and football. Personal and social adjustments were excellent. Past history included no significant disorders except for two fractures of the right leg, one occurring in a fall down stairs and the other as the result of a skiing accident. In neither accident had there been any significant head injury.

A full neurologic evaluation revealed no abnormality. Coordination was quite normal for age. Muscle tone, reflexes, and sensation were all within normal limits. Eye movements were intact, as were the remainder of the cranial nerves. Testing of recent and remote memory revealed no abnormality. He showed considerable insight, personal interest, and concern, appropriate to the testing situation. Cooperation was excellent.

Spontaneous speech was fluent and well articulated, had good melody, and revealed an exceptionally fine vocabulary. Comprehension of spoken language was tested thoroughly and was normal in all spheres. Similarly, repetition of spoken language was entirely normal. There was no demonstrable defect in word-finding ability. He was able to present lengthy lists of words on suggested topics. During sixty-second periods he named 20 animals, 15 makes of automobiles, and 19 words beginning with the letter B, all superior performances.

In reading aloud, his delivery was rapid and smooth, with only occasional omission of a word, most often a grammatical filler, and no paraphasic substitutions. Comprehension of written language was tested using paragraphs followed with either true-false or multiple choice questions. Some paragraphs were from the *Reader's Digest* and others from a reading aptitude test at high school senior/college freshman level. He had no difficulty with any of this material. In contrast to this ease of reading, there was notable difficulty in writing. His script was fairly legible, with small, clumsy letters. When asked to write sentences describing the weather, the profession of his father, or his route to school, the sentences were simple in structure (almost always subject-verb-object) and the vocabulary was elementary, a striking contrast to his spoken vocabulary. When asked to spell specific words, the writing problem became more manifest. He spelled druggist as "drugest," hospitable as "hospitible," yacht as "yought," and telephone as "telaphone."

He could draw a circle, square, and triangle on command, but when he was asked to draw an animal, he merely drew a wavy line with a small circle at one end and called this a snake. He was unable to show the third dimension when asked to draw a box or a cube. His attempts to copy drawings were crude and also failed to demonstrate the third dimension. He correctly performed the mannequin puzzle but this took forty seconds of concentrated effort. He had great difficulty with Koh's block designs, totally failing elementary four-block designs. If a model was made by the examiner and left in view, he copied it successfully but showed "closing-in phenomena" (i.e., the tendency to bring his copy closer and closer to the model). He was able to differentiate right and left on himself after considerable latency and after cuing himself by moving his right hand. If the examiner sat at 90° from the patient and held up one hand, the patient performed randomly in naming the requested hand. He usually chose correctly if the examiner was directly opposite him but made occasional errors and always showed a long latency. He could name only three fingers but could point to the finger named by the examiner. A simple finger-localization test was given. With one hand behind his back and the other on the table in front of him, one of the fingers on the hidden hand was stimulated by the examiner. The patient consistently failed to move the same finger of the exposed hand as requested. Calculations were done poorly and only at the simple rote-memory level. There was difficulty in column placement in both addition and multiplication problems. All calculations, even those in which he produced a correct answer, were done with effort, hesitancy, and uncertainty.

A full Wechsler Adult Intelligence Scale test was performed, showing a verbal score of 131 and a performance score of 101. The verbal score was uneven and depressed by a very low score in arithmetic, a pattern which suggests an even higher level of accomplishment in purely verbal activities. The family and the school authorities were informed of our findings and suggestions were made to both concerning management of his education. In particular, the school was encouraged to accept oral reports and oral test procedures. When last seen, the patient had not only attained appropriate promotion but was ranked in the upper one-third of his class.

In summary, a 12-year-old boy, referred because of threatened school failure, showed superior oral language function and superior comprehension of written material. He manifested distinct abnormalities in writing, calculating, differentiating right from left, localizing his fingers in space, and constructional tasks. The very high level of performance in other cortical functions contrasted sharply with these five failings, the first four of which make up the Gerstmann syndrome. There was neither history nor clinical evidence of brain injury as a source of this syndrome, suggesting, therefore, a probable developmental etiology.

## CASE 2

A 13-year-old white girl was referred to the Aphasia Research Center after examination by two neurologists. These examinations had been suggested by her school because of difficulty in mathematics, contrasting with adequate performance in other subjects. At the time of examination, she was in seventh grade and passing all courses except mathematics.

The patient was a product of artificial insemination and delivered under careful obstetrical care with no complications. Birth weight was 6 lb. 3 oz. The mother noted considerable weight gain during pregnancy and there was some question of a toxemic state at the time of delivery. The patient remained in an incubator for two days and the mother states that the patient had "blue feet." The developmental milestones were appropriate; she walked at 15 months and is said to have talked at an early age.

Family history concerning the father is unobtainable. The mother admits a lifelong difficulty with mathematics but has been able to work as a cashier in a restaurant. The patient has always preferred the right hand for unilateral activities and there is no family history of left-handedness. While the patient has always been considered awkward, she learned to ride a bicycle and to roller skate proficiently at an appropriate age.

Past history was negative for significant head injuries, major surgery, or serious illnesses. There had been no headaches, convulsions, or other neurological symptomatology. She was examined at an early age for thyroid deficiency but no specific abnormality was demonstrated. She spent one year in a special school because of "behavior difficulties." She was asked to leave because she was "so much better than the other children that she was out of place in that setting." Her school record was satisfactory except for the difficulty in arithmetic. She had been receiving high marks in reading up to the time of the present examination.

Careful neurological examination was performed by three neurologists and no definite abnormalities were observed. Several "soft signs" were noted, however. The most pertinent were slowness and awkwardness in performing rapid alternating movements, present bilaterally but more pronounced on the right, some spooning of the extended right hand, and a slight increase in passive tone in the right extremities. There were no abnormalities in reflexes, sensation, gait, vision, or extraocular movement. Mental status evaluation, exclusive of language, suggested that the patient's fund of knowledge was limited, consisting mostly of material associated with her school activities. Formal memory testing demonstrated an adequate ability to learn new material. She intimated a lack of interest in the examination, but with actual testing she became cooperative and at no time did the examiner feel that she performed indifferently.

Her spontaneous speech was at first sparse, but with time she relaxed and finally spoke quite freely. In testing of serial speech she counted and recited the days of the week without difficulty but had trouble reciting the months of the year. She sang with good melody and words. Comprehension tests, including yes-no questions and requests to point to objects in the room and to perform actions, were all carried out well. She could repeat without difficulty. A digit span of five forward was consistently demonstrated. She could name most objects on confrontation but often had difficulty in naming parts of the objects. Evidently she had not known many of the names of the object parts prior to evaluation. Her performance in naming body parts and colors was below anticipated level. She was, however, able to present a list of 19 animal names in a period of sixty seconds.

She read aloud without difficulty, and comprehension of written material was adequate for her age. While she had difficulty understanding written material at the high-school level, she comprehended adequately below this level. Writing, on the other hand, was grossly abnormal, with large, clumsy script. When asked to write a sentence describing what she was going to do later in the day, she made one grammatical error and badly misspelled one of the words. When words were dictated, she made many spelling errors, some of which were phonetic, while others consisted of omissions or reversals of letters.

Right-left orientation was difficult for the patient. She was usually correct on her own body but only after considerable hesitation. She performed randomly when the examiner sat opposite her and asked her to point to his right or left side. Finger identification was also done poorly. She could name only one of the fingers and point to only two of the fingers when the names were given, a marked contrast to her ability to name other body parts. She failed totally at finger-localization tests. Her competence in calculation was extremely low. She was able to write single digits to dictation but when asked to write numbers in the hundreds or thousands, added extra zeros so that 451 was written as 40051. She correctly performed simple addition problems only by counting on her fingers. More complex addition problems were not worked and she was never able to perform subtraction problems. Marked difficulty was seen in construction tests. She put the mannequin puzzle together incorrectly in thirty seconds and was satisfied with the result. She could not perform any of the Koh's block designs unless a model was made for her to copy.

Psychological testing (WAIS) demonstrated a low IQ. The verbal IQ was registered at 79 with the performance IQ at 75. These scores were depressed by the subtests involving arithmetic and construction. It was considered that she could be placed in the dull-normal range if these specially affected areas were omitted.

Following this examination, contact was made with the school authorities and arrangements were made to obviate some of the more significant difficulties. On this basis, she has maintained status in the appropriate class, is doing work satisfactory to the school system and, apparently, will continue education through high school.

In summary, this patient had a learning problem which was noted in the school as a specific difficulty in mathematics. Both clinical impression and psychological testing show a generally dull girl. Evaluation of cortical function revealed the components of the Gerstmann syndrome (right-left disorientation, finger agnosia, dysgraphia, and severe calculation disturbance) plus constructional apraxia. These disabilities apparently accounted for most of her scholastic difficulties. In contrast, oral language and ability to read were at a much higher level. The lack of pertinent neurologic history suggests that this is a developmental defect, although evidence for this is not as strong as in Case 1. Corrective measures within the school have allowed her to continue in an adequate educational program.

## Discussion

The above cases had 5 striking abnormalities: dyscalculia, dysgraphia, right-left disorientation, finger agnosia, and constructional apraxia, of which the first four make up the well-known Gerstmann syndrome. In a series of papers,[1–3] Gerstmann described patients with this clinical combination, noted consistent dominant parietal pathology, and theorized that this symptom combination resulted from a partial autotopagnosia, a defect in recognition of one's own body. Other neurologists soon described cases with similar disorders, confirmed the predominant site of abnormality, but disagreed on the theoretical considerations. Thus, one group[4] suggested apraxia involving the fingers as the basic deficit; others[5,6] suggested a disturbance of spatial orientation, particularly orientation of the body in external space. All agreed on the occurrence of the syndrome and the consistency of dominant parietal pathology, and the Gerstmann syndrome became an accepted tool of neurologic localization.

More recently the existence of the syndrome has been questioned. Heimburger et al.[7] showed that a single symptom from the tetrad could be seen in cases with small lesions located anywhere. All four findings were present only in cases with extensive cerebral damage, invariably accompanied by other symptoms and involving the dominant parietal cortex in about 90%. Benton and co-workers conducted careful studies over many years.[8,9] They showed that the individual components were usually accompanied by other functional abnormalities and failed to demonstrate a high correlation between the four components. Benton concluded that the Gerstmann syndrome was an artifact of biased testing and represented only a chance grouping of symptoms among many produced by a large lesion. In a smaller study, Poeck and Orgass[10] reached similar conclusions and found a high frequency of dysphasia in their cases, suggesting that the Gerstmann tetrad was a manifestation of an actual or latent aphasic condition. Despite the doubts cast on the interpretation of the syndrome, it remains clear that a dominant parietal lesion is probable when all four components are present.

While the interpretation of the adult form of this syndrome may be controversial, the syndrome is not rare. In contrast, there are very few reports of the Gerstmann syndrome in children. Critchley[11] credits a case described by Spillane[12] as the original description of the Gerstmann findings on a developmental basis. Hermann and Norrie,[13] in a study of dyslexic (word-blind) children, noted an increased frequency of difficulty in right-left orientation and finger discrimination but did not mention the other components. They suggested that the dyslexia was developmental and that the Gerstmann syndrome components were part of the same underlying abnormality and concluded that dyslexia was a congenital manifestation of the Gerstmann syndrome. Kinsbourne and Warrington[14] reported 7 children who demonstrated 3 or more of the Gerstmann components, most often associated with other neurological disability. All demonstrated a characteristic pattern on the WAIS, with the verbal score being considerably higher (from 20 to 35 points) than the performance score. The authors considered this a developmental variant of the Gerstmann syndrome which could be either constitutional or posttraumatic, could exist alone or with other neurologic symptomatology, and could cause reading and writing retardation. In a later review, Kinsbourne[15] described this condition as a developmental cognitive deficit which could result from either localized cerebral dysfunction or maturational lag. He again noted reading retardation as a possible accompanying symptom.

Kinsbourne and Warrington noted, however, that serious dyslexia could occur without Gerstmann symptomatology and, conversely, normal reading ability is a possibility in some patients with the full Gerstmann tetrad (one of their cases was an exceptional reader). They concluded that, while the two abnormalities might coexist and influence each other, they should be considered separate disturbances.

The patients presented in this report have all four components of the Gerstmann syndrome plus constructional apraxia. Many authors have noted that constructional apraxia commonly accompanies the Gerstmann syndrome and could be considered an additional component.

We believe that all of the symptoms present in the two patients reported here can be attributed to these five abnormalities. Case 1 demonstrates this most distinctly, an otherwise highly intelligent boy with considerable disability in writing, calculation, and constructional tasks and demonstrable abnormalities in finger discrimination and right-left orientation. To the best of our knowledge, there is no previous report of developmental dysfunction showing the components of the Gerstmann tetrad in an individual of such superior verbal intelligence and, in particular, superior reading ability. This contrast dramatically highlights the specific disabilities producing the depressed Wechsler performance score and serious scholastic difficulties. The second case is less clearcut, but a review of the findings demonstrates that the Gerstmann syndrome deficits are significantly more severe than her other shortcomings. It seem likely that Case 2, with apparent intellectual deficiency overshadowing the specific deficits, may be afflicted with a fairly common variety of learning disorder.

These cases clearly demonstrate that the Gerstmann syndrome variety of learning disability may exist quite independently from dyslexia. Case 1 was an exceptional reader, well above grade level despite serious limitations in both writing and calculation. Even Case 2 had much greater success in reading than in either writing or arithmetic. Thus, in these two cases of developmental Gerstmann syndrome, dyslexia is notably absent. Nonetheless, these children have a disorder which can be classed with the specific learning disorders, both subjects performing far below grade level in selected activities. We would suggest that the developmental Gerstmann syndrome represents a specific learning difficulty which can be easily differentiated from dyslexia. We would stress, also, that severe difficulties in writing and spelling can occur without difficulty in reading. Such cases may be common and erroneously called dyslexic because of the difficulties in spelling and writing.

Very little can be stated concerning the pathology underlying these two cases. Both children are healthy and have no other obvious neurologic abnormality or any history suggesting perinatal or postnatal cerebral disease. In this way, they differ from the cases reported by Kinsbourne and Warrington,[14] of whom 5 had obviously sustained perinatal trauma, 1 had suffered severe septicemia as an infant, and 1 showed considerable accompanying neurologic and behavioral abnormality. The present cases appear to be examples of developmental abnormality, but whether this represents a maturational lag, as suggested by Kinsbourne,[15] can only be answered by additional follow-up. The accepted pathology underlying Gerstmann syndrome in the adult cannot necessarily be attributed to developmental cases. In a recent report, Money[16] noted a frequent difference in verbal and performance subscores in patients with Turner's syndrome (chromosome count 45, X0, female characteristics). In a significant majority, he noted a higher verbal subscore (median, 104.6) than performance (median, 87.6). Unfortunately, the author makes no reference to components of the Gerstmann syndrome or to reading ability in this group. Neither of our patients has this specific genetic abnormality, but the possibility of the existence of some other genetic abnormality can be considered.

Clinically, the developmental Gerstmann syndrome is fairly distinct. Appropriate testing of reading, writing, arithmetic, and constructional skills and attention to right-left orientation and finger discrimination offers a clear picture. A strong difference in WAIS scores, with the verbal score highest, has been seen in most of these cases. Probably there are many cases similar to the two described here which are presently mislabeled as either dyslexia or mental retardation; appropriate testing could place them in the correct diagnostic category.

The desirability of making this diagnosis is apparent from the results in these two cases. Minimal environmental manipulation at home and in school produced beneficial results in both cases. Case 1 rose to the upper one-third of his class after he was allowed to give oral rather than written reports, and his course schedule was shifted to take advantage of his superior reading ability. Case 2 has not done as well, but similar school manipulation has allowed her to remain with her class and there is promise of accomplishing high school graduation. In both situations, informing the school officials of scholastic strengths as well as defects allowed alteration of educational activities to offer maximum opportunity for learning. Just as significant was the psychological benefit obtained by outlining the defect to the families. In both cases, the presence of a specific learning disorder was acceptable and the ensuing support offered to the children was distinctly beneficial.

## Summary

We have presented two cases with an apparent developmental mental syndrome. We call this Gerstmann syndrome because of the presence of the classical tetrad of right-left disorientation, finger agnosia, agraphia, and acalculia. Reading ability was strikingly preserved in both cases. That the findings in these cases actually represent some underlying disorder (i.e., disordered spatial orientation, defective body image, or visuomotor apraxia) is quite possible, but until additional cases have been investigated and fuller explanations are available, we suggest they simply be considered examples of a developmental Gerstmann syndrome.

## References

1. Gerstmann, J.: Fingeragnosie: Eine um schriebene Störung der Orienterung am eigenen Körper, Wien. klin. Wschr. 31:1010, 1924.
2. Gerstmann, J.: Fingeragnosie und isolierte Agraphie, ein neues Syndrom. Z. ges. Neurol. Psychiat. 108:152, 1927.
3. Gerstmann, J.: Zur Symptomatologie der Hirnläsionen im Uebergangsgebeit der unteren Parietal- und mittleren Occipitalwindung. Nervenarzt 3:691, 1931.
4. Hermann, G., and Pötzl, O.: Ueber die Agraphie und Ihre lokaldiagnostischen Beziehungen. Berlin: S. Karger, 1926.
5. Lange, J.: Fingeragnosie und Agraphie. Mschr. Psychiat. Neurol. 76:129, 1930.
6. Stengel, E.: Loss of spatial orientation, constructional apraxia and Gerstmann's syndrome. J. ment. Sci. 90:753, 1944.
7. Heimburger, R., Demyer, W., and Reitan, R.: Implications of Gerstmann's syndome. J. Neurol. Neurosurg. Psychiat. 27:52, 1964.
8. Benton, A.: Right-Left Discrimination and Finger Localization: Development and Pathology. New York: P. B. Hoeber, Inc., 1959.
9. Benton, A.: The fiction of the "Gerstmann syndrome." J. Neurol. Neurosurg. Psychiat. 24:176, 1961.
10. Poeck, K., and Orgass, B.: Gerstmann's syndrome and aphasia. Cortex 2:421, 1966.
11. Critchley, M.: The Parietal Lobes. Baltimore: Williams & Wilkins Co., 1953.
12. Spillane, J.: Disturbances of the body scheme, anosognosia and finger agnosia. Lancet 1:42, 1942.
13. Hermann, K., and Norrie, E.: Is congenital word-blindness a hereditary type of Gerstmann's syndrome? Psychiat. et Neurol. (Basel) 136:59, 1958.
14. Kinsbourne, M., and Warrington, E.: The developmental Gerstmann syndrome. Arch. Neurol. (Chic.) 8:490, 1963.
15. Kinsbourne, M.: Developmental Gerstmann syndrome. Pediat. Clin. N. Amer. 15:771, 1968.
16. Money, J.: Two cytogenetic syndromes: Psychologic considerations. J. psychiat. Res. 2:223, 1964.

This study was supported in part by grant NB-06209 from the National Institute of Neurological Disease and Blindness to Boston University School of Medicine.

# CHAPTER 23

# Disorders of Higher Cortical Functions in Acute Confusional States

*Francois Chédru and Norman Geschwind*

The effects of focal cerebral lesions on language, memory, praxis, visual recognition, visuo-spatial organization, in other words, on all of those behavioral functions generally called the higher cortical functions (H.C.F.), have been studied extensively during the past one hundred years. On the other hand, comparatively little detailed attention has been given to the H.C.F. following diffuse brain lesions and in particular the acute confusional states (A.C.S.).

Lipowski (1967) recently pointed out that no definition of "confusion," "altered states of consciousness," "delirium," or "acute brain syndrome" was universally acceptable. We will not discuss these problems of terminology but will describe what we considered, for the purposes of our study, the principal features of an A.C.S. To us, the main characteristic is a reduction and/or an erratic shifting of attention. Other symptoms occur frequently but are not essential for the diagnosis; these include slowness and sluggishness of response, disorientation for time and space, changes in mood, hallucinations and bilateral slow activity in the E.E.G. The patient in A.C.S. can be lethargic and hypoactive or the opposite, hyperactive and agitated. A.C.S. may appear in head injury, subarachnoid hemorrhage, rapidly increased intracranial pressure, drug intoxication, withdrawal syndromes, acute infections, uremia, hepatic failure, and other types of metabolic disorder. The type of pathogenic agent involved appears to have very little bearing on the clinical picture of A.C.S. (Bonhoeffer, 1912).

In his book on the "symptomatic psychoses," Bonhoeffer mentioned the existence of disorders of writing, of paraphasias, and of ideational apraxia in

Reprinted with permission from Cortex, Masson, S.P.A., Vol. VIII, 1972, pp. 395–411 some patients in A.C.S. Since Bonhoeffer, the rare neuropsychological studies relating to A.C.S. have concerned themselves with certain aspects of language disorder (Curran and Schilder, 1935), temporo-spatial disorientation (Paterson and Zangwill, 1944), the denial of illness (Weinstein and Kahn, 1952a, 1952b), and Gerstmann's syndrome (Juba, 1948; Benton and Abramson, 1952). No study, however, has dealt with the ensemble of alterations of the H.C.F. during A.C.S. We have undertaken such a study for two reasons: first, to attempt to deal with the many questions raised by clinical neurologists regarding the A.C.S.; and second, to try to evaluate from a neuropsychological point of view the relative fragility of the various H.C.F.

This report deals with the results of a neuropsychological evaluation of 24 subjects both during and after an A.C.S. In this way each subject served as his own control. An additional comparison was made between these subjects and a group of normal control subjects.

## Methods

### Subjects

*Pathological groups* The following requirements were set:

a. Reduction and/or shifting of attention of recent onset related to a well-defined toxic or metabolic disorder. The attention disorder was evaluated on the basis of clinical examination.
b. Absence of signs of focal brain lesions and of medical history data pointing to a chronic intellectual deterioration.
c. Age below 60 years.
d. Ability to carry out the test battery. This last condition resulted in our ruling out the most severely confused patients.

Three groups were studied: 1. Patients presenting with "natural A.C.S." (cases 1 to 12); 2. Patients recovering from electroshock therapy (E.C.T.) session (cases 13 to 22); 3. Patients with experimental A.C.S. (cases 23 and 24); the 2 subjects of the third group were, throughout the interview, under the effect of an I.V. barbiturate perfusion which was being given for the induction of surgical anesthesia.

Characteristics of the 24 subjects in regard to age, educational background and etiology are shown in Table 1.

*The control group* These subjects were patients on the internal medical wards who met the criteria (b), (c) and (d) mentioned above and were not confused. No attempt was made to exclude alcoholics. This group was comparable to the pathological patients in regard to age and educational background.

**Procedure**

The neuropsychological examination consisted of the following:

1. The *evaluation of mood*, of *psychomotor activity*, of the subject's *concern* for his *illness* and also of the presence of *confabulations* and *hallucinations*.
2. Ten questions about *orientation* in time and space.
3. Two tests of *attention:* (a) digit span; (b) a test of auditory-motor attention (AMA) based on tests originally developed by Kornetsky, Mirsky, Kessler and Dorff (1959). Letters are presented orally in a random order at a rate of 1 per second; the subject is requested to raise his hand each time he hears the letter A (i.e., 20 times in 80 seconds). The score is based on omissions of A.
4. A study of *language:* (a) spontaneous language. The subject is requested to speak about his job; then he is asked to describe what he would do to change a flat tire; (b) naming: 15 items (5 hospital related, 5 body parts and 5 non-hospital related objects); (c) word list test: listing of names of animals as rapidly as possible. The score is the total number of different animals listed at the end of 1 minute; (d) oral spelling: 4 words; (e) comprehension: 3 orders using grammatical words, similar to commands in the Token test, 3 complex questions using the passive form, the possessive and the comparative form; (f) repetition: 4 sentences; (g) reading: 4 sentences; (h) writing: writing on command and to dictation, and copying of a sentence.

   The verbal output of the subject was recorded on a tape recorder and transcribed.
5. An evaluation of *right-left orientation:* (a) on the subject himself; (b) on the examiner; (c) with the examiner's hands crossed and his fingers interlaced.
6. An evaluation of *finger recognition:* (a) pointing to fingers on command; (b) localization on the subject's own contralateral hand and the examiner's hand of a finger of the other hand, this hand being held behind the subject.
7. *Three simple arithmetical problems:* one addition, one subtraction, one multiplication using 2 digit numbers.
8. *Copying* of a cube and 2 designs from the Bender-Gestalt test.
9. The study of *praxis:* (a) bucco-facial; (b) symbolic movements (e.g., a military salute); (c) transitive movements representing the use of an object (e.g., pretend to use a hammer, a comb) without object; (d) prolonged sequential activity with object manipulation.
10. *The Test of Head:* the subject was asked to imitate non-representational movements performed by the examiner (e.g., pointing to his right ear with his left hand).

11. A study of *visual recognition:* (a) description of the pictures used for the naming test; (b) recognition of hidden figures (Poppelreuter test).
12. *Memory:* (a) remote memory: 6 questions on general information; (b) recent memory: ability to recall 3 words after 10 minutes.
13. Two tests which are considered to evaluate "*Abstract thought*": (a) 6 similarities from the Wechsler-Bellevue test; (b) 5 proverb interpretations with multiple choice (taken from Gorham's Proverbs test).

Except for the word-list test, there was no time limit on any of the tests.

It required approximately 20 minutes for a normal subject to complete the whole test battery. For a confused subject the time required was from 40 to 60 minutes.

The test protocol was presented to the subjects of the second group in several sessions because the A.C.S. following E.C.T. was generally of a short duration.

The order of presentation of tests was randomized for the different patients.

The scoring criteria are summarized in an Appendix at the end of the paper.

## Results

### Quantitative data

The results obtained by the 24 subjects in A.C.S. and out of A.C.S. are shown in Tables 1, 2, and 3. These results can be summarized as follows:

1. 6 of the tests were carried out very poorly during A.C.S. by a large majority of subjects. These tests were: temporo-spatial orientation, the two tests of attention, writing, the word-list test, and the test of Head.
2. 9 tests demonstrated deficits during A.C.S. which were both less severe and less frequent than those in the first category. These tests included: tests of reading and of repetition, of naming, of right-left orientation, of finger recognition, of calculation, of drawing, and of memory, both recent and remote.
3. The rest of the tests showed almost no deficit during A.C.S. These remaining tests included tests of spontaneous speech, comprehension, oral spelling, praxis, visual recognition, and the two tests of abstract thought. Disturbances observed on the tests of spontaneous speech, praxis, and visual recognition were often too mild to be considered abnormal.

The disturbances observed during the A.C.S. were either not seen again or were present with less severity during the second examination following recovery from the A.C.S. Some alterations were to be found mainly in the "natural A.C.S." group, on the following tasks: writing (spelling disorder), word-list test, oral spelling, the test of Head, drawing. In the cases in which these disturbances persisted, we could not be sure if this was due to a minimal and persistent confusion or to an underlying brain lesion.

TABLE 1. Characteristics of the 24 Confused Patients

| *Case no.* | *Age* | *Education* | *Etiology* | *Clinical picture* | *Behavior* | *Disorient.* | *Auditory motor attention* | *Digit span* |
|---|---|---|---|---|---|---|---|---|
| 1 | 42 | III | DT | ACD, GI Bleeding | Ag, Den, Conf | +++ (+) | 0 (0) | ++ (++) |
| 2 | 49 | II | Hep. E. | ACD, PN, Cirrhosis | Leth, Ag | ++ (0) | 0 (0) | ++ (+) |
| 3 | 49 | I | DT | PN, Pneumonia | Leth, Ag | ++ (+) | + (+) | 0 (0) |
| 4 | 52 | III | Hep. E. | PN | Den, Conf | +++ (0) | 0 (0) | + (0) |
| 5 | 40 | I | DT | PN | Leth | + (0) | +++ (++) | + (0) |
| 6 | 49 | III | DT | Cirrhosis | Hall, Den, Conf | +++ (0) | +++ (0) | + (++) |
| 7 | 39 | I | DT | Cirrhosis, PN | Leth | ++ (+) | + (0) | ++ (0) |
| 8 | 53 | I | Wer. E. | Cirrhosis | Leth | ++ (0) | + (+) | 0 (0) |
| 9 | 37 | III | Hep. E. | PN, Acute Liver Dis. | Normal | + (0) | + (0) | +++ (0) |
| 10 | 39 | II | DT | ACD, PN, Cirrhosis | Leth | + (0) | + (0) | 0 (0) |
| 11 | 38 | II | Phenobarbital Intoxication | | Leth | ++ (0) | +++ (+) | ++ (0) |
| 12 | 43 | I | DT | Head Trauma | Leth | ++ (+) | + (+) | 0 (0) |
| 13 | 43 | I | ECT | Psy. Dep. | Leth | ++ (0) | NT | NT |
| 14 | 24 | III | ECT | Schizophrenia | Leth | ++ (0) | NT | NT |
| 15 | 41 | I | ECT | Psy. Dep. | Leth | ++ (0) | NT | NT |
| 16 | 59 | II | ECT | Psy. Dep. | Leth | 0 (0) | NT | NT |
| 17 | 27 | III | ECT | Psy. Dep. | Leth | ++ (0) | NT | NT |
| 18 | 52 | II | ECT | Psy. Dep. | Leth | 0 (0) | NT | NT |
| 19 | 60 | III | ECT | Psy. Dep. | Leth | 0 (0) | NT | NT |
| 20 | 57 | III | ECT | Psy. Dep. | Leth | + (0) | NT | NT |
| 21 | 51 | II | ECT | Psy. Dep. | Leth | ++ (0) | NT | NT |
| 22 | 55 | I | ECT | Psy. Dep. | Leth | ++ (0) | NT | NT |
| 23 | 44 | I | G. Anes. | Herniated Disk | Leth | ++ (0) | + (0) | NT |
| 24 | 37 | III | G. Anes. | Muscle Disease | Leth | ++ (0) | + (0) | NT |

Educational levels were defined as follows: I = subjects with no high school education; II = subjects who had one or more years in high school, but did not graduate; III = high school graduates. DT = delirium tremens. The DT patients were in subacute DT except in case 6 where the DT was acute; Wer. E. = Wernicke encephalopathy; Hep. E. = hepatic encephalopathy; ECT = electroconvulsive therapy; G. Anes. = general anesthesia; ACD = alcoholic cerebellar degeneration; PN = peripheral neuropathy; Psy. Dep. = psychotic depression. Ag. = agressive; Den. = denial of illness; Conf. = confabulations; Leth. = lethargic; Hall. = hallucinations. NT = not tested. In parenthesis are the figures related to the 2nd examination (out of A.C.S.). See Appendix for scoring criteria.

TABLE 2. Performances of A.C.S. Subjects on Some Language-related Tests (Average Degree of Alterations and Number of Ss Demonstrating Abnormal Scores)

| | *Spontaneous speech* | *Naming* | *Word-list* | *Oral spelling* | *Compre-hension* | *Repetition* | *Reading* | *Writing (motor)* | *Writing (spelling)* |
|---|---|---|---|---|---|---|---|---|---|
| Mean impair-ment score | Within normal limits | 0.75 (0.04) | 1.58 (0.50) | 0.46 (0.29) | 0.21 (0.00) | 0.50 (0.00) | 1.08 (0.16) | 1.75 (0.13) | 1.67 (0.30) |
| Percentage of *Ss* performing abnormally | 0 | 50 (4) | 92 (42) | 37 (21) | 12 (0) | 46 (0) | 75 (17) | 92 (12) | 92 (21) |

The impairment score was obtained by assigning 1 to the (+) alteration, 2 to the (++) alteration and 3 to the (+++) alteration, 0 to the normal performances. Mean was computed for the 24 *Ss*. In parentheses are the figures obtained on the 2nd examination (out of A.C.S.).

TABLE 3. Performances of A.C.S. Subjects on Other Aspects of H.C.F.

| | *Right-left orientation* | *Test of Head* | *Finger recognition* | *Calcu-lation* | *Drawing* | *Remote memory* | *Recent memory* | *Similar-ities* | *Proverbs* | *Visual recognition* | *Praxis* |
|---|---|---|---|---|---|---|---|---|---|---|---|
| Mean impair-ment score | 1.08 (0.08) | 2.21 (0.71) | 1.29 (0.08) | 0.87 (0.20) | 1.50 (0.37) | 1.29 (0.29) | 1.54 (0.40) | 0.29 (0.05) | 0.33 (0.16) | Within normal limits[1] | Within normal limits[2] |
| Percentage of *Ss* performing abnormally | 62 (8) | 96 (42) | 58 (8) | 62 (8) | 71 (29) | 64 (18) | 54 (17) | 20 (5) | 20 (10) | | |

See Table 2 for scoring methods.

[1] Mild difficulties on Poppelreuter test.

[2] Use of BPO responses.

The general pattern of the deficits in the 3 different groups was, except for minor variations, quite similar. In the E.C.T. group, the disorders of memory were more marked and disturbances of naming and calculation were less marked.

## Qualitative data

### *Modification of behavior, orientation, and attention*

Most of the *S*s were lethargic. They were strikingly docile and suggestible. Jocularity, similar to the "Witzelsucht" seen in bifrontal disorders, as well as perseveration, were not rare. Mild lack of concern for the illness was the rule. In 3 cases, we observed a complete denial of illness with confabulations quite similar to that reported by Weinstein and Kahn (1952a, 1952b).

Disorientation was especially striking for time (for the day and the month more than for the year). The general tendency was to name a date prior to the date of the interview. When asked to name the location where the current interview was taking place, the patient often gave the name of another hospital situated close to his own home. This type of disorder has been commented on extensively by Weinstein and Kahn (1952a, 1952b). Sometimes he would state that he was either at his own home or at a hotel. It should be noted that responses such as: "I don't know!" were rare for questions regarding orientation, although they were quite frequent for other tasks, for instance naming or memory tests.

The two tests of attention, when they could be evaluated, were in general perturbed, occasionally in isolation from each other.

### *Language*

Verbal production was often "*slurred*": reduction of verbal fluency, alteration of intonation and tonality, often with a monotone, diminution of speech amplitude, and imprecise pronunciation.

*Spontaneous language* was studied especially in groups 1 and 3; in group 2 the degree of verbal fluency was too low for precise study.

The general impression was of normal language. Nonetheless, we were able to note certain peculiarities: (a) Verbal and phonemic "slips of the tongue" were a little more frequent than were seen in normal subjects. (b) Distinct word-finding difficulties were seen, as demonstrated by hesitations, repetitions, circumlocutions or use of one verb for another, especially a vague common word, in place of a more precise low frequency word (e.g., "then I'd . . . then I'd . . . I'd get the bolts . . . loosen the bolts . . . then I loosen the bolts . . . well naturally I'd have the jack into . . . under . . . on under the car . . .").

*Pattern of speech.* The pattern of speech was poorly organized. Its poorly structured aspect was similar to the phenomenon of "parenthetisation" and of "complementation" described by Hécaen, Dubois, and Marcie (1967): a sentence would be interrupted in the middle and another idea produced; suddenly an expression of emotion, for no apparent reason, would appear as if it were "in parentheses"; in addition, the meaning of a sentence could be modified by another sentence beginning with a transition word: "but," "or," "if," or "because."

Despite the area of similarity, the spontaneous language of these subjects in A.C.S. could not be interpreted as similar in all respects to the language of an aphasic subject. Nonetheless there are certain areas of overlap with the language of anomic aphasics.

*Naming.* The naming disorders never resulted in paraphasias except for subject 6. The subjects sought the word with great effort and finally admitted that they did not remember. These disturbances were present for words of low frequency, that is less than 10 per million (on the Thorndike-Lorge Word Count). No difference was noted between the names of objects relating to the hospital, other objects, and of body parts, except for subject 6 who consistently misnamed the items relating to the hospital, thus demonstrating the type of misnaming described by Weinstein and Kahn (1952a, 1952b).

*Reading and repetition.* Both reading and repetition resulted in rare but consistent verbal paraphasias which resembled each other. The word selected in place of the stimulus word, in general, had the following characteristics: it was an English word; it was generally of high frequency (the word, for which a paraphasic substitute was given, was often of low frequency); there were phonemic, and sometimes semantic, similarities to the stimulus word. The sentence retained its grammatical structure, but often lost all meaning, leaving the impression that the subject was paying little attention to the meaning of what he was saying.

Again subject 6 was unique in that he began to produce "jargon" (e.g., he read "the barn swallow captured a plump worm" as "the barn swallow featured a plu . . . a plum working New-Hamshire plum word hand . . . a barn swallow charged the plumber six dollars and work eight million dollars . . . J, H, K, A, L, L, O, M . . . captured a plumgered a plane a plum worth . . . catchin . . . a plum woman who had the fal plump . . .")

*Writing.* Writing was almost always quite defective in its various aspects: motor output (the letters were poorly drawn), spatial organization (the alignment of letters and words was bad), linguistic content (the number of spelling errors was 2 to 3 times those seen in the controls). These disorders are being discussed in detail in another paper (Chédru and Geschwind, 1972).

*Comprehension.* There was virtually no disturbance of comprehension. This may not have been due to the simplicity of the test.

*Word-list.* Disturbance on this test was marked and appeared to be highly correlated with disturbances of attention, i.e., to the AMA Score ($r = 0.57$; $df = 20$; $p < .05$).[1] We consider this disturbance as a good indicator of global mental sluggishness.

[1]The correlation has been calculated for *Ss* 1 to 12 and for 10 other subjects in A.C.S. (natural) who were not included in this study since they had been studied only once (in A.C.S.).

*Right-left orientation*

Disturbances of right-left orientation were seen as hesitation and, in 10 cases, as errors on the examiner.

*Finger recognition*

In finger recognition, hesitations were frequent. In 8 subjects, gross errors were found on the localization test.

*Calculation*

The most frequent calculation errors were those involving the arithmetical procedure of "carry over." In 5 *S*s (with low educational background) the mathematical rule itself seemed to have been forgotten.

*Drawing*

The drawing tests were very frequently carried out poorly. Four subjects were able only to scribble. In those who were able to draw, the following types of abnormalities were noted: (a) wavy lines, reduplication of lines, overlap of lines, or separation of two elements which were contiguous on the model; (b) alteration in the proportions and orientation: the drawings produced by the patients were in general smaller than the model; oblique lines were transformed into horizontal or vertical lines; (c) on the cube there was frequently a loss of three-dimensionality, the *S*s being satisfied with the drawing of a square or a rectangle (but such performances were not rare in the controls). Omission of angles and lines was frequent. Following recovery from the A.C.S., the *S*s performed the drawing tasks better. This improvement was, however, generally incomplete for the drawing of the cube.

All 4 components of the Gerstmann syndrome (i.e., writing difficulty, right-left disorder, disorder of calculation, difficulties in finger localization) were present in 2 subjects in group 2. The disturbances on the drawing test were most marked in those subjects, who had most, or all, of the elements of the Gerstmann syndrome.

*Praxis*

When a subject was asked to demonstrate the use of an object, not being present, he might use a body part to represent the object (BPO responses). Thus the fist was used as a hammer, the index finger as a toothbrush, etc . . . This phenomenon has been described in aphasic subjects (Goodglass and Kaplan, 1963) and in children (Kaplan, 1967). Sometimes the hand was in a correct holding position but was in contact with the body part towards which it was directed, for example, in contact with the cheek in the simulated use of a razor (H + BPO responses). H + BPO responses, on a developmental level, are found to be an intermediary step between BPO responses and correct responses. The rate of BPO and H + BPO responses was significantly higher in 21 patients in A.C.S. Following recovery from A.C.S. patients still demonstrated some abnormalities, particularly H + BPO responses. No other praxic abnormalities were noted.

*Test of Head*

The Test of Head was poorly performed in 23 cases. There were 3 types of error: (a) mirroring of the examiner's movement (e.g., instead of putting his right hand on his left ear, the *S* put his left hand on his right ear); (b) mirroring of the hand but not of the goal of the movement (e.g., left hand on left ear for the movement described above); (c) mirroring of the goal of the movement but with the correct hand (e.g., right hand on right ear). Errors of types (b) and type (c) were the most frequent.

These results may represent an inability to perform a spatial rotation and perhaps also a disturbance of the ability to cross the midline. A recent developmental study has shown that this type of test is in general not correctly carried out until 14 years of age (Wapner and Cirillo, 1968).

*Visual recognition*

The hidden figures test was poorly carried out by 10 subjects, but the accurate description of the pictures used in this test indicate that visual recognition was not a problem.

*Memory*

Tests of recent memory were poorly performed. Since our controls were in the main alcoholics, we may well have underestimated the degree of these alterations in Table 3. Remote memory was more severely affected in group 2 than in the other subjects.

*Similarities*

Similarities and proverb interpretations were very little affected. The rare modifications were always minor, involving no more than 1 out of 6 similarities and 1 out of 5 proverbs.

Throughout all the tasks, the patients in A.C.S. were inattentive and easily distractible. The orders had to be repeated twice or more. Answers were slow. The overall impression was one of "general sluggishness." This sluggishness expressed itself in the length of the interviews of the confused *S*s. Scores would have been very low if time limits had been set for the tasks.

## Discussion

In this study, the following abnormalities appear with relative constancy during A.C.S.

*General disturbances:* disturbances of mood and behavior, disorientation, modification of attitude of concern toward the illness. Although it was not quantitated, slowness, as noted above, was a striking feature of these patients.

*Language disturbances:* mild word finding difficulties, tendency toward verbal paraphasias in repetition and reading tests, slowing of verbal fluency, difficulties in organizing spontaneous speech, and a marked dysgraphia.

*Other cortical function disturbances:* mild spatial disturbances (right-left disorientation and defect on the test of Head), constructional disorder, disturbances in finger recognition, calculation, memory defect. In addition, mild disturbances in visual recognition and minor abnormalities of gestures were found.

We have not observed a deterioration of capabilities on the two tests of "abstract thought." This result is in disagreement with the observations of Curran and Schilder (1935), Paterson (1942), and Zangwill (1945), who reported difficulty in abstraction as well as bizarre ideation in acute confusions. However, the A.C.S. these authors described, were posttraumatic; it is possible that such posttraumatic A.C.S. may be associated with an underlying focal cerebral contusion (frontal or temporal). It must, of course, also be considered as a possibility that some of the more severe patients, whom we excluded because they could not take our battery, might have shown such disorders.

The range of dysfunctions of the H.C.F. was thus limited. We would like to point out those symptoms which we never observed during an A.C.S.: Broca's aphasia, Wernicke's aphasia, pure word deafness, cortical blindness, visual agnosia, severe ideational or ideomotor apraxia.

The results presented here may be considered from a practical point of view. They may aid the clinical neurologist, confronted with a patient with an A.C.S., in avoiding the following errors: (a) the assumption that only a focal cerebral lesion can produce a disturbance of H.C.F., which might lead to the search for a focal lesion which may not be present; (b) the assumption that an A.C.S. can produce any kind of neuropsychological signs, which might lead to the neglect of true focal signs.

The study reported here represents an initial and somewhat gross attempt to systematize the syndrome of A.C.S. It is difficult, at this point, to attempt a systematic interpretation of such a polymorphic syndrome. The following represents an initial tentative step toward such an interpretation.

The alterations in the H.C.F. seen in this study may be considered to be the expression of two types of disturbance:

1. A disorder in which the primary abnormality consists of disturbances in vigilance, in attention, and in retrieval, and could lead to the impression one has of "general mental sluggishness." It would be tempting to attribute these to disorders of subcortical mechanism, in particular, those of the reticular activating system, which is known, for example, to be very sensitive to barbiturates. We cannot exclude at this moment, however, the alternative possibility that these disorders may result from the primary impairment of cortical regions specifically related to these subcortical mechanisms.

2. Another group of disturbances appears at first glance to be suggestive of cortical impairments, in particular spatial disturbances, constructional disorder, difficulties in writing, reading and repetition, and emotional changes. It is conceivable that the regions most involved are the angular gyrus and pre-frontal regions, areas which mature late in terms of myelination (Flechsig, 1901), are richest in polysynaptic connections and are, among cortical regions, the most

sensitive to barbiturates (Brazier and Finesinger, 1945). It is of interest that these highly advanced regions appear to be affected with predilection in some of the chronic cortical degenerative processes, in particular Alzheimer's disease. One must, however, again be cautious, since conceivably these cortical regions might be failing secondary to primary subcortical involvement.

We again wish to stress that in this study we excluded certain patients who could not take our battery. It will be important in the future to study more severely involved patients, to see whether certain features that have been stressed by other authors, do or do not appear, e.g., disorders in abstract thought and ideational apraxia (in the original sense of Liepmann, i.e., impairment in the ability to carry out a well-organized series of acts). It is, however, our belief that the results presented here may aid such further studies.

## Summary

Twenty-four patients with metabolic or toxic disorders of rapid onset, and without focal brain lesion, were selected as "confused" on the basis of an alteration of attention. They were given a short neuropsychological examination, their performances being compared to those of ten controls and to their own after recovering from confusion.

The following disorders were observed: (a) disturbances of mood and behavior, disorientation, unconcern toward illness; (b) mild word-finding difficulties, tendency toward verbal paraphasias in repetition and reading test, slowing of verbal fluency, marked dysgraphia; (c) mild spatial disturbances (right-left recognition; test of Head), constructional apraxia, disturbances in finger recognition and in calculation, memory defect.

Most of the disorders disappeared completely after clearing up of the acute confusional state.

## References

Benton, A. L., and Abramson, L. S. (1952) *Gerstmann symptoms following electroshock treatment,* "Arch. Neurol. Psychiat.," *67,* 248-257.

Bonhoeffer, K. (1912) *Die Psychosen,* in Handbuch der Psychiatrie, 3 Abteilung, I Hafte, Franz Deuticke, Leipzig.

Brazier, M. A. B., and Finesinger, J. E. (1945) *Action of barbiturates on the cerebral cortex,* "Arch. Neurol. Psychiat.," *53,* 51-58.

Chédru, F., and Geschwind, N. (1972) *Writing disturbances in acute confusional states,* "Neuropsychologia," *10,* 343-353.

Curran, F. J., and Schilder, P. (1935) *Paraphasic signs in diffuse lesions of the brain,* "J. Nerv. Ment. Dis.," *82,* 613-636.

Flechsig, P. (1901) *Developmental (myelogenetic) localizations of the cerebral cortex of the human subject,* "Lancet," *2,* 1027-1029.

Goodglass, H., and Kaplan, E. F. (1963) *Disturbances of gesture and pantomime in aphasia,* "Brain," *86,* 703-720.
Hécaen, H., Dubois, J., and Marcie, P. (1967) *Aspects linguistiques des troubles de la vigilance au cours des lésions temporales antéro-internes droite et gauche,* "Neuropsychologia," *5,* 311-328.
Juba, A. (1948) *Über nach Electroshock aufretende korticale Funktionstörungen,* "Schweiz. Arch. Neurol. Psychiat.," *61,* 217-226.
Kaplan, E. F. (1967) *Gestural Representation of Implement Usage: an Organismic Developmental Study,* Ph. D. thesis, Clark University.
Kornetsky, C., Mirsky, A. F., Kessler, E. K., and Dorff, J. E. (1959) *The effects of dextroamphetamine on behavioral deficits produced by sleep loss in humans,* "J. Pharmacol. Exp. Ther.," *127,* 46-50.
Lipowsky, Z. J. (1967) *Delirium, clouding of consciousness and confusion,* "J. Nerv. Ment. Dis.," *145,* 227-255.
Paterson, A. (1942) *Emotional and cognitive changes in post-traumatic confusional states,* "Lancet," *2,* 717-720.
Paterson, A., and Zangwill, O. L. (1944) *Recovery of spatial orientation in traumatic confusional states,* "Brain," *67,* 54-68.
Wapner, S., and Cirillo, L. (1968) *Imitation of a model's hand movement: age changes in transposition of left-right relations,* "Child Devel.," *39,* 887-894.
Weinstein, E. A., and Kahn, R. L. (1952a) *Denial of Illness,* Thomas, Springfield.
Weinstein, E.A., and Kahn, R.L., (1952b) *Non aphasic misnaming in organic brain disease,* "Arch. Neurol. Psychiat.," *67,* 72-79.
Zangwill, O. L. (1945) *Observations on the Rorschach test in two cases of acute concussional head-injury,* "J. Ment. Sci.," *91,* 322-336.

# Appendix

## Scoring Criteria

We considered as normal performances those which were either equal to, or better than, the worst performance of the normal control subjects. Below this value the following evaluation was made: mild alteration (+), moderate alteration (++), severe alteration (+++). Normal performances were marked as (0).

The criteria we used for this evaluation are the following:

*Orientation*: no error: (0); 1 or 2 errors: (+); 3, 4, or 5 errors (++); above 5 errors: (+++).
*Digit span*: 6 digits correctly repeated forward: (0); 5 digits: (+); 4 digits: (++); below 4 digits: (+++).
*A.M.A.*: 0 or 1 omission of A: (0); 2 or 3 omissions: (+); 4 or 5 omissions: (++); more than 5 omissions: (+++).
*Naming*: 0 or 1 error: (0); 2 or 3 errors: (+); 4 or 5 errors: (++); more than 5 errors: (+++).
*Word-list*: 14, or above names of animals in 1 minute: (0); 10 to 13 names: (+); 6 to 9 names: (++); below 9 names: (+++).
*Oral spelling*: 2 mispelled words or less: (0); 3 mispelled words: (+); 4 mispelled words: (+++).
*Comprehension:* 6 correctly understood sentences: (0); 5: (+); 4 or 3: (++); below 3: (+++).

*Repetition*: 0 or 1 error for the whole test: (0); 2 or 3 errors: (+); 4 or 5 errors: (++); above 5 errors: (+++).
*Reading*: no error: (0); 1, 2, 3 errors: (+); 4, 5, 6 errors: (++); above 6 errors: (+++).
*Writing (spelling)*: 0 or 1 spelling error for the whole test: (0); 2 or 3 errors: (+); 4 or 5 errors: (++); more than 5 errors: (+++).
*Writing (motor impairment)*: subjective appreciation by 2 judges on a 4 rate scale (from 0 to +++).
*Right-left orientation*: no error or hesitation on either task: (0); hesitations on either task: (+); errors on the examiner: (++); errors on the subject himself: (+++).
*Finger recognition*: no error or hesitation: (0); hesitations: (+); 1 or 2 errors: (++); above 2 errors: (+++).
*Calculation*: correct data or 1 mild error on the multiplication (i.e., with indication that the rule of the operation was applied): (0); several mild errors: (+); addition and subtraction correct but no preservation of the principle of the multiplication: (++); addition, subtraction incorrect: (+++).
*Drawing*: qualitative appreciations by 2 judges on a point scale from (0) to (+++).
*Head's Test*: 3 or more correctly carried out movements: (0); 2 movements: (+); 1 movement: (++); all movement incorrect: (+++).
*Recent memory:* 1 word retained after 10 minutes: (0); no word retained: (+++).
*Past memory:* 0 or 1 error: (0); 2 or 3 errors: (+); 4 or 5 errors: (++); 6 errors: (+++).
*Similarities:* 4 points out of 12 (Wechsler-Bellevue notation) or more: (0); 3 points: (+); 2 points: (++); below 2 points: (+++).
*Proverbs*: 4 or less misinterpreted proverbs: (0); 5 misinterpreted proverbs: (+++).

Evaluation of spontaneous speech, praxis, and visual recognition was made on a qualitative basis.

Some of the work reported here was supported by Grant NS 06209 from the National Institutes of Health, and by fellowships to Dr. Chédru from the Eli Lilly and Fulbright Foundations.

## CHAPTER 24

# The Borderland of Neurology and Psychiatry: Some Common Misconceptions

*Norman Geschwind*

While it has become fashionable to acknowledge the existence of an area of overlap between neurology and psychiatry, this common ground unfortunately bears more resemblance to a no-man's-land than to an open border. While neurologists tend to mutter darkly about the failure of psychiatrists to be aware of the brain as the organ of the mind, psychiatrists, perhaps somewhat defensively, have stressed their awareness of the whole man, biologic as well as psychologic. Unfortunately, few members of either group have in fact really interested themselves in the borderland area, and too frequently interactions between them are educationally disappointing, whether at the level of mutual consultation or in the interchange of residents for training. Hopefully, this situation will be corrected in the next few years, but until then, both psychiatrists and neurologists will often have to acquire the necessary knowledge themselves.

It is obviously important first to be aware of the magnitude and the difficulties of the problem. There are some who would like to believe that neurologic causes of psychiatric disorder are rare. Neurologic disorders, however, account for at least 30 percent of all first admissions to mental hospitals.[3] Furthermore, even if neurologic causes of psychiatric disorder were uncommon, this would still not justify their neglect, since some of these conditions are treatable. Because of the general lack of interest in this area, misdiagnoses are common. These errors include not only the failure to diagnose neurologic disease causing psychiatric symptoms, but also, far more often than is appreciated, the mistaken diagnosis

---

Reprinted with permission from D.F. Benson and D. Blumer (eds), *Psychiatric Aspects of Neurological Disease*. New York: Grune & Stratton, Inc., A Division of W.B. Saunders, 1975; 1-9.

of untreatable neurologic disorder in patients with reversible psychiatric disease, particularly the late-life depressions. It is not surprising that both types of mistakes are made, since a differential diagnosis can be carried out successfully only if one is aware of both groups of conditions.

Over the years, psychiatric residents occasionally have asked me whether they could not avoid such errors in diagnosis by referring all cases for a neurologic consultation. There are major objections to this policy. First, at this time, too few neurologists are themselves adequately trained in the psychiatric aspects of neurologic disease. Second, it would be a serious error in the management of many psychiatric patients to refer them routinely for neurologic examination, a fact that should not need further emphasis. Just as the psychiatrist must have enough experience and knowledge to decide which patients with somatic complaints need referral to nonpsychiatrists, so he must acquire enough expertise to pick up the signals that make neurologic referral useful. Since this type of referral requires diagnostic skill and medical knowledge, the decision for neurologic referral cannot be delegated to medically untrained personnel, as is sometimes the practice. The psychiatrist also must learn, like any other physician, how to choose and evaluate his consultants, and must be prepared for interchange of ideas with them. He will soon learn that some neurologists will be only too happy to find neurologic disorder in every case referred, while others will be more interested in proving themselves more "psychiatric" than the psychiatrist. He will learn that, in a large number of cases, the neurologist will be as uncertain as he himself as to the presence of organic causation. In other words, the neurologist cannot be expected in every case magically to "rule in" or "rule out" organic disorder with absolute certainty.

It is sometimes argued that psychiatric patients may suffer from physical disorders involving the heart, the lungs, the skin, indeed any organ system. The argument often follows that the brain can simply be regarded as one of a large list of organs that may be affected, and there is no reason why the psychiatrist need be any more expert on the brain than he is on, let us say, gynecologic disorders. I believe, however, that there are reasons why the brain has a very special importance for the psychiatrist. It is, of course, true that many disorders of the nervous system are not different in their psychiatric implications from nonneurologic disorders. One would hardly argue that the behavioral responses of a patient to a peripheral neuropathy would be *directly* affected by the neurologic lesion, and it would be reasonable in such a case to place major emphasis on the past experience of the patient. It may well be reasonable in such a case to speak of "a psychiatric overlay," i.e., the response of the patient to the illness. As we shall see, however, many lesions of the brain directly affect the parts of the nervous system that are involved in emotional behavior and may cause primary behavior disorder. To speak of "overlay" in such a case is misleading.

It must be realized that every behavior has an anatomy. This applies to both elementary and higher-level behaviors. We would accept that, when someone moves his arm, the impulses eventually leading to the movement will be transmitted over delimited, even if multiple, pathways in the nervous system. The same is true if someone speaks and is also true when someone gets angry. There is often the temptation to assume that emotion must be a function of the whole brain. This is, however, not supported by experimental facts. The parts of the brain from which emotional behavior is elicited are limited in extent. One need only cite the extensive physiologic work of Flynn[2] on the regions in which stimulation elicits or inhibits aggression. Thus, stimulation of the lateral hypothalamus leads to aggressive behavior, and its bilateral destruction leads to tameness. When a normal animal learns to respond aggressively to some stimulus, he must carry on this learning by modification of a pathway that eventually will fire the lateral hypothalamus or a small number of related structures. If these structures are destroyed, the animal will not become angry, regardless of his previous life experience. Similarly, destruction of the region of the ventromedial hypothalamus will lead to aggression, regardless of previous experience.

It is clear, therefore, that certain organic lesions can lead to changes in behavior, which in many instances are uninfluenced by the past experience of the animal. Furthermore, one can place lesions so that different emotional responses can be elicited from different parts of the brain[1] which are not connected to each other. Hence, the strategy of "looking at the whole patient," which is often so useful to the psychiatrist in other circumstances, may be actively misleading when certain discharging or destructive lesions of the brain are present.

Neglect of the fact that every behavior has an anatomy may lead in some cases to incorrect psychodynamic explanations of changes in behavior that are not dependent on past experience. One should not, however, make the equally serious error of concluding that, since all behavior takes place in the brain, all disorders of behavior must be organic, a view sometimes expressed in the vivid, but, in my opinion, erroneous aphorism that "behind the crooked thought lies the crooked molecule." No one can deny that learning is one of the major functions of the brain, and it is reasonable to assume that normal learning processes can lead to difficulties in adjustment. To pick a naive example, the child who is taught that dogs are dangerous will have difficulties in ordinary life, but this disadvantageous learning occurs by the same normal mechanism by which he advantageously learns that tigers are dangerous.

Some have argued, as noted above, that since all behavior is a function of the brain, one cannot draw a distinction between "organic" and "functional" disorders. I believe, however, that the organic-functional distinction is valid. A behavior disorder is "functional" if it is learning that has modified the brain by normal physiologic mechanisms; in theory, the functional disorder can be reversed by learning. On the other hand, the organic disorder is one in which the brain structures mediating behavior undergo alterations that reduce partially, or completely, the effects of past experience or new learning. These alterations may consist of destructive or discharging lesions or may consist of biochemical changes affecting impulse transmission or propagation.

It is worth mentioning that, in theory, any behavior disorder, whether organic or functional, can be treated by organic means. On the other hand, many organic disorders cannot be treated by learning methods (in which, of course, I include psychotherapy). Thus, an animal who responds with rage to certain stimuli will lose this response if drugs or surgery put the appropriate regions out of action. But learning cannot affect the activity of areas that are themselves destroyed, or whose necessary afferent pathways are cut off. The fact that organic methods can be used to treat behavior disorders of any etiology is, of course, widely reflected in clinical practice. Perhaps the most widely used form of psychiatric treatment is drug therapy. Each drug probably acts at a limited number of sites in the nervous system, and the use of drugs is in effect chemical, and usually reversible, unlike neurosurgery. The very fact that so much treatment depends on the use of neurally acting agents is another reason for the psychiatrist to be especially aware of the nervous system.

Once the importance of organic causation of a significant minority of psychiatric cases is accepted, the request often follows for some simple method to establish or exclude organic causation. There are, however, no simple methods. If one were to ask a cardiologist for a rule of thumb by which one might diagnose all organic causes of chest pain, he would almost certainly decline to supply it. One must simply learn the clinical pictures of angina, myocardial infarction, dissecting aneurysm, acute pericarditis, rupture of the esophagus, and so on. If simple rules work poorly in the diagnosis of chest or abdominal pain, they must surely be less applicable to that organ of the body that is capable of the widest variety of responses.

Organic causes of behavior disorders are not excluded by a normal elementary neurologic examination. A normal EEG similarly fails to exclude neurologic disease. In fact, in some disorders with striking behavioral change, for example, Alzheimer's disease, the EEG usually remains fully normal. Furthermore, even repeated normal EEGs do not necessarily exclude epilepsy, since the epileptogenic focus may simply be too deep or too distant from the recording electrodes. The lumbar puncture is an extremely useful tool and in general seriously underused in psychiatric circles. I have seen several patients with psychiatric disorders in whom only the presence of abnormalities on lumbar puncture gave away the organic causation. But a normal lumbar puncture does not exclude organic disease. Indeed, even a normal postmortem examination of the brain does not exclude organic causation. One need think not only of obvious disorders, such as drug intoxications, but even of such conditions as Sydenham's chorea, in which most investigators argue that no characteristic pathology has been found.

Another major source of error is the tendency to lump organic disorders into the categories of acute and chronic brain syndromes. These categories are as acceptable for the brain as would be the diagnosis of chronic myocardiopathy for all forms of chronic heart disease. It is obvious that some patients with chronic heart disease have large hearts, while others do not; some are hypertensive, while others have low blood pressure; some have rhythm disorders, while others do not. *Similarly, there is no single feature common to all forms of organic brain disease with behavior disorder.* Memory disorder may be prominent in some cases, but lacking in others. Some patients may be hypomanic, while others are apathetic. The patient with frontal lobe disorder tends to have short-lived shallow anger, which usually disappears rapidly, while the temporal lobe epileptic is likely to justify his anger with elaborate moral arguments and is frequently very slow to forget.

Other sources of error stem from failures on even more elementary levels. There are some psychiatric institutions in which histories are taken by nonmedical personnel, so that certain information is missed. Thus, one patient I saw had a history of episodes of depersonalization, but only slight effort was needed to bring out the fact that these were ushered in by an intense smell of burning rubber. This had been overlooked in a psychiatric hospital where the physician did not take a history, and only later in another hospital, when this information was obtained, was the presumption of temporal lobe epilepsy raised and confirmed.

Another common failure in taking histories or examining patients, even when done by a physician, is the tendency by some to make dynamic interpretations of the patient's behavior right from the initial contact. The possibility of organic diagnosis is almost excluded when the patient is approached in so closed-minded a fashion. It should furthermore be kept in mind that the mere fact that a patient's behavior is concordant with his personality dynamics does not mean that the disorder is psychogenic.

The impression often exists that when organic mental disorder is present, there must be failures in intellectual functioning. This belief is subject to pitfalls in more than one direction. While the presence of true intellectual deficit is an excellent sign of organic behavior disorder, its absence fails to rule it out, and patients with organic disorder may be missed. Patients with frontal lesions, particularly in the early stages, may have striking changes in behavior with no intellectual deficit. Temporal lobe epilepsy with behavioral change is compatible with a distinctly superior level of intellectual performance.

There exists, however, a much greater danger, that of incorrectly diagnosing incurable organic disorder when treatable functional disorder is present. Many patients with functional disorder present with apparent intellectual deficit. This can occur as hysterical pseudodementia, which is not very common. On the other hand, a number of patients suffering from *depression* will present with apparent intellectual failure. English psychiatrists are apparently well aware of this and are more likely to diagnose depression in the aged than many of their American counterparts.[4] The failure to consider this diagnosis is a serious error, since it results in failure to treat a usually reversible disorder. The argument is sometimes advanced that, although some of these patients are depressed, they are also intellectually impaired, and indeed it is often stated that depression itself is the first sign of dementia. My own view, however, is that this is not usually the case and that in general the apparent dementia disappears when the depression is reversed. I recently saw a 75-year-old woman who had been diagnosed as having a progressive dementia because of her gross failures in mental examination; after treatment for depression, she showed perfectly preserved intellectual capacities, and she is representative of many such cases.

Psychological testing is, of course, a tremendously useful tool, but the desire of many people for a simple means of diagnosing organicity often leads to a mistaken confidence in such test findings. Patients with gross organic behavioral disorders may lack any of the so-called signs of organicity. On the other hand, some patients with pseudodementias can be incorrectly diagnosed as showing organic disorder. Psychologic test results are most useful in the context of the entire clinical picture.

There are a few rules that may be helpful. There are patients who may be thought to be cases of manic psychosis who turn out to have disease of the frontal lobe. This occurs classically in general paresis but can occur with other disorders, such as multiple sclerosis or frontal tumors. On the other hand, the ability to maintain a fully classical *agitated* depression almost always excludes organic disease. Apathy is, however, an important feature of many organic disorders and is very frequently misinterpreted as depression. Incontinence of urine or feces is a major danger signal, since it almost never occurs in functional disorders. Neglect of this simple sign has led in my experience to diagnoses that were missed over several months. On the other hand, this sign may lose its usefulness if the patient has been placed on large doses of psychotropic drugs or has recently received electroconvulsive therapy. Another common error is that of misinterpreting the abnormality of emotional expression in patients with bilateral pyramidal disease (so-called pseudobulbar paralysis) as a change in subjective affect, so that the patient may be incorrectly thought to be depressed or euphoric.

The behavioral changes of temporal lobe epilepsy are relevant here. Some physicians have the idea that behavior disorders typically occur only during seizures, and that the patient is amnesic for the episode. The absence of amnesia is often thought to rule out epileptic behavior disorder. This is, however, a misleading rule. The behavioral changes associated with epilepsy are usually present *between* seizures, and behavior disorder occurring only *during* a seizure is rare. Furthermore, in my experience the patient usually remembers acute episodes of anger quite distinctly. The claim of amnesia is often understandably made by the patient when there is a threat of retribution.

The diagnostic difficulties of this borderland area between neurology and psychiatry should not be underestimated. Even expert observers can be misled for months or years. Let me cite only a few illustrative cases.

An atomic physicist on a mission abroad began to develop paranoid ideas about the stealing of atomic secrets. He was returned home, diagnosed as schizophrenic, and hospitalized. After several months he suffered a grand mal seizure. He was seen again in consultation by an expert psychiatrist who felt that the clinical picture was so characteristically schizophrenic that organic causes could be dismissed as the cause of the psychosis. Within a short time, however, when severe headaches developed, the patient was referred for study and a temporal lobe glioblastoma was found.

A hard-driving and very successful business man in his thirties stopped sleeping with his wife shortly after his promotion to vice-president of his company. At his wife's insistence, he went into psychotherapy. It was only several months later that his work performance began to decline, followed by a deterioration in personal cleanliness. These were interpreted as signs of depression, for which the patient was eventually hospitalized. Although he then developed incontinence, the possibility of organic disorder was still not considered until he became stuporous. He was found to have a large subfrontal tumor.

A previously highly successful young officer in the diplomatic corps was returned home because of a loss of interest in his work and a decline in his performance. Despite psychiatric help, he became increasingly apathetic about his work and he was dismissed. He took on a series of successively less attractive jobs and was finally employed keeping pigs. He was repeatedly diagnosed as a character disorder. He eventually developed severe headaches and was found to have a large craniopharyngioma that had compressed the undersurface of his frontal lobe.

A college student sought help because he was afraid that he might attack one of the girls in his classes. He was thought to be preschizophrenic and placed in psychotherapy. Within a year, he had become obviously paranoid and was hospitalized. It was not until about 2 years later that a movement disorder was noticed, although he had not been treated with phenothiazines. He was found to have Huntington's chorea.

The purpose of this chapter has been, to a great extent, a negative one. It has been my intention to point out that disease of the brain is an important and often treatable cause of behavior disorders, which occupies a special place in psychiatry, in terms of both practice and theoretical understanding. I have tried to discourage the notion that simple rules of thumb enable one to separate the organic from the functional. I have also attempted to show that not only is the organic disease erroneously diagnosed as functional, but it is also common to misdiagnose treatable functional disorders as irreversible organic disease. Above all, I have tried to convince the reader that in order to be an effective diagnostician, one must learn the natural course and clinical pictures of the different syndromes, just as one would have to do in any branch of medicine. One must be aware of the different clinical pictures of frontal lobe disorders and temporal lobe epilepsy, of the behavior disorders with which Huntington's chorea may present, or organic causes of tics, of the distinctive behavioral changes in different types of aphasia, of the characteristic pictures of hysterical pseudo-dementia, on the one hand, and of depressive pseudo-dementia on the other, of the psychoses associated with various endocrine diseases. This is only a partial list. The following chapters should provide a useful beginning.

## References

1. Downer, J L de C: Interhemispheric Integration in the Visual Systems, in Mountcastle. V B (ed): Interhemispheric Relations and Cerebral Dominance. Baltimore, Johns Hopkins Press, 1962, pp. 87-100.
2. Flynn J P: The Neural Basis of Aggression in Cats, in Glass, D C (ed): Neurophysiology and Emotion. New York, Rockefeller Univ., 1967, pp 40-59.

3. Malzberg, B: Important Statistical Data About Mental Illness, in Arieti, S (ed): American Handbook of Psychiatry, vol 1. New York, Basic Books, 1959, pp 161-174.
4. Roth, M: Ageing and Mental Diseases of the Aged, in Slater, E, Roth, M (eds): Clinical Psychiatry. London, Bailliéne, Tindall and Cassell, 1969, pp. 533-629.

Some of the work reported here was supported by Grant NS-06209 National Institute of Neurological Diseases and Blindness to the Boston University School of Medicine.

# CHAPTER 25

# Neurological Knowledge and Complex Behaviors

*Norman Geschwind*

Some scholars believe that Cognitive Science is the attempt to achieve in artificial systems what has already been achieved in the brain. Others, by contrast, argue that the study of ideal adaptive mechanisms could go on without reference to the brain. The author points out that the brain may not be the ideal cognitive device because of biological limitations on its capacity. Although it may not be ideal, it is still of major interest to cognitive scientists because of the great interest in the human mind, and, in addition, because at this moment the brain is the most important single reservoir of adaptive mechanisms.

This paper discusses several areas of neuroscience which are likely to shed light on mechanisms of adaptation. The study of simple nervous systems is likely to reveal important design principles of cognitive devices. The study of complex nervous systems will, of course, exert a major influence. The study of such systems leads to certain general principles concerning the neural circuits involved in complex adaptive behaviors: (1) There exist innate specialized systems for the learning of many specific behaviors that at first might appear to be purely cultural. (2) There is no evidence for the existence of any all-purpose computer in the brain. (3) There are many surprising dissociations manifested by the specialized systems in the brain, e.g., a special system for recognition of faces as against other visual patterns. (4) The study of the nervous system enables one to formulate more precise mechanisms for the role of emotion in cognitive function. (5) Some human behaviors can probably be understood poorly or not at all if the neural substrate is not considered. (6) The cognitive systems designed for dealing with attentional processes may be among the most complex neural structures which underlie behavior.

---

Reprinted with permission from *Cognitive Science*. New Jersey: Ablex Publishing Corporation, 1980;4:185-193.

There are certain other properties of brains that should be kept in mind by the cognitive scientists who are studying human behavior: (1) Brains differ from each other in structure, and it is very likely that the strategy for the solution of certain problems differs from person to person. (2) The presence of certain innate cognitive strategies in the brain may prevent that organism from employing other strategies which might be optimal for other problems. (3) Any theory about a particular cognitive strategy will have implications as to the particular mode of breakdown that might be expected after brain lesions. The study of disordered function from brain disease may thus be a valuable way to test certain cognitive theories.

In the months preceding this conference I made a point of asking many of my colleagues for their concept of Cognitive Science. The answers I received were, as one might well expect, remarkably varied, even from some who identified themselves as cognitive scientists. Some argued that it was a new field, whereas one respondent insisted that although he could not define it, the area could not be new since, whatever it was, Helmholtz *must* have practiced it. I soon realized, however, and this realization was, so to speak, punctuated by Professor Simon's elegant opening address, that the novelty of the field was irrelevant. What was important was the novelty of the growing realization that numerous apparently disparate disciplines shared certain concerns in common.

I was equally interested in the response to my second question: If Cognitive Science existed, what did knowledge of the workings of the brain have to do with it? Again the answers were varied. Reading the proceedings of this symposium one finds a similar range of views. There were some who thought that the brain was totally irrelevant, or, worse yet, that the study of nervous mechanisms could only add naive conclusions to befuddle the unwary. Flowers are made of chemicals, but biochemistry exists perfectly happily with the barest nod to floriculture. The brain may be a machine designed for cognitive functions but is hardly the place to study basic principles.

There are, by contrast, others who consciously or otherwise place the brain at the very center of the field. Some would say that ideal cognitive systems are indeed realized,or realizable,in the brain. Others, more extreme, would argue that Cognitive Science will in the end be nothing more than the end product of neurophysiology.

I will, on reflection, accept none of these extreme views, not out of a desire to compromise or from some notion of tolerant intellectual liberalism or distaste for controversy, but simply because none of these arguments convinces me. I hope to make my position clear in the following pages.

If I may borrow from Herbert Simon's presentation, let us accept that Cognitive Science is, above all, a field which concerns itself with strategies of adaptation, particularly to varying and unexpected environmental circumstances.

The realization that the conceptual structure cuts across so many areas should perhaps make us all realize that inspiration may come from areas that appear at first glance to be totally remote. This new society is concerned with psychology, mathematics, computer science, linguistics, philosophy, the social sciences, and, of course, the neurological sciences. But before I deal with the possible role of neurological studies in this hybrid field, let me point out at least two biological fields whose data and theories may in fact have important lessons for Cognitive Science and its concern with systems that can adapt to changes in the environment, and in particular to unexpected changes. How does one design a system to do this? Perhaps the most dramatic example of this type of design is embodied in the immunological systems of the body. How is it that these systems adapt with the most remarkably subtle strategies to environmental alterations that could apparently have never entered into the design of these systems, e.g., immune responses to recently invented chemical structures? There are indeed highly individual responses to thousands of such antigenic substances synthesized only in the past few years. Conversely, many infectious agents, particularly the so-called slow viruses, maintain their infectivity only by ingenious mechanisms which depend precisely on the environments to which they have been subjected. Indeed, immunologists have called attention to the formal similarity of learning and immunological mechanisms.

Another field in which equally remarkable adaptive mechanisms are at play is that of genetics and more broadly the whole process of evolution. Indeed, the existence of genetic codes (I use the plural since we now know that there is no universal code) itself reveals the importance of symbolic systems in biology.

Yet, having pointed out that many biological systems embody cognitive scientific principles, let me hasten to add that I doubt that "*the* brain" is the ideal cognitive device. Indeed, when we say "*the*" brain we imply that there is *only one* model. But we know that brains differ and that some may be far more effective adaptive models than others. Indeed, the problem is further complicated by the fact that some brains adapt well to a certain group of environmental changes but poorly to another group, whereas in other brains the reverse situation may hold. One might even consider the evolution of the brain as a slow progress toward an ideal but nonexistent device.

Why is the brain not ideal? We can only guess. In some instances better paradigms for cognitive tasks have simply never been "wired into" the system by appropriate mutations. But even when superior paradigms are available, not all brains may contain them. The reason for this is probably dependent in major part on the fact that there are many constraints on the brain. It is limited in size at birth by the requirement that it should not exceed the maximum possible diameter of the birth canal. It is limited in final size because it already uses a quarter of the cardiac output. I also suspect that even at its current size not all areas can operate maximally since this would involve increases of blood flow beyond the capacity of the heart in a subject using the rest of his body actively.

The compromises that are made presumably trade superior design in one area for inferior design (one that has too few nerve cells even with the best principles) in another. This distribution of inborn potentials for talent will differ from brain to brain.

If this is true, then the brain may be the *best* device in existence (even this is probably not true in all areas), but it is not the *ideal* device. There is no reason why better devices cannot and will not be built as this field advances. Furthermore, as Duncan Luce has pointed out, there is no reason to assume that the best man-made devices will be similar in design to the best human brains, any more than an airplane's flight is similar to a bird's.

If that is so, then why should the cognitive scientist study the brain and not just the mind? The answer is given away in the very structure of the question. Most cognitive scientists are strongly interested in the human mind, i.e., precisely in the output of a particular accidental device. The field has not yet become a purely mathematical one, but continues to find its major inspiration in behavior. The brain may not be the ideal device, but it is almost certainly at this moment far and away the greatest single reservoir of such adaptive mechanisms. The device comes equipped with hundreds of built-in clever devices designed to maintain certain invariants. Thus, despite a wide range of environmental states, body temperature, food intake, and blood pressure are remarkably constant. Body weight is normally held within an astonishingly narrow range, despite the fact that the machine has no built-in method of directly ascertaining its own weight. Yet these adjustments are only the beginning: It has a remarkable capacity to learn, to store knowledge of changes in the environment, to store knowledge of changes in the strategies followed by others, and to acquire new strategies. Evolution has been a highly effective, if slow, strategy for the development of adaptive cognitive devices, and most of the best ones extant are being carried around in human heads. We are still the best machines for pattern recognition, classification, and for the very talent of design of clever devices.

Despite all this, the position of neural science in relation to cognition remains an uneasy one. Indeed, in this very symposium it is very sparsely represented. And whereas one of the original possible state-of-the-art symposia was to be in the neurosciences, this did not materialize. Some will say that this is because neural science has not delivered the goods. Thus the pioneering attempts of McCulloch and Pitts to correlate detailed neural circuity with function did not succeed, although the more modest attempts of Lettvin and Maturana and Hubel and Wiesel are dramatic examples that such correlates are possible. Our knowledge of the circuity of mammalian brains is extensive, but astonishingly imprecise in the small details. To make this clear, let me point out that there is not a single neuron in the central nervous system of any *mammal* whose connections are fully specified, although such neurons are known in some invertebrates. Despite this fact, the neural sciences and Cognitive Science will perforce be partners. In my view, many of the problems of interfacing the neural sciences with the cognitive sciences are more sociological than scientific, i.e., professional xenophobia and infatuation with one's own discipline are the greatest barriers to adaptation. The average neurological researcher is not likely to be enamored of philosophy, discursive thinking, psychological analysis, or computer models. Conversely, many nonneural cognitive scientists are uncomfortable with the data obtained with the microelectrode from a few neurons or from the derangements in cognitive strategy which follow damage to the nervous system.

Let me now turn to a few, hopefully more precise, indications of how neurological knowledge can contribute to this growing field. Let me briefly indicate an area remote from my own field of major study, that of the study of behavior in relatively simple invertebrate nervous systems. I heard John von Neumann in one of his last lectures point out that there existed invertebrates whose nervous systems contained far fewer units than were present in the primitive calculating machines (as they were still called) of that period. Yet, von Neumann added, these primitive animals were in his view far more complex than these calculating devices, more complex in that he thought it would take more axioms to describe their behavior. Von Neumann's message was clear: There are design principles in these simple nervous systems which will enormously expand our capacities to understand adaptive complexity.

The advantage of these simple systems is obvious. They contain small numbers of nerve cells; and furthermore, the complete connectivity of many of these cells can be specified, and the adaptive ingenuity of many of these organisms is often striking. The possibilities for breeding of genetic variants opens the possibility of experimental tests of theories of mechanisms of strategies of adaptation. At this moment, this field may appear to be far from the major concerns of cognitive science, but my prediction is that it will increasingly be found to be surprisingly relevant.

Let me now turn to some areas nearer to my own central interests. Simon has said in his presentation that when we think we are studying the properties of the nervous system we really may be studying the effects of past history. A little reflection, however, shows that the opposite situation has been equally frequent, when we thought we were studying the effects of experience we were really studying the properties of the nervous system. The adult chimpanzee usually responds to the sight of a snake with fear. The interpretation that immediately comes to mind is that this fear was instilled during development. Yet Hebb showed many years ago that a baby chimpanzee responds with the same brisk fear to his first sight of a snake.

It would in fact be surprising if it were not the case that the brain had many built-in properties. The need for many built-in systems is one of the lessons that the history of the attempts to build intelligent devices, which Simon has so elegantly summarized, has taught cognitive scientists: Any system which has to learn everything it needs is simply too slow and inefficient. The acquisition of motor skills is an excellent example. Children may take years to tie their shoe laces, and even the novice in surgery often takes a remarkably long time to learn to tie knots in sutures. There are, by contrast, complex motor patterns like those of walking that are primarily inborn and are acquired at high speed. In fact, the maturation of an inborn process is often mistaken for learning.

Furthermore, there are some experiments that appear to show learning effects which are, in fact, not really present. Consider the following: Two sets of kittens are raised in the laboratory. In one group the right and left eyes are patched on alternate days so that at no time is the use of both eyes permitted. These animals are compared to controls without eye patches. At six months, it is found that in the first group of animals there are few cells in the visual cortex which respond to binocular stimulation, while in the control group there are many. The apparently obvious conclusion is that the animal who has had binocular stimulation has acquired binocular vision. The elegant experiments of Hubel and Wiesel reveal a different sequence. Cells which respond to binocular stimulation are present in the newborn animal. They are *lost* only if binocular stimulation is not supplied over the following months.

There is of course an experiental effect, but it is the *loss* of a built-in program, rather than the acquisition of a new one. But in some cases it is clear that even the apparent loss of a built-in program is illusory. Consider what happens when for the first time a rat is put into the cage of a cat raised in the laboratory. If the cat has in the past seen rats attacked by other cats, he will almost invariably attack. What happens, however, if the cat has never seen a rat (and has of course never seen one attacked)? As shown by several experiments (e.g., Kuo, 1930; Yerkes and Bloomfield, 1910), about half of the cats do not attack. The remainder, however, do attack. Furthermore, the attack is not random. The cats will, in fact, attack in the same manner as the animal in the wild. They will bite at the neck or turn the rat over so as to bite at the throat.

It is clear therefore that built-in systems for attack are present in the cat, or at least in many cats. There are at least three interpretations as to why certain cats do not attack. The first is that these animals do not have built-in systems and would therefore have had to learn to attack. The second is that innate systems for attack were present but were lost as a result of lack of early experience. The third is that the built-in programs are present but inaccessible. As we will now see, the third interpretation is probably the correct one.

John Flynn of the Yale Medical School has published a dramatic series of experiments on cats who do not attack spontaneously (e.g., Wasman and Flynn, 1962). The animal, with a rat in its cage, receives stimulation through electrodes implanted in the brain. In most locations this stimulation is without effect. If, however, the electrode is in certain locations, e.g., the lateral hypothalamus, the cat will attack. The manner of attack is again similar to that of the wild animal. The attack is specific in its goal, so that the cat does not attack small objects placed in the cage. Furthermore, although a dead stuffed rat is attacked, the attack is less persistent than on a live animal.

These experiments show that the innate program for attack is still present in these animals. In addition, there must be innate perceptual programs which contain models of the anatomy of a rat which determine the specificity not only of the object of attack, but of portions of that object.

We must conclude that there are elaborate preprogrammed systems of analysis and action which can be modified or triggered by experience. Furthermore, even the capacity to learn itself reflects specializations of neural organization:

Whether or not the chimpanzee has language, it is clear that the human learns it better.

The ability to learn is probably not a general one. Instead, there exists systems which have a specialized capacity to learn certain kinds of material. Thus Maureen Dennis of Toronto has studied children with the Sturge-Weber syndrome, a congenital disturbance of the cortex of one side of the brain. Several such children have undergone the total removal of this abnormal cortex from one side of the brain because of uncontrollable seizures. Since these children have all had brain lesions existing from before birth, they tolerate these operations very well, and the types of gross language disorders seen in adults do not occur. Yet even in these cases with very early lesions, Dennis has shown clearly that those who have undergone left decortication employ different strategies in certain linguistic tasks from those of children with early right decortications whose strategies are much closer to those of normal controls.

As I have already indicated, we do not yet have detailed knowledge of neural circuits involved in complex adaptive behaviors. I will, however, list certain general principles illustrated by specific examples. Most of these are based on information from the study of humans who have suffered delimited lesions to their nervous system and have been well studied, although some of these principles are based on experimentation in nonhuman animals.

1. As already noted, *there exist specialized systems for the learning of many behaviors that at first might appear to be purely cultural.* Thus we have known for over 100 years that there are specialized systems for language. We also know that there are systems which deal with recognition of special stimuli, e.g., faces (i.e., systems which are specialized and not designed for the recognition of other types of visual pattern) and for the expression and recognition of emotion.

2. *There is no evidence for the existence of any all-purpose computer.* Instead, there seems to be a multiplicity of systems for highly special tasks, e.g., the systems for facial recognition appear to be separate from those for other visual recognition tasks. Systems for the recognition and production of music appear to be separate from those for language. There is, at present, no good evidence, although counter-evidence is perhaps equally weak, for the existence of a generalized logical deductive capacity.

3. *There are many surprising dissociations,* some of which have already been indicated. There are many others. Thus Japanese patients with reading difficulties acquired as the result of delimited brain damage typically have more difficulty comprehending words written in the apparently simpler syllabary system (*kana*) than in the more elaborate logographic (or ideographic) system (*kanji*) (Sasanuma & Fujimura, 1971). In some Europeans with reading difficulties, the category of written words that is best preserved is that of names of public buildings such as *bank, restaurant,* or *post office.* It is obvious in this case that there is some remarkable interaction between damage to the hardware and past expe-

rience. In this case it appears as if the patient has learned to read words which are attached to their referents (e.g., the words "bank" or "hotel" are usually on the appropriate buildings) in a different or additional way from those which are not (e.g., "telephone," "plate," "if").

4. The study of the nervous system enables one to formulate more precise mechanisms for *the role of emotion in cognitive functions.* I cannot elaborate this in detail here, but I would first point out that the portions of the brain involved in memory functions, e.g., the hippocampus, amygdala, mammillary bodies, etc., are all portions of the limbic system which is clearly involved in emotional activities. Furthermore, MacDonnell and Flynn's (1966) work on aggression in cats again shows that stimulation of specific limbic structures "sets" the animal for increased receptiveness to certain inputs and preparedness for certain outputs. One of the striking effects of many brain lesions is the alteration of these emotional components while rational, calculating functioning may be spared.

5. *Some behaviors can probably be understood poorly or not at all if the neural substrate is not considered.* Thus patients with certain lesions (who suffer from what are called *apraxic* disorders) will show certain remarkable dissociations (Geschwind, 1975). They will fail to carry out certain verbal commands which they understand, whereas they succeed in carrying out others. These patients will fail to salute, to pretend to use a hammer, or throw a ball. They will also fail to pretend how to blow out a match or suck through a straw. On the other hand, they will successfully carry out commands to move the eyes, to stand, to walk, bow, or turn. How do we account for the successful ability to carry out certain movements to verbal command while others fail? Let me point out briefly that the commands for movement which succeed do *not* differ from those which fail in linguistic structure, age of acquisition, or in any measure of complexity. The movements which succeed are those which are mediated by motor systems in the brain other than the contralateral pyramidal system. In other words, there are cognitive systems the understanding of which may depend on knowledge of the specific pattern of realization in the "hardware" of the nervous system.

6. The *most complex* cognitive systems in most brains may be those which deal with *attentional* processes. Simon has stressed the serial features of attention, but I would stress that the parallel features are equally important. An attentional system functions properly only if it combines a central focus with a continuous survey of what is not at the center. The work of Broadbent has illustrated this very well.

Let me now describe some other properties of brains that must be kept in mind by the cognitive scientist who is studying human behavior.

1. There is a tendency to ask, "What is *the* strategy by which a cognitive problem is solved?" But since we know that brains differ from each other in structure, it is very likely that the strategies for solution of certain problems differ

from person to person. Thus patients in whom the corpus callosum is congenitally absent show a marked increase in the size of the anterior commissure. We also know that the brains of left-handers differ on the average from those of right-handers. Thus left-handers have, on the average, less anatomical asymmetry in the brain than right-handers (Galaburda et al., 1978).

2. It is furthermore conceivable that the presence of certain innate cognitive strategies in a brain may prevent that brain from employing other strategies which might be optimal for other problems. This is a situation that evolutionary theory would lead us to expect with considerable frequency. It is even conceivable that disorders such as childhood dyslexia may in some cases be the result of the high development of certain perceptual strategies at the expense of others.

3. Any theory about a cognitive strategy will probably have certain implications as to the particular modes or breakdown that might be expected after brain lesions. This in turn implies that study of disordered cognitive function from brain disease may be a valuable way to test cognitive theories.

Let me close with a prediction and a plea. I believe that the neurological sciences and the study of syndromes of delimited neurological damage will have a continuing major effect on the future development of Cognitive Science. It is well worth recalling that the profound effect of neurology on psychology which has occurred in the past quarter century was not expected by the majority of psychologists. But this influence will not be unilateral. Indeed, I will not be surprised if the influence of cognitive science on the neurological sciences is not greater than the reverse.

Let me now state my plea that the practitioners of both fields take each other seriously. I state this not as the customary exhortation to cooperate, but as the result of the knowledge that the failure not merely to take account of certain neurological data, but even their active suppression, led to the dramatic neglect of important cognitive findings. Thus many of the effects of the destruction of the corpus callosum were elaborately described and well understood theoretically before the First World War. Their neglect was the direct result of the influence of major figures in the history of cognitive psychology such as Karl Lashley, Henry Head, and Kurt Goldstein (Geschwind, 1964). It is tragic that it took until the 1960s to correct this gross error. It would not be fitting for a science whose object is the study of adaptive cognitive strategies to make an equally maladaptive error.

## References

Galaburda, A. M., LeMay, M., Kemper, T. L., & Geschwind, N. Right-left asymmetries in the brain. *Science,* 1978, *199,* 852-856.

Geschwind, N. The paradoxical position of Kurt Goldstein in the history of aphasia. *Cortex,* 1964, *1,* 214-224.

Geschwind, N. The apraxias: Neural mechanisms of disorders of learned movement. *American Scientist,* 1975, *63,* 188-195.

Kuo, Z. Y. The genesis of the cat's response to the rat. *Comp. Psychol.,* 1930, *11,* 1-35.

MacDonnell, M. F., & Flynn, J. P. Control of sensory fields by stimulation of hypothalamus. *Science,* 1966, *152,* 1406-1408.

Sasanuma, S., & Fujimura, O. An analysis of writing errors in Japanese aphasic patients: Kanji versus kana words. *Cortex,* 1971, *8,* 265-282.

Wasman, M., & Flynn, J. P. Directed attack elicited from hypothalamus. *Arch. Neurol.,* 1962, *6* 220-227.

Yerkes, R. M., & Bloomfield, D. Do kittens instinctively kill mice? *Psychol. Bull.,* 1910, *7,* 253-263.

# CHAPTER 26

# Localization in Gerstmann Syndrome

*Richard L. Strub and Norman Geschwind*

## Introduction

In 1924, Joseph Gerstmann reported the case of a 52-year-old woman who had suffered a cerebral vascular insult and was subsequently unable to differentiate the fingers of her hands. This curious clinical sign, described briefly in 1888 by Badel, became a subject of intense interest to Gerstmann and other neurologists interested in the higher cortical functions. Gerstmann, who called the deficit "finger agnosia," believed that the concepts of finger identification and differentiation were critical factors in the development of other higher functions. Over the next 6 years, he reported three additional patients who demonstrated finger agnosia.

With each new case, he observed associated disturbances in cortical functioning; more particularly, right-left disorientation, writing difficulty (*agraphia*) and a calculation defect (*acalculia*) (Gerstmann, 1927, 1930). He regarded these deficits as related to a dissolution of both the morphologic knowledge of the hand and of its highly skilled use in writing and calculation. Although other symptoms were noted in his material, Gerstmann considered that four of the signs—finger agnosia, right-left disorientation, agraphia, and acalculia—formed a distinct constellation. From his pathologic data, he showed that all patients who demonstrated all four symptoms had lesions in the dominant parietal lobe, more specifically, in the region of the angular gyrus and adjacent occipital lobe. Because of the strong correlation of the symptom cluster with focal pathology, Gerstmann considered that the four components formed a genuine symptom cluster; others soon assigned his name as an eponym.

---

Reprinted with permission from A. Kertesz (ed), *Localization in Neuropsychology*. New York: Academic Press, 1983;295-321.

The localizing significance of purely behavioral signs such as aphasia and alexia had been well accepted in clinical practice since the late nineteenth century. Therefore, neurologists quickly accepted Gerstmann's findings as being another behavioral syndrome that could assist them in localizing lesions in the cerebral cortex. Neurologists examining patients at the bedside are usually limited by time in their evaluation of behavior and, therefore, typically make primarily qualitative judgments as to the presence or absence of particular deficits. This is certainly true in the case of the Gerstmann syndrome, as each sign is complicated and even a qualitative assessment of performance is often difficult.

There has been considerable study as well as rather vigorous debate about the Gerstmann syndrome in the past 20 years. In this chapter, we review and comment on the syndrome and its symptoms, we discuss its anatomical and neuropsychological implications, and, hopefully without undue bias, we analyze the controversy that the syndrome has engendered.

## Description of the Syndrome

*The Gerstmann syndrome,* as used in clinical neurology, is a constellation of four distinct behavioral features: finger agnosia, right-left disorientation, agraphia, and acalculia. Each symptom represents a specific disturbance in higher cortical functioning. Although the individual deficits are specific, each is complex and may be elicited by a variety of testing methods. Because of the basic clinical nature of the syndrome, the testing must be applicable for bedside and office examination. We discuss each symptom in detail, but it must be kept in mind that the syndrome can be considered definitely to be present only if all four elements can be shown to be present.

### Finger Agnosia

The pivotal sign in the Gerstmann syndrome is finger agnosia (Gerstmann, 1924). *Finger agnosia* does not mean, as the name implies, that the patient does not recognize fingers as fingers and therefore misidentifies them as, let us say, toes, arms, or toothbrushes; but rather, in Gerstmann's own words, that the patient has a "disability for recognizing, naming, selecting, differentiating, and indicating the individual fingers of either hand, the patient's own as well as those of other persons" (Gerstmann, 1940:398). Gerstmann was the first to stress the significance of this unusual sign, and in Critchley's words his "shrewd and original communication . . . virtually started a new chapter in the story of parietal symptomatology" (Critchley, 1953:203).

In Gerstmann's original patient, and in many patients subsequently reported, the finger recognition problem was pervasive, being present regardless of the method tested. From the definition, however, it is obvious that the faculty of finger recognition is far from a unitary function. Naming, pointing to named fingers, and moving a finger on one hand that corresponds to one that an examiner has moved on his own opposite hand are all quite different functions, each requiring different neuropsychologic mechanisms for successful completion. In some patients, one aspect of finger agnosia may be more prominent than others. At one point in the history of finger gnosis, these separate functions were differentially labeled; "finger aphasia" for the inability to name fingers, "finger apraxia" for the inability to individually move fingers, and so forth (Schilder, 1931). Although such labels emphasize the various aspects of finger agnosia, this proliferation of terms is neither necessary nor practical. One observation that has been made by all clinicians testing finger recognition is that it is the middle three fingers that are most frequently misidentified.

In general, when testing for finger agnosia at the bedside, several methods of examination should be utilized; these are outlined here. Before testing, the examiner must insure that the patient does not have any primary sensory or motor deficit that would adversely influence his performance.

1. Verbal tasks
   a. Finger naming (patient's hand). Ask the patient to name fingers on his own hand pointed to (eyes open) and touched (patient's eyes closed) by examiner.
   b. Comprehension of finger names. Ask the patient to point to fingers on his own hand named by the examiner.
2. Verbal-Nonverbal tasks
   a. Finger naming (examiner's hand and model). Ask patient to name fingers on examiner's hand held opposite the patient in various positions (e.g., palm to patient, back of hand to patient, on table in front of patient, etc.). Also ask patient to name fingers on a line drawing of hand.
   b. Comprehension of finger names (examiner's hand and model). Ask the patient to point to named fingers on examiner's hand and model. Use various orientations of the hand as just suggested.
3. Nonverbal tasks
   a. Imitation of finger movements. Move individual fingers and ask the patient to move the corresponding finger on his own hand. Different hand orientations can be used to make the task progressively more difficult. This can also be done by asking the patient to move fingers on the opposite hand to those moved by the examiner, but this introduces a very strong right-left factor into the task.
   b. Identification of single fingers. Have patient close his eyes, touch one finger, ask patient to open eyes, and ask patient to point to the identical finger on the examiner's hand, patient's other hand, or on a line drawing at a hand.

Kinsbourne and Warrington (1962) have devised several very sophisticated additional tests. They reasoned that finger agnosia represented an inability to appreciate the actual sequence and position of fingers on the hand. They further proposed that, if finger agnosia were truly a single function, testing for it must not be contaminated by either linguistic incompetence (aphasia) or visual perceptive impairment. From this theoretical position, they utilized the following tests that are applicable for bedside testing:

1. The in-between test. The patient's eyes are closed. The examiner touches two fingers on the patient's hand (e.g., ring finger and index finger) and the patient is asked to report how many fingers are in between the two (in this case, 1).
2. Two-point finger test. Eyes closed. The examiner touches two places, either on the same or different fingers. The patient reports whether both touches were on one or two fingers.
3. Matchbox test. Eyes closed. The patient's fingers are touched in two places, either by one box between two fingers or two boxes touching different fingers (only one point of contact for each box). The patient must report if he was touched by one or two boxes.

Despite the wide range of testing methods, patients tend to demonstrate failure on both verbal and nonverbal tests of finger recognition. The correlation of performance on the various verbal tests alone is sufficiently high to consider them as very possibly homogeneous, thereby testing a single function (Poeck and Orgass, 1969).

The nonverbal tasks have a positive correlation with the verbal tests, but the association is not as strong as that among the verbal tests themselves. Kinsbourne and Warrington (1962) found that their own nonverbal tests were consistently failed by their patients who had finger agnosia diagnosed by more conventional means. Not unexpectedly, their tests of finger agnosia were performed more poorly by patients whose performance was less adequate on the routine nonverbal tests. Other investigators have found Kinsbourne's and Warrington's tasks not as useful and question whether such tests are appropriate for testing single-finger recognition as conceived by Gerstmann (Poeck and Orgass, 1969).

One must be careful in testing finger recognition in patients with aphasia, particularly when a verbal comprehension deficit is present. Since the verbal tasks of finger recognition require precise comprehension and naming, the aphasic consistently makes errors on these tests. Several studies clearly have shown this correlation (Poeck and Orgass, 1969; Sauguet, Benton, and Hécaen, 1971). To claim that finger agnosia is merely a manifestation of aphasia is unjustified, however, because there are many cases reported in which finger agnosia is present in the absence of a language disturbance.

From these observations, it is possible to conclude that there is a specific deficit for finger recognition. This varies somewhat, depending on the method of testing and the other deficits manifested by the patient.

Finger agnosia usually is seen in patients with left parietal lesions but has been described with right parietal as well as bilateral lesions. The agnosia is traditionally demonstrable in both hands, although a unilateral variety using nonverbal tests only has been described in the opposite-hand unilateral hemispheric lesions (Gainotti and Tiacci, 1973). Why a generalized dysfunction of finger sense should be found after a focal lesion in the left parietal lobe has been a matter of much speculation. It is thought by some authors that finger agnosia is a restricted aspect of autotopagnosia or failure to appreciate ones topographical body scheme; but finger agnosia usually occurs in isolation from a generalized autotopagnosia. Many theories have attempted to explain the function of finger gnosis but none has adequately explained the phenomenon. Why a left-sided lesion should cause bilateral loss of finger sense is also uncertain. It is well recognized that a left-sided lesion can cause bilateral ideomotor apraxia; therefore, it appears that the left hemisphere is dominant for both sensory knowledge and complex motor performance of both hands (Geschwind, 1975).

### Right-Left Disorientation

Right-left disorientation is a term used to describe a patient's inability to differentiate right from left either on himself or on another. The definition implies that the right-left problem represents a generalized difficulty in applying a spatial concept of lateral orientation to the body rather than merely a linguistic defect in which the labels right and left are misapplied. As with finger agnosia, right-left disorientation is complex, and both verbal and nonverbal testing methods are commonly employed in identifying the defect.

In testing for right-left disorientation, tasks of graded difficulty should be given. Because each question has only two possible answers (i.e., right or left), enough trials must be given to overcome chance factors.

1. Verbal tasks
   a. Naming side indicated by examiner
      1. on patient
      2. on examiner facing patient
      3. on examiner in unusual orientation (e.g., seated sideways with legs crossed; ask patient to identify one foot or knee).
   b. Ask patient to point to body parts on one side of the body named by examiner, (e.g., "point to my right ear")
      1. on patient
      2. on examiner facing patient
      3. on examiner in unusual positions.
   c. Crossed commands. Ask patient to point with specific hand to specific part (e.g., "point to left ear with right hand")
      1. on patient
      2. on examiner facing patient
      3. on examiner in different postures.

2. Nonverbal tests (Head, 1926). With the patient seated opposite the examiner; instruct patient to point to the exact part on his own body that the examiner has pointed to on his (e.g., examiner points to his own right eye and the patient then points to his own right eye). The examiner can also cross his arms or legs and move one part and ask patient to move the similar part.

This series of tests can be administered in a few minutes and can provide the examiner with a comprehensive assessment of the patient's right-left orientation. In mild cases of right-left disorientation, the patient fails only the complex crossed commands. With moderate impairment, the patient consistently fails on tasks with the examiner facing him; with a marked deficit, the patient shows right-left confusion on himself.

Several important factors must be appreciated when interpreting failure on these right-left tasks. One factor is that there are many people in the normal population (including educated people) that have significant difficulties with right-left orientation. Interestingly, this is twice as common in females (17.5%) as in males (8.8%) (Wolf, 1973). A second factor is aphasia. It has been shown repeatedly that aphasic patients usually perform quite poorly on the verbal right-left tasks (Benton, 1979; Dennis, 1976; Sauguet et al., 1971). Accordingly, it is wise to be very cautious in diagnosing right-left disorientation in an aphasic patient unless significant errors are made on nonverbal tasks as well. A third factor is denial. Some patients with denial or unilateral neglect have difficulty with right-left tasks on the basis of a neglected side alone (usually left) (Nielsen, 1938).

Being cognizant of the influencing factors outlined here, it is possible to further analyze the neuropsychologic mechanism involved in right-left discrimination. The major requirement is the development of an autotopographical concept of the body and its inherent right-left symmetry. It is precisely this symmetry that causes confusion; it is a rare patient whose body schema disorientation includes an inability to distinguish nonsymmetrical regions, that is, top from bottom or front from back (Stengel and Vienna, 1944).

During development, the individual initially forms a basic spatial concept of the body and its symmetry. Having done so, he or she is then able to accomplish the more complex operation of reversing and reorienting this right-left symmetry (Benton, 1968). With this higher level of conceptualization of laterality, the individual can correctly identify the right and left of others regardless of their orientation—facing him, walking in the opposite direction, or hanging upside down. It is this spatial conceptualization of right-left that is the essence of right-left orientation. This function, best tested by the nonverbal imitation tasks, can be disturbed by lesions in either right or left hemisphere (Sauguet et al., 1971).

Concomitant with the development of right-left sense, as discussed previously, is the application of verbal labels to the sides of the body. On occasion, errors in right-left orientation are due to the misapplication of the linguistic labels, "right" and "left." This mislabeling can occur by three mechanisms: (a) from aphasia (anomia particularly); (b) because basic spatial disorientation does not allow the individual to appreciate the correct side to label (discussed in this chapter); and (c) a disconnection of the temporoparietal language system that contains the labels from the parieto-occipital tactile-visual system from which the spatial concept of right-left arises. The first and third mechanisms would be seen only in left hemisphere lesions.

### Agraphia

Agraphia is a disorder in the expression of written language that occurs as a result of brain damage (Hécaen and Albert, 1978). As with other complex higher cortical functions, agraphia can be caused by the disruption of a variety of neuropsychologic functions. The patient who is aphasic in speech, for example, almost inevitably is agraphic[1] and produces writing errors that are distinctly aphasic in nature. Some patients who do not demonstrate aphasic speech, however, can exhibit an agraphia that is characterized by misspellings, omissions or intrusions of letters or words, letter or word substitution (paragraphias), syntax errors, and, on occasion, completely nonsensical writing (jargon agraphia). Such cases are classified as *aphasic agraphia.*

There are other examples of agraphia in which the patients are unable to properly align letters and words on the page and may even have difficulty producing recognizable letters. This disorder, often called *spatial agraphia,* appears to be part of a more generalized constructional impairment. Patients with spatial agraphia, unlike many of those with aphasic agraphia, also have a pronounced defect in copying written language.

A third major type of agraphia distinguished by some authors is an *apraxic agraphia.* Not all authors, however, accept this as a separate category. As usually described, the syndrome has the following characteristics: no primary sensory, motor, constructional, or language deficit; yet, the patient is unable to correctly form letters spontaneously or from dictation. The agraphia is due to the loss of the sensory-motor engrams (stored patterns of letters and words) necessary for writing. It is this type of agraphia that is generally felt to be present in patients with the Gerstmann syndrome, however, performance varies (Critchley, 1953; Hécaen and Albert, 1978). In general, most perform more adequately when copying than when writing either spontaneously or from dictation. Spatial problems as well as misspellings due to letter order errors and letter omissions have been described (Kinsbourne and Warrington, 1964). In some patients, a combination of writing errors is demonstrated.

In testing for agraphia, it is important to give the patient material of graded complexity; some patients fail at a very basic level of letter formation whereas others demonstrate their agraphia only in the form of syntax errors in sentence length material.

---

[1]Exceptions to this rule are, at best, extremely rare.

1. Writing to dictation—ask the patient to write letters, numbers, then words, and finally, sentences.
2. Spontaneous writing—have the patient write his name and address, numbers 1–10, the first 10 letters of the alphabet, then the names of objects and finally some sentences (e.g., about the weather, their job, how they would change an automobile tire, etc.).
3. Copying—numbers, letters, words, and sentences.
4. Anagrams or typewriter—if available. Some patients with severe apraxic or spatial agraphia can succeed in composing messages with a typewriter or anagram letters (Valenstein and Heilman, 1979).

Writing is a high-level, complex, cognitive process and a series of steps—each a distinct neuropsychologic function—is required for its successful execution (Luria, 1964, 1966). The individual functions are carried out in separate brain regions and, because of this, a focal cerebral lesion can disturb the writing process in a selective fashion, depending upon the location and extent of the damage.

In the hearing population, written language is predicated upon the auditory-verbal language system. Luria (1966) has demonstrated this by developmental studies. He asked children to write stories but prevented them from vocalizing by having them clench their tongues between their teeth. When thus restricted, the children's writing became grossly agraphic. The written language system in many people appears not to escape fully this reliance on verbal language; therefore, it is likely that in many instances the first step in writing is the mental production of a spoken message. The second step would require the transformation of this verbal phonemic system into a visual-spatial symbolic system. In Western languages, this involves a direct translation into a grapheme or letter-sound system, which is not always fully phonetic. These letters and their combinations become the basic visual-spatial building blocks of the written language system.

Serial ordering is an additional function which obviously is critical in both the phoneme selection of spoken language and the grapheme choice in written language. The actual act of writing requires a third step—the reproduction on paper of the graphemic symbol system. This final step requires a transformation of the visual-spatial symbol into a kinesthetic motor pattern that guides the hand and fingers through the writing motions.

Any lesion producing an aphasia in spoken speech will cause a concomitant agraphia. Left hemisphere posterior temporal lesions and lesions in the peri-Sylvian area posteriorly (supramarginal gyrus) (see Figure 1) will produce a fluent form of aphasia and an aphasic agraphia. If the lesion is more posterior in the parietal lobe (angular gyrus region), spoken language often is spared yet the visual-spatial symbol is deranged; the patient can neither interpret nor reproduce the symbols. This lesion produces an alexia as well as an agraphia (a syndrome discussed in greater detail elsewhere in this volume).

Some authors hypothesize that if a lesion is so placed as to damage the kinesthetic-motor patterns for writing—yet leaves undisturbed both the verbal lan-

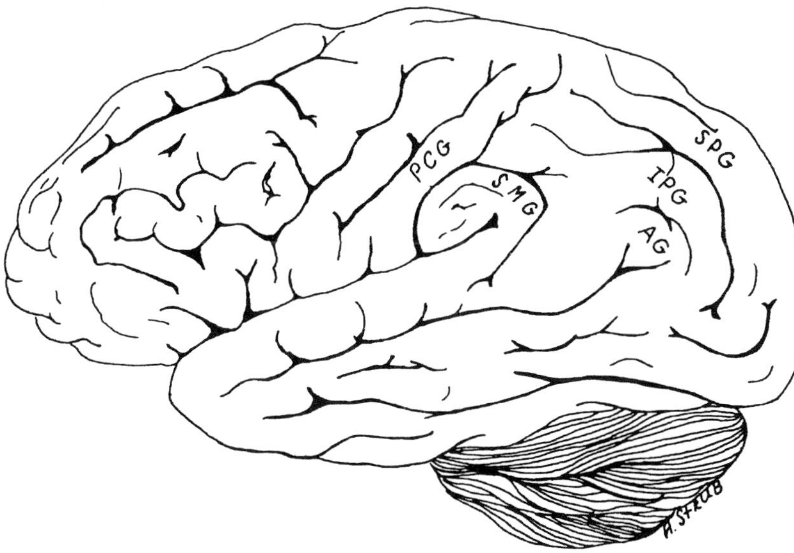


FIGURE 1. Left hemisphere of human brain. Post central gyrus (PCG) (areas 3, 1, 2-Brodmann); supramarginal gyrus (SMG) (area 40–Brodmann); angular (AG) gyrus (area 39–Brodmann); superior and inferior parietal gyri (SPG and IPG), superior parietal lobule (areas 5 and 7–Brodmann).

guage system and the visual-spatial symbolic representation system—a pure agraphia would be produced. This type of agraphia would be an apraxic agraphia, the variety usually described with the Gerstmann syndrome.

The existence of pure agraphia has been debated since Exner (1881) first postulated that an isolated agraphia would be produced by a lesion in the posterior portion of the second frontal gyrus. He contended that a lesion anterior to the hand region of the motor strip could produce a writing disturbance similar to the aphasia described by Broca (a lesion in the third frontal gyrus). The existence of isolated agraphia with frontal lesions continues to be controversal. Hécaen and Consoli (1973) have described some patients with mild, relatively pure agraphias from frontal lesion,s but these have been principally in the third frontal convolution rather than the second. Furthermore, these patients were all left-handers and this may represent a special case.

Lesions in the superior, anterior, and mid parietal area, however, have been reported to produce a pure agraphia (superior and inferior parietal gyrus—Areas 5 and 7) (Basso, Taborelli, and Vignolo, 1978; Russell and Espir, 1961). (See Figure 1.)

It is in this parietal cortex that kinesthetic images for the hand movements necessary for writing are thought to be integrated with the visual-spatial percept of the letters stored in the inferior parietal and parietal-occipital area (angular gyrus and surrounds). Lesions in this area produce, according to some authors, an apraxic agraphia, the type most commonly described in patients with the Gerstmann syndrome. A lesion in this area seems either to destroy the kinesthetic engrams of the graphemes or prevent their integration with the verbal and visual language systems. As patients with Gerstmann syndrome usually can copy much more adequately than they write spontaneously, it is doubtful that there is complete destruction of the sensory-motor engrams.

Several additional aspects of pure agraphia should be mentioned, although these have little relevance to the agraphia seen in the Gerstmann syndrome. Patients with severe constructional impairment, particularly with right or bilateral parietal lesions, often will have a severe spatial agraphia; their writing may either be extremely distorted, or, at times, be reduced to an illegible scrawl. This defect will produce an agraphia that is, in a sense, pure, as there is no aphasia, but the agraphia is more correctly only part of a more generalized constructional defect.

Several individual cases of pure agraphia have been reported. Rosati, De-Bastiani, and Pinna (1979) have described a single case of aphasic agraphia in a right-handed individual with a deep left temporal lesion. This patient had a mild comprehension deficit but demonstrated a severe agraphic disturbance. Assal, Chapuis, and Zander (1970) also reported a patient with a pure agraphia with a left hemisphere insult but of unspecified localization. Also, a rare form of isolated agraphia of the left hand has been described in a right-handed patient with a lesion in the anterior corpus callosum (Geschwind and Kaplan, 1962).

Left-handed patients demonstrate some interesting agraphic syndromes after hemispheric lesions. In general, they may have an agraphia that persists after a widespread aphasic disturbance clears. More specifically, an isolated apraxic agraphia has been described in several left-handed patients with right hemisphere lesions (Heilman, Coyle, Gonyea, and Geschwind, 1973; Valenstein and Heilman, 1979). One of the patients had no aphasia and seemed to have suffered destruction of sensory-motor engrams because he could produce normal written messages on a typewriter.

Chédru and Geschwind (1972) have noted a very high incidence of isolated spatial and aphasic agraphia in patients during acute confusional or delirious states. They comment that writing is a more difficult, less-practiced task that is very delicate and fragile. They raise the possibility that because many patients with pure agraphia have brain tumors, the agraphia they demonstrate may be secondary to the generalized effects of increased intracranial pressure and not the locus of the tumor. This mechanism may well explain many cases of pure agraphia, but it does not account for those seen secondary to stable vascular lesions, stable syndromes after missile wounds, or in the left-handed patient after recovery from a more significant aphasic disturbance.

**Acalculia**

Calculation is a very interesting, complex, cognitive ability. It is built on a set of very rudimentary, innate capacities and has developed to a high level through the use of various symbol systems. There are almost certainly innate functions necessary for the development of the ability to calculate, for example, an innate sense of number, the basic concepts of more and less, and an appreciation of the relationship of parts to the whole. On the other hand, much of the process of calculation is, like language, a culturally learned skill. A number of factors are necessary: first, a symbolic numbering system with some type of ordering as to magnitude; second, a decimal or place value or similar notation; third, a basic set of rules and concepts governing the manipulation of these symbols (e.g., adding, subtracting) and a set of signs to indicate the operations (e.g., +, –, ×). The act of calculation itself refers to this manipulation process.

In the Gerstmann syndrome, a defect in calculating ability or *acalculia* constitutes the fourth and final element. As with the other features of the syndrome, acalculia is a multifaceted abstract and very complex disturbance. Calculation and acalculia have been quite extensively studied and discussed (Grewel, 1952, 1969; Hécaen, Angelergues, and Houllier, 1961; Henschen, 1920) with three main categories of disturbance identified (Hécaen et al., 1961).

The first category is a *spatial acalculia* in which visual spatial impairment prevents the patient from properly organizing figures on the page when carrying out complex written problems. Alignment errors abound and orthographic features are distorted. Although this type of error principally disturbs the performance of complex written problems, complicated oral arithmetic problems requiring mental visualization may also be affected.

The second category of disturbance is a loss of the appreciation of basic arithmetic processes: carrying, borrowing, stepwise computation in complex multiplication, and so forth. This disorder has been labeled *anarithmetria* by Hécaen et al. (1961) and represents the purest form of acalculia.

The third form of acalculia is based on an inability to use the symbolic notation for both numbers and computational signs. This can be aphasic in nature (the patient produces incorrect number substitutions or paraphasias when solving oral calculations). Also, it can take the form of a number-and-sign alexia and agraphia in which the patient is unable to understand and use these written symbols. In one such case, studied by Benson and Denckla (1969), the patient produced both incorrect verbal and written answers to simple problems yet consistently could point to the correct answer from a number display. As is probably true of other cases, actual computational skills are intact although errors in phoneme or grapheme choice prevent the patient from demonstrating his competence.

In severe cases of acalculia, in addition to the deficits discussed, patients also may demonstrate a loss of memory for rote arithmetic tables and some may even lose their basic number concepts.

The acalculia in the Gerstmann syndrome has not received extensive study and there does not seem to be any agreement as to the type of calculation abnormality exhibited by the patients. Gerstmann (1940) felt it was a basic defect in arithmetic operations (anarithmetria) that, in severe cases, would manifest itself as a failure to understand number sequence and decimal value. Hécaen and Albert (1978) agree. Critchley (1953), on the other hand, considered it to be primarily a parietal or spatial acalculia which was evident most prominently on written calculation. Kinsbourne and Warrington (1962) observed a combination of errors: computational, spatial, and symbolic. They felt that automatic rote problems were least affected.

Since the exact nature of the acalculia in the Gerstmann syndrome is not well formulated, the evaluation of calculating ability should be comprehensive.

1. Counting—have the patient count up to 30 (errors do not often show up in simple one-digit numbers).
2. Assessing number concept—ask the patient which two numbers or stacks of coins is larger, and so on. Unfortunately, this type of testing requires verbal instructions and may show errors based on failure to comprehend complex relational, grammatical forms.
3. Translation of number concept into verbal and written symbol:
    a. Ask patient to tell and write down the number of objects shown to him (e.g., fingers, coins, etc.)
    b. Ask patient to read numbers and hold up the number of fingers indicated.
4. Oral calculations—start with rote sums and proceed to subtraction, multiplication, division, and then to complex calculations (e.g., 38 + 56). If incorrect answers are given, see if the patient can write or point to correct answer in a display or list of numbers.
5. Written calculations—use the same hierarchy suggested in Number 4. Vary signs and difficulty. Dictate problems for the patient to write and provide written examples.

Lesions in almost any region of the cortex can produce a disturbance in calculation; therefore, localization based on the presence of acalculia alone is impossible. There are, however, certain aspects of calculation errors that indicate damage in more defined areas of the cortex. Spatial acalculia is almost always associated with a parietal lesion, with right parietal lesions being more likely to produce a severe defect than left. Aphasic, agraphic, or alexic calculation problems are seen with lesions of the speech-dominant hemisphere. Anarithmetria usually is seen in bilateral disease but also can be seen with left parietal involvement. In the Gerstmann syndrome, the type of acalculia is uncertain so it is difficult to attach any specific localization significance to that specific symptom in isolation.

**Discussion of the Syndrome**

It is these four behavioral signs that constitute the classic Gerstmann syndrome. The diagnosis should not be made unless all four elements are present; to speak of a partial Gerstmann syndrome only serves to muddy already turbid waters. One problem that arises when assessing any behavioral sign is the specification of the quality or severity of failure necessary before a patient is considered to be suffering from a deficit in the corresponding function. Operational definitions have been devised that include quantitative cut-off scores on extensive test batteries. On the other hand, the presence of the four behavioral signs can often be satisfactorily ascertained at the bedside. If an adequate sample of behavior is obtained using the various modes of testing outlined, the diagnosis can be made, in most instances, without great difficulty.

In a medical syndrome, ideally, the principal symptoms or signs of the syndrome should be present in isolation or at least stand out clearly against any other behavioral or neurologic signs. In the Gerstmann syndrome, this luxury is seldom if ever enjoyed. In cases of the full Gerstmann syndrome, it is very common to find other accompanying signs; some, particularly constructional impairment, nearly always present; others, alexia, color agnosia, and right hemianopia, are found less frequently. Anomic aphasia is very commonly present but can be quite mild; and, as we have noted, aphasia may be totally absent. Despite the fact that associated symptoms are present to varying degrees, this does not detract from the localizing significance of the full syndrome as we discuss in the following section.

## Localization

In the many cases of the Gerstmann syndrome described in the literature, the overwhelming majority of patients have had a lesion involving the left parietal lobe (Table 1). Not unexpectedly, a patient with bilateral parietal or diffuse brain disease also can show the full syndrome. Rarely have cases been reported with right hemisphere lesions, and these have either been in left-handed patients or in patients whose right parietal lesion was a large tumor with widespread dysfunction from raised intracranial pressure. In general, a right-handed patient presenting with a full Gerstmann syndrome is very likely to have a left parietal lesion. In the study by Heimburger, Demyer, and Reitan (1964), 95% of the patients with the full syndrome had a left parietal lesion.

The syndrome has its greatest utility when other, more strongly, localizing signs are not present. The presence of significant aphasia in a right-handed patient, for example, very quickly and certainly identifies a left hemisphere lesion regardless of the presence or absence of finger agnosia. But the demonstration of the Gerstmann signs in a nonaphasic patient can be of great clinical value. The syndrome can be present in a progressive lesion such as a tumor or noted only as

TABLE 1. Cases of Full Gerstmann Reported in Literature

| *Author* | *Case No.* | *Hemisphere* | *Location and Type of Lesion* |
|---|---|---|---|
| Gerstmann (1924) | 1 | L | Angular gyrus—vascular |
| Herrmann and Pötzl (1926) | 2 | R | Angular gyrus—second occipital gyrus (ambidextrous patient) |
| Gerstmann (1927, 1930) | 1 | L | Parieto-occipital—tumor |
| | 2 | L | Parieto-occipital—vascular |
| Lange (1930) | | L | Parieto-occipital—temporal |
| Lange (1933) | | L | Parietal |
| Mussio-Fournier and Rawak (1934) | | L | Hemisphere—tumor |
| Muncie (1935) | 1 | L | Parieto-occipital—Tumor |
| | 2 | | Bilateral |
| Nielsen (1938) | 1 | L | Hemisphere—posterior, metastatic tumors |
| Olsen and Ruby (1941) | | L | Parietal—vascular |
| Stengel and Vienna (1944) | | | Bilateral—vascular |
| Arbuse (1947) | | L | Parieto-occipital—tumor |
| Critchley (1953) | 35118 | L | Parietal tumor |
| | C. S. | L | Parietal tumor |
| | J. W. | L | Hemisphere vascular |
| | 32579 | L | Parietal tumor |
| | 22019 | L | Parietal vascular |
| | 25140 | L | Hemisphere vascular |
| | L. B.-J. | L | Temporoparietal—tumor |
| | A. P. | | Bilateral—vascular |
| | 23452 | | Bilateral parietal—vascular |
| | F. E. W. | | Bilateral atrophy |
| | 24033 | | Bilateral parieto-occipital vascular |
| | 12621 | L | Bilateral—vascular |
| | 36459 | L | Angular gyrus—tumor |
| | 35427 | L | Hemisphere—tumor |
| Russell and Espir (1961) | 68 | L | Anterior superior parietal—missle |
| Kinsbourne and Warrington (1962) | 1 | | Bilateral atrophy |
| | 2 | | Bilateral atrophy |
| | 3 | | Bilateral atrophy |
| | 4 | | Bilateral atrophy |
| | 5 | L & R | Multiple sclerosis |
| | 6 | L | Degeneration |
| | 7 | L | Posterior parietal—tumor |
| | 8 | L | Parieto-occipital—tumor (left-handed) |
| | 9 | R | Parieto-temporal—vascular (left-handed) |

*continued*

TABLE 1. Cases of Full Gerstmann Reported in Literature (continued)

| *Author* | *Case No.* | *Hemisphere* | *Location and Type of Lesion* |
|---|---|---|---|
| Heimburger et al. (1964) | 23 cases | | |
| *Statistical study showing* | 78% | L | Posterior |
| | 13% | | Bilateral |
| | 9% | R | Hemisphere (large tumor, no comment as to handedness) |
| Poeck and Orgass (1966) | 4 cases | | All left hemisphere or bilateral |
| Benson and Denckla (1969) | 1 | L | Posterior parietal—vascular |
| | 2 | L | Posterior parietal—tumor |
| Kinsbourne and Rosenfield (1974) | 1 | L | Posterior parietotemporal vascular |
| Strub and Geschwind (1974) | 1 | | Bilateral atrophy |
| Hrbek (1977) | 1 | L | Upper-mid parietal—tumor |
| | 2 | L | Parietal—tumor |
| | 3 | L | Hemisphere—tumor |
| | 4 | L | Parietotemporal—hemorrhage |
| | 5 | L | Pareital—vascular |
| | 6 | L | Inferior parietal—vascular |
| | 7 | L | Anterior—mid parie |
| | 8 | L | Parietotemporal—trauma |
| | 9 | L | Parietal—not well-localized encephalitis |
| | 10 | L | Inferior parietal—vascular |
| | 11 | | Bilateral atrophy |
| | 12 | L | Temporal—tumor (transient symptoms) |
| | 13 | L | Temporal hemorrhage |
| | 14 | L | Frontotemporal—tumor |
| | 15 | L | Frontotemporal—tumor |
| | 17 | | Diffuse embolization |
| Kertesz (1979) | 1 | L | Parietal—vascular |
| | 2 | L | Parietal—vascular |
| | 3 | L | Parietal—aneurysm |
| | 4 | L | Parietal—hemorrhage |
| | 5 | | Unspecified—trauma |
| | 6 | L | Parietal—tumor |
| | 7 | L | Parietal—tumor |
| | 8 | L | Parietal—tumor |
| | 9 | | Bilateral—tumor |
| Rosati et al. (1979) | 1 | L | Parietotemporo-occipital—tumor |
| Roeltgen et al. (1983) | 1 | L | Parietal—infarct |

| | | |
|---|---|---|
| Total | L Hemisphere | 68 |
| | Bilateral | 20 |
| | R Hemisphere | 4 |
| | Either L or Bilateral | 4 (Poeck & Orgass, 1969) |
| | | 96 |

a more significant deficit is regressing. This latter group is no less interesting scientifically yet is of less obvious clinical usefulness.

Of theoretical interest has been the attempt to localize the lesion more discretely within the left parietal lobe. Although of no great additional clinical importance, such an exercise may help us to further understand the complex functioning of the parietal lobe. We disagree with Critchley (1953) that any attempt at more discrete localization is "a vain and unpromising task." Some of the pathologic material may allow a certain degree of regional localization within the left parietal lobe and can supply indication for further research.

Gerstmann (1930, 1940) felt that the lesion involved the angular gyrus (Figure 1) and contiguous second occipital convolution. Heimburger et al. (1964) agreed that the angular gyrus was involved, but not in all cases. They also described some cases in which a lesion restricted to this gyrus did not produce the syndrome. Judging from their data, damage to the angular gyrus is neither essential nor sufficient for the appearance of the syndrome. It should be noted that all their patients with the four Gerstmann signs had large lesions which invariably produced a picture of widespread neurologic dysfunction. Specific localization data for their cases are not reported but their conclusions are well founded.

In a missile wound case reported by Russell and Espir (1961), a severe, nonaphasic Gerstmann syndrome was described with a lesion in the mid and superior left parietal lobe, somewhat superior to, but including, the angular gyrus (Case 68). Hrbek (1977), in an extensive discussion of the syndrome with a description of 17 personally collected cases, argues that the necessary lesion is on the border between supramarginal gyrus and superior parietal lobule. Roeltgen, Sevush, and Heilman (1983) have reported a case of a pure Gerstmann syndrome (all four components and no evidence of aphasia or constructional impairment) in which the lesion was in the superior angular gyrus that extended into the supramarginal gyrus and minimally into the inferior parietal gyrus (inferior portion of the superior parietal lobule).

From a review of the reported cases, it appears that the most likely lesion to produce the Gerstmann syndrome is posteriorly placed in the parietal lobe, in the angular gyrus as suggested originally by Gerstmann, but extending into the superior parietal lobule (superior and inferior parietal gyrus) rather than into occipital lobe. Such a lesion seems to produce the syndrome in its least contaminated form. This high lesion, such as the one described by Russell and Espir (1961, Case 68), Kertesz (1979, cases 1 and 7), and Roeltgen, Sevush, and Heilman (1983) is well away from the classic language zone and therefore produces neither aphasia nor alexia. Constructional impairment is present in all but the case of Roeltgen, Sevush, and Heilman (1983) and seems almost inexorably associated with the classic four components of the syndrome. It is clear that many patients will show evidence of aphasia because the language zone is quite close and frequently involved.

It is true, and not too surprising, that most lesions of the left parietal lobe will not produce the Gerstmann syndrome but will show other interesting and important neurologic and behavioral signs. This is a separate issue entirely and in no way negates the utility, and certainly not the existence, of the syndrome.

## Discussion

### Pathophysiology and Neuropsychology of the Syndrome

From an analysis of the symptomatology and a description of pathologic data, it is evident that the Gerstmann syndrome represents a complex multifaceted disturbance of dominant parietal function. The basis of the neuropsychologic deficits have been debated and various attempts have been made to establish a single unifying mechanism to explain all findings. Gerstmann attempted to show that a basic disturbance in body schema could explain the entire syndrome. The principal features of finger agnosia and right-left disorientation are aspects of a spatial knowledge of the body, particularly the hand. However, to associate calculation ontogenetically with counting on the fingers and writing with a physiologic differentiation of the fingers may be stretching the concept of body scheme beyond its definition.

Stengel and Vienna (1944) believed that the defect in constructional ability was the basic disturbance. Constructional impairment is admittedly commonly seen with the syndrome, and Stengel's case could certainly be explained on the basis of constructional impairment alone. There are, however, many other cases that clearly would not support this hypothesis.

Poeck and Orgass (1966) propose that the Gerstmann syndrome merely reflects a more generalized language disturbance or aphasia. Aphasia often is present because of the propinquity of the language zone to the angular gyrus and superior parietal lobule. An aphasic will demonstrate agraphia and may show difficulty on verbal testing of finger identification, right-left, and calculation. The syndrome produced is often an artifactual Gerstmann syndrome but not as it is commonly understood. We disagree with Poeck and Orgass and also Russell (1963) that to separate the Gerstmann symptoms from an aphasic disorder is an artificial exercise. Agraphia and acalculia are certainly language-related, but the concepts of body schema embodied in finger agnosia and right-left sense are very likely distinctly spatial and may not be related to language except through the verbal method of testing.

Kinsbourne and Warrington (1964) suggest that the Gerstmann syndrome is basically a disorder of spatiotemporal sequencing. The correct ordering of fingers on the hand, letters in the word, numbers in the continuum, and sides of the body are directly related to spatial and temporal ordering. This is an appealing hypothesis as ordering is a common feature; yet, it may merely reflect a basic analytic function ascribed to the entire left hemisphere. Thus, a common underlying feature may be present but may, in fact, actually be too general a function to be classified as a unifying mechanism.

In our view, there is, at present, no single underlying neuropsychologic defect that can explain the four cardinal symptoms seen in the Gerstmann syndrome. The parietal lobe is a complex and very highly developed region of cortex in which visual, tactile, and auditory-sensory information is processed and stored (Luria, 1966). It is in the parietal lobe that cross-modal associations are probably formed between the sense modalities. Complex kinesthetic patterns also are developed and stored in the parietal lobe; these, in turn, guide highly skilled and complex motor activity. It is obvious that the parietal lobe has many diverse functions and that any lesion will (in all likelihood) disrupt several separate yet interlocking cortical systems. Depending on the exact location and extent of the lesion and the peculiarities of the individual brain in which the lesion occurs, a variety of symptoms and symptom clusters may be seen. In some patients, a specific left parietal lesion will produce a clinical picture of the Gerstmann syndrome. Careful analysis of the individual symptoms and localization data gives us a realistic understanding of the pathophysiology of the symptom complex and allows us to postulate the region of the dominant parietal most likely to be involved (Hrbek, 1977). It seems that a lesion involving the symbolic system of the angular gyrus and kinesthetic system of the superior parietal lobule can produce, in relatively isolated fashion, the four signs of the Gerstmann syndrome accompanied by constructional impairment.

## Criticism of the Syndrome

In recent years, the Gerstmann syndrome has been assailed on several fronts. To some, it is an enigma (Critchley, 1966); to others, a fiction (Benton, 1961, 1977; Heimburger et al., 1964; Poeck and Orgass, 1966). Since the syndrome has engendered so much controversy in the recent literature, we feel that the principal arguments should be aired to make the reader aware of the issues surrounding the controversy.

Some investigators have argued that the syndrome is intrinsically a part of a broader aphasic disorder (Poeck and Orgass, 1966). In support of this view, Critchley (1966, 1970) speaks of latent, or preaphasia, as a possible explanation of many of the symptoms. We discussed this issue earlier in the chapter and summarize here.

It is true that many individuals with significant aphasia will—because of their aphasia—be unable adequately to perform the more complex tasks described by Gerstmann. The Gerstmann syndrome may be seen in patients with only mild aphasia, in which the Gerstmann components are severe and cannot, therefore, be accounted for by the aphasia. In such a case, it would be unjustified to consider the syndrome as resulting from aphasia. There are, of course, cases of the syndrome in which no aphasia has been demonstrated, evidence that substantially negates the argument that the syndrome is actually part of an aphasic disorder. The question of a latent or preaphasia in this context is somewhat cryptic. Whereas it is true that many functions tested in the Gerstmann components have drawn to a greater or lesser extent on verbal language during development, it seems illogical to call on language errors to explain this syndrome in a clinically nonaphasic patient.

A second issue revolves around a basic misunderstanding about the concept of a syndrome as used in clinical medicine. It has been stated that the correlation among the Gerstmann components is weak and that individual components are more strongly correlated with other deficits (Benton, 1961). Benton (1961) and others state that it is, therefore, not a syndrome at all. We believe, however, that this analysis is based on a fundamental misunderstanding of what traditionally is meant by a syndrome.

The essence of a medical syndrome is that a collection of signs or symptoms, when all present, indicate the presence of a specific disease. The correlation between elements in a syndrome can be low, high, or in between. Thus, the combination of hoarseness, nystagmus, a Horner's syndrome, pain loss on one side of the face and on the opposite side of the body would lead to the diagnosis of an infarction in the lateral medulla, most commonly as a result of an occlusion in the posterior inferior cerebellar artery or in the vertebral artery from which it springs. It is obvious that, if one were to study a great number of patients, one would find a very low correlation between hoarseness and nystagmus, or between a Horner's syndrome and either of these.

Indeed, a syndrome is most useful as a diagnostic tool precisely when the elements usually are not found together. When they are found together, this strongly points to some special pathological process. Furthermore, the lateral medullary syndrome is composed of elements not based on a disturbance of some common physiological foundation but on proximity of anatomical systems. Other syndromes, in particular, those based on some underlying pathologic disturbance, do have symptoms which have a common pathophysiology, that is, the components of Addison's syndrome or of congestive heart failure. The anatomic studies have shown that the Gerstmann syndrome does predict—with high accuracy—damage to the left parietal lobe and, because of this, the Gerstmann syndrome qualifies as a true clinical syndrome.

A final and very important criticism of the Gerstmann syndrome is that the four elements of the syndrome are not seen in isolation from other neurologic and behavioral findings. Many authors, including Gerstmann himself, have noted that their patients demonstrate associated symptoms. The major point of the criticism is that Gerstmann arbitrarily chose the four elements from personal bias, and might just as easily have chosen another cluster of left parietal symptoms. Certainly, this is a valid point. It is clear, however, that Gerstmann chose his four components very well since, in fact, they do predict left parietal disease with high accuracy. Future research can discover whether there is some other constellation that is even more strongly predictive. There are many interesting behavioral deficits associated with dominant parietal lesions and clinical neurologists (as well as psychologists) should be aware of them. One would hope that, through increased study of cases, a variety of focal behavioral syndromes can be identified. Because of the many functions performed by the dominant parietal lobe, it is obvious that a number of typical syndromes have evolved and will continue to do so. The syndrome of alexia with agraphia with or without anomic aphasia is one well-established example. Unfortunately, much time has been spent in the last 20 years seeking to discredit or support the Gerstmann syndrome rather than establishing the validity of other behavioral syndromes associated with parietal disease.

In conclusion, we can say that Gerstmann made a definite contribution to the study of higher cognitive functioning and that his syndrome is still of clinical value. We would, however, strongly agree with Benton (1961) that many investigators, in their adherence to the four classic symptoms, have often prejudiced their clinical observations and not given adequate attention to other behavioral signs of parietal disease. At this point, it seems far better to end the condemnation or praise of the syndrome and let time place it in its proper perspective in the field of neurobehavior.

## References

Arbuse, D. I. (1947). The Gerstmann Syndrome. Case report and review of the literature. *Journal of Nervous and Mental Disease, 105,* 359–371.

Assal, G., Chapuis, G., & Zander, E. (1970). Isolated writing disorders in a patient with stenosis of the left internal carotid artery. *Cortex, 6,* 241–248.

Badal, J. (1888). Contribution à l'étude des cécités psychiques; alexie, agraphe, hémianope inférieure, trouble du sens de l'espace. *Archives Ophthalmologie (Paris), 8,* 97–117.

Basso, A., Taborelli, A., & Vignolo, A. (1978). Dissociated disorders of speaking and writing in aphasia. *Journal of Neurology, Neurosurgery and Psychiatry, 41,* 556–563.

Benson, D. F., & Denckla, M. B. (1969). Verbal paraphasia as a source of calculation disturbance. *Archives of Neurology (Chicago), 21,* 96–102.

Benton, A. L. (1961). The fiction of the "Gerstmann syndrome." *Journal of Neurology, Neurosurgery and Psychiatry, 24,* 176–181.

Benton, A. L. (1968). Right-left discrimination. *Pediatric Clinics of North America, 15,* 747–758.

Benton, A. L. (1977). Reflections on the Gerstmann Syndrome. *Brain and Language, 4,* 45–62.

Benton, A. L. (1979). Body schema disturbances: Finger agnosia and right-left disorientation. In K. M. Heilman & E. Valenstein (Eds.), *Clinical neuropsychology.* London & New York: Oxford University Press, pp. 141–158.

Chédru, F., & Geschwind, N. (1972). Writing disturbances in acute confusional states. *Neuropsychologia, 10,* 343–353.

Critchley, M. (1953). *The parietal lobes.* London: Arnold.

Critchley, M. (1966). The enigma of Gerstmann's syndrome. *Brain, 89,* 183–198.

Critchley, M. (1970). *Aphasiology and other aspects of language.* London: Arnold.

Dennis, M. (1976). Dissociated naming and locating of body parts after left anterior temporal lobe resection: An experimental case study. *Brain and Language, 3,* 147–163.

Exner, S. (1881). *Untersuchungenüber die Lokalisation der Funktionen in der Grosshirnrinde des Menschen.* Vienna: W. Braumuller.

Gainotti, G., & Tiacci, C. (1973). The unilateral forms of finger agnosia. *Confinia Neurologia, 35,* 271–284.

Gerstmann, J. (1924). Fingeragnosie: Eine umschriebene Störung der Orientierung am eigenen Körper. *Wiener Klinische Wochenschrift, 37,* 1010–1012.

Gerstmann, J. (1927). Fingeragnosie und isolierte Agraphie, ein neues Syndrom. *Zeitschrift fuer die Gesamte Neurologie und Psychiatrie, 108,* 381–402.

Gerstmann, J. (1930). Zur Symptomatologie der Hirnläsionen im Uebergangsgbeit der unteren Parietal und mittleren Occipitalwindung. *Nervenarzt, 3,* 691–695.

Gerstmann, J. (1940). Syndrome of finger agnosia, disorientation for right and left, agraphia and acalculia. *Archives of Neurology and Psychiatry, 44,* 398–408.

Geschwind, N. (1975). The apraxia: Neural mechanisms of disorders of learned movement. *American Scientist, 63,* 188–195.

Grewel, F. (1952). Acalculia. *Brain, 75,* 397–407.

Grewel, F. (1969). The acalculia. In P. G. Vinken & G. W. Bruyn (Eds.), *Handbook of clinical neurology* (Vol. 4). Amsterdam: North-Holland, pp. 181–194.

Head, H. (1926). *Aphasia and kindred disorders of speech* (Vol. 1). London & New York: Cambridge University Press, pp. 157–158.

Hécaen, H., Angelergues, R., & Houllier, S. (1961). Les variétés cliniques des acalculies au cours des lésions retro-rolandiques: Approche statistique du problème. *Revue Neurologique, 105,* 85–103.

Hécaen, H., & Albert, M. L. (1978). *Human neuropsychology.* New York: Wiley.

Hécaen, H., & Consoli, S. (1973). Analyse des troubles du langage au cours des lésions de l'aire de Broca. *Neuropsychologia, 11,* 377–388.

Heilman, K. M., Coyle, J. M., Gonyea, E. F., & Geschwind, N. (1973). Apraxia and agraphia in a left-hander. *Brain, 96,* 21–28.

Heimburger, R. F., Demyer, W., & Reitan, R. M. (1964). Implications of Gerstmann's syndrome. *Journal of Neurology, Neurosurgery and Psychiatry, 27,* 52–57.

Henschen, S. E. (1920). *Klinische und anatomische Beritrage zur Pathologie des Gehirns.* Stockholm: Nordiska Bokhandel'n.

Herrmann, G., & Pötzl, O. (1926). *Über die Agraphie und ihre lokaldiagnostischen Beziehungen.* Basel: Karger.

Hrbek, V. (1977). Pathophysiologic interpretation of Gerstmann's syndrome. Definition of new broader syndrome of interparietal disconnection. Their value for topical diagnostics of lesions in the dominant cerebral hemisphere. *Acta Univde l'aire de Broca. Neuropsychologia, 11,* 377–388.

Kertesz, A. (1979). *Aphasia and associated disorders: Taxonomy, localization, and recovery.* New York: Grune & Stratton, pp. 211–229.

Kinsbourne, M., & Rosenfield, D. B. (1974). Agraphia selective for written spelling. *Brain and Language, 1,* 215–225.

Kinsbourne, M., & Warrington, E. K. (1962). A study of finger agnosia. *Brain, 85,* 47–66.

Kinsbourne, M., & Warrington, E. K. (1964). Disorders of spelling. *Journal of Neurology, Neurosurgery and Psychiatry, 27,* 224–228.

Lange, J. (1930). Fingeragnosie und Agraphie (ein psychopathologische studie). *Monatsschrift fuer Psychiatrie und Neurologie, 76,* 129–188.

Lange, J. (1933). Probleme der Fingeragnosie. *Zeitschrift fuer die Gesamte Neurologie und Psychiatrie, 147,* 594–610.

Luria, A. R. (1964). Neuropsychology in the local diagnosis of brain damage. *Cortex, 1,* 3–18.

Luria, A. R. (1966). *Higher cortical functions in man.* New York: Basic Books.

Muncie, E. (1935). Finger Agnosia (Gerstmann). *Bulletin of the Johns Hopkins Hospital, 57,* 330–342.

Mussio-Fournier, J. C., & Rawak, F. (1934). Glioblastome de l'hémisphère gauche avec syndrome de Gerstmann. *Revue Neurologique, 2,* 681–685.

Nielsen, J. M. (1938). Gerstmann Syndrome: Finger agnosia, agraphia, confusion of right and left and acalculia. *Archives of Neurology and Psychiatry, 39,* 536–560.

Olsen, C. W., & Ruby, C. (1941). Anosognosia and autotopagnosia. *Archives of Neurology and Psychiatry, 46,* 340–345.

Poeck, K., & Orgass, B. (1966). Gerstmann's syndrome and aphasia. *Cortex, 2,* 421–439.

Poeck, K., & Orgass, B. (1969). An experimental investigation of finger agnosia. *Neurology, 19,* 801–807.

Roeltgen, D. P., Sevush, S., & Heilman, K. M. (1983). Pure Gerstmann's syndrome from a focal lesion. *Archives of Neurology (Chicago), 40,* 46–47.

Rosati, G., & DeBastiani, P. (1979). Pure agraphia: A discrete form of aphasia. *Journal of Neurology, Neurosurgery and Psychiatry, 42,* 266–269.

Rosati, G., DeBastiani, P., & Pinna, L. (1979). La sindrome di Gerstmann: Considerazioni su un caso. *Rivista di Neurologia, 49,* 205–218.

Russell, W. R. (1963). Some anatomical aspects of aphasia. *Lancet, 1,* 1173–1177.

Russell, W. R., & Espir, M. L. E. (1961). *Traumatic aphasia.* London & New York: Oxford University Press.

Sauguet, J., Benton, A. L., & Hécaen, H. (1971). Disturbances of the body schema in relation to language impairment and hemisphere locus of lesion. *Journal of Neurology, Neurosurgery and Psychiatry, 34,* 496–501.

Schilder, P. (1931). Fingeragnosie, Fingerapraxie, Fingeraphasie. *Nervenartz, 4,* 625–629.

Stengel, E., & Vienna, M. D. (1944). Loss of spatial orientation, constructional apraxia and Gerstmann's syndrome. *Journal of Mental Science, 90,* 753–760.

Strub, R. L., & Geschwind, N. (1974). Gerstmann syndrome without aphasia. *Cortex, 10,* 378–387.

Valenstein, E., & Heilman, K. M. (1979). Apraxic agraphia with neglect induced paragraphia. *Archives of Neurology (Chicago), 36,* 506–508.

Wolf, S. M. (1973). Difficulties in right-left discrimination in a normal population. *Archives of Neurology (Chicago), 29,* 128–129.

# CHAPTER 27

# Anatomical Localization in Clinical Neuropsychology

*Antonio R. Damasio and Norman Geschwind*

The resurgence of behavioral neurology in the sixties had a major focus on the structural basis of the higher brain functions, and the introduction and development of modern methods of brain imaging have revived interest in the anatomical correlates of behavioral disorders. In the ten years since the introduction of computerized tomography (CT), and especially since the appearance of third and fourth generation scanners which permit the visualization of fine anatomical detail, it has become possible not only to replicate classic anatomical studies in larger series of patients, but to add numerous new features to the anatomical mapping of neuropsychological syndromes, and even to describe the anatomical correlates of previously uncharted disorders. The current development of nuclear magnetic resonance imaging (MRI) promises further advances in this direction, while the techniques of positron emission tomography (PET) and single photon emission tomography (SPET), complement the structural findings with important functional data.

The net result of these developments is that the study of the behavioral correlates of focal lesions in humans, the method that has perhaps single-handedly contributed more than any other to the field of brain-behavior relationships, is once again a valid and productive means of gathering information on brain structure and function. The theoretical limitations and the pitfalls of the method have, however, not changed. The procedural constraints required to make its use valid are as necessary as ever, and the appropriate interpretation of results still depends on thorough neurological competence. In the first part of this chapter

---

Reprinted with permission from P.J. Vinken, G.W. Bruyn, and H.L. Klawans (eds), *Handbook of Clinical Neurology. Volume 1 (45): Clinical Neuropsychology.* Amsterdam: Elsevier Science Publishers B.V., 1985; 7-22.

we discuss some of these methodological problems. In the later sections we have presented two areas as illustrative of the power of localizing studies.

## Problems in Anatomical Localization

By far the most common types of criticism of the lesion method have been based on (a) the inappropriate attribution of a lost function to the locus of a lesion, and (b) exceptions to and inconsistencies of anatomical localization. The first of these reflects problems of interpretation. Only an uninformed or naive thinker can believe that Wernicke regarded the area which came to carry his name as the site where the full process of auditory comprehension took place; yet, Wernicke and many of his most important followers have been accused of precisely that belief. No effort should be spared to make it clear that the effects of a circumscribed locus of damage can be understood only by taking into account that the healthy brain tissue that has been destroyed was a component of a neural network, the activity of which mediates the normal function; and furthermore, that to understand post-lesion alterations in function one must take into account changes in other parts of that network.

The argument regarding exceptions and inconsistencies in localization depends, as usually stated, on invalid assumptions. No one can disagree with the assertion that exceptions or inconsistencies demand attention. In some instances they lead to the realization that the asserted localization is incorrect, and thus serve the same function that discrepant data serve in every branch of science. All too often, however, the argument is advanced that the existence of discrepancies shows that the very concept of localization of function is untenable. Implicit in this argument is the belief that a particular localization is acceptable only if it is universally valid. This odd assumption would lead to the conclusion that ulnar nerve lesions could not produce differing patterns of sensory loss in different cases, rejecting the possibility of individual variations. It is clear that, in order to establish a valid correlation between disordered behavior and the site of anatomical brain damage related to it, it is necessary to take into account a large number of factors, the principal of which are: (a) the nature of the pathological process, (b) the size of the lesion, (c) the speed of the pathological process, (d) the timing of the anatomical and behavioral observations, (e) individual variations in neurological organization, and (f) the age, level of education, sex, and premorbid psychological and social factors of the individual under study. Experimental studies of lesions in nonhuman species amply document both the importance of such factors and their neurological mechanisms, and reading of the classical masters of localization will uncover awareness of these issues, even if, in the hundred and twenty years since Broca described his first patient with aphasia, few studies have taken into account many of these factors. Yet, in spite of imperfect methodology, the consistency of many findings has been overwhelming, and it has been possible to draw strong conclusions about some relations between brain structure and behavior. Although critics of anatomical localization constantly emphasize the exceptional instances which deviate from those conclusions, it is by far the regularity and consistency of the correlations that is striking, considering that more often than not they can be verified. In fact, the mere consideration of the frequency of individual variations in the factors enumerated above makes it surprising that so many strong associations have been established. With improvements in methodology the accuracy of localization and the capacity to account for discrepant instances are likely to improve steadily.

## Nature of pathology

*Cerebral vascular disease.* Lesions caused by cerebral vascular disease are appropriate for anatomical localization, especially those caused by non-hemorrhagic infarction. In many respects some non-hemorrhagic infarctions are equivalent to the acute lesions that an investigator can make in an experimental animal in a laboratory setting and are—in some instances—superior, since the complications of anesthesia and surgery do not play an interfering role. Like an experimental lesion, a stroke suddenly produces damage in a previously normal brain with standard anatomical organization while, as we will indicate, tumors often grow in embryonic cell nests reflecting anomalous brain organization. Even in the acute phase, provided they are of limited size, strokes usually do not have much surrounding edema and therefore do not shift brain structures to any great extent. Nonetheless, even in such 'ideal' instances, some factors must be taken into account before a one-to-one relationship is established between lesion and dysfunction. For instance, patients with fresh cerebrovascular disease sometimes have other lesions, previously or simultaneously acquired. On the other hand, some cases with multiple lesions are especially important for two reasons: (1) They can provide clues as to how a system reacts to successive losses. When a new lesion appears in a patient who has undergone careful study of an earlier one, the situation can come close to the staged lesion experiment in the laboratory; properly utilized, such instances are of great importance. (2) A particularly important point is that combinations of lesions can produce effects which do not result from either lesion in isolation, and can thus give important clues as to both normal functional organization and mechanisms of recovery after lesions. Destruction of the splenium alone does not lead to an inability to comprehend written language, yet the combination of a splenial lesion with an occipital one frequently does so.

Hemorrhagic infarctions raise problems of interpretation although they are by no means insurmountable. In most patients, during the acute phase, blood can behave as a space-occupying lesion and cause dysfunction in adjoining structures. But as the healing process proceeds this is no longer the case and a more cautious correlation is possible.

It is sometimes stated that vascular lesions are unacceptable because the brain is almost invariably riddled with other lesions or suffers from general low level ischemia. While multiple strokes certainly do occur in some cases, a very large proportion of patients with cerebrovascular disease do not suffer a second stroke. Pathological study confirms that a very large proportion of patients have suffered only a single stroke.

*Brain tumors.* Localization based on brain tumors can be hazardous. The prediction of the locus of lesion purely for clinical purposes works well in the majority of instances, but research investigations based on this material must take into account the variable mechanism of mass action of tumors. For instance, meningiomas may act by compressing the brain from without, by producing edema, by the elicitation of seizures or, rarely, by causing vascular disturbances. Disordered function may result from disturbances in an area far larger than that which the tumor overlies. Gliomas, on the other hand, can grow even to massive size in the midst of neurons without actually damaging them, and may cause fewer signs than a vascular lesion of similar size and location. Seizures or regional vascular steal syndromes may confound the picture, giving rise to dysfunction in areas distant from the lesion.

Surgical ablations performed to excise tumors may provide excellent material for behavioral correlation. Some of these cases may actually be ideal, especially when the surgery is performed to remove large meningiomas that have impinged on nearby healthy brain tissue.

Some further factors must be considered in evaluating the effects of tumors. When growth is slow one may have a situation comparable to that of experimental staged lesions which often produce much less impairment than total lesions of the same extent produced in one stage. Some tumors arise from areas malformed in utero which often lead to alteration of the pattern of the brain. Tumors which have grown very slowly since early life may produce as little impairment as other childhood lesions despite extensive damage.

*CNS infection.* Instances of CNS infection and inflammatory disease rarely constitute good material for anatomical investigation, but herpes simplex encephalitis is an exception. Survivors of this devastating illness have well-defined and stable lesions, for the most part confined to structures of the limbic system.

*Cerebral anoxia* is another example of usually unsuitable pathology although there are conspicuous exceptions. Severity and distribution of damage, even if it falls in relatively predictable patterns of cellular vulnerability, is dependent on the type and duration of anoxic insult and on the method and vigor of the ensuing treatment.

*Head injury.* Although there is a definite association between patterns of closed head injury and damage to certain areas of the brain, the material from head injury is mostly unsuitable for detailed localization. It is almost always impossible for investigation purposes to exclude the presence of additional damage and dysfunction caused by trauma or by its consequences. Bilateral damage caused by contrecoup injury is especially common. Some authors state that penetrating brain wounds provide superb material for localization because they produce clean, well-defined lesions. This, however, reflects unawareness of the pathological findings in most such cases, including gross brain distortion, edema, and infection.

*Surgery for epilepsy.* Surgery for epilepsy can often provide excellent material for localization, but two general problems must be considered. In the first place, the patients have previous neurological disease that leads to the surgery and often have a variety of accompanying factors related to the disease such as learning disorders, complex psychological reaction to their morbid condition, drug toxicity, etc. In a very large proportion of cases, the majority in many series, the lesions date back to childhood or prenatal life, thus leading to all the complications of early lesions. Secondly, the surgery may cause lesions in locations other than the planned site of the surgery. Thus split-brain subjects who typically have early lesions and long standing epilepsy, often suffer damage to extracallosal structures, e.g., the medial frontal lobes and the fornices. Even the most careful and observant surgeon may not be able to see the true extent of the pathology, particularly when the craniotomy is small. As any pathologist knows, even at post mortem, intact meninges can prevent visualization of a lesion which may be quite obvious after the meninges are stripped.

### Location and size of lesion

The location and the size of a lesion are inseparable factors. Any cerebral lesion may involve loci in predominantly gray matter or white matter, or both, and a larger lesion hence encompasses a larger number of loci. In addition, size can have its independent effects. A large lesion of whatever nature can, by its space-occupying action or by surrounding edema, displace cerebral contents and shift them across the midline, or downward, or upward, leading to a variety of cerebral herniation syndromes. The net effect is the creation of dysfunction in areas which were not primarily involved by the lesion, by a variety of mechanical, vascular, and metabolic mechanisms. Lack of awareness of such potential effects can lead to major errors in localization, especially when the localization is made purely on the basis of clinical signs without post-mortem or neuroimaging information. By far the most common example of this problem is the appearance, in cases with large lesions of one hemisphere, of ipsilateral motor signs such as hemiparesis, tremor, or rigidity, caused by compression of the contralateral midbrain against the tentorium.

### Other factors

The *time elapsed since the onset of lesion,* even if the causative process is static, is of crucial importance. In most lesions caused by cerebral vascular disease, the process of repair runs its course within the first four weeks, and beyond the second month most of these lesions are stable. The adaptation of the patient to the associated behavioral defects, and the spontaneous or acquired mechanisms of compensation may, however, continue actively beyond that period, depending on a variety of individual differences in brain organization and on psychological and social circumstances.

The roles of *age* and *level of education* are generally well known, but some points deserve comment. It is well known that extensive unilateral lesions of the language areas in childhood are typically followed by excellent, if not perfect recovery, which is attributable to a shift of the language zones. Yet it is not uncommon to find that excision of a lesion that dates back to childhood, in one of the usual language cortices (e.g., for epilepsy), causes only transient aphasia or no aphasia. Such cases are often cited as evidence against standard teachings on localization. Similarly, the possibility that many early lesions lead to reorganization is overlooked, leading to incorrect conclusions regarding the applicability of the post-surgical effects to standard patterns of brain organization.

*Sex* may also be of major importance. There is uncontrovertible evidence that the vulnerability to a variety of diseases is sex-related. It is also likely that certain aspects of brain organization related to higher forms of behavior are sexually dimorphic; this may well account for differences of localization in relation to certain behaviors.

Even within the same sex, varying *endocrine factors during fetal and childhood development* probably lead to remarkable differences in the anatomical and functional organization of the brain, perhaps most markedly in relation to such processes as language and affect. Our understanding of those variations is elementary and the clinical indices of such variation are imperfect, e.g., handedness or the lateralization of performance in dichotic listening. These variations will demand more attention in the future and it is reasonable to suspect that they play a role in the consistency or inconsistency of anatomical clinical correlations.

*Epileptic lesions* can lead to an alteration in nervous system pathways. Despite this fact many authors overlook the possibility that *surgery* in cases with long-standing epilepsy may produce deviant results, especially when the epilepsy is the result of a childhood lesion.

## Neuroimaging methods

It is not appropriate to discuss here the complex methodology necessary for appropriate neuroimaging studies, but because most lesion studies are and will be based on some form of neuroimaging, some comments are in order. In the first place, the technical quality of the principal neuroimaging method, computerized tomography, has changed by leaps and bounds in the first decade of its existence. The quality of a technically satisfactory fourth generation CT scan bears little resemblance to images obtained only five years ago, because of improved resolution and reduction of artifacts in areas of interface between high and low X-ray absorption. Furthermore, with improved techniques of reconstruction it is now possible, with cuts of appropriate thickness, to visualize a lesion from virtually any angle and thus establish definitively the extent of damage. Second, as knowledge of CT neuroanatomy has grown, experienced individuals have become able to chart lesions with remarkable accuracy, as confirmed later by post-mortem studies. Third, it has come to be realized the timing of CT is of essence, especially in well-studied cases of vascular disease. Thus, as many as half of the CTs obtained within the first 24 hours may be normal, while CTs obtained within the second week will not only demonstrate the lesion clearly but will also show, in scans with contrast, the phenomenon of gray matter enhancement (GME) in which cortical gyri or nuclear gray masses will be depicted with precision. CTs obtained beyond the fourth week can add further data, but these must be interpreted with caution: certain changes, e.g., retraction of brain structures caused by scar tissue, can lead to false lucencies in the vicinity of the lesion. The study of the CT scan requires competence and care in every respect similar to that necessary for pathological study at post mortem, and is fraught with much the same pitfalls and limitations. It must be stressed that in many respects CT does not measure up to a detailed post-mortem examination, e.g., there is no way of guaranteeing the intactness of tissue surrounding a lesion. Small lesions below the resolution power of CT may not show up, and, in certain types of damage there can be loss of vulnerable neurons in a specific region without actual collapse of the surrounding structure. Informed neurological judgment is essential on each case used for anatomical localization, so that neglect of damage undetected by CT will not lead to an incorrect localization. The refinement of such methods as SPET, PET, and, in the future, MRI may help to reduce this problem by providing measures of cerebral metabolism and cerebral blood flow which complete the structural picture obtained by CT.

We have devoted considerable space to the problems of establishing correct localization for both clinical and research purposes for several reasons. In the first place, many clinicians have almost abandoned consideration of all the clinical data in favor of total reliance on the remarkable new imaging methods without awareness of the possible errors and impossibilities of such a policy. The situation is unfortunately often equally poor in the investigative literature. While journals publishing studies on brain and behavior will often insist, justifiably, on the most rigid standards in the use and interpretation of statistical methods, they will often accept anatomical data uncritically, without equivalent attention to pitfalls and misinterpretations.

## Visual Disorders

### Pure alexia

The fundamental understanding of the anatomical basis of the syndrome of pure alexia (alexia without agraphia), comes from the post-mortem studies of Déjerine (1892) and, more recently, that of Geschwind and Fusillo (1966). Reading was impaired acutely, while writing (spontaneously and to dictation), oral spelling, and nonverbal visual recognition were intact. The anatomical analysis of the post mortem findings led to the conclusion that a lesion in the left occipital lobe is capable of interrupting the flow of information from both the left and right visual cortices to the language cortex of the dominant temporoparietal region. The lesion thus creates both an *intra*hemispheric and *inter*hemispheric disconnection that prevents the language areas from being informed of verbal information conveyed by visual means. The precise mechanism which caused the disconnection in each of these cases was, however, different. In the case of Déjerine, the patient was able to see in both visual fields, although the right visual field was achromatopsic, i.e., deprived of color perception. The left visual cortex was still operating normally, as far as form vision was concerned, and the blockage of information which prevented reading in the right visual field thus took place beyond the left visual cortex, in a pathway capable of bringing visuo-verbal information to the language cortex. Information flow from the right visual cortex was blocked, in the Déjerine case, by damage to fibers coming out of the splenium of the corpus callosum and coursing in the direction of the left language areas. Déjerine pointed out that one single lesion could parsimoniously disrupt both pathways. That lesion was located in the vicinity of the occipital horn of the left ventricle, destroying a variety of components of white matter connections (Déjerine 1892).

In the patient described by Geschwind and Fusillo (1966), the mechanism was the same but the site of disconnection was different. The patient had a complete right homonymous hemianopia, i.e., *no* visual information arrived in his left visual cortex. He thus depended entirely on visual information from his right visual cortex for seeing both nonverbal and verbal stimuli. A lesion located anywhere along the pathway that conveys information from the right visual cortex to the left language areas would be capable of rendering this patient alexic. A major lesion was found in the splenium of the corpus callosum which entirely prevented any information from coursing *inter*hemispherically. The flow of information within the right hemisphere was maintained and the patient thus had normal visual perception and recognition of nonlinguistic material.

A variety of lesions can, therefore, cause the syndrome of pure alexia, provided they achieve both an intrahemispheric and interhemispheric disconnection. Study of a large series of patients with systematic CT and behavioral analyses has confirmed this thesis (Damasio and Damasio 1983; Greenblatt 1983). In many cases the CT lesion is the same as that found by Déjerine. The lesion, most often of vascular origin but occasionally produced by a tumor or an inflammatory process involving the white matter of the dominant occipital lobe, is located within what we have termed the *paraventricular* area, i.e., the region behind, beneath, and beside the occipital horn of the dominant lateral ventricle. The optic radiations sustain partial damage, and in some cases none at all, so that there is either a right upper quadrant field defect or complete absence of hemianopia. In patients with a right upper field defect, the lower portion of the field has a defect in color perception; in those without any right form vision defect, the right field may be achromatopsic. These patients have no difficulty whatsoever in naming colors in the entirely normal left visual field.

In another group of cases one finds by CT the pathology described by Geschwind and Fusillo. Both white matter and extensive portions of the occipital cortex perish. The primary visual cortex, the optic radiations, and a sizeable sector of the inferior visual association cortex and subjacent white matter are damaged. The natural continuation of the splenium of the corpus callosum in the occipital lobe, the *forceps major,* is destroyed. These patients have a complete right homonymous hemianopia. In their visually intact left visual field, where they can see both form *and* color, they have a defect in the naming of colors and in pointing to colors when given their names. This color-naming defect is generally known as color anomia and occasionally as color agnosia. The presence of this defect constitutes the major difference between patients of this type and the Déjerine type, the latter being able to name colors normally in the intact left visual field.

In the patient of Geschwind and Fusillo, the lesion went beyond the occipital lobe and occipito-temporal region, encompassing the more rostral, medial portion of the temporal lobe, and thus involving the parahippocampal gyrus and the underlying hippocampal formation. The presence of this lesion explained the appearance of a major amnesia, predominantly for verbal material. We have studied a similar patient, who showed a comparable lesion on CT (Damasio and Damasio 1983). This extension of the lesion is found in some but not all cases who have the same form of occipital lobe pathology.

### Color naming defects

This disorder appears to be the result of a visual-verbal disconnection comparable to that which causes pure alexia. The fact that pure alexia can occur without color anomia, and color anomia without pure alexia, indicates that the site of disconnection is different in the two cases. On the basis of a review of published post-mortem data and study of a new series of cases, we concluded that color anomia occurs only when visual information is restricted to the left visual field, i.e., when a right homonymous hemianopia is present. In addition, the lesion must involve the cortex of the occipito-temporal transition zone, so that the cortical regions which lie immediately beneath the splenium of the corpus callosum are involved (Damasio and Damasio 1983). We believe that the latter cortex and its connections are essential for normal color naming. These structures, like those which can cause alexia, depend for blood supply on the posterior cerebral artery. It is thus not surprising that sizable lesions compromise both functions, although an infarction confined to the territory of one arterial branch can impair only one of them.

### Visual agnosia

The term visual agnosia has been used to cover a variety of disorders with different physiopathological mechanisms. It was often used simply to describe any patient who failed to name a visual stimulus correctly, in the face of apparently normal spontaneous language, and in the absence of obvious visual disorder. Lissauer introduced a division between *associative* and *apperceptive* forms of agnosia. In the first form, perception was clearly intact as evidenced by the ability to match the stimulus correctly to an identical one in a group, or to draw it correctly. In the apperceptive form, despite normal acuity and full visual fields, the patients failed the matching and drawing tasks because of severe high level perceptive impairment. We believe that the apperceptive forms of visual agnosia are not real disorders of recognition, but rather the consequence of disordered visuospatial perception (most patients with Balint syndrome have a disturbance of this type).

The associative forms, in turn, were also broken down into two groups. One set of patients failed to name a visual stimulus (in the presence of normal spontaneous speech) and might also fail to select it from a group when the name is offered by the examiner, yet showed clear evidence of correct recognition by other tests. Thus the patient might correctly match one stimulus to another nonidentical one of the same class (e.g., two keys of quite different form). Furthermore he might respond correctly to it, e.g., a patient who denies recognizing a glass of water and cannot describe its use, yet, when thirsty picks up the glass and drinks from it. This set of patients is best categorized under another classical but neglected term, i.e., optic aphasia. A clear example is the failure to name colors or choose them by name which may accompany pure alexia. The mechanism appears to be the result of a visual-verbal disconnection, with the preservation of other associations of the stimulus. Optic aphasia might be regarded as a limited form of visual agnosia in which only verbal associations are lost. The other set of patients with visual associative agnosia is the one to which we believe the term visual agnosia should be reserved, i.e., for patients who—despite intact spontaneous language and correct perception—still fail to show evidence of normal recognition, i.e., previously familiar visual stimuli no longer arouse the appropriate learned associations. The disorder goes beyond the inability to name an object or face, since nonverbal recognition is itself affected. The patient is able to perceive an object or face as a visual form, but cannot recall the appropriate associated memories, e.g., its function and purpose, its association with the viewer, and the temporal aspects of that association. A patient with visual agnosia is not capable of naming on the basis of visual information alone. The patient will fail, for example, to respond correctly to a stimulus, e.g., if given a nail and a piece of wood, he will not pick up a hammer from a group. It is likely in our view that this type of failure implies damage to or lack of access by a visual stimulus to an area which contains what might be called a 'template system' of various categories of objects, against which incoming percepts are 'matched.' The lesion may (a) prevent access to that system, or (b) destroy it, or else (c) block the downstream activation that template matching would produce (Damasio et al. 1982b).

The most dramatic and also most common type of visual agnosia is prosopagnosia, in which there is failure not only of recognition of previously familiar faces, but also of other stimuli that, like faces, are *visually ambiguous*, i.e., belong to a group in which many *different* members are structurally *similar.* (By contrast, in a visually distinctive group *different* members have *different* structures.) Most patients with prosopagnosia are able to achieve a generic recognition of stimuli, i.e., they are able to recognize a face as a face, a car as a car, but cannot place a particular stimulus in its special personal, historical, perspective.

A second form is visual object agnosia. Most patients with visual object agnosia also have prosopagnosia, but, in addition, they cannot arrive at even the generic recognition of stimuli, e.g., confronted with a pen, they will not name the object and can neither state nor demonstrate its use. Needless to say, they have no notion whether the object belongs to them.

The fundamental relation between the visual agnosias and damage in the central visual system has been obvious since the turn of the century. Nonetheless, CT studies have contributed importantly to understanding of the anatomical underpinnings of these disorders. In the first place, these studies have confirmed that bilateral lesions are an absolute prerequisite for true visual agnosia. Lesions of either the left or the right occipital lobe alone fail to produce prosopagnosia, although they can be associated with pure alexia or a specific visuospatial processing defect respectively. The bilateral lesions of visual agnosia are often accompanied by appropriate visual field defects. Secondly, the subcalcarine sector is always damaged in agnosia, i.e., lesions must be present in the inferior occipital or occipito-temporal region, where they compromise structures in the ventral component of the visual association cortex. Thirdly, the lesions have to be functionally symmetrical, i.e., must be within the same sector on both sides, even though they are rarely, if ever, mirror images (Damasio et al. 1982b).

The anatomical relationship between visual agnosia and pure alexia deserves comment. In reality, pure alexia can perhaps be regarded as a limited form of visual agnosia that selectively impairs the recognition of words and often also of letters, as individual visual stimuli. Nonetheless, the location of the functional disconnection causing alexia is not necessarily the one at which the functional disconnection that causes visual agnosia operates. The evidence for this comes from one of our patients with prosopagnosia, with bilateral occipito-temporal lesions, who can read normally. The analysis of the findings in this case is most revealing: the lesion in the occipito-temporal region spares the paraventricular area that we consider essential for the production of pure alexia. Thus, the visual-verbal connectivity essential for the process of reading is kept intact while the connections that appear essential for recognition of other visual stimuli is interrupted.

## Achromatopsia

The term achromatopsia designates a disturbance of color perception which may be of peripheral (retinal) or central origin. In this section, we will deal with central achromatopsia, i.e., caused by lesions in the central visual system. The first descriptions of achromatopsia are contemporaneous with those of pure alexia and visual agnosia. As noted above, Déjerine's (1892) patient had achromatopsia in the right visual field. In the original description of Verrey (1888), there was hemiachromatopsia but without alexia. This disorder can affect half of the visual field or both visual fields. The hemiachromatopsias are caused by unilateral lesions while the full field achromatopsias are related to bilateral lesions (the latter generally accompanied by prosopagnosia). Furthermore, the lesions associated with achromatopsia, like those with visual agnosia, are generally located in the inferior occipital lobe or occipito-temporal region, i.e., below the calcarine fissure. Whether or not this is always the case remains to be clarified, although the association has held in the majority of cases (Meadows 1974b; Green and Lessell 1977; Damasio et al. 1980).

We are currently trying to establish the exact lesion necessary for permanent achromatopsia. We suspect that the lesion must be located in a fairly caudal position in the inferior visual association cortex, because in several of our patients in which the lesion was located in the rostral end of the association cortex there was no achromatopsia.

It is important to emphasize that achromatopsia can appear only when the primary visual cortex and the optic radiations are spared, i.e., when basic information for form vision is still being processed. Damage to primary visual cortex or to optic radiations leads to visual loss. Achromatopsia is almost always caused by infarction in the territory of the posterior cerebral artery. The calcarine branch must be patent, and the area involved corresponds to the distribution of an inferior occipital branch. Cerebrovascular disease often performs the perfect natural experiment, damaging either visual association cortex or subjacent white matter pathways without injuring optic radiations or primary visual cortex. Far more often the experiment is imperfect and damage overlaps the two sectors. In this instance, the portion of the field that loses form vision cannot possibly be achromatopsic, but often an interesting combination is seen, i.e., the upper quadrant has lost form vision, while the inferior quadrant of the same hemifield maintains form vision but loses color vision. This can occur because form vision for the upper and lower quadrants is dependent on the inferior and superior visual association cortices respectively, while color vision depends on the inferior visual association cortex alone (Damasio et al. 1980).

The separation between form and color vision which these findings have shown must be present in humans, has also been noted in animal studies. Zeki has described an area in the peristriate cortex of the rhesus monkey in which cells respond quite specifically to color stimuli (Zeki 1973, 1977), while Livingstone and Hubel have now identified strongly color-coded cells in the primary visual cortex of the monkey, which are regularly interspersed with non-color sensitive cells. The color-coded cells connect directly with cells in the association cortex which in turn also alternate with non-color sensitive ones. These color sensitive units can be stained selectively with cytochrome oxidase (Livingstone and Hubel 1984).

## Disorders of visuospatial analysis (Balint syndrome)

The Balint syndrome is an acquired disturbance of the ability to perceive the visual field as a whole, leading to the unpredictable perception of only parts of it (simultanagnosia). The disturbance is accompanied by an impairment of target-pointing under visual guidance (optic ataxia), and by an inability to shift gaze towards new visual stimuli (sometimes called ocular apraxia). The eponym is used when patients present the three cardinal manifestations: visual disorientation (simultanagnosia), optic ataxia, and ocular apraxia. Both visual disorientation and optic ataxia can occur by themselves. Ocular apraxia is always accompanied by either optic ataxia or visual disorientation. The patients may have visual field defects (inferior quadrant cuts) but these do not play a role in the pathogenesis of the syndrome, since in many patients the visual fields are intact.

In our experience, the complete Balint syndrome is associated with bilateral damage in the occipito-parietal regions. There is involvement of area 7 (superior parietal lobule), mesially or dorso-laterally, although the adjoining area 19 and sometimes part of area 39 (angular gyrus) may be also involved. The lesions are often quite symmetrical but may be of different size. They are generally the result of infarction in the borderzone (watershed) between the anterior and posterior cerebral artery territories, most commonly as the result of sudden hypotension. Most patients with Balint syndrome are elderly, have premorbid cerebrovascular disease and are thus especially vulnerable to severe systemic blood pressure drop. The presence of Balint syndrome in a patient with cerebrovascular disease is thus indicative of a type of stroke different from those causing the agnosias or pure alexia. The Balint syndrome can be caused also by bilateral metastases, which may be asymmetrical, in the occipito-parietal region.

These damaged areas correspond to structures that, in the monkey, have been found to contain visuo-motor neurons related to the detection of stimuli in the peripheral visual field and to the visual guidance of the arm and hand in space (Mountcastle et al. 1975).

## Astereopsis

Stereopsis is the ability to discriminate depth on the basis of *binocular* visual information. Due to the spatial separation of the eyes, the two dimensional projections of objects occupy slightly different positions on the right and left retinas and this disparity is the source of stereopsis. Stereopsis is one mechanism of depth perception, but there are others which depend upon *monocular* information obtained from image contours, texture, apparent size of familiar objects, interposition of near and far, linear perspective, and monocular parallax.

Current research indicates that structures in the occipito-parietal region may be crucial for normal stereopsis. Astereopsis has not been found with unilateral lesions of this area, but bilateral lesions which also cause Balint syndrome, have led to this defect.

## Neglect

When a patient fails to orient to or identify a stimulus appearing in one of the hemispaces, or when he fails spontaneously to move the limbs on one side in the absence of sensory disturbance or weakness, he is likely to have neglect. Hemi-inattention, true hemispatial neglect, and hemiakinesia, are closely related manifestations. In general, neglect is associated with focal lesions of one of the cerebral hemispheres, although damage in the diencephalon or mesencephalon can also lead to neglect (Heilman 1979).

Patients with hemi-inattention fail to orient to, report, or respond to visual and tactile stimuli, contralateral to their focal lesion. They may deny, especially shortly after onset, that the contralateral limbs are their own. Lesions in the parietal lobe are the ones most commonly associated with inattention, but in some cases the lesions are confined to the frontal region either dorsolaterally or medially but persistent severe hemi-inattention is usually associated with parietal lesions.

Lesions of the right parietal lobe more commonly produce neglect than lesions of the left parietal lobe. In addition, the evidence suggests that the magnitude and persistence of inattention are more marked with right than with left lesions. Lesions outside the cortex can also be associated with inattention, e.g., unilateral lesions of the basal ganglia.

Extinction to simultaneous stimulation, both visual and tactile, is an example of inattention that often persists after patients recover their ability to orient or manipulate objects in the contralateral, previously neglected field. In general, the lesions associated with this phenomenon are the same. On occasion, a paradoxical form of extinction has been noted, i.e., an extinction on the same side as the lesion. It is possible that in relation to the somatosensory system paradoxical extinction is especially associated with frontal and basal ganglia loci of damage. As is well known, paradoxical extinction in the auditory system, as shown by dichotic listening tests, is seen primarily with damage to the inter-hemispheric pathways, i.e., with lesions of either the mid-corpus callosum or of the callosal fibers in the parietal regions in which the interauditory pathways travel (Sparks and Geschwind 1968; Damasio and Damasio 1979).

Hemi-spatial (or visuo-spatial) neglect, is another facet of the same unilateral neglect. On occasion, patients who can attend to new stimuli presented in either visual space, may copy only one half of a model or may draw only half of an object they are asked to reproduce from memory. This phenomenon is far more common with right than with left hemisphere lesions. The phenomenon can be quantified by having the patient cross out each line in an array on a page.

Hemi-akinesia is another form of neglect. It is generally contralateral to the causative lesion, but it may be seen ipsilaterally or bilaterally. The primary loci related to hemi-akinesia are the mesial frontal lobes, including the cingulate gyrus and supplementary motor areas, and the neostriatal portion of the basal ganglia and the motor thalamus.

## Language Disorders

### The new aphasia syndromes

Some of the syndromes of aphasia which could not previously be assigned to any of the categories of the Boston Diagnostic Aphasia Examination have been found to be associated with lesions of the basal ganglia and thalamus of the dominant hemisphere. Damasio et al. (1982a) noted that damage to the head of the caudate, the anterior aspect of the putamen and the anterior limb of the capsule is, in the absence of cortical lesions, often associated with these aphasias. Naeser et al. (1982) arrived at much the same localization, although they emphasized the putaminal component of the lesion. Some of these patients have fluent speech, others nonfluent, but most have disturbed auditory comprehension and produce semantic paraphasias. Almost invariably they have right hemiparesis, at least in the acute stage, and disturbances of articulation. It is possible that more than one syndrome exists, as Naeser believes, correlated with the exact placing of the lesion along an anteroposterior dimension. It is also too early to comment on the relative severity of these aphasias in comparison with the more typical ones related to predominantly cortical lesions. Our impression is that these atypical aphasias are generally milder and recover more rapidly.

In earlier studies, Hier et al. (1977) and Alexander and Lo Verme (1980) had found atypical aphasias following hemorrhages of the basal ganglia in hypertensive patients. Those cases share some features with the ones discussed above but also had disturbances of attention. Because of their space occupying nature, those large hemorrhagic lesions did not permit a precise anatomical correlation. The same reservations apply to the cases of atypical aphasia with hemorrhages in the thalamus. The clinical characteristics of those cases are variable, although they are generally suggestive of transcortical sensory aphasia (Mohr 1975; Cappa and Vignolo 1979). A similar picture has been noted in patients with nonhemorrhagic infarctions of the thalamus (Graff-Radford et al. 1984). These patients have normal repetition, and speech is commonly sparse, hypophonic, and paraphasic. Auditory comprehension is impaired.

The mechanisms which lead to the disturbances of speech and language in cases in which the cortex is definitely spared, must differ in some respects from those of the cortical aphasias. In the case of the basal ganglia it appears that the neostriatal lesions impair not only a major motor re-entrant circuit (neostriatum → pallidum → motor thalamus → premotor and motor cortices), but may also influence the function of the premotor, prefrontal, and auditory cortices crucial to normal language processing. There is ample evidence from neuroanatomical studies in higher primates that the auditory cortex projects strongly to the head of the caudate (Van Hoesen et al. 1981; Damasio and Van Hoesen 1982). The caudate exerts influence on frontal structures (via pallidal and thalamic relays) which, in turn, are strongly associated with the language cortices (Damasio 1983). Recent evidence from PET and SPET studies supports this point (Damasio et al. 1984; Benson 1984).

The mechanics at play in lesions of the thalamus probably involve the disorder of attentional mechanisms which accompanies most lesions in this structure. It is likely, however, that some nuclear components of the thalamus are especially devoted to language processing. Support for this hypothesis comes from a study by Galaburda and Eidelberg (1982), in which an asymmetry of thalamic nuclei connected to temporo-parietal structures was noted in human brains (the left nuclei being larger than the right).

## Wernicke's aphasia

Wernicke's aphasia is characterized by fluent paraphasic speech, poor repetition, and an auditory comprehension deficit. In most cases the lesions involve Wernicke's area although the amount of involvement is variable. The exact extent of Wernicke's area, damage necessary to produce in most cases a permanent severe Wernicke's aphasia, is still not known. It must include at a minimum Brodmann's area 22, lying in the posterior aspect of the left superior temporal gyrus. The primary left auditory cortex (areas 41, 42) need not necessarily be involved. The lesion often extends into the lower parietal lobe, especially into the angular gyrus (Brodmann's area 39), and into the posterior and inferior temporal lobe (the second and third temporal gyri), in which areas 37, 21, 20, and 37 are located (Damasio 1981). The extension of the lesion into other areas is variable and accompanies the presence or absence of associated disturbances, e.g., constructional disorder and acalculia. In cases with vascular lesions, there is infarction or hemorrhage in the territory of the posterior temporal branches of the middle cerebral artery. The perfusion zone of the angular gyrus artery may be involved as well. On occasion, the lesions may be exclusively subcortical and act by disrupting the input and output of an otherwise intact auditory association cortex. The consistency of the anatomical findings in patients with the syndrome of Wernicke's aphasia is remarkable.

## Conduction aphasia

Conduction aphasia shares a defect in repetition with both Wernicke's and Broca's aphasia. But unlike the situation in Wernicke's aphasia, auditory comprehension is relatively well preserved and the speech is far more fluent than in a Broca's aphasia. This entity was at one time almost entirely ignored in many classification systems. Although the existence of the syndrome has now generally become accepted, the questions as to the existence of an equally distinctive anatomical correlate rested on only few studies, e.g., the findings of Kleist (1962), Geschwind (1965), and Benson et al. (1973). Recently CT findings on a large number of cases have confirmed that conduction aphasia is usually associated with lesions, located between the area regularly damaged in Wernicke's aphasia and the area commonly associated with Broca's aphasia and its variants. In some instances, the lesion is located in the lower parietal region (the supramarginal gyrus, consisting primarily of Brodmann's field 40), and involves the underlying white matter extensively. In other instances, the lesion involves a part of the auditory and insular cortices and the white matter underlying both, sparing the supramarginal gyrus. In such instances the lesion spares most of Wernicke's area while consistently involving the primary auditory cortex. Finally, in some specimens, the lesion encompasses all of these sites: the supramarginal, auditory, and insular cortices (Kertesz et al. 1979; Damasio and Damasio 1980). These findings led to the conclusion that, both neuropsychologically and anatomically, conduction aphasia is an intermediate syndrome. The complete or partial sparing of Wernicke's area is certainly the reason for the remarkably preserved auditory comprehension, while the sparing of Broca's area probably explains the fluency of speech. In all likelihood, the lesion in conduction aphasia impairs structures necessary for the transfer of auditory information to the motor system, a step required for the complex act of repeating accurately a sentence provided by the examiner. Those structures include not only the classical arcuate fasciculus, an important long association tract which is part of the superior longitudinal fasciculus and travels in the depth of the parieto-frontal operculum, but also an additional system of auditory-motor connections which travel underneath the insula, in the extreme and external capsules.

### Broca's aphasia

The characteristic features of Broca's aphasia are non-fluent aphasic speech and poor repetition. Auditory comprehension as tested at the bedside is remarkably preserved, although the performance of standard auditory comprehension tests is often impaired. A controversy on the issue of the pathological basis of Broca's aphasia was the topic of the debates between Pierre Marie and Jules Déjerine at the Société de Médicine of Paris in 1908. In essence, Broca and his followers believed that lesions of the foot of the third frontal gyrus were sufficient to cause this form of aphasia, while Marie and others argued that the lesion had to be more extensive. Occasional instances of Broca's aphasia in which no lesion could be found in Broca's area and cases with lesions in Broca's area without the typical picture of Broca's aphasia prolonged the controversy to our times.

Broca's description of Leborgne's lesion had been made entirely from inspection of the lateral surface of the left hemisphere, since the brain was never sectioned. He stated that the third left frontal gyrus was damaged and he proposed that area as the seat of the faculty of articulate language. On the other hand, Marie contended that the lesion involved not only the third frontal gyrus but also the insula and basal ganglia, as well as Wernicke's area itself. On Broca's side, Déjerine argued that the lesion spared both Wernicke's area and the basal ganglia. Recent CT studies finally revealed the limits of the lesion in Leborgne's case. CT cuts of Leborgne's brain, obtained in the horizontal level of Déjerine's classical cerebral sections, revealed that the lesion unequivocally spared Wernicke's area, as Broca and Déjerine had claimed, but that there was major involvement of the basal ganglia and insular cortex (Castaigne et al. 1980).

More recently Mohr (1976) has proposed that damage to the inferior frontal gyrus alone, causes a transient period of mutism but not a marked linguistic defect. A larger area of damage involving most of the frontal operculum and insula is associated with a more severe disturbance characterized by persistent mutism, verbal stereotypes, and agrammatism. Findings from other studies (Naeser et al. 1978; Damasio et al. 1979; Kertesz et al. 1979; Damasio 1981) support the contention that the effective lesion for Broca's aphasia extends beyond the third frontal convolution.

Current CT evidence thus supports the notion that Broca's aphasia is related to damage of the anterior language zone, and that it is not, as Marie would have it, the result of a combination of lesions in Wernicke's area and in the motor system. The controversy clearly stems from the fact that the anatomo-clinical correlation in this syndrome is not as consistent as in Wernicke's aphasia.

Let us note that the recent data on the minimum lesion necessary for producing Broca's aphasia in most cases, have often been misinterpreted as showing that 'a Broca's area lesion does not produce Broca's aphasia.' It is correct to say that there were arguments in the past as to the extent of the lesion necessary to produce a Broca's aphasia, and it is now clear that there is an anterior language zone which is larger than the region postulated by many authors, including Broca himself. Let us also comment that the minimum area is larger than the anterior language region as mapped by cortical stimulation. This probably reflects two facts: (1) cortical stimulation is done with low current intensities so as to avoid stimulation of distant structures; but this of necessity leads to failure to ascertain the full extent of high threshold units which may well be wider than that of low threshold ones; (2) cortical zones around the area of excitable speech cortex may be potentially capable of participation in language after damage to the central speech region.

## Transcortical motor aphasia (TMA)

Patients with TMA have remarkably preserved repetition. Speech output is generally non-fluent but in some instances can be fluent. Auditory comprehension is generally intact but in the less fluent cases can be disturbed. The original cases of transcortical aphasia had been diagnosed and the disorder related to a hypothesized anatomic locus well before the first post mortem studies were reported. It was, in general, believed that transcortical motor aphasia was caused by lesions located anteriorly and superiorly to Broca's area. Studies with radionuclide scans (Rubens 1975; Kertesz et al. 1977) supported this localization and suggested that not only lateral frontal lesions but also mesial frontal lesions could be associated with TMA. CT study has modified some of these views. Most instances of TMA occur with lesions of the lateral frontal lobe which spare Broca's area at least in part, i.e., located in the left premotor region. In vascular cases the damage is often located in the border zone between the anterior and middle cerebral artery territories. In some instances, however, the lesions are exclusively subcortical, located deep in the frontal lobe, anteriorly and superiorly to the left frontal horn, i.e., infarctions in the deep aspect of the border zone between the anterior and middle cerebral vascular territories.

Patients with lesions in the mesial aspect of the frontal lobe, which involve the supplementary motor area, the cingulate gyrus, or both, have TMA only in the sense that repetition is normal and spontaneous speech is lacking. This syndrome is one of mutism and akinesia. The behavior of these cases is entirely different from that of TMA patients in that they show no intent to communicate, by word or by gesture, and have a marked disturbance of affect and emotion. It is true that they have little or no spontaneous speech, along with comparatively good comprehension and preserved repetition, but the essential feature is that drive to communicate, not just to speak, is disturbed. There is no evidence that language processing is altered, and, with recovery, the patients produce grammatically correct speech, without lexical or syntactical errors. The lesions are located in mesial limbic system cortices and not in lateral regions of neocortex, and the disorder is motor and affective but not primarily linguistic.

A similar but often more persistent syndrome has been described in patients with surgical callosal disconnection. This is caused, in our view, by damage to the mesial cortex, probably bilaterally in the longlasting cases. This can be due to direct surgical trauma of the mesial brain surface, especially as the result of retraction, or to damage in the same regions as a result of damage to veins. Those surgeons who make large craniotomies, use the operating microscope, and meticulously avoid sacrificing veins appear to have a much lower rate of this complication. Another possible mechanism is sectioning of the bidirectional interconnections of the cingulate and supplementary area, which course in the anterior portion of the body of the callosum.

### Transcortical sensory aphasia (TSA)

Patients with transcortical sensory aphasias have remarkably intact repetition but major impairments of auditory comprehension and naming. The lesion spares the primary auditory cortex and part or all of Wernicke's area but involves the inferior temporal cortices, especially in area 37. In some cases it involves visual association cortex (lateral aspect) and the subjacent white matter underneath (Damasio 1981). The lesions are thus quite distinct from those seen in the other fluent aphasias (Wernicke's and conduction aphasia). The lesions associated with transcortical sensory aphasia are generally the result of infarcts in the posterior border zone, i.e., in the territory supplied by terminal branches of both the middle and posterior cerebral arteries.

### Global aphasia

Patients with global aphasia have severely limited, non-fluent speech, poor repetition, and markedly impaired comprehension. CT has confirmed that the usual basis for the most devastating of the aphasias in an extensive lesion involving all of the language areas located in the perisylvian territory of the left hemisphere, i.e., the territories supplied by cortical and lenticulostriate branches of the middle cerebral artery. CT has shown that the lesions need not be contiguous, i.e., a lesion in Broca's area combined with another in Wernicke's, can cause global aphasia.

## References

Alexander, M. P. and S. R. Lo Verme: Aphasia after left hemispheric intracerebral hemorrhage. Neurology 30 (1980) 1193–1202.

Benson, D. F.: Positron emission tomography in aphasia. Semin. Neurol. (1984) in press.

Benson, D. F., W. A. Sheremata, R. Buchard, J. Segarra, D. Price and N. Geschwind: Conduction aphasia. Arch. Neurol. 28 (1973) 339–46.

Cappa, S. F. and L. A. Vignolo: 'Transcortical' features of aphasia following left thalamic hemorrhage. Cortex 15 (1979) 121–30.

Castaigne, P., F. Lhermitte, J. L. Signoret and R. Abelanet: Déscription et étude scannographique du cerveau de Leborgne (la découverte de Broca). Rev. Neurol. 136 (1980) 563–83.

Damasio, A.: Central achromatopsia. Neurology 31 (1981a) 920–921.

Damasio, H.: Cerebral localization of the aphasias. In: M. T. Sarno (Ed.), Acquired Aphasia. New York, Academic Press (1981b) 27–50.

Damasio, A.: Language and the basal ganglia. Trends Neurosci. 6 (1983) 442–444.

Damasio, H. and A. Damasio: 'Paradoxic' ear extinction in dichotic listening: Possible anatomic significance. Neurology 29 (1979) 644–653.

Damasio, H. and A. Damasio: The anatomical basis of conduction aphasia. Brain 103 (1980) 337–350.

Damasio, A. and H. Damasio: The anatomical basis of pure alexia. Neurology 33 (1983) 1573–1583.

Damasio, H., A. Damasio, K. Hamsher and N. Varney: CT scan correlates of aphasia and allied disorders. Neurology 29 (1979a) 572.

Damasio, H. and G. W. Van Hoesen: Anatomical basis of some subcortical aphasias. Neurology 32 (1982) 95.

Damasio, A., J. McKee and H. Damasio: Determinants of performance in color anomia. Brain and Language 7 (1979b) 74–85.

Damasio, A., T. Yamada, H. Damasio, J. Corbett and J. McKee: Central achromatopsia: behavioral, anatomic and physiologic aspects. Neurology 30 (1980) 1064–1071.

Damasio, A., H. Damasio, M. Rizzo, N. Varney and F. Gersh: Aphasia with nonhemorrhagic lesions in the basal ganglia and internal capsule. Arch. Neurol. 39 (1982a) 15–20.

Damasio, A., H. Damasio and G. W. Van Hoesen: Prosopagnosia: anatomic basis and behavioral mechanisms. Neurology 32 (1982b) 331–41.

Damasio, H., P. Eslinger and H. Adams: Aphasia following basal ganglia lesions: New evidence. Semin. Neurol. 4 (1984) 151–161.

Déjerine, J.: Contribution a l'étude anatomo-pathologique et clinique des différentes variétés de cécité verbale, Mém. Soc. Biol. 4 (1892) 61–90.

Galaburda, A. M. and D. Eidelberg: Symmetry and asymmetry in the human posterior thalamus. Part 1: Cytoarchitectonic analysis in normal persons. Arch. Neurol. 39 (1982) 325–32.

Geschwind, N.: Disconnexion syndromes in animals and man. Brain 88 (1965) 237–294.
Geschwind, N. and M. Fusillo: Color-naming defects in association with alexia. Arch. Neurol. 15 (1966) 137–146.
Graff-Radford, N., P. Eslinger, T. Yamada and A. Damasio: Nonhemorrhagic infarction of the thalamus: Behavioral, anatomical and physiologic correlates. Neurology 34 (1984) 14–23.
Green, G. J. and S. Lessell: Acquired cerebral dyschromatopsia. Arch. Ophthalmol. 95 (1977) 121–128.
Greenblatt, S.: Localization of lesions in alexia. In: A. Kertesz (Ed.), Localization in Neuropsychology. New York, Academic Press (1983).
Heilman, K.: Neglect and related disorders. In: K. M. Heilman and A. Valenstein (Eds), Clinical Neuropsychology. New York, Oxford University Press (1979) 268–307.
Hier, D. B., K. R. Davis, E. P. Richardson et al.: Hypertensive putaminal hemorrhage. Dev. Neurol. Behav. Pediatr. 1 (1977) 54–57.
Kertesz, A., D. Lesk and P. McCabe: Isotope location of infarcts in aphasia. Arch. Neurol. 34 (1977) 590–601.
Kertesz, A., W. Harlock and R. Coates: Computer tomographic localization, lesion size, and prognosis in aphasia and nonverbal impairment. Brain and Language 8 (1979) 34–50.
Kleist, K.: Sensory Aphasia and Amusia (Transl.). London. Pergamon Press (1962).
Livingstone, M. S. and D. H. Hubel: Anatomy and physiology of a color system in the primate visual cortex. J. Neurosci. 4 (1984) 309–356.
Meadows, J. C.: The anatomical basis of prosopagnosia. J. Neurol. Neurosurg. Psychiatry 37 (1974a) 489–501.
Meadows, J. C.: Disturbed perception of colors associated with localized cerebral lesions. Brain 97 (1974b) 615–632.
Mohr, J. P.: Broca's area and Broca's aphasia. In: H. Whitaker (Ed.), Studies in Neurolinguistics. New York, Academic Press (1976) 201–236.
Mohr, J. P., W. C. Watters and G. W. Duncan: Thalamic hemorrhage and aphasia. Brain and Language 2 (1975) 3–17.
Mohr, J. P., J. Leicester, L. T. Stoddard and M. Sidman: Right hemianopia with memory and color deficits in circumscribed left posterior cerebral artery territory infarction. Neurology 21 (1971) 1104.
Mountcastle, V. C., J. C. Lynch and A. Georgopoulos: Posterior parietal association cortex of the monkey: Command functions for operations within extrapersonal space. J. Neurophysiol. 38 (1975) 871–908.
Naeser, M. A. and R. W. Hayward: Lesion localization in aphasia with cranial computed tomography and the Boston diagnostic aphasia exam. Neurology 28 (1978) 545–551.
Naeser, M. A., M. P. Alexander, N. Helm-Estabrooks, H. L. Levine, S. A. Laughlin and N. Geschwind: Aphasia with predominantly subcortical lesion sites: Description of three capsular/putaminal aphasia syndromes. Arch. Neurol. 39 (1982) 2–14.
Rubens, A. B.: Aphasia with infarction in the territory of the anterior cerebral artery. Cortex 11 (1975) 239–250.
Sparks, R. and N. Geschwind: Dichotic listening in man after section of neocortical commissures Cortex 4 (1968) 3–16.
Van Hoesen, G. W., E. H. Yeterian and R. Lavizzo-Mourey: Widespread cortico-striate projections from temporal cortex of the rhesus monkey. J. Comp. Neurol. 199 (1981) 205–219.

Verrey, D.: Hemiachromatopsie droite absolue. Arch. Ophtalmol. (Paris) 8 (1888) 289–300.
Zeki, S. M.: Colour coding in rhesus monkey prestriate cortex. Brain Res. 53 (1973) 422–427.
Zeki, S. M.: Colour coding in the superior temporal sulcus of rhesus monkey visual cortex. Proc. R. Soc. Lond. (Biol.) 197 (1977) 195–223.

This study was supported by NINCDS Grant P01 NS 19632-01 (A.R.D.) and supported in part by grants from the NIH (NS-06209), The Orton Research Fund, and the Essel Research Fund, to the Department of Neurology and Dana Research Laboratories, Beth Israel Hospital, Boston; Department of Neurology, Harvard Medical School; and Boston University Aphasia Research, VA Hospital, Boston (N.G.).

# Norman Geschwind's Bibliography


## 1955

Geschwind, N, and Simpson, JA. Procaine Amide in the Treatment of Myotonia. Brain, 1955; 78, 81-91.

## 1956

Walton, JN, Geschwind, N, and Simpson, JA. Benign Congenital Myopathy with Myasthenic Features. J Neurol Neurosurg Psychiatry, 1956; 1, 224-231.

## 1957

Schmitt, FO, and Geschwind, N. The Axon Surface. Progress in Biophysics. 1957; 8, 165-215.

## 1960

Geschwind, N, and Segal, JR. Colors of All Hues from Binocular Mixing of Two Colors. Science, 1960; 131, 608.

## 1962

Random Reports: Human Split-Brain Syndromes. N Engl J Med, 1962; 266, 1013 (published anonymously with Edith Kaplan).

*Geschwind, N. The Anatomy of Acquired Disorders of Reading. In J Money (ed.), *Reading Disability*. Baltimore: Johns Hopkins Press, 1962, pp. 115-129.

*Geschwind, N, and Kaplan, E. A Human Cerebral Deconnection Syndrome: A Preliminary Report. Neurology, 1962; 12, 675-685.

## 1964

Geschwind, N and Howes, D. Quantitative Studies of Aphasic Language. In D Rioch and E Weinstein (eds.), *Disorders of Communication. Proceedings of Association for Research in Nervous and Mental Diseases*. Baltimore: Williams & Wilkins, 1964, pp. 229-244.

*Geschwind, N, and Fusillo, MG. Color-Naming Defects in Association with Alexia. Trans Am Neurol Assoc, 1964; 89, 172-176 (see also 1966).


---

*articles appearing with this book

Geschwind, N. Skeletal Muscle Cramps in Proceedings of Veterans Administration Symposium on Skeletal Muscle Hypertonia. Clin Pharmacol Ther (Suppl.), 1964; 5, 859-863.

Geschwind, N. The Development of the Brain and the Evolution of Languag. In CIJM Stuart (ed.), *Monograph Series on Languages and Linguistics*, Vol. 17. Washington, DC: George Washington University Press, 1964, pp. 155-169.

*Geschwind, N. Non-Aphasic Disorders of Speech. Int J Neurol, 1964; 4(3), 207-214.

*Geschwind, N. The Paradoxical Position of Kurt Goldstein in the History of Aphasia. Cortex, 1964; 1, 214-224.

## 1965

Geschwind, N. Alexia and Color-Naming Disturbance. In G Ettlinger (ed.), *Ciba Foundation Symposium on the Functions of the Corpus Callosum.* London: Churchill, 1965, pp. 95-100.

Geschwind, N. Disconnexion Syndromes in Animals and Man. I. Brain; 1965; 88(2), 237-294.

Geschwind, N. Disconnexion Syndromes in Animals and Man. II. Brain, 1965; 88(3), 585-644.

Geschwind, N. Il Problema del Linguaggio in Rapporto allo Sviluppo Filogenetico del Cervello [The Problem of Language in Relation to the Phylogenetic Development of the Brain]. Sist Nerv, 1965; 6, 411-419.

Geschwind, N. The Test of Time. VIII: Aphasia. Boston Med Q, 1965; 16, 129-130.

*Sherwin, I, Geschwind, N, and Abramowicz, A. Language-Induced Epilepsy. Trans Am Neurolog Assoc, 1965; 90, 182-188 (see also 1967).

## 1966

Geschwind, N. Carl Wernicke, The Breslau School and The History of Aphasia. In EC Carterette (ed.), *Brain Function, Volume III: Speech, Language, and Communication.* Berkeley: University of California Press, 1966, pp. 1-16.

Geschwind, N, and Fusillo, M. Color-Naming Defects in Association with Alexia. Arch Neurol, 1966; 15(2), 137-146.

## 1967

Benson, DF, and Geschwind, N. Shrinking Retrograde Amnesia. J Neurol Neurosurg Psychiatry, 1967; 30(6), 539-544.

Geschwind N. Neurological Foundations of Language. In HR Mykelbust (ed.) *Progress in Learning Disabilities*, Vol. 1. Grune & Stratton, New York, 1967, pp. 182-198.

Geschwind, N, and Sherwin, I. Language Induced Epilepsy. Arch Neurol, 1967; 16(1), 25-31.

Geschwind, N. Brain Mechanisms Suggested by Studies of Interhemispheric Connections. In F Darley and C Millikan (eds.), *Brain Mechanisms Underlying Speech and Language.* New York: Grune & Stratton, 1967, pp. 103-108.

Geschwind, N. Hydrocephalus. Lancet 1967; I:1330 (letter).

Geschwind, N. The Apraxias. In EW Straus and RM Griffith (eds.), *Phenomenology of Will and Action.* Pittsburgh: Duquesne University Press, 1967, pp. 91-102.

Geschwind, N. The Neural Basis of Language. In K and S Salzinger (eds.), *Research in Verbal Behavior and Some Neurological Implications.* New York: Academic Press, 1967, pp. 423-427.

*Geschwind, N. The Varieties of Naming Errors. Cortex, 1967; 3, 97-112.
*Geschwind, N. Wernicke's Contribution to the Study of Aphasia. Cortex, 1967; 3, 449-463.

### 1968

Behan, PO, Geschwind, N, Lamarche, JB, Lisak, RP, and Kies, MW. Delayed Hypersensitivity to Encephalitogenic Protein in Disseminated Encephalomyelitis. Lancet, 1968; 2(576), 1009-1012.
Benson, DF, and Geschwind, N. Cerebral Dominance and Its Disturbances. Pediatr Clin North Am, 1968; 15(3), 759-769.
Geschwind, N, and Levitsky, W. Human Brain: Left-Right Asymmetries in Temporal Speech Region. Science, 1968; 161(837), 186-187.
Geschwind, N, Quadfasel, FA, and Segarra, JM. Isolation of the Speech Area. Neuropsychology, 1968; 6, 327-340.
Geschwind, N. The Mechanism of Normal Pressure Hydrocephalus. Neurol Sci, 1968; 7(3), 481-493.
Levitsky, W, and Geschwind, N. Asymmetries of the Right and Left Hemisphere in Man. Trans Am Neurol Assoc, 1968; 93, 232-233.
Sparks, R, and Geschwind, N. Dichotic Listening in Man After Sectioning of Neocortical Commissures. Cortex, 1968; 4, 3-16.

### 1969

*Benson, DF and Geschwind, N. The Alexias. In PJ Vinken and GW Bruyn (eds.), *Handbook of Clinical Neurology*, Vol. 4. Amsterdam: North-Holland, 1969, pp. 112-140.
Geschwind, N, and Segarra, JM. Sensory Radicular Neuropathy (Denny-Brown's Disease), Dementia and Seizures. In S Locke (ed.), *Modern Neurology.* Boston: Little, Brown & Company, 1969, pp. 509-513.
Geschwind, N. Anatomy and the Higher Functions of the Brain. In RS Cohen and MW Wartofsky (eds.), *Boston Studies in the Philosophy of Science*, Vol. IV. Dordrecht-Holland: D Reidel, 1969, pp. 98-136.
Geschwind, N. Problems in the Anatomical Understanding of the Aphasias. In AL Benton (ed.), *Contributions to Clinical Neuropsychology.* Chicago: Aldine, 1969, pp. 107-128.
Geschwind, N. The Apraxias and Agnosias. In GA Talland, and NC Waugh (eds.), *The Pathology of Memory.* New York: Academic Press, 1969, pp. 3-8.
Geschwind, N. The Work and Influence of Wernicke. In RS Cohen and MW Wartofsky (eds.), *Boston Studies in the Philosophy of Science*, Vol. IV. Dordrecht-Holland: D Reidel, 1969, pp. 1-33.

### 1970

*Benson, DF, and Geschwind, N. Developmental Gerstmann Syndrome, Neurology, 1970; 20(3), 293-298.
Geschwind, N. Disturbances of Language, Perception and Memory. In CS Keefer and RW Wilkins (eds.), *Medicine: Essentials of Clinical Practice.* Boston: Little, Brown & Company, 1970, pp. 973-980.
Geschwind, N. Intermodal Equivalence of Stimuli in Apes. Science, 1970; 168(936), 1249.

Geschwind, N. Language Disturbances in Cerebrovascular Disease. In A Benton (ed.), *Behavioral Changes in Cerebrovascular Disease.* New York: Harper & Row, 1970, pp. 29-36.

Geschwind, N. Some Differences Between Human and Other Primate Brains. In LE Jarrard (ed.), *Cognitive Processes of Nonhuman Primates.* New York: Academic Press, 1970, pp. 149-154.

Geschwind, N. The Clinical Syndromes of the Cortical Connections. In D Williams (ed.), *Modern Trends in Neurology.* London: Butterworths, 1970, pp. 29-40.

Geschwind, N. The Organization of Language and the Brain. Science, 1970; 170(961), 940-944.

Heilman, KM, Pandya, DN, and Geschwind, N. Trimodal Inattention Following Parietal Lobe Ablations. Trans Am Neurol Assoc, 1970; 95, 259-261.

## 1971

*Geschwind, N. Aphasia. N Engl J Med, 1971; 284, 654-656.

Geschwind, N. Focal Disturbances of Higher Nervous Function. In P Beeson and W McDermott (eds.), *Textbook of Medicine.* Philadelphia: WB Saunders, 1971, pp. 99-102.

Heilman, KM, Pandya, DN, Karol, EA, and Geschwind, N. Auditory Inattention. Arch Neurol, 1971; 24(4), 323-325.

Heilman, KM, Safran, A, and Geschwind, N. Closed Head Trauma and Aphasia. J Neurol Neurosurg Psychiatry, 1971; 34(3), 265-269.

Kertesz, A, and Geschwind, N. Patterns of Pyramidal Decussation and Their Relationship to Handedness. Arch Neurol, 1971; 24(4), 326-332.

## 1972

Chedru, F and Geschwind, N. Writing Disturbances in Acute Confusional States. Neuropsychology, 1972; 10(3), 343-353.

*Chedru, F, and Geschwind, N. Disorders of Higher Cortical Functions in Acute Confusional States. Cortex, 1972; 8(4), 395-411.

Geschwind, N. Anatomical Evolution and the Human Brain. Orton Soc Bull, 1972; 22, 7-13.

Geschwind, N. Cerebral Dominance and Anatomic Asymmetry. N Engl J Med, 1972; 287(4), 194-95.

Geschwind, N. Disorders of Higher Cortical Function in Children. Clin Proc Child Hosp Nat Med Cent, 1972; 28, 262-272.

Geschwind, N. Language and the Brain. Sci Am, 1972; 226(4), 76-83.

Geschwind, N. Review of "Traumatic Aphasia" by AR Luria. Language, 1972; 48, 755-763.

## 1973

Behan, PO, and Geschwind, N. The Ophthalmoplegic Form of the Guillain-Barre-Syndrome: An Immunologic Study. Acta Ophthalmol, 1973; 51(4), 529-542.

Benson, DF, Sheremata, WA, Bouchard, R, Segarra, JM, Price, D, and Geschwind, N. Conduction Aphasia: A Clinicopathological Study. Arch Neurol, 1973; 28(5), 339-346.

*Geschwind, N. Effects of Temporal-Lobe Surgery on Behavior. N Engl J Med, 1973; 289(9), 480-481.

Geschwind, N. El Lenguaje Escrito y sus Desordenes. In A Caceres (ed.), *Lenguaje y Audicion* Lima: Editorial Juridica, 1973, pp. 49-56.

Geschwind, N. Progressive Personality Changes and Hemiparesis in a Middle-Aged Man. MT Southgate (ed.), Clinical Pathological Conference. JAMA, 1973; 225, 143-153.

Geschwind, N. The Brain and Language. In GA Miller, (ed.), *Communication, Language and Meaning*. New York: Basic Books, 1973, pp. 61-72.

Heilman, KM, Coyle, JM, Gonyea, EF, and Geschwind, N. Apraxia and Agraphia in a Left-Hander. Brain, 1973; 96(1), 21-28.

Sabin, TD and Geschwind, N. The Neurological Examination. In VH Mark (ed.), *Practice of Surgery*. Maryland: Harper & Row, 1973, pp. 1-48.

## 1974

Geschwind, N. Clinical Experience and Interpretation. In EW Straus (ed.), *Language and Language Disturbances*. Pittsburgh: Duquesne University Press, 1974, pp. 111-122.

Geschwind, N. Late Changes in the Nervous System: an Overview. In D Stein, and J Rosen (eds.), *Plasticity and Recovery of Function in the Central Nervous System*. New York: Academic Press, 1974, pp. 467-508.

Geschwind, N. The Anatomical Basis of Hemispheric Differentiation. In JG Beaumont and S Dimond (eds.), *Hemisphere Function in the Human Brain*. London: Paul Elek, 1974, pp. 7-24.

Heilman, KM, Gonyea, EF, and Geschwind, N. Apraxia and Agraphia in a Right-Hander. Cortex, 1974; 10, 284-288.

Strub, R, and Geschwind, N. Gerstmann Syndrome Without Aphasia. Cortex, 1974; 10(4), 378-387.

*Waxman, SG, and Geschwind, N. Hypergraphia in Temporal Lobe Epilepsy. Neurology, 1974; 24(7), 629-636.

## 1975

Benson, DF, and Geschwind, N. Psychiatric Conditions Associated with Focal Lesions in the Nervous System. In S Arieti (ed.), *American Handbook of Psychiatry*, Vol. 4. New York: Basic Books, 1975, pp. 208-243.

Geschwind, N, and Richardson, EP, Jr. A 77-Year-Old Woman with a Gait Disorder and Confusion. Clinical Pathological Conference. N Engl J Med, 1975; 231(6), 852-857.

Geschwind, N, and Strub, R. Gerstmann Syndrome Without Aphasia: A Reply to Poeck and Orgass. Cortex, 1975; 11(3), 296-298.

*Geschwind, N. Language and Cerebral Dominance. In DB Tower (ed.), *The Nervous System*, Vol. 2. New York: Raven Press, 1975, pp. 433-439.

Geschwind, N. Le Concept de Disconnexion: L'histoire d'une Idee Banale Mais Importante. Symposium on Corpus Callosum, Lyon, France, (May 1974), 1975, pp. 11-15.

Geschwind, N. Preservation of Axial Movements to Verbal Command in Cases of Apraxia or Comprehension Deficit. Symposium on Corpus Callosum, Lyon, France, (May, 1974), 1975, pp. 301-316.

Geschwind, N. The Apraxias: Neural Mechanisms of Disorders of Learned Movement. Am Sci, 1975; 63(2), 188-195.

*Geschwind, N. The Borderland of Neurology and Psychiatry: Some Common Misconceptions. In DF Benson, and D Blumer (eds.), *Psychiatric Aspects of Neurological Disease.* New York: Grune & Stratton, 1975, pp. 1-9.

Geschwind, N. The Clinical Setting of Aggression in Temporal Lobe Epilepsy. In WS Fields and WH Sweet (eds.), *The Neural Basis for Violence and Aggression.* St. Louis: WH Green, 1975, pp. 273-284.

Heilman, KM, Schwartz, HD, and Geschwind, N. Defective Motor Learning in Ideomotor Apraxia. Neurology, 1975; 25(11), 1018-1020.

LeMay, M, and Geschwind, N. Hemispheric Differences in the Brains of Great Apes. Brain Behav Evol, 1975; 11(1), 48-52.

Ross, ED, Jossman, PB, Bell, B, Sabin, T, and Geschwind, N. Musical Hallucinations in Deafness. JAMA, 1975; 231(6), 620-622.

*Waxman, SG and Geschwind, N. The Interictal Behavior Syndrome of Temporal Lobe Epilepsy. Arch Gen Psychiatry, 1975; 32(12), 1580-1586.

### 1976

Goodglass, H and Geschwind, N. Language Disorders (Aphasia). In EC Carterette and MP Friedman (eds.), *Handbook of Perception, Vol. VII: Language and Speech.* New York: Academic Press, 1976, pp. 390-428.

Mesulam, MM and Geschwind, N. Disordered Mental States in the Postoperative Period. Urol Clin North Am, 1976; 3(2), 199-215.

Mesulam, MM, Waxman, SG, Geschwind, N, and Sabin, TD. Acute Confusional States with Right Middle Cerebral Artery Infarctions. J Neurol Neurosurg Psychiatry, 1976; 39(1), 84-89.

Waxman, SG, Brill, MH, Geschwind, N, Sabin, TD, and Lettvin, JY. Probability of Conduction Deficit as Related to Fiber Length in Random-Distribution Models of Peripheral Neuropathies. Neurol Sci, 1976; 29(1), 39-53.

### 1977

Geschwind N. Dysplasia, Dyspraxia and Disorders of the Body Image. In DA Rottenberg and FH Hochberg (eds.), *Neurology Classics in Modern Translation.* New York: RH Hafner Press, 1977, pp. 129-130.

Geschwind, N. Behavioral Change in Temporal Lobe Epilepsy (editorial). Arch Neurol, 1977; 34(8), 453.

Geschwind, N. Insensitivity to Pain in Psychotic Patients (letter). N Engl J Med, 1977; 296(25), 1480.

*Geschwind, N. Introduction to Conference on Psychiatric Complications in the Epilepsies: Current Research and Treatment. McLean Hosp J (Special Issue), June 1977, 6-8.

Mesulam, MM, Van Hoesen, GW, Pandya, DN, and Geschwind, N. Limbic and Sensory Connections of the Inferior Parietal Lobule (Area PG) in the Rhesus Monkey: A Study with a New Method for Horseradish Peroxidase Histochemistry. Brain Res, 1977; 136(3), 393-414.

Rubens, AB, Geschwind, N, Mahowald, MW, and Mastri, A. Posttraumatic Cerebral Hemispheric Disconnection Syndrome. Arch Neurol, 1977; 34(12), 750-755.

Schoene, WC, Carpenter, S, Behan, PO, and Geschwind, N. "Onion Bulb" Formations in the Central and Peripheral Nervous System in Association with Multiple Sclerosis and Hypertrophic Polyneuropathy. Brain, 1977; 100(4), 755-773.

### 1978

Galaburda, AM, LeMay, M, Kemper, TL, and Geschwind, N. Right-Left Asymmetries in the Brain. Science, 1978; 199(4331), 852-856.

*Galaburda, AM, Sanides, F, and Geschwind, N. Human Brain Cytoarchitectonic Left-Right Asymmetries in the Temporal Speech Region. Arch Neurol, 1978; 35(12), 812-817.

Geschwind, N. Anatomical Asymmetry as the Basis for Cerebral Dominance. Federation Proc, 1978; 37(9), 2263-2266.

Geschwind, N. Organic Problems in the Aged: Brain Syndromes and Alcoholism. Discussion. Geriatr Psychiatry, 1978; 11(2), 161-166.

LeMay, M and Geschwind, N. Asymmetries of the Human Cerebral Hemispheres. In E Zurif and A Caramazza (eds.), *The Acquisition and Breakdown of Language: Parallels and Divergencies.* Baltimore: Johns Hopkins Press, 1978, pp. 311-328.

Mesulam, MM and Geschwind, N. On the Possible Role of Neocortex and its Limbic Connections in Attention and Schizophrenia. In LC Wynne (ed.), *The Nature of Schizophrenia.* New York: John Wiley, 1978, pp. 161-166.

Mesulam, MM, and Geschwind, N. On the Possible Role of Neocortex and Its Limbic Connections in the Process of Attention and Schizophrenia: Clinical Cases of Inattention in Man and Experimental Anatomy in Monkey. Psychiatr Res, 1978; 14, 249-259.

### 1979

Geschwind, N, and Kondo, K. Corticosteroid Therapy and Tourette Syndrome (letter). Ann Neurol, 1979; 5(5), 495.

Geschwind, N, Galaburda, A, and LeMay, M. Morphological and Physiological Substrates of Language and Cognitive Development. In R Katzman (ed.), *Congenital and Acquired Cognitive Disorders Research Publication: Research in Nervous and Mental Diseases, Vol. 57.* New York: Raven Press, 1979, pp. 31-42.

Geschwind, N. Anatomical and Functional Specialization of the Cerebral Hemispheres in the Human. Bull Mem Acad R Med Belg, 1979; 134(6), 286-297.

Geschwind, N. Anatomical Foundations of Language and Dominance. In CL Ludlow and ME Doran-Quine (eds.), *The Neurological Bases of Language Disorders in Children: Methods and Directions for Research.* Washington, DC: US Government Printing Office, 1979, pp. 145-157.

Geschwind, N. Asymmetries of the Brain—Newer Developments. Orton Soc Bull, 1979; 29, 67-73.

Geschwind, N. Behavioral Changes in Temporal Lobe Epilepsy (Editorial). Psycho Med, 1979; 9(2), 217-219.

Geschwind, N. In Rebuttal: Where Would We Be Without Clinical Research? Wellesley, 1979; 7, 22-27.

Geschwind, N. Occasional Notes. "Wings"—A Neurologist at the Theater. N Engl J Med, 1979; 300(10), 569-571.

Geschwind, N. Specializations of the Human Brain. Sci Amer, 1979; 241(3), 180-199.

Swadlow, HA, Geschwind, N, and Waxman, SG. Commissural Transmission in Humans (letter). Science, 1979; 204(4392), 530-531.

## 1980

Galaburda, AM, and Geschwind, N. The Human Language Areas and Cerebral Asymmetries. Rev Med Suisse Romande, 1980; 100(2), 119-128.

Geschwind, N, and Putnam, JJ. L'Aphasie de Broca: Le Phenix Neurologique [Broca's Aphasia: The Neurologic Phoenix]. Rev Neurol, 1980; 136(10), 585-589.

Geschwind, N, Shader, RI, Bear, D, North, B, Levin, K, and Chetham, D. Case 2: Behavioral Changes with Temporal Lobe Epilepsy: Assessment and Treatment. J Clin Psychiatry, 1980; 41(3), 89-95.

Geschwind, N. Carotid Endarterectomy in Transient Cerebral Ischemia (letter). N Engl J Med, 1980; 302(25), 1423-1424.

Geschwind, N. Language and Communication in the Elderly: an Overview. In LK Obler and ML Albert (eds.), *Language and Communication in the Elderly.* Lexington: DC Heath, 1980, pp. 205-209.

*Geschwind, N. Neurological Knowledge and Complex Behaviors. Cognit Sci, 1980; 4, 185-193.

Geschwind, N. On the Other Hand. Sciences, September 1980.

Geschwind, N. Some Comments on the Neurology of Language. In D Caplan (ed.), *Biological Studies of Mental Processes.* Cambridge: MIT Press, 1980, pp. 301-319.

Swadlow, HA, Waxman, SG, and Geschwind, N. Small-Diameter Nonmyelinated Axons in the Primate Corpus Callosum. Arch Neurol, 1980; 37(2), 114-115.

## 1981

Ansara A, Geschwind N, Galaburda A, Albert M, Gartrell, eds. *Reading Ability in Boys and Girls: Sex Differences in Dyslexia.* Towson, MD: Orton Dyslexia Society, 1981.

Galaburda, AM and Geschwind, N. Anatomical Asymmetries in the Adult and Developing Brain and Their Implications for Function. In LA Barnes (ed.), *Advances in Pediatrics.* Chicago: Year Book Medical, 1981, pp. 271-292.

Geschwind, N. A Reaction to the Conference on Sex Differences and Dyslexia. In A Ansara, N Geschwind, A Galaburda, M Albert, and N Gartrell (eds.), *Sex Differences in Dyslexia.* Towson: The Orton Dyslexia Society, 1981, pp. xiii-xviii.

Geschwind, N. Foreword. In F Boller and E Frank (eds.), *Sexual Dysfunction in Neurological Disorders.* New York: Raven Press, 1981, pp. xi-xiii.

Geschwind, N. Hemispheric Specialization: Biological Foundations. In S Katsuki, T Tsubaki, and Y Toyokura (eds.), *Proceedings of the 12th World Congress of Neurology, International Congress Series, No. 568S.* Amsterdam: Elsevier, 1981, pp. 3-11.

Geschwind, N. Is the March of Science Always Upward? J Med Lyon, 1981; 62, 97-102.

Geschwind, N. Linguistic Distinctions in Aphasia. Contemp Psychol, 1981; 26, 833-834.

Geschwind, N. Linguistic Distinctions in Aphasia. Review of M. Coltheart, K Patterson, JC Marshall (eds.), *Deep Dyslexia.* (London: Routledge & Kegan Paul, 1980).

Geschwind, N. Nature of the Decussated Innervation of the Sternocleidomastoid Muscle (letter). Ann Neurol, 1981; 10(5), 495.

Geschwind, N. Neurological Knowledge and Complex Behaviors. In DA Norman (ed.), *Perspectives on Cognitive Science.* NJ: Ablex Publishing, 1981, pp. 27-35.

Geschwind, N. The Significance of Lateralization in Nonhuman Species. Behav Brain Sci, 1981; 4, 26-27.

LeMay, MJ and Geschwind, N. Morphological Cerebral Asymmetries in Primates. In B Preilowski and HC Engele (eds.), *Is There a Cerebral Hemispheric Asymmetry in Non-Human Primates?* Symposium at VII Congress International Primatological Society, Bangalore, India, January 1979. Tuebingen, Germany: Bruno Preilowski, 1981, pp. 9-25.

## 1982

Eidelberg, DM, Galaburda, AM, and Geschwind, N. Cerebral Asymmetries: Implications for the Lateralization of Language Function, Handedness, and Vision. In S Lessell and JTW van Dalen (eds.), *Neuro-Ophthalmology*, Vol. 2. Amsterdam: Excerpta Medica, 1982, pp. 108-125.

Galaburda AM, Geschwind N. Dyslexia Update. Neurol Neurosurg Update, 1982; 3(33), 1-8.

*Geschwind, N, Behan, P. Left-handedness: Association with Immune Disease, Migraine, and Developmental Learning Disorder. Proc Nat Acad Sci USA, 1982; 79(16), 5097-5100.

Geschwind, N. Anatomical and Pharmacological Asymmetries in the Cerebral Hemispheres. In H Akimoto, H Kazamatsuri, M Seino, and A Ward, Jr. (eds.), *Advances in Epileptology. XIIIth Epilepsy International Symposium.* New York: Raven Press, 1982, pp. 379-383.

Geschwind, N. Aphasia Part 1: Examination of the Aphasic Patient. Neurol Neurosurg Update, 1982; 3(6).

Geschwind, N. Aphasia Part 2: Diagnosis, Prognosis, and Treatment. Neurol Neurosurg Update, 1982; 3(7).

Geschwind, N. Derek-Ernest Denny-Brown 1901-1981. J Neurol Sci, 1982; 53(1), 137-139.

Geschwind, N. Disorders of Attention: A Frontier in Neuropsychology. Philos Trans R Soc Lond B Biol Sci, 1982; 298(1089), 173-185.

Geschwind, N. Focal Disturbances of Higher Nervous Function. In JB Wyngaarden and LH Smith (eds.), *Textbook of Medicine.* Philadelphia: WB Saunders, 1982, pp. 1935-1940.

Geschwind, N. Immunological Associations of Cerebral Dominance. Abstracts of the First International Congress on Neuroimmunology, Stresa Italy. J Neuroimmunol, (Suppl. 1), 1982, S7.

Geschwind, N. Samuel Torrey Orton. Ann Dyslexia. 1982; 32, 9-11.

Geschwind, N. Why Orton Was Right. Ann Dyslexia. 1982; 32, 13-30.

Herzog, AG, Russell, V, Vaitukaitis, JL, and Geschwind, N. Neuroendocrine Dysfunction in Temporal Lobe Epilepsy. Arch Neurol, 1982; 39(3), 133-135.

LeMay, M, Billig, MS, and Geschwind, N. Asymmetries of the Brains and Skulls of Nonhuman Primates. In E Armstrong and D Falk (eds.), *Primate Brain Evolution: Methods and Concepts.* New York: Plenum Press, 1982, pp. 263-278.

Naeser, MA, Alexander, MP, Helm-Estabrooks, N, Levine, HL, Laughlin, SA, and Geschwind, N. Aphasia with Predominantly Subcortical Lesion Sites: Description of Three Capsular/Putaminal Aphasia Syndromes. Arch Neurol, 1982; 39(1), 2-14.

Sackeim, HA, Greenberg, MS, Weiman, AL, Gur, RC, Hungerbuhler, JP, and Geschwind, N. Hemispheric Asymmetry in the Expression of Positive and Negative Emotions. Neurologic Evidence. Arch Neurol, 1982; 39(4), 210-218.

Sherman, GF, Galaburda, AM, and Geschwind, N. Neuroanatomical Asymmetries in Non-Human Species. Trends Neurosci, 1982; 5, 5097-5100.

## 1983

Geschwind N. Genetics: Fate, Chance, and Environmental Control. In CL Ludlow and JR Cooper (eds.) *Genetic Aspects of Speech and Language Disorders.* New York: Academic Press, 1983, pp. 21-33.

Geschwind, N. Biological Foundations of Language and Hemispheric Dominance. In M Studdert-Kennedy (ed.), *Psychobiology of Language.* Cambridge: MIT Press, 1983, pp. 62-68.

Geschwind, N. Fondements Biologiques de la Specialisation Hemispherique [Biological Foundations of Hemispheric Specialization]. Rev Neurol, 1983; 139(1), 11-14.

Geschwind, N. Interictal Behavioral Changes in Epilepsy. Epilepsia, 1983; 24 (Suppl. 1), S23-S30.

Geschwind, N. Leitungsstorungen. In C Hopf, K Poeck, and H Schliack (eds.), *Neurologie in Praxis und Klinik*, Vol. 1. New York: Stultgard, 1983, pp. 71-77.

Geschwind, N. Pathogenesis of Behavior Change in Temporal Lobe Epilepsy. In AA Ward, Jr., JK Penry, and D Purpura (eds.), *Epilepsy.* New York: Raven Press, 1983, pp. 355-370.

Geschwind, N. Pathogenesis of Behavior Change in Temporal Lobe Epilepsy. Research Publications—Association for Research in Nervous and Mental Diseases, Vol. 61, 1983, pp. 355-370.

Geschwind, N. The Organization of the Living Brain. In J Miller (ed.), *States of Mind.* London: British Broadcasting Corporation, 1983, pp. 116-134.

Judd, T, Gardner, H, and Geschwind, N. Alexia without Agraphia in a Composer. Brain, 1983; 106 (Pt 2), 435-457.

*Strub, RL and Geschwind, N. Localization in Gerstmann Syndrome. In A Kertesz (ed.), *Localization in Neuropsychology.* New York: Academic Press, 1983, pp. 295-321.

Waxman, SG, and Geschwind, N. Major Morbidity Related to Hypothermia in Multiple Sclerosis. Ann Neurol, 1983; 13(3), 348.

## 1984

Alexander, MP, and Geschwind, N. Dementia in the Elderly. In ML Albert (ed.), *Clinical Neurology of Aging.* Oxford: Oxford University Press, 1984, pp. 254-276.

*Damasio, AR, and Geschwind, N. The Neural Basis of Language. In WM Cowan, EM Shooter, CF Stevens, and RF Thompson (eds.), *Annual Review of Neuroscience.* Palo Alto: Annual Reviews, 1984, pp. 127-147.

Geschwind, N and Behan, PO. Laterality, Hormones and Immunity. In N Geschwind and AM Galaburda (eds.), *Cerebral Dominance: The Biological Foundations.* Cambridge: Harvard University Press, 1984, pp. 211-224.

Geschwind, N, and Galaburda, AM (eds.) *Cerebral Dominance: The Biological Foundations.* Cambridge: Harvard University Press, 1984.

Geschwind, N. Cerebral Dominance in Biological Perspective. Neuropsychologia, 1984; 22(6), 675-683.

Geschwind, N. Clinician-Scientists (letter). Science, 1984; 224(4646), 239.

Geschwind, N. D.E. Denny-Brown, Faculty of Medicine Memorial Minute. Harvard University Gazette, 79 (21:4), 1984.

Geschwind, N. Developmental Implications of the Biological Foundations of Cerebral Dominance. Discuss Neurosci, 1984; 1(2), 102-106.

Geschwind, N. Dostoievsky's Epilepsy. In D Blumer (ed.), *Psychiatric Aspects of Epilepsy.* Washington, DC: American Psychiatric Press, 1984, pp. 325-334.

Geschwind, N. Immunological Associations of Cerebral Dominance. In PO Behan and F Spreafico (eds.), *Neuroimmunology.* New York: Raven Press, 1984, pp. 451-461.

Geschwind, N. Review of *Les Gauchers* by Henry Hecaen. Trends Neurosci, 1984; 7, 346.

Geschwind, N. The Biology of Cerebral Dominance: Implications for Cognition. Cognition, 1984; 17(3), 193-208.

Geschwind, N. The Neglect of Advances in the Neurology of Behavior. In R Duncan and M Weston-Smith (eds.), *The Encyclopaedia of Medical Ignorance.* Oxford: Pergamon Press, 1984, pp. 9-15.

Geschwind, N. The Riddle of the Left-Hand. Medical and Health Annual, *Encyclopaedia Britannica*, 1984, pp. 38-51.

Herskowitz, J, Rosman, NP, and Geschwind, N. Seizures Induced by Singing and Recitation. A Unique Form of Reflex Epilepsy in Childhood. Arch Neurol, 1984; 41(10), 1102-1103.

Herzog, AG, Seibel, MM, Schomer, D, Vaitukaitis, J, and Geschwind, N. Temporal Lobe Epilepsy: An Extrahypothalamic Pathogenesis for Polycystic Ovarian Syndrome? Neurology, 1984; 34(10), 1389-1393.

### 1985

Behan, P and Geschwind, N. Dyslexia, Congenital Anomalies, and Immune Disorders: The Role of the Fetal Environment. Ann NY Acad Sci, 1985; 457, 13-18.

Behan, WM, Behan, PO, and Geschwind, N. Anti-Ro Antibody in Mothers of Dyslexic Children (letter). Dev Med Child Neurol, 1985; 27(4), 538-540.

*Damasio, AR, and Geschwind, N. Anatomical Localization in Clinical Neuropsychology. In PJ Vinken, GW Bruyn, and HL Klawans (eds.), *Handbook of Clinical Neurology Vol. I (45): Clinical Neuropsychology.* Amsterdam: Elsevier Science, 1985, pp. 7-22.

Freeman, RL, Galaburda, AM, Cabal, RD, and Geschwind, N. The Neurology of Depression Cognitive and Behavioral Deficits with Focal Findings in Depression and Resolution After Electroconvulsive Therapy. Arch Neurol, 1985; 42(3), 289-291.

Galaburda, AM, Sherman, GF, Rosen, GD, Aboitiz, F, and Geschwind, N. Developmental Dyslexia: Four Consecutive Patients with Cortical Anomalies. Ann Neurol, 1985; 18(2), 222-233.

*Geschwind, N, and Damasio, AR. Apraxia. In PJ Vinken, GW Bruyn, and HL Klawans (eds.), *Handbook of Clinical Neurology Vol. I (45): Clinical Neuropsychology.* Amsterdam: Elsevier Science, 1985, pp. 423-432.

*Geschwind, N, and Galaburda, AM. Cerebral Lateralization Biological Mechanisms, Associations, and Pathology: I. A Hypothesis and a Program for Research. Arch Neurol, 1985; 42(6), 428-459.

*Geschwind, N, and Galaburda, AM. Cerebral Lateralization Biological Mechanisms, Associations, and Pathology: II. A Hypothesis and a Program for Research. Arch Neurol, 1985; 42(6), 521-552.

*Geschwind, N, and Galaburda, AM. Cerebral Lateralization Biological Mechanisms, Associations, and Pathology: III. A Hypothesis and a Program for Research. Arch Neurol, 1985; 42(6), 634-654.

Geschwind, N. Mechanisms of Change After Brain Lesions. Ann NY Acad Sci, 1985; 457, 1-11.

Sherman, GF, Galaburda, AM, and Geschwind, N. Cortical Anomalies in Brains of New Zealand Mice: A Neuropathologic Model of Dyslexia? Proc Natl Acad Sci USA, 1985; 82(23), 8072-8074.

## 1986

Healey, JM, Liederman, J, and Geschwind, N. Handedness Is Not a Unidimensional Trait. Cortex, 1986; 22(1), 33-53.

Helm-Estabrooks, N, Yeo, R, Geschwind, N, Freedman, M, and Weinstein, C. Stuttering: Disappearance and Reappearance with Acquired Brain Lesions. Neurology, 1986; 36(8), 1109-1112.

Herzog, AG, Seibel, MM, Schomer, DL, Vaitukaitis, JL, and Geschwind, N. Reproductive Endocrine Disorders in Men with Partial Seizures of Temporal Lobe Origin. Arch Neurol, 1986; 43(4), 347-350.

Herzog, AG, Seibel, MM, Schomer, DL, Vaitukaitis, JL, and Geschwind, N. Reproductive Endocrine Disorders in Women with Partial Seizures of Temporal Lobe Origin. Arch Neurol, 1986; 43(4), 341-346.

## 1987

Schachter, SC, Ransil, BJ, and Geschwind, N. Associations of Handedness with Hair Color and Learning Disabilities. Neuropsychology, 1987; 25(1B), 269-276.

## 1989

Mullally, WJ, Ronthal, M, Huff, K, and Geschwind, N. Chronic Confusional State. NJ Med, 1989; 86(7), 541-544.

# Index